D0061887

The
Rehabilitation
Specialist's
Handbook

The Rehabilitation Specialist's Handbook

Jules M. Rothstein, Ph.D., P.T.

Professor and Head
Department of Physical Therapy
University of Illinois at Chicago
and
Chief of Physical Therapy Services
University of Illinois Hospital
Chicago, Illinois

Serge H. Roy, Sc.D., P.T.

Senior Research Associate
Research Assistant Professor
NeuroMuscular Research Center
Boston University
Boston, Massachusetts

Steven L. Wolf, Ph.D., F.A.P.T.A.

Professor and Director of Research
Department of Rehabilitation Medicine
and
Associate Professor
Department of Anatomy and Cell Biology
Emory University School of Medicine
Atlanta, Georgia

 F. A. DAVIS Company • Philadelphia

Printed in the United States of America

Last digit indicates print number: 10 9 8 7 6

NOTE: As new scientific information becomes available through basic and clinical research, recommended treatments and drug therapies undergo changes. The author(s) and publisher have done everything possible to make this book accurate, up-to-date, and in accord with accepted standards at the time of publication. The authors, editors, and publisher are not responsible for errors or omissions or for consequences from application of the book, and make no warranty, expressed or implied, in regard to the contents of the book. Any practice described in this book should be applied by the reader in accordance with professional standards of care used in regard to the unique circumstances that may apply in each situation. The reader is advised always to check product information (package inserts) for changes and new information regarding dose and contraindications before administering any drug. Caution is especially urged when using new or infrequently ordered drugs.

Library of Congress Cataloging-in-Publication Data

Rothstein, Jules M.
   The rehabilitation specialist's handbook / Jules M. Rothstein, Serge H. Roy, Steven L. Wolf.
      p.   cm.
   Includes bibliographical references and index.
   ISBN 0-8036-7629-8 (hardbound : alk. paper)
   1. Physical therapy — Handbooks, manuals, etc. 2. Rehabilitation — Handbooks, manuals, etc. I. Roy, Serge H., 1949– . II. Wolf, Steven L. III. Title.
   [DNLM: 1. Physical Therapy — handbooks. 2. Rehabilitation — handbooks.   WB 39 R847r]
   RM735.3.R68   1990
   DNLM/DLC
   for Library of Congress   90-14090
                                                              CIP

Dedication

A 4-year labor of love necessitates certain obsessive compulsive behaviors which, in our cases, were directed toward the birth and nurturing of this book. As a result, we often ignored the callings of those who still, remarkably, love us to this day. For all the late dinners, broken promises, and unannounced sojourns, we are indebted to the unfaltering support and encouragement of our families. In the warmth of their caring about our obsession we found strength and sustenance.

We dedicate this book to our supportive wives: Marilyn Rothstein, Caroline Roy and Lois Wolf, and to our children: Katherine and Jessica Rothstein; Lindsay and Renee Roy; and Josh and Adam Wolf. We pray that they will take as much pride in their husbands and fathers as we take in them and in this book, our newest baby.

Preface

Most people sympathize with the plight of the female elephant who carries her young for a 1-year gestational period. We hope that they will be similarly sympathetic to the authors of this volume. For some of us, this book has been gestating for considerably more than a decade. This volume was conceived by two of us (JMR and SHR) shortly after we graduated from Physical Therapy School. We realized that there had to be a better way to carry around useful information than on an ever-growing collection of index cards. In our first year out of school we actually began to write some sample pages, some of which have even found their way into this final version. Professional and family obligations, however, soon made completion of the book impossible.

The manuscript pages lay on our shelves yellowing and collecting dust until the project was resurrected in early 1987. The third member of our writing team (SLW) heard of the idea and quickly joined our effort. He helped reshape our original outline and became a motivating force in bringing our idea into reality. The project then proceeded because of our collective belief that this book is needed. And it proceeded because of the extraordinary support of our publisher F. A. Davis, and especially the tireless efforts of the unrelenting, brow-beating Allied Health Editor, and our friend, Jean-François Vilain. During later stages of development, the survival of the book was assured because of the nurturing of F. A. Davis' ever-patient production manager, Herb Powell.

Now that we have told you how this book came to be, we need to explain what this book is all about. The information needed by rehabilitation professionals is extraordinary. The diversity of information defies anyone's memory. Certainly chest physical therapists should know the positions for postural drainage, but if these techniques are hardly used, they may easily be forgotten. Similarly, someone who conducts electro-diagnostic testing should know normal and abnormal conduction values, but many of us do not routinely conduct such tests. Our understanding of such a report would be essentially impossible unless these values are known. This book is designed to provide the information clinicians need.

We have collected information and organized it so that the busy clinician has a quick source of information. The design of the book allows clinicians to carry the book with them so that it is always available. For example, we can imagine portability being particularly useful when someone needs to know how to communicate with a Spanish speaking patient. Because clinicians can carry the book with them, all that is needed is to look up the table listing translations.

We have attempted to do more than just collect information and reprint it. We organized material into tables and figures to facilitate clinical practice. For example, by looking up the name of a muscle in the alphabetized listing you can read about the function of the muscle, the origin and insertion, and the innervation (both the nerve and the root). Or, if you want to know what muscles externally rotate the humerus you can look at the table that lists muscles by function and see in that same table the innervation (both the nerve and the root).

This book is not meant to replace reference books. We provide information that clinicians need in a succinct form. Because we recognize that clinicians may need additional information we have listed references at the end of each section. These references are not necessarily the sources we have used for our material. The references are there because we believe they are useful resources that can be used to obtain more information. Because we wanted to guide the reader to useful sources and not inundate them we have kept the reference lists very small.

We have attempted to cover many areas in this book. There are some things that we have not attempted. We have walked a fine line in judging what to include. This is a quick reference volume, a compendium of useful and frequently used information. We have tried to present this information clearly and to present what readers will find useful, not just what we believe in or endorse. Realizing that we could not simply be passive conduits, we made some decisions. We have omitted treatment protocols and evaluation procedures that have yet to be validated. Whenever possible we make clear that we are conveying ideas from other sources, but we know that in choosing whose words we repeated we made decisions which we hope are good and responsible.

Only the reader can judge whether we have made clinical practice easier. We hope that we have. We also hope that by providing a source of information we have made it easier for clinicians to deliver a higher level of care. Every imaginable effort has been made to check the accuracy of our information and to organize it for efficient use. We hope we have kept errors to a minimum and have anticipated all the needs of clinicians. If your needs are not met, or if you find errors, please let us know. The content of future editions will be dictated by the responses and needs of our readers.

Contributors

Three authors are listed for this book but in reality many people contributed. Nora Donohue, P.T., developed the materials in the areas of cardiology and pulmonary care. In addition, she served as a consultant for many other areas. Dan L. Riddle, P.T., developed some of the materials in orthopaedics and consulted for other sections. Terrence Karselis, M.T. (A.S.C.P.) provided the section on instrumentation. Joan Edelstein, P.T., developed most of the materials in the sections on prosthetics and orthotics. Thomas P. Mayhew, O.T., P.T., had the unenviable task of reading and commenting on the entire manuscript. He also contributed to various sections, particularly those containing anatomical and neuroanatomical information. The extraordinary efforts of these people made this book possible.

Major Sections

Musculoskeletal Anatomy, Orthopaedics, and Orthopaedic Therapy

THE SKULL

Anterior (Frontal) View

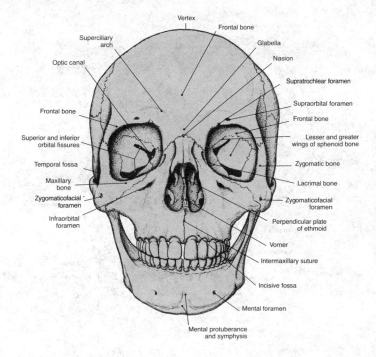

Vertex

Frontal bone

Glabella

Nasion

Superciliary arch

Optic canal

Supratrochlear foramen

Supraorbital foramen

Frontal bone

Frontal bone

Lesser and greater wings of sphenoid bone

Superior and inferior orbital fissures

Zygomatic bone

Temporal fossa

Lacrimal bone

Maxillary bone

Zygomaticofacial foramen

Zygomaticofacial foramen

Perpendicular plate of ethmoid

Infraorbital foramen

Vomer

Intermaxillary suture

Incisive fossa

Mental foramen

Mental protuberance and symphysis

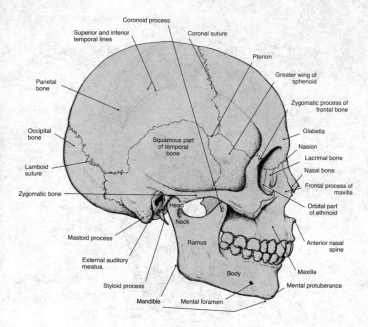

THE SKULL

Interior View — Looking Laterally from the Midline

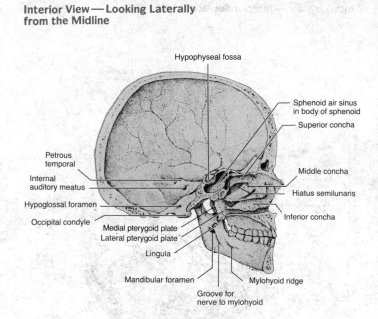

Hypophyseal fossa

Sphenoid air sinus in body of sphenoid

Superior concha

Petrous temporal

Internal auditory meatus

Hypoglossal foramen

Occipital condyle

Middle concha

Hiatus semilunaris

Inferior concha

Medial pterygoid plate

Lateral pterygoid plate

Lingula

Mandibular foramen

Mylohyoid ridge

Groove for nerve to mylohyoid

Interior View — Inferior Surface

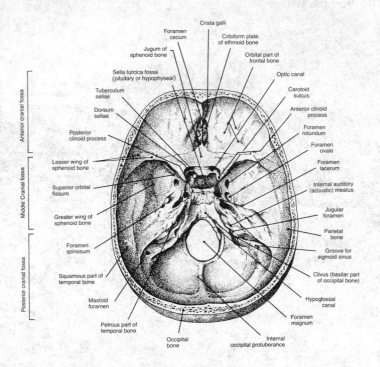

THE SKULL

Inferior Base

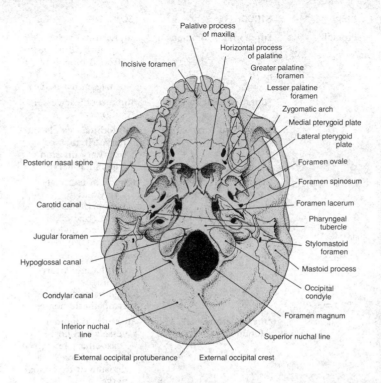

Palative process of maxilla

Horizontal process of palatine

Incisive foramen

Greater palatine foramen

Lesser palatine foramen

Zygomatic arch

Medial pterygoid plate

Lateral pterygoid plate

Posterior nasal spine

Foramen ovale

Foramen spinosum

Carotid canal

Foramen lacerum

Pharyngeal tubercle

Jugular foramen

Stylomastoid foramen

Hypoglossal canal

Mastoid process

Condylar canal

Occipital condyle

Inferior nuchal line

Foramen magnum

Superior nuchal line

External occipital protuberance

External occipital crest

OPENINGS IN THE SKULL AND THEIR CONTENTS (By View)

VIEW	STRUCTURE	CONTENTS
Frontal	Supraorbital foramen	Supraorbital vessels, supraorbital nerve (frontal branch of ophthalmic division of trigeminal nerve)
	Supratrochlear foramen	Supratrochlear vessels and nerve
	Infraorbital foramen	Infraorbital vessels and nerve (branch of maxillary division of trigeminal nerve)
	Zygomaticofacial foramen	Branch of lacrimal artery and zygomaticofacial nerve (branch of maxillary division of trigeminal nerve)
Orbital	Optic canal	Optic nerve, ophthalmic artery, meninges, ophthalmic plexus of sympathetic nerves
	Anterior ethmoidal foramen	Anterior ethmoidal vessels and nerve (nasociliary branch of ophthalmic division of trigeminal nerve)
	Posterior ethmoidal foramen	Posterior vessels and nerve (nasociliary branch of ophthalmic division of trigeminal nerve)
	Nasolacrimal canal	Nasolacrimal duct
	Infraorbital foramen	Infraorbital nerve and vessels

VIEW	STRUCTURE	CONTENTS
	Superior orbital fissure (lateral to origin of the lateral rectus muscle)	Lacrimal nerve, frontal nerve, trochlear nerve, meningeal branch of lacrimal artery, orbital branch of middle meningeal artery, sympathetic branches from the carotid plexus
	Superior orbital fissure (between the heads of the lateral rectus muscle)	Superior and inferior ophthalmic veins, oculomotor nerve, nasociliary nerve, abducens nerve
Posterior	Mastoid foramen	Emissary vein connecting sigmoid sinus to the posterior auricular vein
Lateral	External auditory meatus	Air
	Tympanomastoid fissure	Auricular branch of vagus nerve
	Alveolar canals	Posterior superior alveolar nerves
	Infraorbital fissure	Infraorbital nerve and vessels
	Zygomaticofacial foramen	Branch of lacrimal artery and zygomaticofacial nerve (branch of maxillary division of trigeminal)
	Zygomaticotemporal foramen	Zygomaticotemporal nerve of the mandibular division of the trigeminal nerve

continued

VIEW	STRUCTURE	CONTENTS
Inferolateral	Pterygomaxillary fissure	Maxillary artery to infratemporal fossa artery
Anterior wall	Inferior orbital fissure	Connects with orbit
Inferior wall	Greater palatine canal	To posterior surface of hard palate
	Foramen rotundum	Connects with middle cranial fossa and allows for passage of maxillary division of the trigeminal nerve
Superior wall	Pterygoid canal	Connects foramen lacerum via root of pterygoid process (vessel and nerve of pterygoid canal)
	Pharyngeal canal (palatinovaginal)	Connects with posterior opening of nose
Medial wall	Sphenopalatine foramen	Connects with superior meatus of nose
Inferior	Incisive foramen	Greater palatine artery, nasopalatine nerve
	Greater palatine foramen	Greater palatine artery and nerve
	Palatinovaginal canal	Pharyngeal branches of pterygopalatine (pharyngeal canal) ganglion and third portion of maxillary artery
	Foramen spinosum	Middle meningeal artery

VIEW	STRUCTURE	CONTENTS
	Foramen ovale	Mandibular division of trigeminal nerve, motor root of mandibular nerve, accessory meningeal artery, lesser superficial petrosal nerve, emissary veins connecting cavernous sinus to pterygoid venous plexus
	Foramen magnum	Spinal roots of accessory nerve, two vertebral arteries, medulla oblongata, two posterior spinal arteries, one anterior spinal artery, sympathetic plexuses about vertebral arteries, tonsil of cerebellum
	Posterior condylar canal	Emissary vein connecting sigmoid sinus to suboccipital venous plexus
	Anterior condylar canal	Hypoglossal nerve, emissary veins connecting meningeal veins to pharyngeal venous plexus
	Stylomastoid foramen	Facial nerve

continued

VIEW	STRUCTURE	CONTENTS
	Jugular foramen	
	Anterior compartment	Inferior petrosal sinus
	Middle compartment	Glossopharyngeal, vagus, and accessory nerves
	Posterior compartment	Sigmoid sinus to internal jugular vein
	Tympanic canaliculus	Tympanic branch of glossopharyngeal nerve
	Carotid canal	Internal carotid artery, sympathetic carotid plexus, emissary vein connecting cavernous sinus to pharyngeal plexus
	Caroticotympanic canaliculi	Branches of carotid sympathetic plexus, tympanic branches of internal carotid artery
	Foramen lacerum	Meningeal branch of ascending pharyngeal artery, emissary vein connecting cavernous sinus to pharyngeal plexus, internal carotid artery, sympathetic plexus, deep petrosal nerve (from otic sympathetic plexus), greater petrosal nerve (parasympathetic from facial nerve)

VIEW	STRUCTURE	CONTENTS
	Canal for auditory tube (eustachian tube)	Temporal bone between tympanic plate and petrosal portion of temporal bone
	Petrotympanic fissure	Chorda tympani nerve of facial nerve
Internal		
Anterior cranial fossa	Foramen cecum	Emissary vein connecting superior sagittal sinus to veins of nose
	Cribriform plate of ethmoid bone	Filaments of olfactory nerve
Middle cranial fossa	Optic canal	Optic nerve, ophthalmic artery, meninges, ophthalmic plexus of sympathetic nerves
	Superior orbital fissure (lateral to origin of the lateral rectus muscle)	Lacrimal nerve, frontal nerve) trochlear nerve, meningeal branch of lacrimal artery, orbital branch of middle meningeal artery, sympathetic branches from the carotid plexus
	Superior orbital fissure (between the heads of the lateral rectus muscle)	Superior and inferior ophthalmic veins, oculomotor nerve, nasociliary nerve, abducens nerve

continued

VIEW	STRUCTURE	CONTENTS
	Foramen rotundum	Connects with middle cranial fossa and allows for passage of maxillary division of the trigeminal nerve
	Foramen ovale	Mandibular nerve of trigeminal nerve, motor root of mandibular division, accessory meningeal artery, lesser superficial petrosal nerve, emissary veins connecting cavernous sinus to pterygoid verous plexus
	Foramen spinosum	Middle meningeal artery
	Foramen lacerum	Meningeal branch of ascending pharyngeal artery, emissary vein connecting cavernous sinus to pharyngeal plexus, internal carotid artery, sympathetic plexus, deep petrosal nerve (from otic sympathetic plexus), greater petrosal nerve (parasympathetic from facial nerve)

VIEW	STRUCTURE	CONTENTS
	Pterygoid canal	Nerve of pterygoid canal (formed by greater and deep petrosal nerves), artery of pterygoid canal (branch of maxillary artery)
Posterior cranial fossa	Foramen magnum	Spinal roots of accessory nerve, two vertebral arteries, medulla oblongata, two posterior spinal arteries, one anterior spinal artery, sympathetic plexuses about vertebral arteries, tonsil of cerebellum
	Anterior condylar canal	Hypoglossal nerve, emissary veins connecting meningeal veins to pharyngeal venous plexus
	Posterior condylar canal	Emissary vein connecting sigmoid sinus to suboccipital venous plexus
	Mastoid foramen	Emissary vein connecting sigmoid sinus to the posterior auricular vein
	Jugular foramen Anterior compartment	Inferior petrosal

continued

VIEW	STRUCTURE	CONTENTS
	Middle compartment	Glossopharyngea vagus, and accessory nerves
	Internal auditory meatus	Motor and sensory roots of facial nerve, vestibulocochlear nerve
	Opening of aqueduct of vestibule	Endolymphatic duct
Mandible	Mandibular foramen	Inferior alveolar vessels and nerve (mandibular division of trigeminal)
	Mental foramen	Mental vessels and nerve (mandibular division of trigeminal)
	Mylohyoid groove	Mylohyoid vessels and mylohyoid nerve (mandibular division of trigeminal)
	Mandibular notch	Vessels to masseter muscle and nerve to masseter (mandibular division of trigeminal)

Reference

1. Clemente, CD (ed): Gray's Anatomy, ed. 30. Lea & Febiger, Philadelphia, 1985.

THE VERTEBRAL COLUMN

Lateral and Anterior Views

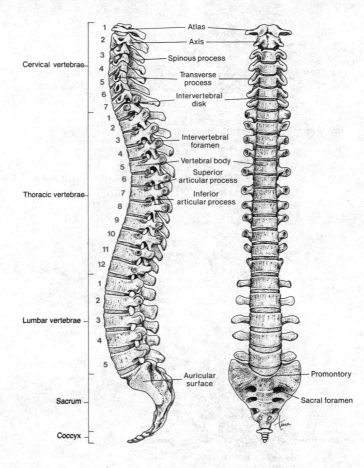

Cervical vertebrae
1
2
3
4
5
6
7

Atlas
Axis
Spinous process
Transverse process
Intervertebral disk

Thoracic vertebrae
1
2
3
4
5
6
7
8
9
10
11
12

Intervertebral foramen
Vertebral body
Superior articular process
Inferior articular process

Lumbar vertebrae
1
2
3
4
5

Auricular surface

Sacrum

Coccyx

Promontory
Sacral foramen

CERVICAL VERTEBRAE

Superior Views

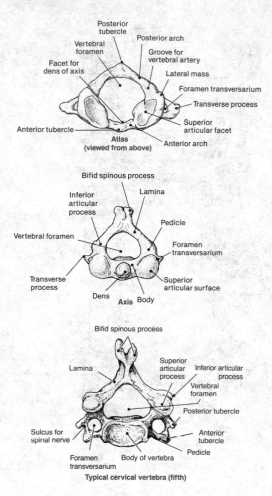

Posterior tubercle
Vertebral foramen
Facet for dens of axis
Posterior arch
Groove for vertebral artery
Lateral mass
Foramen transversarium
Transverse process
Superior articular facet
Anterior tubercle
Anterior arch

Atlas
(viewed from above)

Bifid spinous process
Inferior articular process
Lamina
Vertebral foramen
Pedicle
Foramen transversarium
Transverse process
Superior articular surface
Dens **Axis** Body

Bifid spinous process
Lamina
Superior articular process
Inferior articular process
Vertebral foramen
Posterior tubercle
Anterior tubercle
Pedicle
Sulcus for spinal nerve
Foramen transversarium
Body of vertebra

Typical cervical vertebra (fifth)

VERTEBRAE

Superior Views

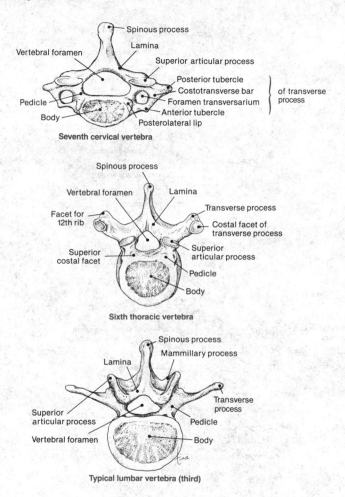

Spinous process
Lamina
Vertebral foramen
Superior articular process
Posterior tubercle
Costotransverse bar
Foramen transversarium
Anterior tubercle
Posterolateral lip
Pedicle
Body

of transverse process

Seventh cervical vertebra

Spinous process
Vertebral foramen
Lamina
Facet for 12th rib
Transverse process
Costal facet of transverse process
Superior costal facet
Superior articular process
Pedicle
Body

Sixth thoracic vertebra

Spinous process
Mammillary process
Lamina
Transverse process
Superior articular process
Pedicle
Vertebral foramen
Body

Typical lumbar vertebra (third)

Anterior and Posterior Views

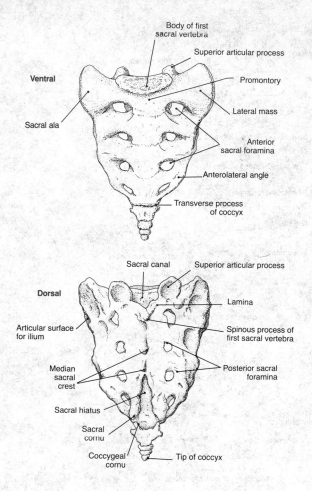

Body of first
sacral vertebra

Superior articular process

Ventral

Promontory

Lateral mass

Sacral ala

Anterior
sacral foramina

Anterolateral angle

Transverse process
of coccyx

Sacral canal

Superior articular process

Dorsal

Lamina

Articular surface
for ilium

Spinous process of
first sacral vertebra

Median
sacral
crest

Posterior sacral
foramina

Sacral hiatus

Sacral
cornu

Coccygeal
cornu

Tip of coccyx

THE THORACIC CAGE

Anterior View

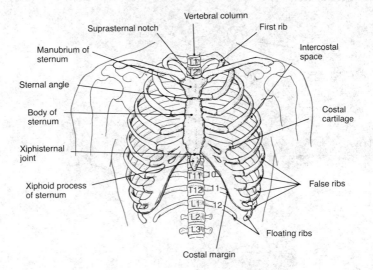

Vertebral column

Suprasternal notch

First rib

Manubrium of sternum

Intercostal space

Sternal angle

Body of sternum

Costal cartilage

Xiphisternal joint

Xiphoid process of sternum

False ribs

Floating ribs

Costal margin

COSTOVERTEBRAL AND
COSTOSTERNAL ARTICULATIONS

Lateral View

Superior articular process

Articular surface for tubercle of rib

Transverse processes of vertebrae

Tubercle of rib

Angle of rib

Body

Articular surface for head of rib

Body of vertebra

Intervertebral disk

Head of rib

Neck of rib

Costal groove

Sternum

Costal cartilage

T4

T5

5

THE CLAVICLE

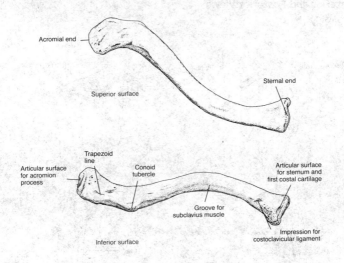

Acromial end

Sternal end

Superior surface

Trapezoid line

Articular surface for acromion process

Conoid tubercle

Articular surface for sternum and first costal cartilage

Groove for subclavius muscle

Impression for costoclavicular ligament

Inferior surface

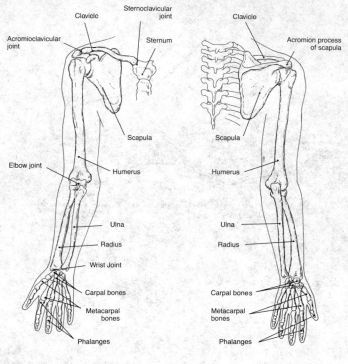

Anterior surface

Posterior surface

THE SCAPULA

Costal and Dorsal Surfaces

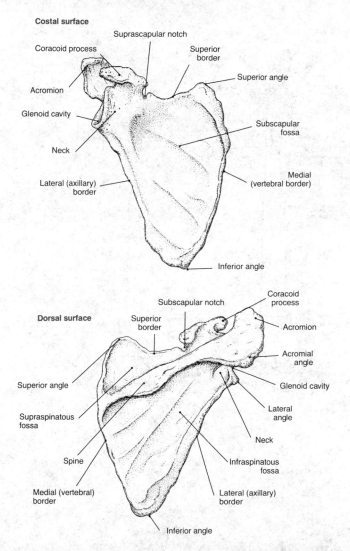

Costal surface

Coracoid process
Suprascapular notch
Superior border
Superior angle
Acromion
Glenoid cavity
Subscapular fossa
Neck
Lateral (axillary) border
Medial (vertebral border)
Inferior angle

Dorsal surface
Subscapular notch
Coracoid process
Superior border
Acromion
Acromial angle
Superior angle
Glenoid cavity
Supraspinatous fossa
Lateral angle
Neck
Spine
Infraspinatous fossa
Medial (vertebral) border
Lateral (axillary) border
Inferior angle

THE HUMERUS

Ventral and Dorsal Surfaces

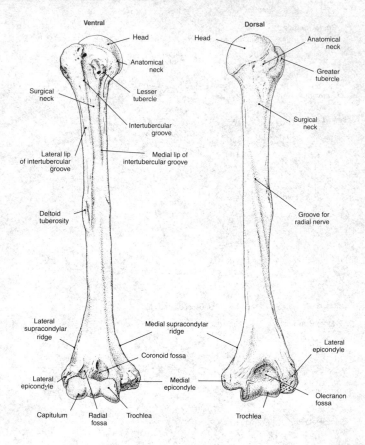

Ventral

- Head
- Anatomical neck
- Surgical neck
- Lesser tubercle
- Intertubercular groove
- Lateral lip of intertubercular groove
- Medial lip of intertubercular groove
- Deltoid tuberosity
- Lateral supracondylar ridge
- Medial supracondylar ridge
- Coronoid fossa
- Lateral epicondyle
- Medial epicondyle
- Capitulum
- Radial fossa
- Trochlea

Dorsal

- Head
- Anatomical neck
- Greater tubercle
- Surgical neck
- Groove for radial nerve
- Lateral epicondyle
- Olecranon fossa
- Trochlea

THE RADIUS AND ULNA

Ventral Surface

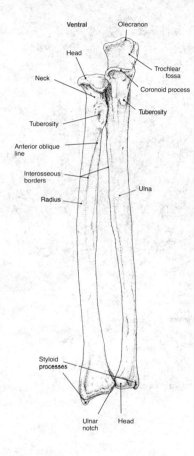

Ventral

Olecranon

Head

Trochlear fossa

Neck

Coronoid process

Tuberosity

Tuberosity

Anterior oblique line

Interosseous borders

Ulna

Radius

Styloid processes

Ulnar notch

Head

THE HAND

Palmar Surface

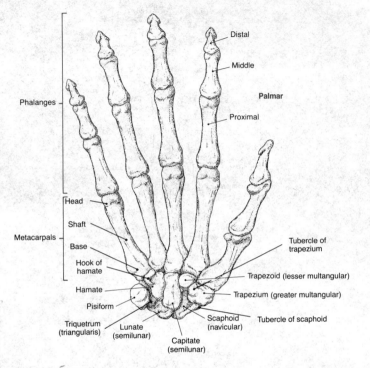

Phalanges
- Distal
- Middle
- **Palmar**
- Proximal

Metacarpals
- Head
- Shaft
- Base
- Hook of hamate
- Hamate
- Pisiform

Triquetrum (triangularis)
Lunate (semilunar)
Capitate (semilunar)
Scaphoid (navicular)
Tubercle of scaphoid
Trapezium (greater multangular)
Trapezoid (lesser multangular)
Tubercle of trapezium

See table Articulations of the Hand.

ARTICULATIONS OF THE HAND

Articulations of the Carpal Bones Proximal Row

BONE	NUMBER OF ARTICULATIONS	ARTICULATES WITH
Scaphoid (navicular)	Five	Radius, trapezium, trapezoid, capitate, lunate
Lunate (semilunar)	Five	Radius, capitate, hamate, scaphoid, trapezium
Triquetrum (triangularis)	Three	Lunate, pisiform, hamate (separated from the ulna by the triangular articular disk)
Pisiform	One	Triquetrum

Articulations of the Carpal Bones Distal Row

BONE	NUMBER OF ARTICULATIONS	ARTICULATES WITH
Trapezium (greater multangular)	Four	Scaphoid, first and second metacarpals, trapezoid
Trapezoid (lesser multangular)	Four	Scaphoid, second metacarpal, capitate, trapezium
Capitate	Seven	Scaphoid, lunate, second, third, and fourth metacarpals, trapezoid, hamate
Hamate	Five	Lunate, fourth and fifth metacarpals, triquetrum, capitate

Articulations of the Metacarpal Bones

First: trapezium, proximal phalanx

Second: trapezium, trapezoid, capitate, third metacarpal, proximal phalanx

Third: capitate, second and fourth metacarpals, proximal phalanx

Fourth: capitate, hamate, third and fifth metacarpals, proximal phalanx

Fifth: hamate, fourth metacarpal, proximal phalanx

THE LOWER QUARTER

Anterior and Posterior Views

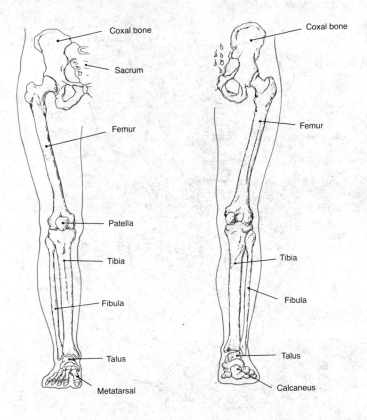

Coxal bone

Sacrum

Femur

Patella

Tibia

Fibula

Talus

Metatarsal

Coxal bone

Femur

Tibia

Fibula

Talus

Calcaneus

THE PELVIC GIRDLE

Ventral Surfaces of the Female Pelvis and the Male Pelvis

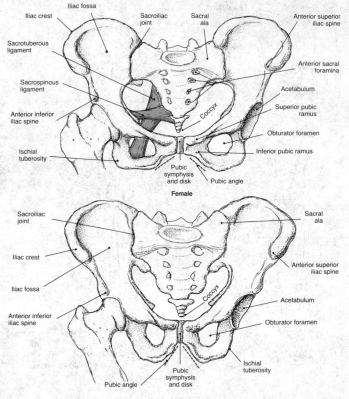

Female

Male

COMPARISONS OF THE MALE
AND FEMALE PELVES

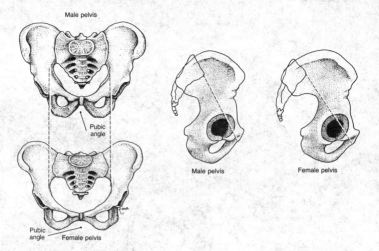

Male pelvis

Pubic
angle

Pubic
angle — Female pelvis

Male pelvis

Female pelvis

The female pelvic outlet is larger than the male. The pubic angle on the female pelvis forms a more obtuse angle than does that of the male pelvis.

THE PELVIS

Lateral Surface

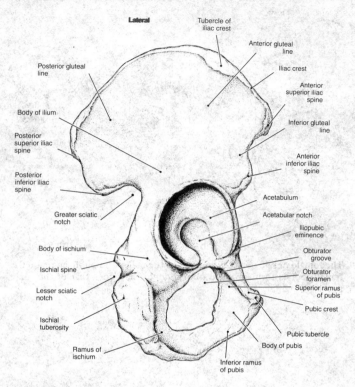

Lateral

Tubercle of
iliac crest

Anterior gluteal
line

Iliac crest

Anterior
superior iliac
spine

Inferior gluteal
line

Anterior
inferior iliac
spine

Acetabulum

Acetabular notch

Iliopubic
eminence

Obturator
groove

Obturator
foramen

Superior ramus
of pubis

Pubic crest

Pubic tubercle

Body of pubis

Inferior ramus
of pubis

Posterior gluteal
line

Body of ilium

Posterior
superior iliac
spine

Posterior
inferior iliac
spine

Greater sciatic
notch

Body of ischium

Ischial spine

Lesser sciatic
notch

Ischial
tuberosity

Ramus of
ischium

THE PELVIS

Medial Surface

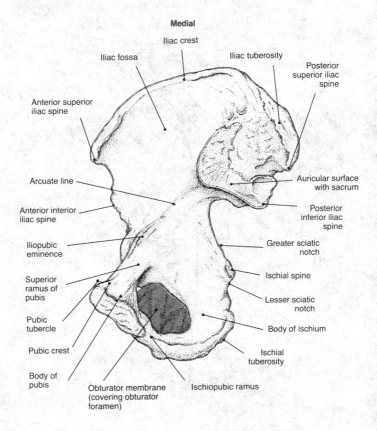

Medial

Iliac crest

Iliac fossa

Iliac tuberosity

Posterior superior iliac spine

Anterior superior iliac spine

Arcuate line

Auricular surface with sacrum

Anterior interior iliac spine

Posterior inferior iliac spine

Iliopubic eminence

Greater sciatic notch

Superior ramus of pubis

Ischial spine

Pubic tubercle

Lesser sciatic notch

Pubic crest

Body of ischium

Body of pubis

Ischial tuberosity

Obturator membrane (covering obturator foramen)

Ischiopubic ramus

THE FEMUR

Ventral Surface

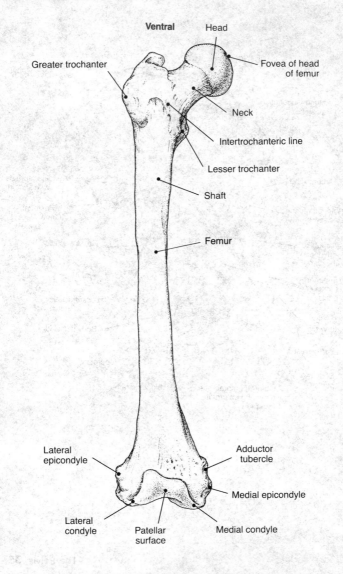

Ventral

Head

Greater trochanter

Fovea of head of femur

Neck

Intertrochanteric line

Lesser trochanter

Shaft

Femur

Lateral epicondyle

Adductor tubercle

Medial epicondyle

Lateral condyle

Patellar surface

Medial condyle

THE FEMUR

Dorsal Surface

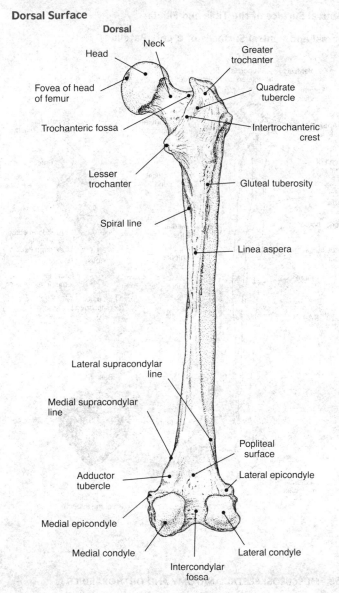

Dorsal

Head

Neck

Greater trochanter

Fovea of head of femur

Quadrate tubercle

Trochanteric fossa

Intertrochanteric crest

Lesser trochanter

Gluteal tuberosity

Spiral line

Linea aspera

Lateral supracondylar line

Medial supracondylar line

Popliteal surface

Adductor tubercle

Lateral epicondyle

Medial epicondyle

Medial condyle

Lateral condyle

Intercondylar fossa

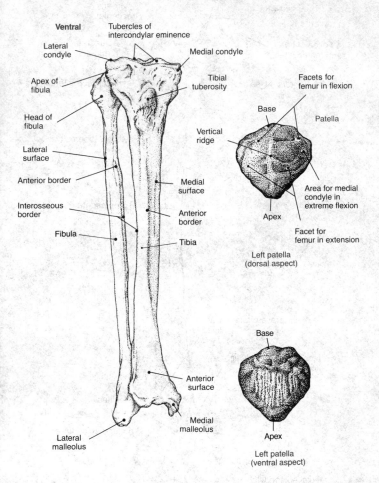

Ventral

Tubercles of intercondylar eminence

Lateral condyle

Medial condyle

Apex of fibula

Tibial tuberosity

Head of fibula

Facets for femur in flexion

Base

Patella

Vertical ridge

Lateral surface

Anterior border

Medial surface

Interosseous border

Anterior border

Area for medial condyle in extreme flexion

Apex

Fibula

Tibia

Facet for femur in extension

Left patella (dorsal aspect)

Anterior surface

Base

Medial malleolus

Lateral malleolus

Apex

Left patella (ventral aspect)

THE FOOT

Lateral and Medial Views

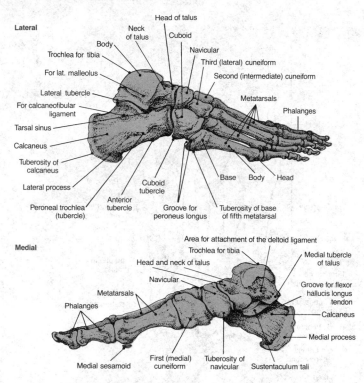

Lateral

- Head of talus
- Neck of talus
- Body
- Cuboid
- Navicular
- Third (lateral) cuneiform
- Second (intermediate) cuneiform
- Trochlea for tibia
- For lat. malleolus
- Lateral tubercle
- For calcaneofibular ligament
- Tarsal sinus
- Calcaneus
- Tuberosity of calcaneus
- Lateral process
- Peroneal trochlea (tubercle)
- Anterior tubercle
- Cuboid tubercle
- Groove for peroneus longus
- Tuberosity of base of fifth metatarsal
- Metatarsals
- Phalanges
- Base
- Body
- Head

Medial

- Area for attachment of the deltoid ligament
- Trochlea for tibia
- Medial tubercle of talus
- Head and neck of talus
- Navicular
- Groove for flexor hallucis longus tendon
- Metatarsals
- Calcaneus
- Phalanges
- Medial process
- Medial sesamoid
- First (medial) cuneiform
- Tuberosity of navicular
- Sustentaculum tali

See Table Articulations of the Foot.

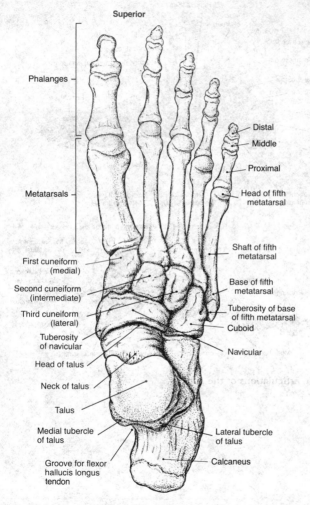

Superior

Phalanges

Distal

Middle

Proximal

Head of fifth metatarsal

Metatarsals

Shaft of fifth metatarsal

First cuneiform (medial)

Base of fifth metatarsal

Second cuneiform (intermediate)

Tuberosity of base of fifth metatarsal

Third cuneiform (lateral)

Cuboid

Tuberosity of navicular

Navicular

Head of talus

Neck of talus

Talus

Medial tubercle of talus

Lateral tubercle of talus

Groove for flexor hallucis longus tendon

Calcaneus

See Table Articulations of the Foot, page 42.

THE FOOT

Inferior View

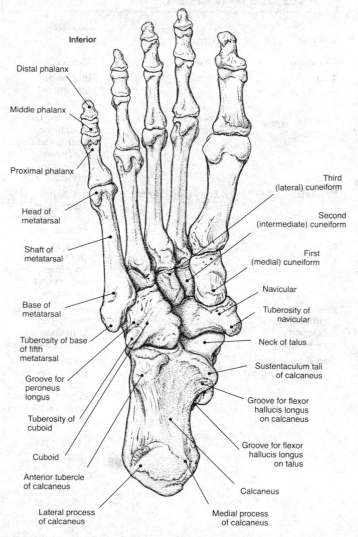

Inferior

Distal phalanx

Middle phalanx

Proximal phalanx

Head of
metatarsal

Shaft of
metatarsal

Base of
metatarsal

Tuberosity of base
of fifth
metatarsal

Groove for peroneus
longus

Tuberosity of
cuboid

Cuboid

Anterior tubercle
of calcaneus

Lateral process
of calcaneus

Third
(lateral) cuneiform

Second
(intermediate) cuneiform

First
(medial) cuneiform

Navicular

Tuberosity of
navicular

Neck of talus

Sustentaculum tali
of calcaneus

Groove for flexor
hallucis longus
on calcaneus

Groove for flexor
hallucis longus
on talus

Calcaneus

Medial process
of calcaneus

See Table Articulations of the Foot, page 42.

ARTICULATIONS OF THE FOOT

Articulations of the Tarsal Bones

BONE	NUMBER OF ARTICULATIONS	ARTICULATES WITH
Calcaneus	Two	Talus, cuboid
Talus	Four	Tibia, fibula, calcaneus, navicular
Cuboid	Four (sometimes five)	Calcaneus, lateral cuneiform, fourth and fifth metatarsal, sometimes navicular
Navicular	Four (sometimes five)	Talus, three cuneiforms, sometimes cuboid
Medial cuneiform (first cuneiform)	Four	Navicular, intermediate cuneiform, first and second metatarsal
Intermediate cuneiform (second cuneiform)	Four	Navicular, medial and lateral cuneiforms, second metatarsal
Lateral cuneiform (third cuneiform)	Six	Navicular, intermediate cuneiform, cuboid, second, third, and fourth metatarsals

Articulations of the Metatarsal Bones

First: second metatarsal, contains grooves for two sesamoids, medial cuneiform, proximal phalanx

Second: first and third metatarsals, three cuneiforms, proximal phalanx

Third: second and fourth metatarsals, lateral cuneiform, cuboid, proximal phalanx

Fourth: third and fourth metatarsals, lateral cuneiform, cuboid, proximal phalanx

Fifth: fourth metatarsal, cuboid, proximal phalanx

TYPES OF FRACTURES

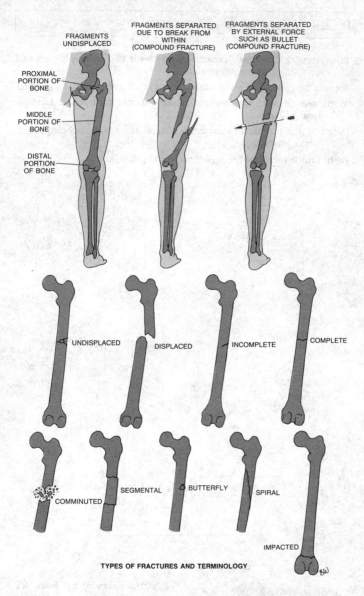

FRAGMENTS
UNDISPLACED

FRAGMENTS SEPARATED
DUE TO BREAK FROM
WITHIN
(COMPOUND FRACTURE)

FRAGMENTS SEPARATED
BY EXTERNAL FORCE
SUCH AS BULLET
(COMPOUND FRACTURE)

PROXIMAL
PORTION OF
BONE

MIDDLE
PORTION OF
BONE

DISTAL
PORTION
OF BONE

UNDISPLACED

DISPLACED

INCOMPLETE

COMPLETE

COMMINUTED

SEGMENTAL

BUTTERFLY

SPIRAL

IMPACTED

TYPES OF FRACTURES AND TERMINOLOGY

SALTER'S FRACTURE CLASSIFICATION

According to Salter, to describe a fracture completely, you must identify the site, extent, configuration, relationship of the fracture fragments to each other, the relationship of the fracture fragments to the external environment, and the presence or absence of complications.

Site

Classification. Diaphyseal, metaphyseal, epiphyseal, or intra-articular. A dislocation occurring in conjunction with a fracture is a fracture dislocation.

Extent

Classification. Complete or incomplete. Types of incomplete fractures are crack, hairline, buckle, and green-stick fractures.

Configuration

Classification. Complete fractures can have a transverse, oblique, or spiral arrangement. If there are more than two fragments, the fracture is a comminuted fracture.

Relationship of the Fracture Fragments to Each Other

Classification. Fragments can be either displaced or nondisplaced. When the fragments are displaced, they can be shifted sideways, angulated, rotated, distracted, overriding, or impacted.

Relationship of the Fracture Fragments to the External Environment

Classification. Closed or open. A closed fracture is one in which the skin in the area of the fracture is intact. An open fracture is one in which the skin in the area of the fracture is not intact. The fracture fragment may have penetrated the skin, or an object may have penetrated the skin to cause the fracture. Closed fractures are also called *simple fractures* and open fractures are also called *compound fractures*.

Complications

Classification. Complicated or uncomplicated. A complicated fracture is one that results in either a local or systemic complication due to the fracture or the treatment of the fracture. An uncomplicated fracture is one that does not immediately result in a local or systemic complication and heals uneventfully.

Reference

1. Salter, RB: Textbook of Disorders and Injuries of the Musculoskeletal System, ed. 2. Williams & Wilkins, Baltimore, 1983.

CLASSIFICATION SYSTEM USED FOR JOINTS

Fibrous

syndesmosis: A union via cordlike ligamentous fibers.

suture: Aligning the growing edges of two bones with thin, fibrous tissue.

gomphosis: Tooth and periodontal membrane (membranous union).

Cartilaginous

synchondrosis: Residual cartilage plate between two bones.

symphysis: Two bones united by a coating of fibrocartilage and reinforced.

Synovial

Plane

arthrodial: Gliding articulations with flat surfaces.

amphiarthrodial: Bony articulating surfaces connected by a cartila-

synarthrodial: Skeletal articulations are maintained by a continuous intervening cartilage, fibrous tissue, or bone.

Uniaxial

ginglymus: hinge.

trochoid: pivot.

Biaxial

Allows circumduction.

   condyloid: Ball and socket without rotation.

   ellipsoid: Oval and socket.

Multiaxial

True ball and socket.

Reference

1. Clemente, CD (ed): Gray's Anatomy, ed. 30. Lea & Febiger, Philadelphia, 1985.

CLASSIFICATIONS OF THE JOINTS OF THE BODY

(in alphabetical order)

JOINT	CLASSIFICATION
Acromioclavicular	Arthrodial
Ankle	Ginglymus
Atlantoaxial	Trochoid and arthrodial
Calcaneocuboid	Arthrodial
Capitate and hamate with scaphoid and lunate	Condyloid
Carpometacarpal	Condyloid
Cranial bones	Sutures
Distal carpal bones	Arthrodial
Elbow	Ginglymus
Hip	Multiaxial
Intercarpal joints	Arthrodial
Intermetatarsal	Arthrodial
Interphalangeal	Ginglymus
Knee	Ginglymus
Manubrium and sternum	Symphysis
Metacarpophalangeal	Condyloid
Metatarsophalangeal	Condyloid
Proximal carpal bones	Arthrodial
Pubic rami	Symphysis
Radioulnar (middle)	Syndesmosis
Radioulnar (proximal and distal)	Trochoid
Sacrococcygeal	Amphiarthrodial
Sacroiliac	Synchondrosis
Shoulder	Multiaxial
Sphenoid-ethmoid	Synchondrosis
Sternoclavicular	Double arthrodial
Sternocostal	Arthrodial
Subtalar	Arthrodial
Talocalcaneonavicular	Arthrodial
Tarsometatarsal	Arthrodial

JOINT	CLASSIFICATION
Teeth and surrounding membrane	Gomphosis
Temporomandibular	Ginglymus and arthrodial
Tibiofibular	Arthrodial
Tibiofibular with interosseous membrane	Syndesmosis
Tubercles and necks of ribs	Arthrodial
Vertebral arches	Arthrodial and syndesmosis
Vertebral column with cranium	Condyloid
Vertebral bodies	Amphiarthrodial
Wrist (radiocarpal)	Condyloid

OSTEOLOGY AND ARTHROLOGY: JOINTS AND THEIR CLASSIFICATIONS

Anterior View

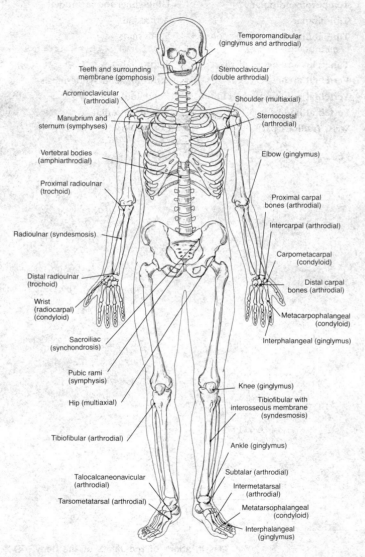

Temporomandibular (ginglymus and arthrodial)

Teeth and surrounding membrane (gomphosis)

Sternoclavicular (double arthrodial)

Acromioclavicular (arthrodial)

Shoulder (multiaxial)

Manubrium and sternum (symphyses)

Sternocostal (arthrodial)

Vertebral bodies (amphiarthrodial)

Elbow (ginglymus)

Proximal radioulnar (trochoid)

Proximal carpal bones (arthrodial)

Intercarpal (arthrodial)

Radioulnar (syndesmosis)

Carpometacarpal (condyloid)

Distal radioulnar (trochoid)

Distal carpal bones (arthrodial)

Wrist (radiocarpal) (condyloid)

Metacarpophalangeal (condyloid)

Sacroiliac (synchondrosis)

Interphalangeal (ginglymus)

Pubic rami (symphysis)

Knee (ginglymus)

Hip (multiaxial)

Tibiofibular with interosseous membrane (syndesmosis)

Tibiofibular (arthrodial)

Ankle (ginglymus)

Subtalar (arthrodial)

Talocalcaneonavicular (arthrodial)

Intermetatarsal (arthrodial)

Tarsometatarsal (arthrodial)

Metatarsophalangeal (condyloid)

Interphalangeal (ginglymus)

OSTEOLOGY AND ARTHROLOGY: JOINTS AND THEIR CLASSIFICATIONS

Posterior View

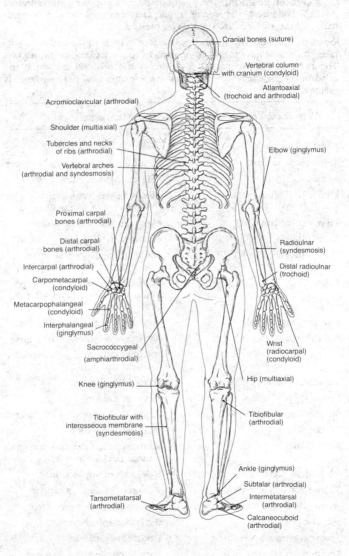

Cranial bones (suture)

Vertebral column with cranium (condyloid)

Atlantoaxial (trochoid and arthrodial)

Acromioclavicular (arthrodial)

Shoulder (multiaxial)

Tubercles and necks of ribs (arthrodial)

Vertebral arches (arthrodial and syndesmosis)

Elbow (ginglymus)

Proximal carpal bones (arthrodial)

Radioulnar (syndesmosis)

Distal carpal bones (arthrodial)

Distal radioulnar (trochoid)

Intercarpal (arthrodial)

Carpometacarpal (condyloid)

Metacarpophalangeal (condyloid)

Interphalangeal (ginglymus)

Sacrococcygeal (amphiarthrodial)

Wrist (radiocarpal) (condyloid)

Knee (ginglymus)

Hip (multiaxial)

Tibiofibular with interosseous membrane (syndesmosis)

Tibiofibular (arthrodial)

Ankle (ginglymus)

Subtalar (arthrodial)

Tarsometatarsal (arthrodial)

Intermetatarsal (arthrodial)

Calcaneocuboid (arthrodial)

CLOSE-PACKED AND LOOSE-PACKED POSITIONS FOR THE JOINTS

Definitions of Terms

close-packed position: The position in which opposing joint surfaces are fully congruent, the area of contact between joint surfaces is maximal, and the surfaces are tightly compressed.

loose-packed position: The position in which opposing joint surfaces are not congruent and some parts of the articular capsule are lax. The maximum loose packed position is the position in which the capsule and ligaments are most lax and separation of joint surfaces is greatest.

Close-packed position of joints (in alphabetical order)	
JOINT	CLOSE-PACKED POSITION
Acromioclavicular	Shoulder abducted to 30 degrees
Ankle	Maximal dorsiflexion
Elbow (radiohumeral)	Elbow flexed 90 degrees, 5 degrees of supination
Elbow (ulnohumeral)	Maximal elbow extension
Facet (spine)	Maximal extension
Glenohumeral	Maximal shoulder abduction and lateral rotation
Hip	Maximal extension of the hip and maximal medial rotation of the hip
Interphalangeal (fingers)	Maximal extension of IP joints
Interphalangeal (toes)	Maximal extension of IP joints
Knee	Maximal extension and maximal lateral rotation
Metacarpophalangeal (thumb)	Maximal opposition
Metacarpophalangeal (fingers)	Maximal flexion
Metatarsophalangeal (toes)	Maximal extension of MP joints
Midtarsal	Maximal supination
Radiocarpal	Maximal extension and maximal ulnar deviation
Radioulnar (distal)	5 degrees of supination
Radioulnar (proximal)	5 degrees of supination
Sternoclavicular	Maximal shoulder elevation
Subtalar	Maximal supination
Tarsometatarsal	Maximal supination
Temporomandibular	Teeth clenched

Maximum Loose-packed Positions of Joints (in alphabetical order)

JOINT	LOOSE-PACKED POSITION
Acromioclavicular	Shoulder in anatomical position
Ankle	10 degrees of plantar flexion
Carpometacarpal	Anatomical position of the wrist
Elbow (radiohumeral)	Anatomical position
Elbow (ulnohumeral)	70 degrees of elbow flexion, 10 degrees of supination
Facet (spine)	Midway between flexion and extension
Glenohumeral	55 degrees of shoulder abduction, 30 degrees of horizontal adduction
Hip	30 degrees of hip flexion, 30 degrees of hip abduction, and slight lateral rotation of the hip
Interphalangeal (fingers)	Slight flexion of IP joints
Interphalangeal (toes)	Slight flexion of IP joints
Knee	25 degrees of knee flexion
Metacarpophalangeal	Slight flexion of MCP joints
Metatarsophalangeal	Midrange position
Midtarsal	Midrange position
Radiocarpal	Anatomical position relative to flexion and extension with slight ulnar deviation
Radioulnar (distal)	10 degrees of supination
Radioulnar (proximal)	70 degrees of elbow flexion, 35 degrees of supination
Sternoclavicular	Shoulder in anatomical position
Subtalar	Midrange position
Tarsometatarsal	Midrange position
Temporomandibular	Mouth slightly open

References

1. Warwick, R and Williams, PL: Gray's Anatomy, ed 35. WB Saunders, Philadelphia, 1973 (for definitions).
2. Magee, DJ: Orthopedic Physical Assessment. WB Saunders, Philadelphia, 1987.

MAJOR LIGAMENTS AND THEIR FUNCTIONS

(by regions)

Upper Quarter (proximal to distal)		
JOINT	**LIGAMENT**	**FUNCTION**
Shoulder girdle	Coracoclavicular	Binds the clavicle to the coracoid process
	Costoclavicular	Binds the clavicle to the costal cartilage of the first rib
Shoulder joint	Coracohumeral	Strengthens the upper portion of the joint capsule
	Glenohumeral	Reinforces the anterior aspect of the joint capsule
	Coracoacromial	Protects the superior aspect of the joint
Elbow joint	Annular	Holds the head of radius in position
	Ulnar collateral	Restricts medial displacement of the elbow joint
	Radial collateral	Restricts lateral displacement of the elbow joint
Wrist	Volar and dorsal radioulnar	Holds the distal ends of the radius and ulna in place
	Flexor and extensor retinacula	Holds tendons against fingers
	Interosseous	Binds the carpal bones together
	Dorsal and volar collateral	Connects articulations between the rows of carpal bones
Fingers	Volar and collateral interphalangeal	Prevents displacement of the interphalangeal joints

JOINT	LIGAMENT	FUNCTION
Ischium	Sacrospinous	Runs from sacrum to ischial spine to create the greater sciatic foramen
	Sacrotuberous	Runs from the sacrum to the ischial tuberosity and prevents the sacrum from tilting excessively; creates lesser sciatic foramen
Pubis	Transverse	Converts the acetabular notch into a foramen
	Superior pubic	Holds the pubic bones together
	Arcuate pubic	Holds the pubic bones together
Hip joint	Ligamentum teres	Carries nutrient vessels into the head of the femur
	Transverse	Holds the femoral head in place
	Iliofemoral	Limits extension of the hip joint
	Ischiofemoral	Limits anterior displacement of the hip joint
	Pubofemoral	Limits extension of the hip joint
Knee joint	Medial collateral	Stabilizes the medial aspect of the knee joint (tibial-femoral articulation)

Cont. on the following page(s)

JOINT	LIGAMENT	FUNCTION
Knee Joint (cont'd)	Lateral collateral	Stabilizes the lateral aspect of the knee joint (tibial-femoral articulation)
	Medial and lateral menisci	Cartilages that provide stability and cushioning to the tibial-femoral articulation
	Anterior cruciate	Prevents backward sliding of the femur and hyperextension of the knee
	Posterior cruciate	Prevents forward sliding of the femur
	Oblique and arcuate popliteal	Provides lateral and posterior support to the knee joint
Ankle joint	Deltoid	Provides stability between the medial malleolus, navicular, talus, and calcaneus
	Anterior and posterior talofibular	Secures the fibula to the talus
	Calcaneofibular	Secures the fibula to the calcaneus
Intertarsal joints	Long plantar	Provides a groove for the peroneus longus tendon and runs from the calcaneus to the metatarsals

JOINT	LIGAMENT	FUNCTION
	Calcaneonavicular	Supports the head of the talus between the navicular and the calcaneus
Tarsometatarsal joints	Dorsal and plantar interosseus	Limits movement of the tarsal bones
Intermetatarsal joints	Dorsal and plantar metatarsal	Limits movement of the metatarsal bones
Metatarsophalangeal	Plantar and transverse metatarsal	Holds the metatarsophalangeal joints in place

Vertebral (caudal to cephalad)		
JOINT	LIGAMENT	FUNCTION
Vertebral column	Iliolumbar	Provides stability between L4–L5 and the iliac crest
	Interspinous	Limits movement between the spinous processes
	Lateral odontoid	Stabilizes the odontoid process of the axis with respect to the occipital condyles
	Lateral occipitoatlantal	Stabilizes the transverse processes of the atlas and the jugular processes of the occipital bone
	Sacroiliac	Consists of two ligaments that hold the sacrum to the ilium
	Flava	Holds adjacent lamina together
	Nuchae	Runs from C7 to the occipital bone for reinforced neck stability; limits movement between cervical spinous processes
	Anterior and posterior longitudinal	Provides reinforcement and strengthens the vertebral bodies and disks

Reference

1. Clemente, CD (ed): Gray's Anatomy, ed. 30. Lea & Febiger, Philadelphia, 1985.

GRADING OF LIGAMENTOUS SPRAINS

Grade I: Microscopic tearing of the ligament with no loss of function.

Grade II: Partial disruption or stretching of the ligament with some loss of function.

Grade III: Complete tearing of the ligament with complete loss of function.

Reference

1. Zarins, B and Boyle, J: Knee ligament injuries. In Nicholas, AJ and Hershman, EB (eds): The Lower Extremity and Spine in Sports Medicine. CV Mosby, St. Louis, 1986.

HUGHSTON CLASSIFICATION SYSTEM FOR QUANTIFYING KNEE JOINT LAXITY

1+: 0 to 5 millimeters of joint separation.

2+: 5 to 10 millimeters of joint separation.

3+: Greater than 10 millimeters of joint separation.

Reference

1. Hughston, JC, et al: Classification of knee ligament instabilities. Part 1: The medial compartment and cruciate ligaments. J Bone Joint Surg 58A: 159, 1976.

CLASSIFICATION OF KNEE LIGAMENT INJURIES ACCORDING TO O'DONOGHUE

Mild (first degree): A few fibers of the ligament are damaged; there is no loss of the strength of the ligament. Little treatment is necessary. Treatment is only for relief of symptoms.

Moderate (second degree): A definite tear in some component of the ligament with loss of strength of the ligament. There is no wide separation of the fibers. Treatment is primarily to protect the ligament.

Severe (third degree): Ligament is torn completely and no longer functions. There is potentially a wide separation of fragments of the ligament. Treatment is to restore ligament continuity.

Reference

1. O'Donoghue, DH: Treatment of Injuries to Athletes, ed. 3. WB Saunders, Philadelphia, 1976.

TERMS USED TO DESCRIBE POSITIONAL DEFORMITIES

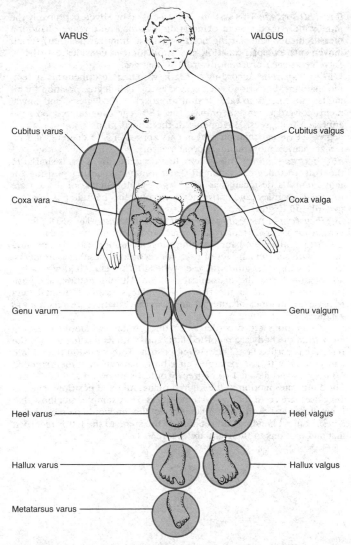

VARUS

VALGUS

Cubitus varus

Cubitus valgus

Coxa vara

Coxa valga

Genu varum

Genu valgum

Heel varus

Heel valgus

Hallux varus

Hallux valgus

Metatarsus varus

The figure above shows varus deformities (on the left) and valgus deformities (on the right) as they occur at various limb segments.

SYSTEMS FOR NOTATING AND RECORDING ROM MEASUREMENTS

0 to 180 system: This system, first described by Silver, is probably the most widely used system of notating and recording range of motion measurements. The starting position (the anatomical position) for all movements except pronation and supination is considered to be 0. Movements then proceed toward 180 degrees.

180 to 0 system: According to Clark, who first described this system, the anatomical position is designated as the 180-degree position for all joints. Movements toward flexion approach 180 degrees, and movements toward extension or past the 180-degree or neutral position approach 0 degrees. Movements in the frontal plane also approach 0 degrees. External rotation movements approach 180 degrees, and internal rotation movements approach zero.

360-degree system: This system, first described by West, is similar to the 180- to 0-degree system in that the neutral starting position for most joints is designated as 180 degrees. Movements of flexion are toward 0 degrees, and movements beyond the neutral position are toward 360 degrees.

SFTR system of recording range of motion values: The SFTR (abbreviation for sagittal, frontal, transverse, and rotation) system combines the 0 to 180 method for notating range-of-motion (ROM) measurements with a systematic set of rules for recording these measurements. The following rules guide the use of the SFTR system. All joint motions are measured from the anatomical position. All joint motions and positions are recorded in the three basic planes (sagittal, frontal, and transverse). Motions of internal and external rotation are recorded as rotations.

All motions are recorded with three numbers. Motions leading away from the body are recorded first, and motions leading toward the body are recorded last. The starting position is recorded in the middle and is usually 0. For example, an elbow that can be hyperextended 10 degrees and flexed 140 degrees would be recorded as S 10-0-140. The *S* indicates motion in the sagittal plane. All fixed positions, such as ankyloses, are recorded with two numbers. For example, an elbow that is ankylosed at a position of 30 degrees of flexion would be recorded as S 0-30. Lateral bending and rotation of the spine to the left is recorded first and motions to the right are recorded last.

References

1. Silver, D: Measurement of the range of motion in joints. J Bone Joint Surg 21:569, 1923.
2. Clark, WA: A system of joint measurement. J Orthop Surg 2:687, 1920.
3. West, CC: Measurement of joint motion. Arch Phys Med 26:414, 1945.
4. Gerhardt, JJ and Russe, OA: International SFTR Method of Measuring and Recording joint Motion. Huber, Bern, 1975.
5. Gerhardt, JJ: Clinical measurements of joint motion and position in the neutral-zero method and SFTR: Basic principles. Int Rehab Med 5:161–164, 1983.

Normal Range of Motion (in degrees) According to Various Authors*

JOINT	AAOS	BOONE AND AZEN	CLARK	CMA	DANIELS AND WORTHINGHAM	DORINSON AND WAGNER	ESCH AND LEPLEY	GERHARDT AND RUSSE	HOPPENFELD	JAMA	KAPANDJI	KENDALL AND McCREARY	WIECHEC AND KRUSEN
Shoulder													
Flexion	180	167	130	170	—	180	170	170	—	150	180	180	180
Extension	60	62	80	30	50	45	60	50	45	40	50	45	45
Abduction	180	184	180	170	—	180	170	170	180	150	180	180	180
Internal rotation	70	69	90†	60†	90	90	80	80	55	40†	95	70	90
External rotation	90	104	40†	80†	90	90	90	90	45	90†	80	90	90
Horizontal abduction	—	45	—	—	—	—	—	30	—	—	—	—	—
Horizontal adduction	135	140	—	—	—	—	—	135	—	—	—	—	—

Elbow													
Flexion	150	143	150	135	160	145	150	150	150	150	145	145	135
Radioulnar													
Pronation	80	76	50	75	90	80	90	80	90	80	85	90	90
Supination	80	82	90	85	90	70	90	90	90	80	90	90	90
Wrist													
Flexion	80	76	80	70	90	80	90	60	80	70	85	80	60
Extension	70	75	70	65	90	55	70	50	70	60	85	70	55
Radial deviation	20	22	15	20	25	20	20	20	20	20	15	20	35
Ulnar deviation	30	36	30	40	65	40	30	30	30	30	—	35	75
Hip													
Flexion	120	122	120	110	125	125	130	125	135	100	120	125	120
Extension	30	10	20	30	15	50	45	15	30	30	30	10	45
Abduction	45	46	55	50	45	45	45	45	50	40	30	45	45
Adduction	30	27	45	30	0	20	15	15	30	20	30	10	—
Internal rotation	45	47	20	35	45	30	33	45	35	40	30	45	—
External rotation	45	47	45	50	45	50	36	45	45	50	60	45	—

Cont. on the following page(s)

Normal Range of Motion (in degrees) According to Various Authors* *Continued*

JOINT	AAOS	BOONE AND AZEN	CLARK	CMA	DANIELS AND WORTHING-HAM	DORINSON AND WAGNER	ESCH AND LEPLEY	GERHARDT AND RUSSE	HOPPEN-FELD	JAMA	KAPANDJI	KENDALL AND MCCREARY	WIECHEC AND KRUSEN
Knee													
Flexion	135	143	145	135	130	140	135	130	135	120	160	140	135
Ankle													
Plantar Flexion	50	56	50	50	45	45	65	45	50	40	50	45	55
Dorsiflexion	20	13	15	15	—	20	10	20	20	20	30	20	30
Subtalar Joint													
Inversion	35	37	—	35	—	50	30	40	—	30	52	35	—
Eversion	15	26	—	20	—	20	15	20	—	20	30	20	—

*References for the normal values are: American Academy of Orthopaedic Surgeons: Joint Motion: Method of Measuring and Recording. AAOS, Chicago, 1965; Boone, DC and Azen, SP: Normal range of motion in male subjects. J Bone Joint Surg 61A:756, 1979; Clark, WA: A system of joint measurement. J Orthop Surg 2:687, 1920; Commission of California Medical Association and The Industrial Accident Commission of the State of California: Evaluation of Industrial Disability. Oxford University Press, New York, 1960; Daniels, L and Worthingham, C: Muscle Testing: Techniques of Manual Examination, ed 3. WB Saunders, Philadelphia, 1972; Dorinson, SM and Wagner, ML: An exact technique for clinically measuring and recording joint motion. Arch Phys Med 29:468, 1948; Esch, D and Lepley, M: Evaluation of Joint Motion: Methods of Measurement and Recording. University of Minnesota Press. Minneapolis, 1974; Gerhardt, JJ and Russe, OA: International SFTR Method of Measuring and Recording Joint Motion. Huber, Bern, 1975; Hoppenfeld, S: Physical Examination of the Spine and Extremities. Appleton-Century-Crofts, New York, 1976; Journal of the American Medical Association: A guide to the evaluation of permanent impairment of the extremities and back. JAMA (special edition) 1, 1958; Kapandji, IA: Physiology of the Joints, Vols 1 and 2, ed 2. Churchill Livingstone, London, 1970; Kendall, FP and McCreary, EK: Muscles, Testing and Function, ed 3. Williams & Wilkins, Baltimore, 1983; and Wiechec, FJ and Krusen, FH: A new method of joint measurement and a review of the literature. Am J Surg 43:659, 1939.

†Measurements obtained with the shoulder in 0 degrees of abduction.

SUMMARY OF THE RELIABILITY OF GONIOMETRIC MEASUREMENTS OBTAINED IN A CLINICAL SETTING

The values can be interpreted as the percent agreement associated with multiple measurements; for instance, an ICC of 0.95 means 95 percent agreement and 5 percent error associated with the measurement between or within therapists. Unless otherwise indicated the statistic used to calculate the intraclass correlation coefficient (ICC) was formula (1,1) of Shrout and Fleiss. N indicates the number of subjects measured to obtain the ICC.

Intratester Reliability			
JOINT	MOTION	ICC	N
Shoulder	Flexion	0.98	100
	Extension	0.94	100
	Abduction	0.98	100
	Horizontal abduction	0.91	100
	Horizontal adduction	0.96	100
	External rotation	0.98	100
	Internal rotation	0.94	100
Elbow	Extension	0.95*	24
	Flexion	0.95*	24
Knee	Extension	0.95*	24
	Flexion	0.98*	24
Ankle	Subtalar neutral	0.77	100
	Inversion (unref.)	0.74	100
	Eversion (unref.)	0.75	100
	Dorsiflexion	0.90	100
	Plantarflexion	0.86	100

*These ICC values were calculated using a less conservative form of the ICC than the other ICC values listed in the table.

†These measurements were not referenced back to the subtalar neutral position.

Cont. on the following page(s)

JOINT	MOTION	ICC	N
Shoulder	Flexion	0.88	50
	Extension	0.27	50
	Abduction	0.85	50
	Horizontal abduction	0.29	50
	Horizontal adduction	0.37	50
	External rotation	0.90	50
	Internal rotation	0.48	50
Elbow	Extension	0.94*	12
	Flexion	0.93*	12
Knee	Extension	0.70*	12
	Flexion	0.85*	12
Ankle	Subtalar neutral	0.25	50
	Inversion (unref.)	0.32	50
	Eversion (unref.)	0.17	50
	Dorsiflexion	0.50	50
	Plantarflexion	0.72	50

*These ICC values were calculated using a less conservative form of the ICC than the other ICC values listed in the table.

These measurements were not referenced back to the subtalar position.

References

1. Shoulder — Riddle, DL, Rothstein, JM, and Lamb, RL: Goniometric reliability in a clinical setting: Shoulder measurements. Phys Ther 67:668, 1985.
2. Elbow and knee — Rothstein, JM, Miller, PJ, and Roettger, RF: Goniometric reliability in a clinical setting: Elbow and Knee measurements. Phys Ther 63:1611, 1983.
3. Foot and ankle — Elveru, R, Rothstein, JM, and Lamb, RL: Goniometric reliability in a clinical setting: Subtalar and ankle measurements. Phys Ther 68:672, 1988.
4. Shrout, PE, Fleiss, JL: Intraclass correlations: Uses in assessing rater reliability. Psychol Bull 86:420–428, 1979.

MUSCLES LISTED ALPHABETICALLY

The muscles of the body are listed in alphabetical order. The functions, secondary functions, origins, and insertions are listed for the major muscles.

abdominals: See individual listings for the obliquus externus abdominis, obliquus internus abdominis, and rectus abdominis.

abductor digiti minimi of the hand: *Function*—abducts the fifth finger; *secondary function*—flexes the fifth finger; *origin*—pisiform bone, the tendon of flexor carpi ulnaris; *insertion*—ulnar side of the base of the proximal phalanx of the little finger; *innervation*—ulnar nerve, C8–T1.

abductor digiti minimi of the foot: *Function*—abducts the small toe; *origin*—medial and lateral processes of the calcaneal tuberosity, the plantar aponeurosis, and intermuscular septum; *insertion*—the lateral side of the proximal phalanx of the fifth toe; *innervation*—lateral plantar nerve, S2–S3.

abductor hallucis: *Function*—abducts and flexes the great toe; *origin*—the flexor retinaculum, calcaneal tuberosity, plantar aponeurosis, and intermuscular septum; *insertion*—the medial side of the base of the proximal phalanx of the great toe; *innervation*—medial plantar nerve, L5–S1.

abductor pollicis brevis: *Function*—abducts the thumb; *origin*—the flexor retinaculum, scaphoid, and trapezium; *insertion*—the radial side of the proximal phalanx at the base of the thumb; *innervation*—median nerve, C8–T1.

abductor pollicis longus: *Function*—abducts and extends the thumb; *secondary function*—abducts the wrist; *origin*—the middle third of the posterior surface of the radius, posterior surface of the ulna, and interosseous membrane; *insertion*—the radial side of the base of the first metacarpal bone; *innervation*—radial nerve, C6–C7.

adductor brevis: *Function*—adducts and flexes the thigh; *secondary function*—rotates the thigh medially; *origin*—the external aspect of the body and inferior ramus of the pubis; *insertion*—by an aponeurosis to the line from the greater trochanter to the linea aspera of the femur; *innervation*—obturator nerve, L2–L4.

adductor hallucis: *Function*—adducts the great toe; *origin*—the oblique head arises from the second, third, and fourth metatarsal bones, and the transverse head arises from the plantar ligaments of the third, fourth, and fifth toes; *insertion*—the lateral sesamoid bone and base of the first phalanx of the large toe; *innervation*—lateral plantar nerve, S2–S3.

adductor longus: *Function*—adducts and flexes the thigh; *secondary function*—rotates the thigh medially; *origin*—the pubic crest and symphysis; *insertion*—by an aponeurosis to the middle third of the linea aspera of the femur; *innervation*—obturator nerve, L2–L4.

adductor magnus: *Function*—adducts the thigh; *secondary function*—upper fibers flex and rotate the thigh medially, and lower fibers extend and rotate the thigh laterally; *origin*—the inferior ramus of the pubis, the ramus of ischium, and the inferolateral aspect of the ischial tuberosity; *insertion*—by an aponeurosis to the linea aspera and adductor tubercle of the femur; *innervation*—obturator nerve, L2–L4, and tibial portion of the sciatic nerve, L2–L4.

adductor pollicis: *Function*—adducts the thumb; *origin*—the oblique head arises from the capitate, bases of the second and third metacarpals, and the palmar carpal ligaments, and the transverse head arises from the distal two thirds of the palmar surface of the third metacarpal; *insertion*—fibers converge into a tendon containing a sesamoid bone that attaches to the ulnar side of the base of the proximal phalanx of the thumb; *innervation*—ulnar nerve, C8–T1.

anal sphincter (external): *Function*—closes the anal canal and orifice; *innervation*—S4 and inferior rectal branch of the pudendal nerve.

anal sphincter (internal): *Function*—assists external sphincter in an involuntary manner; *innervation*—sympathetic and sacral parasympathetic fibers by way of inferior mesenteric and hypogastric plexuses.

anconeus: *Function*—extends the forearm; *origin*—posterior surface of the lateral epicondyle of the humerus; *insertion*—lateral side of the olecranon and the proximal fourth of the posterior shaft of the ulna; *innervation*—radial nerve, C7–C8.

anterior deltoid: See deltoid.

articularis genus: *Function*—retracts the synovial membrane of the knee joint proximally (cephalad); *origin*—the anterior surface of the distal shaft of the femur; *insertion*—the upper part of the synovial membrane of the knee joint; *innervation*—femoral nerve, L3–L4.

aryepiglotticus: *Function*—closes the glottal opening; *innervation*—recurrent laryngeal branches of the vagus nerve.

arytenoid (arytenoideus): *Function*—closes glottal opening; *innervation*—recurrent laryngeal branches of the vagus nerve.

auricularis anterior: *Function*—draws auricula forward and upward; *innervation*—temporal branches of the facial nerve.

auricularis posterior: *Function*—draws auricula backward; *innervation*—posterior auricular branches of the facial nerve.

auricularis superior: *Function*—draws auricula upward; *innervation*—temporal branches of the facial nerve.

biceps brachii: *Function*—flexes the arm (the long head), flexes the forearm (both heads), and supinates the forearm; *origin*—the short head arises from the coracoid process, and the long head arises from the supraglenoid tubercle at the apex of the glenoid cavity; *insertion*—radial tuberosity of the radius; *innervation*—musculocutaneous nerve, C5–C6.

biceps femoris (long head): *Function*—flexes and laterally rotates the leg and extends and laterally rotates the thigh; *origin*—the ischial tuberosity and sacrotuberous ligament; *insertion*—head of the fibula and lateral condyle of the tibia; *innervation*—tibial portion of the sciatic nerve, S1–S3.

biceps femoris (short head): *Function*—flexes and laterally rotates the leg; *origin*—the lateral lip of the linea aspera of the femur; *insertion*—the head of the fibula and the lateral condyle of the tibia; *innervation*—peroneal portion of the sciatic nerve, L5–S2.

brachialis: *Function*—flexes the forearm; *origin*—the distal half of the anterior surface of the humerus; *insertion*—the tuberosity of the ulna and the coronoid process; *innervation*—musculocutaneous, C5–C6, and radial nerve (for sensory only).

brachioradialis: *Function*—flexes the forearm; *origin*—the proximal two thirds of the lateral supracondylar ridge of the humerus; *insertion*—styloid process of the radius; *innervation*—radial nerve, C5–C6.

buccinator: *Function*—compresses the cheek (assists in mastication); *origin*—the alveolar process of the maxillary bone, pterygomandibular raphe, and the buccinator ridge of the mandible; *insertion*—orbicularis oris; *innervation*—buccal branches of the facial nerve.

bulbospongiosus (bulbocavernosus): *Function*—empties the canal of the urethra and in the female reduces the orifice of the vagina; *innervation*—perineal branch of pudendal nerve, S2–S4.

chondroglossus: See hyoglossus.

ciliaris: *Function*—draws the ciliary process centrally and relaxes the suspensory ligaments of the lens, changing the convexity of the lens; *innervation*—short ciliary nerves.

coccygeus: *Function*—brings the coccyx ventrally; *innervation*—pudendal plexus including S4–S5.

constrictor inferior: See inferior constrictor.

constrictor medius: See middle constrictor.

constrictor superior: See superior constrictor.

coracobrachialis: *Function*—flexes and adducts the arm; *origin*—coracoid process of the scapula; *insertion*—middle of the medial surface of the humerus; *innervation*—musculocutaneous nerve, C6–C7.

corrugator supercilii: *Function*—draws the eyebrow down and medially; *origin*—superciliary arch of the frontal bone; *insertion*—skin over the middle third of the supraorbital margins; *innervation*—temporal and zygomatic branches of the facial nerve.

cremaster: *Function*—in the male draws testes up, and in the female draws labial folds up toward the superficial inguinal ring; *innervation*—genital branch of the genitofemoral nerve.

cricoarytenoideus lateralis: See lateral cricoarytenoid.

cricoarytenoideus posterior: See posterior cricoarytenoid.

cricothyroid (cricothyroideus): *Function*—tightens the vocal cords; *innervation*—internal laryngeal nerve of the vagus nerve.

deltoid: (see individual listings for anterior, middle, and posterior): *Function*—abducts the arm; *secondary function*—ventral fibers rotate the arm medially, and dorsal fibers rotate the arm laterally; *innervation*—axillary nerve, C5–C6.

deltoid (anterior): *Function*—flexes the arm; *origin*—the lateral third of the clavicle; *insertion*—the deltoid tuberosity of the lateral aspect of the humerus; *innervation*—axillary nerve, C5–C6.

deltoid (middle): *Function*—abducts the arm; *origin*—superior surface of the acromion; *insertion*—deltoid tuberosity of the lateral aspect of the humerus; *innervation*—axillary nerve, C5–C6.

deltoid (posterior): *Function*—extends the arm; *origin*—spine of the scapula; *insertion*—deltoid tuberosity of the lateral aspect of the humerus; *innervation*—axillary nerve, C5–C6.

depressor anguli oris: *Function*—depresses the angle of mouth; *origin*—oblique line of the mandible; *insertion*—skin at the angle of the mouth; *innervation*—mandibular and buccal branches of the facial nerve.

depressor labii inferioris: *Function*—draws the lower lip down and back; *origin*—oblique line of the mandible; *insertion*—skin of the lower lip; *innervation*—mandibular and buccal branches of the facial nerve.

depressor septi: *Function*—draws the ala of the nose downward; *innervation*—buccal branches of the facial nerve.

diaphragm: *Function*—draws the central tendon downward and forward during inspiration to increase the volume and decrease the pressure within the thoracic cavity and also decreases the volume and increases the pressure within abdominal cavity; *origin*—xiphoid process, costal cartilages of the lower six ribs, and lumbar vertebrae; *insertion*—central tendon; *innervation*—phrenic nerve, C3–C5.

digastricus (anterior belly): *Function*—brings hyoid bone forward; *innervation*—mylohyoid nerve from the inferior alveolar branch of the mandibular division of the trigeminal nerve.

digastricus (posterior belly): *Function*—brings hyoid bone backward; *innervation*—facial nerve.

dilator pupillae: *Function*—dilates the pupil; *innervation*—sympathetic efferents from the superior cervical ganglion.

dorsal interossei of the hand: See interossei.

dorsal interossei of the foot: See interossei.

extensor carpi radialis brevis: *Function*—extends the wrist; *secondary function*—abducts the wrist; *origin*—lateral epicondyle of the humerus, the radial collateral ligament of the elbow, and its covering aponeurosis; *insertion*—dorsal surface of the base of the third metacarpal; *innervation*—radial nerve, C6–C7.

extensor carpi radialis longus: *Function*—extends and abducts the wrist; *origin*—distal one third of the lateral supracondylar ridge of the humerus; *insertion*—radial side of the base of the second metacarpal; *innervation*—radial nerve, C6–C8.

extensor carpi ulnaris: *Function*—extends and adducts the wrist; *origin*—lateral epicondyle; *insertion*—tubercle on the medial side of the base of the fifth metacarpal; *innervation*—radial nerve, C6–C8.

extensor digiti minimi: *Function*—extends the fifth finger; *origin*—common extensor tendon; *insertion*—extensor hood (dorsal digital expansion) of the fifth digit; *innervation*—radial nerve, C6–C8.

extensor digitorum: *Function*—extends the fingers; *secondary function*—extends the wrist; *origin*—lateral epicondyle of the humerus by a common extensor tendon; *insertion*—middle and distal phalanges of second through fifth digits; *innervation*—radial nerve, C6–C8.

extensor digitorum brevis: *Function*—extends the proximal phalanges of the great toe and the adjacent three toes; *origin*—superolateral surface of the calcaneus; *insertion*—the first phalanx of the great toe and the tendons of the extensor digitorum longus; *innervation*—deep peroneal nerve, L5–S1.

extensor digitorum longus: *Function*—extends the proximal phalanges of the four toes; *secondary function*—dorsiflexes, abducts, and everts the foot; *origin*—lateral condyle of the tibia, the proximal three fourths of the anterior surface of the fibula, and interosseous membrane; *insertion*—middle and distal phalanges of second through fifth digits; *innervation*—deep peroneal nerve, L4–S1.

extensor hallucis longus: *Function*—extends the proximal phalanx of the great toe; *secondary function*—dorsiflexes, adducts, and inverts the foot; *origin*—middle two fourths of the medial surface of the fibula; *insertion*—dorsal aspect of the base of the distal phalanx of the great toe; *innervation*—deep peroneal nerve, L4–S1.

extensor indicis: *Function*—extends the index finger; *secondary function*—abducts the index finger; *origin*—the posterior surface of the ulnar and interosseous membrane; *insertion*—the extensor hood of the index finger; *innervation*—radial nerve, C6–C8.

extensor pollicis brevis: *Function*—extends the proximal phalanx of the thumb; *origin*—posterior surface of the radius and interosseus membrane; *insertion*—dorsal surface of the base of the proximal phalanx of the thumb; *innervation*—radial nerve, C6–C7.

extensor pollicis longus: *Function*—extends the second phalanx of the thumb; *origin*—middle third of the posterior surface of the shaft of the ulna; *insertion*—base of the distal phalanx of the thumb; *innervation*—radial nerve, C6–C8.

external intercostals: See intercostales externi.

external oblique: See obliquus externus abdominis.

extrinsic muscles of the eye: See levator palpebrae superioris, obliquus inferior, obliquus superior, rectus inferior, rectus lateralis, rectus medialis, and rectus superior.

flexor carpi radialis: *Function*—flexes and abducts the wrist; *origin*—common flexor tendon from the medial epicondyle of the humerus; *insertion*—the palmar surface of the base of the second metacarpal; *innervation*—median nerve, C6–C7.

flexor carpi ulnaris: *Function*—flexes and adducts the wrist; *origin* —one head arises from the common flexor tendon of the medial epicondyle of the humerus, and the other head arises from the medial margins of the olecranon, and the proximal two thirds of the posterior border of the ulna; *insertion*—the pisiform bone and fifth metacarpal; *innervation*—ulnar nerve, C8–T1.

flexor digiti minimi brevis of the foot: *Function*—flexes the proximal phalanx of small toe; *origin*—plantar surface of the base of the fifth metatarsal; *insertion*—lateral side of the base of the proximal phalanx of the fifth toe; *innervation*—lateral plantar nerve, S2–S3.

flexor digiti minimi brevis of the hand: *Function*—flexes the fifth finger; *origin*—the hamulus (hook) of the hamate and the flexor retinaculum; *insertion*—ulnar side of the base of the proximal phalanx of the little finger; *innervation*—ulnar nerve, C8–T1.

flexor digitorum accessorius: See quadratus plantae.

flexor digitorum brevis: *Function*—flexes the second phalanges of the four toes; *origin*—medial process of the tuberosity of the calcaneus, the plantar aponeurosis, and intermuscular septa; *insertion*— the tendons divide and attach to both sides of the middle phalanges of the second through fifth toes; *innervation*—medial plantar nerve, L5–S1.

flexor digitorum longus: *Function*—flexes the four toes; *secondary function*—plantar flexes the ankle and flexes, adducts, and inverts the foot; *origin*—posterior surface of the tibia; *insertion*—distal phalanges of the second through fifth toes; *innervation*—tibial nerve, L5–S1.

flexor digitorum profundus: *Function*—flexes the distal phalanx of each finger; *secondary function*—flexes the more proximal phalanges of each finger and flexes the wrist; *origin*—the proximal three fourths of the anterior and medial surfaces of the ulna, interosseous membrane, and a depression on the medial side of the coronoid process; *insertion*—palmar surface of the base of the distal phalanx of the second through fifth digits; *innervation*—median and ulnar nerves, C8–T1.

flexor digitorum superficialis: *Function*—flexes the second phalanx of each finger; *secondary function*—flexes the first phalanx of each finger and flexes the wrist; *origin*—medial epicondyle of the humerus by the common flexor tendon, intermuscular septa, medial side of the coronoid process, and anterior border of the radius from the radial tuberosity to the insertion of the pronator teres; *insertion*—tendons divide and insert into the sides of the shaft of the middle phalanx of the second through fifth digits; *innervation*—median nerve, C7 – C8.

flexor hallucis brevis: *Function*—flexes the proximal phalanx of the great toe; *origin*—medial part of the plantar surface of the cuboid, lateral cuneiform, and medial intermuscular septum; *insertion*—the tendon divides and attaches to the sides of the base of the proximal phalanx of the hallux (a sesamoid bone is usually in each of the attachments); *innervation*—medial plantar nerve, L5 – S1.

flexor hallucis longus: *Function*—flexes the distal (second) phalanx of the great toe; *secondary function*—flexes, adducts, and inverts the foot; *origin*—the inferior two thirds of the posterior surface of the fibula, the distal part of the interosseous membrane, posterior crural intermuscular septum, and fascia; *insertion*—the plantar aspect of the base of the distal phalanx of the great toe; *innervation*—tibial nerve, L5 – S2.

flexor pollicis brevis: *Function*—flexes the proximal phalanx of the thumb and adducts the thumb; *origin*—the superficial head arises from the distal border of the flexor retinaculum and the tubercle of the trapezium, and the deep head arises from the trapezoid and capitate; *insertion*—the superficial head attaches by a tendon containing a sesamoid bone to the radial side of the base of the proximal phalanx of the thumb, and the deep head attaches by a tendon that unites with the superficial head on the sesamoid bone and base of the first phalanx; *innervation*—superficial head: median nerve, C8 – T1; deep head: ulnar nerve, C8 – T1.

flexor pollicis longus: *Function*—flexes the second phalanx of the thumb; *origin*—the grooved anterior surface of the radius, interosseous membrane; *insertion*—the palmar surface of the base of the distal phalanx of the thumb; *innervation*—median nerve, C8 – T1.

gastrocnemius: *Function*—plantar flexes the foot and flexes the leg; *origin*—the medial head arises from the posterior part of the medial femoral condyle, and the lateral head arises from the lateral surface of the lateral femoral condyle; *insertion*—both heads form a tendon that joins the tendon of the soleus to form the tendocalcaneus, which inserts on the posterior surface of the calcaneus; *innervation*—tibial nerve, S1 – S2.

gemelli (superior and inferior): *Function*—laterally rotates the extended thigh and abducts the flexed thigh; *origin*—the superior gemellus arises from the dorsal surface of the spine of the ischium, and the inferior gemellus arises from the upper part of the tuberosity of the ischium; *insertion*—both the superior and inferior attach to the medial surface of the greater trochanter; *innervation*—superior gemellus: nerve to obturator internus, L5 – S2; inferior gemellus: nerve to quadratus femoris, L4 – S1.

genioglossus: *Function*—protrudes or retracts the tongue and elevates the hyoid bone; *innervation*—hypoglossal nerve.

geniohyoid: *Function*—brings the hyoid bone anteriorly; *innervation*—branch of first cervical nerve via the hypoglossal nerve.

gluteus maximus: *Function*—extends and laterally rotates the thigh; *origin*—posterior gluteal line of the ilium, iliac crest, aponeurosis of the erector spinae, dorsal surface of the lower part of the sacrum, side of the coccyx, sacrotuberous ligament, and intermuscular fascia; *insertion*—the iliotibial tract of the fascia lata and the gluteal tuberosity of the femur; *innervation*—inferior gluteal nerve, L5–S2.

gluteus medius: *Function*—abducts and medially rotates the thigh; *secondary function*—anterior portion flexes the thigh, and the posterior portion extends the thigh; *origin*—outer surface of the ilium between the iliac crest and the posterior gluteal line, anterior gluteal line, and fascia; *insertion*—the lateral surface of the greater trochanter; *innervation*—superior gluteal nerve, L4–S1.

gluteus minimus: *Function*—abducts and medially rotates the thigh; *origin*—outer surface of the ilium between the anterior and inferior gluteal lines, and the margin of the greater sciatic notch; *insertion*—the ridge laterally situated on the anterior surface of the greater trochanter; *innervation*—superior gluteal nerve, L4–S1.

gracilis: *Function*—adducts the thigh; *secondary function*—flexes the leg and rotates the tibia medially; *origin*—thin aponeurosis from the medial margins of the lower half of the body of the pubis and the whole of the inferior ramus; *insertion*—proximal part of the medial surface of the tibia, below the tibial condyle and just proximal to the tendon of the semitendinosus; *innervation*—obturator nerve, L2–L3.

hamstrings muscles: See biceps femoris, semitendinosus, semimembranosus.

hyoglossus and chondroglossus: *Function*—depresses the side of tongue and retracts the tongue; *innervation*—hypoglossal nerve.

iliacus: *Function*—flexes the thigh; *origin*—superior two thirds of the iliac fossa and the upper surface of the lateral part of the sacrum; *insertion*—fibers converge with tendon of the psoas major; *innervation*—femoral nerve, L2–L3.

iliocostalis (cervicis, thoracis, lumborum): See individual muscles.

iliocostalis cervicis: *Function*—extends the vertebral column and bends it to one side; *origin*—angles of the third through sixth ribs; *insertion*—posterior tubercles of the transverse processes of the fourth, fifth, and sixth cervical vertebrae; *innervation*—dorsal primary divisions of the spinal nerves.

iliocostalis lumborum: *Function*—extends the vertebral column and bends it to one side and draws the ribs down; *origin*—the broad erector spinae tendon from the median sacral crest, spines of the lumbar and lower thoracic vertebrae, and iliac crest; *insertion*—inferior borders of the angles of the lower six or seven ribs; *innervation*—dorsal primary divisions of the spinal nerves.

iliocostalis thoracis: *Function*—extends the vertebral column, bends it to one side, and draws the ribs down; *origin*—upper borders of the angles of the lower six ribs; *insertion*—upper borders of the angles of the upper six ribs; *innervation*—dorsal primary divisions of the spinal nerves.

inferior constrictor: *Function*—narrows the pharynx for swallowing; *innervation*—pharyngeal plexus and the external laryngeal and recurrent nerves.

inferior gemellus: See gemelli.

inferior oblique: See obliquus inferior.

inferior rectus: See rectus inferior.

infraspinatus: *Function*—lateral rotation of the arm; *secondary function*—the upper fibers abduct and the lower fibers adduct the arm; *origin*—medial two thirds of the infraspinatus fossa; *insertion*—middle impression (facet) on the greater tubercle of the humerus; *innervation*—suprascapular nerve, C5–C6.

intercostal muscles: See intercostales externi and intercostales interni.

intercostales externi: *Function*—elevates the ribs to increase the volume of the thoracic cavity; *origin*—inferior border of the rib above; *insertion*—superior border of the rib below; *innervation*—intercostal nerves.

intercostales interni: *Function*—elevates the ribs to decrease the volume of the thoracic cavity; *origin*—floor of the costal grooves; *insertion*—upper border of the rib below; *innervation*—intercostal nerves.

internal intercostals: See intercostales interni.

internal oblique: See obliquus internus abdominis.

interossei of the foot (dorsal): *Function*—abducts the toes; *secondary function*—flexes the proximal phalanges and extends the distal phalanges; *origin*—arise via two heads from the adjacent sides of two metatarsal bones; *insertion*—bases of the proximal phalanges and to the dorsal digital expansions, the first reaching the medial side of the second toe and the other three passing to the lateral sides of the second, third, and fourth toes; *innervation*—lateral plantar nerve, S2–S3.

interossei of the foot (plantar): *Function*—adduct the third through fifth digits; *secondary function*—flexes proximal phalanges and extends the distal phalanges; *origin*—bases and medial sides of the third, fourth, and fifth metatarsal bones; *insertion*—medial sides of the bases of the proximal phalanges of the same toes and into their dorsal digital expansions; *innervation*—lateral plantar nerve, S2–S3.

interossei of the hand (palmar): *Function*—adducts fingers; *secondary function*—flexes the metacarpophalangeal joints and extends the interphalangeal joints; *origin*—with the exception of the first, each of the four arises from the entire length of the metacarpal bone of one finger, and the first interosseus arises from the ulnar side of the palmar surface of the base of the first metacarpal bone; *insertion*—the first interosseus inserts into a sesamoid bone on the ulnar side of the proximal phalanx of the thumb and into the thumb's dorsal digital expansion, and the remaining three interossei pass to the dorsal digital expansion of the same digit; *innervation*—ulnar nerve, C8–T1.

interossei of the hand (dorsal): *Function*—abducts the fingers; *secondary function*—flexes the metacarpophalangeal joints and extends the interphalangeal joints; *origin*—adjacent sides of two metacarpal bones; *insertion*—bases of the proximal phalanges and extensor hoods (dorsal digital expansions); the first interossei is attached to the radial side of the proximal phalanx of the index finger, the second and third interossei are attached to the middle finger, the second to the radial side, and the third to the ulnar side, and the fourth interossei attaches to the dorsal digital expansion of the ring finger; *innervation*—ulnar nerve, C8–T1.

intertransversarii: *Function*—bends the vertebral column laterally; *origin*—transverse processes of the vertebrae; *insertion*—adjacent transverse processes; *innervation*—anterior, lateral, and posterior branches of the ventral primary divisions of the spinal nerves.

ischiocavernosus: *Function*—in the male compresses the crus of the penis and in the female compresses the crus of the clitoris; *innervation*—perineal branch of the pudendal nerve, S2–S4.

lateral cricoarytenoid: *Function*—narrows the glottis; *innervation*—recurrent laryngeal nerve of the vagus nerve.

lateral pterygoid: *Function*—opens the jaw, protrudes the mandible, and moves the mandible from side to side; *origin*—the upper head arises from the infratemporal surface and infratemporal crest of the greater wing of the sphenoid bone, and the lower head arises from the lateral surface of the lateral pterygoid plate; *insertion*—depression on the front of the neck of the mandible, articular capsule, and disk of the temporomandibular joint; *innervation*—lateral pterygoid nerve of the mandibular division of the trigeminal nerve.

lateral rectus: See rectus lateralis.

latissimus dorsi: *Function*—adducts, extends, and medially rotates the arm; *origin*—spines of the lower six thoracic vertebrae, posterior layer of the thoracolumbar fascia, and posterior part of the crest of the ilium; *insertion*—bottom of the intertubercular sulcus of the humerus; *innervation*—thoracodorsal nerve, C6–C8.

levator anguli oris: *Function*—raises the angle of the upper lip; *innervation*—buccal branches of the facial nerve.

levator ani iliococcygeus: *Function*—supports and raises the pelvic floor and resists any increase in intra-abdominal pressure; *innervation*—pudendal plexus, including S3–S5.

levator ani pubococcygeus: *Function*—brings the anus toward the pubis and constricts it; *innervation*—pudendal plexus, including S3–S5.

levator labii superioris: *Function*—elevates the upper lip; *innervation*—buccal branches of the facial nerve.

levator labii superioris alaeque nasi: *Function*—elevates the upper lip and dilates the naris; *innervation*—buccal branches of the facial nerve.

levator palpebrae superioris: *Function*—raises the upper eyelid; *innervation*—oculomotor nerve.

levator scapulae: *Function*—elevates the scapula; *secondary function*—rotates the scapula downward; *origin*—transverse processes of the atlas and axis and posterior tubercles of the transverse processes of the third and fourth cervical vertebrae; *insertion*—medial border of the scapula between the superior angle and the spine; *innervation*—C3–C4 and frequently the dorsal scapular nerve, C5.

levator veli palatini: *Function*—elevates the soft palate; *innervation*—pharyngeal plexus of the accessory nerve.

levatores costarum: *Function*—raises the ribs to increase the thoracic cavity and extends the vertebral column, bending it laterally with slight rotation to opposite side; *origin*—the ends of the transverse processes of the seventh cervical and first to eleventh thoracic vertebrae; *insertion*—the upper edge and external surfaces of the rib immediately below the vertebrae, from which it takes origin between the tubercle and the angle; *innervation*—intercostal nerves.

longissimus capitis: *Function*—extends the head and bends it to the same side, rotating the face to that side; *origin*—transverse processes of the upper four or five thoracic vertebrae; *insertion*—posterior margin of the mastoid process; *innervation*—dorsal primary divisions of spinal nerves.

longissimus cervicis: *Function*—extends the vertebral column and bends it to one side while drawing the ribs down; *origin*—the transverse processes of the upper four or five thoracic vertebrae; *insertion*—posterior tubercles of the transverse processes of C2–C6; *innervation*—dorsal primary divisions of spinal nerves.

longissimus thoracis: *Function*—extends the vertebral column and bends it to one side while drawing the ribs down; *origin*—the whole length of the posterior surfaces of the transverse processes of the lumbar vertebrae; *insertion*—to the tips of the transverse processes of all the thoracic vertebrae and lower nine or ten ribs; *innervation*—dorsal primary divisions of spinal nerves.

longus capitis: *Function*—flexes head; *origin*—the anterior tubercles of the transverse processes of the third, fourth, fifth, and sixth cervical vertebrae; *insertion*—the inferior surface of the basilar part of the occipital bone; *innervation*—branches of spinal nerves C1–C3.

longus colli: *Function*—flexes the neck with slight cervical rotation; *origin*—superior oblique portion arises from the anterior tubercles of the transverse processes of the third, fourth, and fifth cervical vertebrae, inferior oblique portion arises from the anterior surfaces of the first two thoracic vertebrae, and vertical portion arises from the antero-lateral surface of the bodies of the first three thoracic and last three cervical vertebrae; *insertion*—superior oblique portion inserts on the tubercle of the atlas, inferior oblique portion inserts on the anterior tubercles of the transverse processes of the fifth and sixth cervical vertebrae, and vertical portion inserts into the anterior surface of the bodies of the second through fourth cervical vertebrae; *innervation*—ventral branches of the C2–C6 spinal nerves.

lower trapezius: See trapezius.

lumbricals of the foot: *Function*—flexes the proximal phalanges and extends the distal phalanges of the four toes; *origin*—tendons of the flexor digitorum longus; *insertion*—the extensor hoods (dorsal digital expansions) on the proximal phalanges of the second through fifth digits; *innervation*—first lumbrical is by the medial plantar nerve, L5–S1, and second through fourth lumbricals by the lateral plantar nerve, S2–S3.

lumbricals of the hand: *Function*—flexes the metacarpophalangeal joints and extends the interphalangeal joints; *origin*—tendons of the flexor digitorum profundus; *insertion*—lateral margins of the extensor hoods (dorsal digital expansions) of the second through fifth digits; *innervation*—first and second lumbricals by the median nerve, C8–T1, and third and fourth lumbricals by the ulnar nerve, C8–T1.

masseter: *Function*—closes the jaw; *origin*—zygomatic process of the maxilla and from the anterior two thirds of the lower border of the zygomatic arch; *insertion*—angle and ramus of the mandible; *innervation*—masseteric branch of the mandibular division of the trigeminal nerve.

medial pterygoid: *Function*—closes the jaw; *origin*—medial surface of the lateral pterygoid plate and the pyramidal process of the palatine bone; *insertion*—posterior part of the medial surfaces of the ramus and angle of the mandible; *innervation*—medial pterygoid branch of the mandibular division of the trigeminal nerve.

medial rectus: See rectus medialis.

mentalis: *Function*—raises and protrudes the lower lip and wrinkles the chin; *origin*—incisive fossa of the mandible; *insertion*—skin of the chin; *innervation*—mandibular and buccal branches of the facial nerve.

middle constrictor: *Function*—narrows the pharynx for swallowing; *innervation*—pharyngeal plexus.

middle deltoid: See deltoid.

multifidus: *Function*—extends the vertebral column and rotates it toward opposite side; *origin*—the sacral portion arises from the posterior superior iliac spine and the dorsal sacroiliac ligaments, the lumbar portion arises from the mamillary processes, the thoracic portion arises from all thoracic transverse processes, and the cervical portion arises from the articular processes of the lower four vertebrae; *insertion*—the whole length of the spine of the vertebrae above; *innervation*—dorsal primary divisions of the spinal nerves.

musculus uvulae: *Function*—elevates the uvula; *innervation*—pharyngeal plexus of the accessory nerve.

mylohyoid: *Function*—raises the hyoid bone and tongue; *innervation*—mylohyoid nerve of the mandibular division of the trigeminal nerve.

nasalis: *Function*—enlarges the opening of nares; *innervation*—buccal branches of the facial nerve.

obliques: See obliquus externus abdominis and obliquus internus abdominis.

obliquus capitis inferior: *Function*—rotates the atlas and turns the head to the same side; *origin*—spine of the axis; *insertion*—transverse process of the atlas; *innervation*—dorsal primary ramus of the suboccipital nerve.

obliquus capitis superior: *Function*—extends and bends the head laterally; *origin*—transverse process of the atlas; *insertion*—occipital bone between the superior and inferior nuchal lines; *innervation*—dorsal primary ramus of the suboccipital nerve.

obliquus externus abdominis: *Function*—compresses the abdominal contents, flexes the vertebral column, and rotates the column to bring forward the shoulder on the same side as the active muscle; *origin*—the inferior borders of the lower eight ribs; *insertion*—the iliac crest, aponeurosis; *innervation*—intercostal nerves, T7–T12.

obliquus inferior: *Function*—elevates, abducts, and rotates the eye laterally; *innervation*—oculomotor nerve.

obliquus internus abdominis: *Function*—compresses abdominal contents, flexes the vertebral column, and rotates the column to bring the shoulder forward on the side opposite from the active muscle; *origin*—lateral two thirds of the upper surface of the inguinal ligament, iliac crest, and thoracolumbar fascia; *insertion*—posterior fibers pass upward and laterally to the inferior borders of the lower three or four ribs, the inguinal ligament fibers attach to the crest of the pubis, and the remainder of the fibers end in an aponeurosis that forms the linea alba; *innervation*—branches of the intercostal nerves from T8–T12 and the iliohypogastric and ilioinguinal branches of L1.

obliquus superior: *Function*—depresses, abducts, and rotates the eye laterally; *innervation*—trochlear nerve.

obturator externus: *Function*—laterally rotates the thigh; *origin*—rami of the pubis, ramus of the ischium, and medial two thirds of the outer surface of the obturator membrane; *insertion*—trochanteric fossa of the femur; *innervation*—obturator nerve, L3–L4.

obturator internus: *Function*—laterally rotates the thigh; *secondary function*—abducts when the thigh is flexed; *origin*—internal surface of the anterolateral wall of the pelvis and the obturator membrane; *insertion*—medial surface of the greater trochanter; *innervation*—nerve to obturator internus, L5–S2.

occipitofrontalis: *Function*—draws scalp back to raise the eyebrows and wrinkles forehead; *origin*—superior nuchal line of the occipital bone and intermuscular attachments with the orbicularis oculi; *insertion*—galea aponeurotica; *innervation*—temporal and posterior auricular branches of the facial nerve.

omohyoid: *Function*—draws the hyoid bone downward; *innervation*—ansa cervicalis containing fibers of C1–C3.

opponens digiti minimi: *Function*—abducts, flexes, and laterally rotates the fifth finger; *origin*—hamulus (hook) of the hamate bone and flexor retinaculum; *insertion*—whole length of the ulnar margin of the fifth metacarpal bone; *innervation*—ulnar nerve, T1.

opponens pollicis: *Function*—abducts, flexes, and medially rotates the thumb; *origin*—the ridge of the trapezium and the flexor retinaculum; *insertion*—whole length of the lateral border of the metacarpal bone of the thumb; *innervation*—median nerve (sometimes by branch of the ulnar nerve), C8–T1.

orbicularis oculi: *Function*—closes the eyelids; *innervation*—temporal and zygomatic branches of the facial nerve.

orbicularis oris: *Function*—closes the lips; *innervation*—buccal branches of the facial nerve.

palatoglossus: *Function*—elevates the posterior tongue and constricts the fauces; *innervation*—pharyngeal plexus of the accessory nerve.

palatopharyngeus: *Function*—constricts the fauces and closes off the nasopharynx; *innervation*—pharyngeal plexus of the accessory nerve.

palmar interossei of the foot: See interossei.

palmar interossei of the hand: See interossei.

palmaris brevis: *Function*—wrinkles the skin of the ulnar side of the palm; *origin*—the flexor retinaculum and palmar aponeurosis; *insertion*—dermis on the ulnar border of the hand; *innervation*—ulnar nerve, C8–T1.

palmaris longus: *Function*—flexes the hand; *origin*—arises from the common flexor tendon on the medial epicondyle of the humerus; *insertion*—palmar aponeurosis; *innervation*—median nerve, C6–C7.

pectineus: *Function*—flexes and adducts the thigh; *secondary function*—rotates the thigh medially; *origin*—pecten of the pubis; *insertion*—along a line leading from the lesser trochanter to the linea aspera; *innervation*—femoral, obturator, or accessory obturator nerves, L2–L4.

pectoralis major: *Function*—flexes and adducts the arm; *secondary function*—rotates the arm medially; *origin*—anterior surface of the sternal half of the clavicle, anterior surface of the sternum as low as the attachment of the cartilage of the sixth rib, from the cartilages of all true ribs, and from the aponeurosis of the obliquus externus abdominis; *insertion*—lateral lip of the intertubercular sulcus of the humerus; *innervation*—medial and lateral pectoral nerves, C5–T1.

pectoralis minor: *Function*—rotates the scapula downward and forward; *secondary function*—raises third, fourth, and fifth ribs; *origin*—third, fourth, and fifth ribs; *insertion*—medial border of the coracoid process; *innervation*—medial pectoral nerve, C8–T1.

peroneus brevis: *Function*—everts and abducts the foot; *secondary function*—plantar flexes the foot; *origin*—distal two thirds of the lateral surface of the fibula and the crural intermuscular septa; *insertion*—tubercle on the base of the fifth metatarsal bone on its lateral side; *innervation*—superficial peroneal nerve, L4–S1.

peroneus longus: *Function*—everts and abducts the foot; *secondary function*—plantar flexes the foot; *origin*—head and proximal two thirds of the lateral surface of the fibula and the crural intermuscular septa; *insertion*—lateral side of the base of the first metatarsal bone and the medial cuneiform; *innervation*—superficial peroneal nerve, L4–S1.

peroneus tertius: *Function*—abducts, dorsiflexes, and everts the foot; *origin*—lower (distal) third of the anterior surface of the fibula and crural intermuscular septum; *insertion*—dorsal surface of the base of the fifth metatarsal bone; *innervation*—deep peroneal nerve, L5–S1.

piriformis: *Function*—laterally rotates and abducts thigh; *origin*—anterior sacrum, gluteal surface of the ilium, capsule of the sacroiliac joint, and sacrotuberous ligament; *insertion*—upper border of the greater trochanter of the femur; *innervation*—sacral plexus, S1.

plantar interossei: See interossei.

plantaris: *Function*—flexes the leg, plantar flexes the foot; *origin*—distal linea aspera (lower part of the lateral supracondylar line) and from the oblique popliteal ligament; *insertion*—inserts with the tendocalcaneus into the calcaneus; *innervation*—tibial nerve, L4–S1.

platysma: *Function*—retracts and depresses the angle of the mouth; *innervation*—cervical branch of the facial nerve.

popliteus: *Function*—flexes the leg, rotates the leg (tibia) medially; *origin*—lateral condyle of the femur and arcuate popliteal ligament; *insertion*—medial two thirds of the triangular area above the soleal line on the posterior surface of the tibia; *innervation*—tibial nerve, L4–S1.

posterior cricoarytenoid: *Function*—opens the glottis; *innervation*—recurrent laryngeal nerve of the vagus nerve.

posterior deltoid: See deltoid.

procerus: *Function*—wrinkles the nose and draws the medial eyebrow downward; *origin*—fascia covering the lower part of the nasal bone; *insertion*—skin over the lower part of the forehead between the eyebrows; *innervation*—buccal branches of the facial nerve.

pronator quadratus: *Function*—pronates the forearm; *origin*—the oblique ridge on the distal part of the anterior surface of the shaft of the ulna; *insertion*—distal fourth of the anterior border and surface of the shaft of the radius; *innervation*—median nerve, C8–T1.

pronator teres: *Function*—pronates the forearm; *origin*—the humeral head arises from the common flexor tendon on the medial epicondyle of the humerus, and the ulnar head arises from the medial side of the coronoid process of the ulna; *insertion*—the rough area midway along the lateral surface of the radial shaft; *innervation*—median nerve, C6–C7.

psoas major: *Function*—flexes the thigh; *secondary function*—flexes the lumbar vertebrae and bends them laterally; *origin*—transverse processes of all the lumbar vertebrae, bodies, and intervertebral disks of the lumbar vertebrae; *insertion*—lesser trochanter of the femur; *innervation*—lumbar plexus, L2–L3.

psoas minor: *Function*—flexes the pelvis and the lumbar vertebrae; *origin*—sides of the bodies of the twelfth thoracic and first lumbar vertebrae and from the disk between them; *insertion*—pecten pubis (pectineal line) and the iliopectineal eminence; *innervation*—lumbar plexus, L1.

pyramidalis: *Function*—tightens the linea alba; *origin*—pubic crest; *insertion*—linea alba; *innervation*—branch of twelfth thoracic nerve.

quadratus femoris: *Function*—rotates the thigh laterally; *origin*—the ischial tuberosity; *insertion*—quadrate tubercle of the femur; *innervation*—nerve to quadratus femoris, L4–S1.

quadratus lumborum: *Function*—laterally flexes the lumbar vertebral column; *origin*—iliolumbar ligament and the iliac crest; *insertion*—inferior border of the last rib and transverse processes of the first four lumbar vertebrae; *innervation*—T12–L3 (or L4).

quadratus plantae (flexor digitorum accessorius): *Function*—flexes the distal phalanges of the third through fifth digits; *origin*—a medial head arises from the medial concave surface of the calcaneus, and a lateral head arises from the lateral border of the calcaneus and long plantar ligament; *insertion*—tendons of the flexor digitorum longus; *innervation*—lateral plantar nerve, S2–S3.

quadriceps femoris: See rectus femoris, vastus lateralis, vastus intermedius, vastus medialis.

rectus abdominis: *Function*—flexes the vertebral column, tenses the anterior abdominal wall, and assists in compressing the abdominal contents; *origin*—crest of the pubis; *insertion*—fifth, sixth, and seventh costal cartilages; *innervation*—T7–T12 and ilioinguinal (L-1) and iliohypogastric nerves, (T12-L1).

rectus capitis anterior: *Function*—flexes the head; *origin*—anterior surface of the lateral mass of the atlas; *insertion*—basilar part of the occipital bone in front of the occipital condyle; *innervation*—fibers from cervical nerve of C1 and C2.

rectus capitis lateralis: *Function*—bends the head laterally; *origin*—upper surface of the transverse process of the atlas; *insertion*—inferior surface of the jugular process of the occipital bone; *innervation*—fibers from cervical nerves C1–C2.

rectus capitis posterior major: *Function*—extends and rotates the head to the same side; *origin*—spine of the axis; *insertion*—lateral part of the inferior nuchal line of the occipital bone; *innervation*—dorsal ramus of C1 (suboccipital nerve).

rectus capitis posterior minor: *Function*—extends the head; *origin*—the tubercle on the posterior arch of the atlas; *insertion*—medial part of the inferior nuchal line of the occipital bone; *innervation*—dorsal ramus of C1 (suboccipital nerve).

rectus femoris: *Function*—flexes the thigh and extends the leg; *origin*—by two heads, from the anterior inferior iliac spine, and a reflected head from the groove above the acetabulum; *insertion*—base of the patella; *innervation*—femoral nerve, L2–L4.

rectus inferior: *Function*—depresses, adducts, and rotates the eye medially; *innervation*—oculomotor nerve.

rectus lateralis: *Function*—abducts the eye; *innervation*—abducens nerve.

rectus medialis: *Function*—adducts the eye; *innervation*—oculomotor nerve.

rectus superior: *Function*—elevates, adducts, and rotates the eye medially; *innervation*—oculomotor nerve.

rhomboid major: *Function*—adducts the scapula; *secondary function*—rotates the scapula down; *origin*—spines of the second through fifth thoracic vertebrae and supraspinous ligaments; *insertion*—medial border of the scapula between the root of the spine and the inferior angle; *innervation*—dorsal scapular nerve, C5.

rhomboid minor: *Function*—adducts the scapula; *secondary function*—rotates the scapula down; *origin*—lower part of the ligamentum nuchae and from the spines of the seventh cervical and first thoracic vertebrae; *insertion*—the triangular smooth surface at the medial end of the spine of the scapula; *innervation*—dorsal scapular nerve, C5.

risorius: *Function*—retracts the angle of the mouth; *origin*—parotid fascia; *insertion*—skin at the angle of the mouth; *innervation*—mandibular and buccal branches of the facial nerve.

rotatores: *Function*—extends vertebral column and rotates it toward the opposite side; *origin and insertion*—each of the rotatores connects the upper and posterior part of the transverse process of one vertebra to the lower border and lateral surface of the spine of the one or two vertebrae above; *innervation*—dorsal primary divisions of the spinal nerves.

salpingopharyngeus: *Function*—elevates the nasopharynx; *innervation*—pharyngeal plexus.

sartorius: *Function*—flexes, abducts, and laterally rotates the thigh, and also flexes and rotates the tibia medially; *origin*—anterior superior iliac spine and the notch below the anterior superior iliac spine; *insertion*—upper part of the medial surface of the tibia anterior to the gracilis; *innervation*—femoral nerve, L2–L3.

scalenus anterior: *Function*—raise the first rib; *origin*—anterior tubercles of the transverse processes of the third, fourth, fifth, and sixth cervical vertebrae; *insertion*—scalene tubercle on the inner border of the first rib; *innervation*—branches from the anterior rami of C5–C6.

scalenus medius: *Function*—raises the first rib; *origin*—transverse process of the atlas and the posterior tubercles of the transverse processes of the lower six cervical vertebrae; *insertion*—upper surface of the first rib; *innervation*—branches from the anterior rami of C3–C8.

scalenus posterior: *Function*—raises the second rib; *origin*—posterior tubercles of the transverse processes of the fourth, fifth, and sixth cervical vertebrae; *insertion*—second rib; *innervation*—ventral primary rami of C6–C8.

semimembranosus: *Function*—flexes the leg and extends the thigh; *secondary function*—medially rotates the flexed leg; *origin*—ischial tuberosity; *insertion*—medial tibial condyle; *innervation*—tibial portion of the sciatic nerve, L5–S2.

semispinalis capitis: *Function*—extends the head and rotates it toward opposite side; *origin*—transverse processes of the upper six or seven thoracic and the seventh cervical vertebrae; *insertion*—medial part of the area between the superior and inferior nuchal lines of the occipital; *innervation*—dorsal primary divisions of cervical nerves.

semispinalis cervicis: *Function*—extends the vertebral column and rotates it toward opposite side; *origin*—transverse processes of the upper five or six thoracic vertebrae; *insertion*—spines of the cervical vertebrae; *innervation*—dorsal primary divisions of spinal nerves.

semispinalis thoracis: *Function*—extends the vertebral column and rotates it toward opposite side; *origin*—transverse processes of the sixth to the tenth thoracic vertebrae; *insertion*—spines of the upper four thoracic and lower two cervical vertebrae; *innervation*—dorsal primary divisions of spinal nerves.

semitendinosus: *Function*—flexes the leg and extends the thigh; *secondary function*—medially rotates the flexed leg; *origin*—ischial tuberosity; *insertion*—upper part of the medial surface of the tibia behind the attachment of the sartorius and below that of the gracilis; *innervation*—tibial portion of the sciatic nerve, L5–S2.

serratus anterior: *Function*—rotates the scapula upward and abducts the scapula; *origin*—outer surfaces of the upper eight or nine ribs; *insertion*—costal aspect of the medial border of the scapula; *innervation*—long thoracic nerve, C5–C7.

serratus posterior inferior: *Function*—draws the ribs down and out; *origin*—spines of the lower two thoracic and upper two lumbar vertebrae; *insertion*—inferior borders of the lower four ribs; *innervation*—ventral primary divisions of T9–T12.

serratus posterior superior: *Function*—raises the ribs to increase the size of the thoracic cavity; *origin*—lower part of the ligamentum nuchae and the spines of the seventh cervical and the upper two thoracic vertebrae; *insertion*—upper borders of the second, third, fourth, and fifth ribs; *innervation*—ventral primary divisions of T1–T4.

soleus: *Function*—plantar flexes the foot; *origin*—head and proximal third of the posterior surface of the fibula, and from the soleal line and middle third of the medial border of the tibia; *insertion*—joins the tendon of gastrocnemius to form tendocalcaneus inserting on the calcaneus; *innervation*—tibial nerve, S1–S2.

sphincter pupillae: *Function*—constricts the pupil; *innervation*—motor root of the ciliary ganglion from the oculomotor nerve.

sphincter urethrae: *Function*—compresses the urethra; *innervation*—perineal branch of the pudendal nerve, S2–S4.

spinalis (capitis, cervicis, thoracis): *Function*—extends the vertebral column; *origin*—arises from the spines of vertebrae in each region; *insertion*—inserts on vertebral spines a few segments above; *innervation*—dorsal primary divisions of the spinal nerves.

splenius capitis: *Function*—brings the head and neck posteriorly and laterally with some rotation; *origin*—lower half of the ligamentum nuchae, the spine of the seventh cervical vertebra, and the spines of the upper three or four thoracic vertebrae; *insertion*—occipital bone inferior to the superior nuchal line, and the mastoid process of the temporal bone; *innervation*—dorsal primary divisions of the middle cervical roots.

splenius cervicis: *Function*—brings the head and neck posteriorly and laterally with some rotation; *origin*—spines of the third to sixth thoracic vertebrae; *insertion*—posterior tubercles of the transverse processes of the upper two cervical vertebrae; *innervation*—dorsal primary divisions of the lower cervical roots.

stapedius: *Function*—pulls the head of the stapes posteriorly to increase tension of fluid in ear; *innervation*—tympanic branch of the facial nerve.

sternocleidomastoid (sternomastoid): *Function*—rotates the head; *origin*—upper part of the anterior surface of the manubrium sterni and medial third of the clavicle; *insertion*—mastoid process of the temporal bone; *innervation*—spinal part of the accessory nerve.

sternohyoid: *Function*—draws the hyoid bone inferiorly; *innervation*—branches of ansa cervicalis hypoglossi, including fibers from C1–C3.

sternomastoid: See sternocleidomastoid.

sternothyroid: *Function*—draws the larynx downward; *innervation*—branches of ansa cervicalis hypoglossi, including fibers from C1–C3.

styloglossus: *Function*—retracts and elevates the tongue; *innervation*—hypoglossal nerve.

stylohyoid: *Function*—elevates and retracts the hyoid bone; *innervation*—facial nerve.

stylopharyngeus: *Function*—elevates and dilates the pharynx; *innervation*—glossopharyngeal nerve.

subclavius: *Function*—depresses and pulls forward (anteriorly) the lateral end of the clavicle; *origin*—the junction of the first rib and its costal cartilage; *insertion*—groove on inferior surface of middle third of the clavicle; *innervation*—nerve to subclavius, C5–C6.

subscapularis: *Function*—medially rotates the arm; *secondary function*—flexes, extends, abducts, and adducts the arm, depending on the arm position; *origin*—medial two thirds of subscapular fossa; *insertion*—lesser tubercle of the humerus; *innervation*—upper and lower subscapular nerves, C5–C6.

superior constrictor: *Function*—narrows the pharynx for swallowing; *innervation*—pharyngeal plexus.

superior gemellus: See gemelli.

superior oblique: See obliquus superior.

superior rectus: See rectus superior.

supinator: *Function*—supinates the forearm; *origin*—lateral epicondyle of the humerus and the supinator crest of the ulna; *insertion*—lateral surface of the proximal third of the radius; *innervation*—radial nerve, C6.

supraspinatus: *Function*—abducts the arm; *secondary function*—flexes and laterally rotates the arm; *origin*—medial two thirds of the supraspinatus fossa; *insertion*—superior facet of the greater tubercle of the humerus; *innervation*—suprascapular nerve, C5.

temporalis: *Function*—closes the jaw, and the posterior portion retracts the mandible; *origin*—temporalis fossa; *insertion*—medial surface, apex, anterior, and posterior borders of the coronoid process and the anterior border of the ramus of the mandible; *innervation*—anterior and posterior deep temporal nerves of the mandibular division of the trigeminal nerve.

temporoparietalis: *Function*—draws the skin backward over temples and wrinkles the forehead; *innervation*—temporal branches of the facial nerve.

tensor fasciae latae: *Function*—flexes and abducts the thigh; *secondary function*—medially rotates the thigh; *origin*—outer lip of the iliac crest and the lateral surface of the anterior superior iliac spine; *insertion*—iliotibial tract; *innervation*—superior gluteal nerve, L4–S1.

tensor tympani: *Function*—draws the tympanic membrane medially to increase tension on the membrane; *innervation*—mandibular division of the trigeminal nerve through the otic ganglion.

tensor veli palatini: *Function*—stretches the soft palate; *innervation*—trigeminal nerve.

teres major: *Function*—adducts and extends the arm; *secondary function*—medially rotates the arm; *origin*—dorsal surface of the inferior angle of the scapula; *insertion*—medial lip of the intertubercular sulcus of the humerus; *innervation*—lower subscapular nerve, C5–C6.

teres minor: *Function*—laterally rotates the arm; *secondary function*—adducts the arm; *origin*—proximal two thirds of the lateral border of the scapula; *insertion*—inferior facet of the greater tubercle of the humerus; *innervation*—axillary nerve, C5.

thyroarytenoid (thyroarytenoideus): *Function*—relaxes the vocal cords; *innervation*—recurrent laryngeal nerve of the vagus nerve.

thyroepiglotticus: *Function*—depresses the epiglottis; *innervation*— recurrent laryngeal nerve of the vagus nerve.

thyrohyoid (thyroidens): *Function*—brings the hyoid bone inferiorly or raises the thyroid cartilage; *innervation*—fibers from C1.

tibialis anterior: *Function*—dorsiflexes, adducts, and inverts foot; *origin*—lateral condyle and proximal half of the lateral surface of the tibial shaft; *insertion*—medial cuneiform and the base of the first metatarsal bone; *innervation*—deep peroneal nerve, L4–S1.

tibialis posterior: *Function*—plantar flexes, adducts, and inverts the foot; *origin*—posterior surface of the tibia and fibula; *insertion*— tuberosity of the navicular, the three cuneiforms, cuboid, and the bases of the second, third, and fourth metatarsals; *innervation*—tibial nerve, L5–S1.

transversus abdominis: *Function*—compresses the abdomen to assist in defecation, emesis, parturition, and forced expiration; *origin*— lateral third of the inguinal ligament, iliac crest, and the lower costal cartilages; *insertion*—primarily to the linear alba; *innervation*— branches of T7–T12, iliohypogastric and ilioinguinal nerves.

transversus menti: *Function*—depresses the angle of the mouth; *innervation*—mandibular and buccal branches of the facial nerve.

transversus perinei profundus: *Function*—compresses the urethra; *innervation*—perineal branch of the pudendal nerve.

transversus perinei superficialis: *Function*—fixes the central tendinous part of the perineum; *innervation*—perineal branch of the pudendal nerve.

transversus thoracis: *Function*—brings the ventral ribs downward to decrease the size of the thoracic cavity; *origin*—distal third of the posterior surfaces of the body of the sternum and the xiphoid process; *insertion*—lower borders of the costal cartilages of the second, third, fourth, fifth, and sixth ribs; *innervation*—intercostal nerves.

trapezius: *Function*—lower trapezius draws the scapula down, middle trapezius adducts the scapula, and upper trapezius draws the scapular upward; *origin*—medial third of the superior nuchal line of the occipital bone, external occipital protuberance, ligamentum nuchae, seventh cervical and all the thoracic vertebral spinous processes, and the corresponding supraspinous ligaments; *insertion*—lateral third of the clavicle, acromion process, and spine of the scapula; *innervation*—spinal part of accessory nerve.

triceps brachii: *Function*—extends the forearm; *origin*—the long head arises from the infraglenoid tubercle of the scapula, the lateral head arises from the posterior surface of the shaft of the humerus along an oblique line above the radial groove, and the medial head arises from the posterior surface of the shaft of the humerus below the radial groove; *insertion*—upper surface of the olecranon process of the ulna; *innervation*—radial nerve, C7–C8.

upper trapezius: See trapezius.

vastus intermedius: *Function*—extends the leg; *origin*—anterior and lateral surfaces of the proximal two thirds of the femoral shaft; *insertion*—patella, with some fibers passing over to blend with the ligamentum patellae; *innervation*—femoral nerve, L2–L4.

vastus lateralis: *Function*—extends the leg; *origin*—by a broad aponeurosis to the proximal part of the intertrochanteric line, anterior and inferior borders of the greater trochanter, lateral lip of the gluteal tuberosity, and the proximal half of the lateral lip of the linea aspera; *insertion*—lateral border of the patella; *innervation*—femoral nerve, L2–L4.

vastus medialis: *Function*—extends the leg; *origin*—distal part of the intertrochanteric line, spiral line, medial lip of the linea aspera, and the medial intermuscular septum; *insertion*—medial border of the patella; *innervation*—femoral nerve, L2–L4.

vocalis: *Function*—closes the glottis; innervation recurrent laryngeal branch of the vagus nerve.

zygomaticus major: *Function*—draws angle of mouth upward and backward; *origin*—zygomatic bone in front of the zygomaticotemporal suture; *insertion*—angle of the mouth; *innervation*—buccal branches of the facial nerve.

zygomaticus minor: *Function*—forms the nasolabial furrow; *origin*—lateral surface of the zygomatic bone immediately behind the zygomaticomaxiallary suture; *insertion*—muscular substance of the upper lip; *innervation*—buccal branches of the facial nerve.

Reference

1. Clemente, CD (ed): Gray's Anatomy, ed 30. Lea & Febiger, Philadelphia, 1985.

MUSCLES CLASSIFIED BY FUNCTION

**Nerves and Innervating Roots
Are in Parentheses**

For a more detailed description of muscle action, look under the muscle's name in the reference (alphabetized) list of muscles. Here muscles are listed in the order of their relative importance in contributing to the movement listed.

Muscles That Move or Stablize the Scapula			
ADDUCTION	ABDUCTION	UPWARD ROTATION	DOWNWARD ROTATION
Trapezius (spinal part of accessory nerve, sensory branches C3 – C4)	Serratus anterior (long thoracic nerve, C5 – C7	Upper trapezius (spinal accessory nerve, sesnsory branches C3 – C4)	Lower trapezius (spinal accessory nerve, sensory branches, C3 – C4)
		Serratus anterior (long thoracic nerve, C5 – C7)	Rhomboid major (dorsal scapular nerve, C5)
			Rhomboid minor (dorsal scapular nerve, C5)
			Levator scapulae (branches of C3 and C4, also frequently by the dorsal

Cont. on the following page(s)

ADDUCTION	ABDUCTION	UPWARD ROTATION	DOWNWARD ROTATION
			scapular nerve, C5)
			Pectoralis minor (medial pectoral nerve, C8–T1)

Muscles That Are Primarily Active at the Glenohumeral Joint			
EXTENSION	**FLEXION**	**ABDUCTION**	**ADDUCTION**
Latissimus dorsi (thoracodorsal nerve, C6–C8)	Pectoralis major (medial and lateral pectoral nerves, C5–T1)	Middle deltoid (axillary nerve, C5–C6)	Latissimus dorsi (thoracodorsal nerve, C6–C8)
Triceps brachii long head (radial nerve, C7–C8)	Anterior deltoid (axillary nerve, C5–C6)	Supraspinatus (suprascapular nerve, C5)	Pectoralis major (medial and lateral pectoral nerves, C5–T1)
Posterior deltoid (axillary nerve, C5–C6)	Supraspinatus (suprascapular nerve, C5)	Infraspinatus upper fibers C5 (suprascapular nerve, C5–C6)	Teres major (lower subscapular nerve, C5–C6)
Teres major (lower subscapular nerve, C5–C6)	Biceps brachii (musculocutaneous nerve, C5–C6)		Triceps brachii long head (radial nerve, C7–8)
Subscapularis (upper and lower subscapular nerves, C5–C6)	Coracobrachialis (musculocutaneous nerve, C6–C7)		Teres minor (axillary nerve, C5)
	Subscapularis (upper and lower subscapular nerves, C5–C6)		Infraspinatus lower fibers (suprascapular nerve, C5–C6)

Cont. on the following page(s)

Muscles That Are Primarily Active at the Glenohumeral Joint *Continued*	
MEDIAL ROTATION	LATERAL ROTATION
Latissimus dorsi (thoracodorsal nerve, C6–C8)	Deltoid dorsal fibers (axillary nerve, C5–C6)
Pectoralis major (medial and lateral pectoral nerves, C5–T1)	Infraspinatus (suprascapular nerve, C5–C6)
Subscapularis (upper and lower subscapular nerves, C5–C6)	Supraspinatus (suprascapular nerve, C5)
Teres major (lower subscapular nerve, C5–C6)	Teres minor (axillary nerve, C5)
Deltoid ventral fibers (axillary nerve, C5–C6)	

Muscles of the Elbow and Radioulnar Joints

EXTENSION	FLEXION	SUPINATION	PRONATION
Triceps brachii long head (radial nerve, C7–C8)	Biceps brachii (musculocutaneous nerve, C5–C6)	Biceps brachii (musculocutaneous nerve, C5–C6)	Pronator teres (median nerve, C6–C7)
Anconeus (radial nerve, C7–C8)	Brachialis (musculocutaneous nerve, C5–C6 and radial nerve for sensory)	Supinator (radial nerve, C6)	Pronator quadratus (median nerve, C8–T1)
	Brachioradialis (radial nerve, C5–C6)		

Cont. on the following page(s)

Muscles of the Wrist

EXTENSION

Extensor carpi radialis
  longus (radial nerve,
  C6–C8)

Extensor carpi radialis
  brevis (radial nerve,
  C6–C7)

Extensor carpi ulnaris
  (radial nerve, C6–C8)

Extensor digitorum (radial
  nerve, C6–C8)

FLEXION

Flexor carpi radialis
  (median nerve, C6–C7)

Flexor carpi ulnaris (ulnar
  nerve, C8–T1)

Palmaris longus (median
  nerve, C6–C7)

Flexor digitorum
  superficialis (median
  nerve, C7–C8)

Flexor digitorum
  profundus (median and
  ulnar nerves, C8–T1)

ABDUCTION

Flexor carpi radialis
  (median nerve, C6–C7)

Extensor carpi radialis
  longus (radial nerve,
  C6–C8)

Extensor carpi radialis
  brevis (radial nerve,
  C6–C7)

Abductor pollicis longus
  (radial nerve, C6–C7)

Extensor pollicis longus
  (radial nerve, C6–C8)

Extensor pollicis brevis
  (radial nerve, C6–C7)

ADDUCTION

Flexor carpi ulnaris (ulnar
  nerve, C8–T1)

Extensor carpi ulnaris
  (radial nerve, C6–C8)

Muscles that Move the Fingers			
EXTENSION	FLEXION	ABDUCTION	ADDUCTION
Extensor digitorum (radial nerve, C6–C8)	Flexor digitorum superficialis (median nerve, C7–C8)	Dorsal interossei (ulnar nerve, C8–T1)	Palmar interossei, (ulnar nerve, C8–T1)
Extensor indicis (proprius) (radial nerve, C6–C8)	Flexor digitorum profundus (median and ulnar nerves, C8–T1)	Abductor digiti minimi (ulnar nerve, C8–T1)	
Extensor digiti minimi (radial nerve, C6–C8)	Flexor digiti minimi (ulnar nerve, C8–T1)	Opponens digiti minimi (ulnar nerve, T1)	
Lumbricals (1 and 2 by median nerve, C8–T1; 3 and 4 by ulnar nerve, C8–T1)	Opponens digiti minimi (ulnar nerve, T1)	Extensor indicis (radial nerve, C6–C8)	
Interossei (dorsal and palmar, IP extension) (ulnar nerve, C8–T1)	Lumbricals (1 and 2 by median nerve, C8–T1; 3 and 4 by ulnar nerve, C8–T1)		
	Interossei (dorsal and palmar, MP flexion) (ulnar nerve, C8–T1)		

Cont. on the following page(s)

Muscles that Move the Thumb

EXTENSION	FLEXION	ABDUCTION	ADDUCTION
Extensor pollicis longus (radial nerve, C6–C8)	Flexor pollicis longus (median nerve, C8–T1)	Abductor pollicis longus (radial nerve, C6–C7)	Adductor pollicis (ulnar nerve, C8–T1)
Extensor pollicis brevis (radial nerve, C6–C7)	Flexor pollicis brevis (median nerve to superficial head, C8–T1; ulnar nerve to deep head, C8–T1)	Abductor pollicis brevis (median nerve, C8–T1)	Opponens pollicis (median nerve and sometimes by a branch of the ulnar, C8–T1)
	Opponens pollicis (median nerve and sometimes by a branch of the ulnar, C8–T1)		Flexor pollicis longus (median nerve, C8–T1)
			Flexor pollicis brevis (median nerve to superficial head, C8–T1; ulnar nerve to deep head, C8–T1)

Lower Extremity

Muscles that Move the Hip

FLEXION	EXTENSION	ABDUCTION	ADDUCTION	MEDIAL ROTATION	LATERAL ROTATION
Psoas major (lumbar plexus, L2–L3)	Gluteus maximus (inferior gluteal nerve, L5–S2)	Gluteus medius (superior gluteal nerve, L4–S1)	Adductor magnus (obturator nerve, L2–L4; tibial portion of sciatic nerve, L2–L4)	Gluteus medius (superior gluteal nerve, L4–S1)	Gluteus maximus (inferior gluteal nerve, L5–S2)
Psoas minor (lumbar plexus, L1)	Gluteus medius (posterior portion) (superior gluteal nerve, L4–S1)	Gluteus minimus (superior gluteal nerve, L4–S1)	Gracilis (obturator nerve, L2–L3)	Gluteus minimus (superior gluteal nerve, L4–S1)	Sartorius (femoral nerve, L2–L3)
Iliacus (femoral nerve, L2–L3)	Biceps femoris (long head) (tibial portion of sciatic nerve, S1–S3)	Piriformis (sacral plexus, S1)	Adductor longus (obturator nerve, L2–L4)	Tensor fasciae latae (superior gluteal nerve, L4–S1)	Piriformis (sacral plexus, S1)
Sartorius (femoral nerve, L2–L3)	Semimembranosus (tibial portion of sciatic nerve, L5–S2)	Obturator internus (nerve to obturator internus, L5–S2)	Adductor brevis (obturator nerve, L2–L4)	Adductor longus (obturator nerve, L2–L4)	Obturator internus (nerve to obturator internus, L5–S2)
Rectus femoris (femoral nerve, L2–L4)			Pectineus (femoral, obturator, or accessory obturator nerves, L2–L4)	Pectineus (femoral, obturator, or accessory obturator nerves, L2–L4)	Gemellus superior (nerve to obturator internus, L5–S2)
Pectineus (femoral, obturator, or accessory obturator nerves, L2–L4)					

Cont. on the following page(s)

Muscles that Move the Hip *Continued*

FLEXION	EXTENSION	ABDUCTION	ADDUCTION	MEDIAL ROTATION	LATERAL ROTATION
Gluteus medius (anterior portion) (superior gluteal nerve, L4–S1)	Semitendinosus (tibial portion of sciatic nerve, L5–S2)			Adductor brevis (obturator nerve, L2–L4)	Adductor magnus (lower portion) (obturator nerve, L2–L4; tibial portion of sciatic nerve, L2–L4)
Gluteus minimus (superior gluteal nerve, L4–S1)	Adductor magnus (lower portion) (obturator nerve, L2–L4; tibial portion of sciatic nerve, L2–L4)			Adductor magnus (upper portion) (obturator nerve, L2–L4; tibial portion of sciatic nerve, L2–L4)	Gemellus inferior (nerve to quadratus femoris, L4–S1)
Adductor longus (obturator nerve, L2–L4)	Piriformis (sacral plexus, S1)				Obturator externus (obturator nerve, L3–L4)
Adductor brevis (obturator nerve, L2–L4)	Obturator internus (nerve to obturator internus, L5–S2)				
Adductor magnus (upper portion) (obturator nerve, L2–L4; tibial portion of sciatic nerve, L2–L4)					

Muscles of the Knee

FLEXION	EXTENSION	MEDIAL ROTATION OF THE TIBIA	LATERAL ROTATION OF THE TIBIA
Biceps femoris (long head: tibial portion of sciatic nerve, S1–S3; and short head: peroneal portion of sciatic nerve, L5–S2)	Rectus femoris (femoral nerve, L2–L4)	Sartorius (femoral nerve, L2–L3)	Biceps femoris (long head: tibial portion of sciatic nerve, S1–S3; and short head: peroneal portion of sciatic nerve, L5–S2)
Semitendinosus (tibial portion of sciatic nerve, L5–S2)	Vastus medialis (femoral nerve, L2–L4)	Gracilis (obturator nerve, L2–L3)	
Semimembranosus (tibial portion of sciatic nerve, L5–S2)	Vastus intermedius, (femoral nerve, L2–L4)	Semitendinosus (tibial portion of sciatic nerve, L5–S2)	
Gastrocnemius (tibial nerve, S1–S2)	Vastus lateralis (femoral nerve, L2–L4)	Semimembranosus (tibial portion of sciatic nerve, L5–S2)	
Plantaris (tibial nerve, L4–S1)	Articularis genus (femoral nerve, L3–L4)		
Sartorius (femoral nerve, L2–L3)			

continued

Muscles that Move the Ankle and Subtalar Joints

DORSIFLEXION	PLANTAR FLEXION	INVERSION	EVERSION	ADDUCTION	ABDUCTION
Tibialis anterior (deep peroneal nerve, L4–S1)	Gastrocnemius (tibial nerve, S1–S2)	Tibialis posterior (tibial nerve, L5–S1)	Peroneus longus (superficial peroneal nerve, L4–S1)	Tibialis anterior (deep peroneal nerve, L4–S1)	Extensor digitorum longus (deep peroneal nerve, L4–S1)
Extensor hallucis longus (deep peroneal nerve, L4–S1)	Soleus (tibial nerve, S1–S2)	Flexor digitorum longus (tibial nerve, L5–S1)	Peroneus brevis (superficial peroneal nerve, L4–S1)	Tibialis posterior (tibial nerve, L5–S1)	Peroneus longus (superficial peroneal nerve, L4–S1)
Extensor digitorum	Flexor hallucis longus (tibial nerve, L5–S2)	Flexor hallucis longus (tibial nerve, L5–S2)	Peroneus tertius (deep peroneal	Flexor hallucis longus (tibial nerve, L5–S2)	Peroneus brevis (superficial
	Flexor digitorum longus (tibial				

longus (deep peroneal nerve, L4–S1)
Peroneus tertius (deep peroneal nerve, L5–S1)

nerve, L5–S1)
Tibialis posterior (tibial nerve, L5–S1)
Plantaris (tibial nerve, L4–S1)
Peroneus longus (superficial peroneal nerve, L4–S1)
Peroneus brevis (superficial peroneal nerve, L4–S1)

Tibialis anterior (deep peroneal nerve, L4–S1)
Extensor hallucis longus (deep peroneal nerve, L4–S1)

nerve, L5–S1)
Extensor digitorum longus (deep peroneal nerve, L4–S1)
Extensor digitorum brevis (deep peroneal nerve, L5–S1)

Flexor digitorum longus (tibial nerve, L5–S2)
Extensor hallucis longus (deep peroneal nerve, L5–S1)

peroneal nerve, L4–S1)
Peroneus tertius (deep peroneal nerve, L5–S1)

Cont. on the following page(s)

Muscles that Move the Toes			

EXTENSION	FLEXION	ABDUCTION	ADDUCTION
Extensor digitorum longus (deep peroneal nerve, L4–S1)	Flexor digitorum longus (tibial nerve, L5–S1)	Abductor hallucis (medial plantar nerve, L5–S1)	Adductor hallucis (lateral plantar nerve, S2–S3)
Extensor hallucis longus (deep peroneal nerve, L4–S1)	Flexor hallucis longus (tibial nerve, L5–S2)	Abductor digiti minimi (lateral plantar nerve, S2–S3)	Dorsal interossei (lateral plantar nerve, S2–S3)
Extensor digitorum brevis (deep peroneal nerve, L5–S1)	Flexor digitorum brevis (medial plantar nerve, L5–S1)	Plantar interossei (lateral plantar nerve, S2–S3)	
Lumbricals (distal IP extension) (first lumbrical by medial plantar nerve, L5–S1; and second through fourth lumbricals by the lateral plantar nerve, S2–S3)	Flexor hallucis brevis (medial plantar nerve, L5–S1)		
Interossei, dorsal and plantar (IP extension) (lateral	Lumbricals (MTP flexion) (first lumbrical by medial plantar nerve, L5–S1; and second through fourth lumbricales by the lateral plantar nerve, S2–S3)		

Muscles that Move the Toes *Continued*

EXTENSION	FLEXION	ABDUCTION	ADDUCTION
plantar nerve, S2–S3)	Interossei (MTP flexion) (lateral plantar nerve, S2–S3)		
	Flexor digiti minimi (lateral plantar nerve, S2–S3)		
	Quadratus plantae (lateral plantar nerve, S2–S3)		

References

1. Clemente, CD (ed): Gray's Anatomy, ed 30. Lea & Febiger, Philadelphia, 1985.
2. Pact, V, Sirotkin-Roses, M, and Beatus, J: The Muscle Testing Handbook. Little, Brown & Co, Boston, 1984.

MUSCLES CLASSIFIED BY REGION

Muscles are listed by body region. See the alphabetized reference list of muscles for descriptions that include function, innervation, origin, and insertion.

Muscles of the External Ear
Auricularis anterior
Auricularis posterior
Auricularis superior

Muscles of Facial Expression
Buccinator
Corrugator supercilii
Depressor anguli oris
Depressor labii inferioris
Depressor septi
Levator anguli oris
Levator labii superioris
Levator labii superioris alaeque
  nasi
Levator palpebrae superioris
Mentalis
Nasalis
Occipitofrontalis
Orbicularis oculi
Orbicularis oris
Platysma
Procerus
Risorius
Temporoparietalis
Transversus menti
Zygomaticus major
Zygomaticus minor

Muscles of Mastication
Buccinator
Lateral pterygoid
Masseter
Medial pterygoid
Temporalis

Muscles of the Eye
Ciliaris
Dilator pupillae
Levator palpebrae superioris
Obliquus inferior (inferior
  oblique)
Obliquus superior (superior
  oblique)
Rectus inferior (inferior rectus)
Rectus lateralis (lateral rectus)
Rectus medialis (medial rectus)

Rectus superior (superior rectus)
Sphincter pupillae

Muscles of the Internal Ear
Stapedius
Tensor tympani

Muscles of the Tongue
Chondroglossus
Genioglossus
Hyoglossus
Palatoglossus
Styloglossus

Muscles of the Palate
Levator veli palatini
Musculus uvulae
Palatoglossus
Palatopharyngeus
Tensor veli palatini

Muscles of the Pharynx
Inferior constrictor (constrictor
  inferior)
Middle constrictor (constrictor
  medius)
Palatopharyngeus
Salpingopharyngeus
Stylopharyngeus
Superior constrictor (constrictor
  superior)

Muscles of the Larynx
Aryepiglotticus
Arytenoid (arytenoideus)
Cricothyroid (cricothyroideus)
Lateral cricoarytenoid
  (cricoarytenoideus lateralis)
Posterior cricoarytenoid
  (cricoarytenoideus posterior)
Thyroarytenoid
  (thyroarytenoideus)
Thyroepiglotticus
Vocalis

Muscles of the Neck
Digastricus (anterior and
  posterior bellies)

Geniohyoid
Longus capitis
Longus colli
Mylohyoid
Omohyoid
Rectus capitis anterior
Rectus capitis lateralis
Scalenus anterior
Scalenus medius
Scalenus posterior
Sternohyoid
Sternothyroid
Stylohyoid
Thyrohyoid

Muscles Behind the Cranium
Obliquus capitis inferior
Obliquus capitis superior
Rectus capitis posterior major
Rectus capitis posterior minor

Muscles of the Back
Iliocostalis cervicis
Iliocostalis lumborum
Iliocostalis thoracis
Intertransversarii
Longissimus capitis
Longissimus cervicis
Longissimus thoracis
Multifidus
Rotatores
Semispinalis capitis
Semispinalis cervicis
Semispinalis thoracis
Spinalis capitis
Spinalis cervicis
Spinalis thoracis
Splenius capitis
Splenius cervicis

Muscles of the Thorax
Diaphragm
Innermost intercostals
Intercostales externi (external
    intercostals)
Intercostales interni (internal
    intercostals)
Levatores costarum
Serratus anterior
Serratus posterior inferior
Serratus posterior superior
Transversus thoracis

**Muscles of the
    Abdominal Region**
Cremaster
Obliquus externus abdominis
    (external oblique)
Obliquus internus abdominis
    (internal oblique)
Rectus abdominis
Transversus abdominis

Muscles of the Pelvis
Coccygeus
Levator ani iliococcygeus
Levator ani pubococcygeus

Muscles of the Perineum
Anal sphincter (external)
Anal sphincter (internal)
Bulbospongiosus
    (bulbocavernosus)
Ischiocavernosus
Sphincter urethrae
Transversus perinei profundus
Transversus perinei superficialis

**Muscles Connecting the
    Trunk or the Head to the
    Scapula**
Levator scapulae
Lower trapezius
Pectoralis minor
Rhomboid major
Rhomboid minor
Serratus anterior
Sternocleidomastoid
    (sternomastoid)
Upper trapezius

Muscles of the Shoulder
Deltoid (anterior, middle,
    posterior)
Infraspinatus
Latissimus dorsi
Pectoralis major
Subscapularis
Supraspinatus
Teres major
Teres minor

Muscles of the Arm
Biceps brachii
Brachialis
Coracobrachialis
Triceps brachii

Muscles of the Forearm
Abductor pollicis longus
Anconeus
Brachioradialis
Extensor carpi
  radialis brevis
Extensor carpi
  radialis longus
Extensor carpi ulnaris
Extensor digiti minimi
Extensor digitorum
Extensor indicis
Extensor pollicis brevis
Extensor pollicis longus
Flexor carpi radialis
Flexor carpi ulnaris
Flexor digitorum profundus
Flexor digitorum superficialis
Flexor pollicis longus
Palmaris longus
Pronator quadratus
Pronator teres
Supinator

Muscles of the Hand
Abductor digiti minimi
Abductor pollicis brevis
Adductor pollicis
Flexor digiti minimi
Flexor pollicis brevis
Interossei (dorsal and palmar)
Lumbricales
Opponens digiti minimi
Opponens pollicis
Palmaris brevis

Muscles of the Iliac Region
Iliacus
Psoas major
Psoas minor
Quadratus lumborum

Muscles of the Thigh
Adductor brevis
Adductor longus
Adductor magnus
Articularis genus

Biceps femoris
Gemelli (superior and inferior)
Gluteus maximus
Gluteus medius
Gluteus minimus
Gracilis
Obturator externus
Obturator internus
Pectineus
Piriformis
Rectus femoris
Sartorius
Semimembranosus
Semitendinosus
Tensor fasciae latae
Vastus intermedius
Vastus lateralis
Vastus medialis

Muscles of the Leg
Extensor digitorum longus
Extensor hallucis longus
Flexor digitorum longus
Flexor hallucis longus
Gastrocnemius
Peroneus brevis
Peroneus longus
Peroneus tertius
Plantaris
Popliteus
Soleus
Tibialis anterior
Tibialis posterior

Muscles of the Foot
Abductor digiti minimi
Abductor hallucis
Adductor hallucis
Extensor digitorum brevis
Flexor digiti minimi brevis
Flexor digitorum brevis
Flexor hallucis brevis
Interossei (dorsal and plantar)
Lumbricales
Quadratus plantae (flexor
  digitorum accessorius)

Reference

1. Clemente, CD (ed): Gray's Anatomy, ed 30. Lea & Febiger, Philadelphia, 1985.

MANUAL MUSCLE TESTING POSITIONS

There are two major texts on muscle testing: Kendall, FP and McCreary, EK: Muscles, Testing and Function, ed 3. Williams & Wilkins, Baltimore, 1983, and Daniels, L and Worthingham, C: Muscle Testing: Techniques of Manual Examination, ed 5. WB Saunders, Philadelphia, 1986. Each suggests different positions for testing. See manual muscle testing grading scales for differences in how they grade muscles. To facilitate testing patients once they have been positioned, the following table lists the positions suggested by the two texts.

Supine Position

DANIELS AND WORTHINGHAM

Neck flexion — all tests

Trunk flexion — all tests

Trunk rotation — all tests except poor

Elevation of pelvis — all tests

Hip flexion — poor, trace, and zero

Hip abduction — poor, trace, and zero

Hip lateral rotation — poor, trace, and zero

Hip adduction — poor, trace, and zero

Medial rotation — poor, trace, and zero

Knee extension — trace and zero

Ankle plantar flexion — normal, good, and fair

Ankle dorsiflexion — trace and zero

Subtalar inversion — poor, trace, and zero

Subtalar eversion — poor, trace, and zero

Toes — all tests

Scapular abduction — normal, good, and fair

Cont. on the following page(s)

KENDALL AND McCREARY

Toe extensors

Toe flexors

Tibialis anterior

Tibialis posterior

Peroneals

Tensor fasciae latae

Sartorius

Iliopsoas

Abdominals

Neck flexors

Finger flexors

Finger extensors

Thumb muscles

Wrist extensors

Wrist flexors

Supinators

Pronators

Biceps brachii

Brachioradialis

Triceps brachii — supine test

Pectoralis major — upper part

Pectoralis major — lower part

Pectoralis minor

Shoulder medial rotators — supine test

DANIELS AND
WORTHINGHAM

Scapular upward rotation —
normal, good, and fair

Scapular elevation — poor,
trace, and zero

Shoulder flexion — trace and
zero

Shoulder abduction — poor,
trace, and zero

Shoulder horizontal abduction
— normal, good, and fair

Elbow flexion — poor, trace,
and zero

Forearm muscles — all tests

Wrist muscles — all tests

Finger muscles — all tests

Thumb muscles — all tests

KENDALL AND McCREARY

Teres minor

Infraspinatus

Shoulder lateral rotators —
supine test

Serratus anterior

Anterior deltoid — supine test

Prone Position

DANIELS AND
WORTHINGHAM

Neck extension — all tests

Trunk extension — all tests

Hip extension — all tests except
poor

Knee flexion — all tests except
poor

Scapular adduction — normal,
good, and fair

Scapular downward rotation —
normal, good, and fair

Scapular elevation — poor,
trace, and zero

KENDALL AND McCREARY

Gastrocnemius

Plantaris

Soleus

Hamstrings — medial and lateral

Gluteus maximus

Neck extensors

Back extensors

Quadratus lumborum

Latissimus dorsi

Lower trapezius

Middle trapezius

DANIELS AND
WORTHINGHAM

Scapular adduction with
downward rotation — normal,
good, and fair

Scapular depression with
adduction — all tests

Shoulder extension — all tests

Shoulder horizontal abduction
— normal, good, and fair

Shoulder lateral rotation — all
tests

Shoulder medial rotation — all
tests

KENDALL AND McCREARY

Rhomboids

Posterior deltoid — prone test

Triceps brachii — prone test

Teres major

Shoulder medial rotators —
prone test

Shoulder lateral rotators —
prone test

Side Lying Position

DANIELS AND WORTHINGHAM

Hip flexors — poor

Hip extensors — poor

Hip abductors — normal, good, and
fair

Hip abductors from the flexed
position — normal, good, and fair

Hip adduction — normal, good, and
fair

Knee flexors — poor

Knee extensors — poor

Ankle plantar flexors — poor, trace,
and zero

Subtalar inversion — normal, good,
and fair

Subtalar eversion — normal, good,
and fair

KENDALL AND McCREARY

Gluteus medius

Gluteus minimus

Hip adductors

Lateral abdominals

DANIELS AND WORTHINGHAM

Trunk rotation — poor

Hip flexion — normal, good, and fair

Hip flexion with abduction and rotation — normal, good, and fair

Hip abduction from the flexed position — poor, trace, and zero

Hip lateral rotation — normal, good, and fair

Hip medial rotation — normal, good, and fair

Knee extension — normal, good, and fair

Ankle dorsiflexion with subtalar inversion — normal, good, fair, and poor

Subtalar inversion — fair

Scapular abduction with upward rotation — poor, trace, and zero

Scapular adduction with downward rotation — poor, trace, and zero

Scapular adduction — poor, trace, and zero

Scapular elevation — normal, good, and fair

Shoulder flexion — normal, good, and fair

Shoulder abduction — normal, good, and fair

Shoulder horizontal abduction — poor, trace, and zero

Shoulder horizontal adduction — poor, trace, and zero

Elbow flexion — normal, good, and fair

KENDALL AND McCREARY

Quadriceps femoris

Hip medial rotators

Hip lateral rotators

Hip flexors — group test

Deltoid — all parts

Coracobrachialis

Upper trapezius

Serratus anterior — preferred test

DANIELS AND
WORTHINGHAM   KENDALL AND McCREARY

Forearm muscles (with forearm
  and hand resting on table) —
  all tests

Wrist muscles (with forearm
  and hand resting on table) —
  all tests

Finger muscles (with forearm
  and hand resting on table) —
  all tests

Thumb muscles (with forearm
  and hand resting on table) —
  all tests

Standing Position

DANIELS AND WORTHINGHAM   KENDALL AND McCREARY

Elevation of the pelvis — alternate   Serratus anterior
  position for fair test   Ankle plantar flexors
Ankle plantar flexors — normal,
  good, and fair

GRADING SYSTEMS FOR MANUAL MUSCLE TESTING

Manual muscle testing has been used to describe the performance of muscles and muscle groups. Two major texts describe different forms of testing and grading. The tests and the grading scales are described here without modification.

Grading System of Daniels and Worthingham

Daniels and Worthingham describe three aspects of muscular performance as the basis for their grading scale.
1. The amount of resistance that can be given to a muscle, or group of muscles, causing a movement.
2. The ability of a muscle, or a group of muscles, to move a limb segment through part of a range of motion working against gravity or horizontal to the gravitational vector.
3. Whether there is evidence of a muscle contraction.

They further describe the use of pluses and minuses to modify their grading system. A plus or minus is applied depending upon the resistance that is felt by the examiner. According to Daniels and Worthingham, this determination is part of the judgment call that an examiner makes. They also state, however, that when grading is based on the range of motion a muscle takes a limb segment in opposition to gravity, there are distinct criteria for pluses and minuses. If less than half of the range is completed "against gravity," they suggest giving the lower grade (presumably as compared to the resistance felt) and adding a plus. They also suggest giving the higher grade with a minus if more than half of the movement is made but full range of motion did not occur.

normal and good grades: These, according to Daniels and Worthingham, are judgment calls that an examiner can make by either comparing an affected limb to a nonaffected (contralateral) limb or by using an experiential model. Resistance for these grades can be applied either at the end of a range of motion or throughout the range of motion.

fair grades: Grades of fair appear to be given when a muscle or muscle group moves a limb segment in direct opposition to the line of gravity (the gravitational vector) through a complete range of motion.

poor grades: Muscles are tested for grades of poor by positioning limb segments so that they will be moved horizontally with respect to gravity, decreasing the force needed by the muscle to overcome gravity. A poor grade is obtained when the limb segment can be moved through a complete range of motion in this position. Poor grades may also be given when there is partial movement through a range of motion against gravity.

trace and zero grades: A zero grade represents an absence of an observable (or palpable) contraction, whereas a trace grade is given when some form of contraction is present.

Grading System of Kendall and McCreary

The system of muscle testing first described by Florence and Henry Kendall differs from that suggested by Daniels and Worthingham in several fundamental aspects. These differences affect the grading scales. The Kendalls describe specific positions for testing, and these are usually not at the end of a range of motion. In describing each muscle test, the Kendalls do not describe gravity-dependent positions. In addition, almost all tests are isometric. However, gravity is mentioned in the grading scale. Presumably, there is the option for the tester to allow the subject to move voluntarily into the test position.

Although Kendall and McCreary provide a table of equivalence between their "percentage-based" grading system and those used by others, there is no clear evidence of equivalence. The scale that appears here is modified from that of Kendall and McCreary. Although muscle test grades are expressed as percentages, it should be noted that they are just names, that is, the scale is ordinal and should not be considered ratio scaled. Grades are based on the resistance the examiner feels.

Kendall and McCreary discourage use of the term *resistance* because they believe it means a force is being applied that resists motion. Because they suggest allowing a person to move into a position before the examiner applies resistance, they prefer the term *pressure* and describe the pressure applied in testing. The following uses the more common term of *resistance*.

GRADE	TEST
100%	This grade is given when a person can hold his or her limb segment against gravity and the maximum resistance given by the examiner, or when a person can move the limb segment into a test position (which is against gravity) and hold against maximum resistance.
95%	This grade is not described in detail. Presumably it is given when resistance is less than that for 100% and greater than that for 90%.
90%	This grade is given when all the criteria for 100% are met by the person, but he or she can hold against only "moderate resistance." The term *moderate resistance* is not defined.
80%	This grade is not described in detail. Presumably it is given when resistance is less than that for 90% and greater than that for 70%.
70%	This grade is given when all the criteria for 100% are met by the person, but the person can hold against only "minimum resistance." The term *minimum resistance* is not defined.
60%	This grade is not described in detail. Presumably it is given when resistance is less than that for 70% and greater than that for 50%.

GRADE	TEST
50%	This grade is given when a person can hold the test position against gravity or when a person can move into the test position and hold it against gravity.
40%	This grade is given when a person cannot hold a limb segment in the test position because the force of gravity causes him or her to release slowly, or the grade may be given when the person cannot move to the test position and needs assistance with the last part of the motion or when the person can move to the test position only if gravity is eliminated.
30%	Two methods of awarding this grade are described: if the person can move the limb segment into the position (Kendall and McCreary use the term *arc*) in a gravity-lessened position or the examiner, based on the assistance given in the gravity-maximized position, estimates what would have happened in a gravity-minimized condition. A 30% grade means the examiner gave or anticipated giving "moderate assistance."
20%	This grade is given using criteria similar to that used for a 30% contraction, but in this case more than "moderate assistance" is needed.
10%	When there is no visible movement of a limb segment but a contraction may be seen or palpated, then a grade of 10% is given.
5%	This grade is not described in detail. Presumably this grade is given when there is less of a contraction than is seen with a 10% contraction.
0%	No contraction is felt or seen in the muscle.

References

1. Daniels, L and Worthingham C: Muscle Testing: Techniques of Manual Examination, ed 5. WB Saunders, Philadelphia, 1986.
2. Kendall, FP and McCreary, EK: Muscles, Testing and Function, ed 3. Williams & Wilkins, Baltimore, 1983.

ORTHOPAEDIC TESTS

The following table lists orthopaedic tests by body region and the pathology to be tested. For details on each test, consult the list of orthopaedic tests.

BODY REGION AND PATHOLOGY (regions are listed from cephalad to caudal)	TEST
Cervical Region	
Dural irritation	L'hermitte's sign
Nerve root lesions	Brachial plexus tension test
	Distraction test
	Foraminal compression test
	Shoulder abduction test
	Shoulder depression test
	Valsalva test
(Vascular compression)	Vertebral artery test
Shoulder	
Anterior shoulder dislocation	Apprehension test
Biceps tendon instability	Impingement sign (also tests the supraspinatus)
	Ludington's test (for ruptured biceps tendon)
	Speed's test (biceps test) (for bicipital tendonitis)
	Transverse humeral ligament test
	Yergason's test (for bicipital tendonitis)
Neurovascular compression syndromes	Adson maneuver (for thoracic outlet syndrome)
	Allen maneuver (for thoracic outlet syndrome)
	Halstead maneuver (for thoracic outlet syndrome)
	Costoclavicular syndrome test (for thoracic outlet syndrome)
	Hyperabduction syndrome test
	Suprascapular nerve entrapment test
Posterior shoulder dislocation	Apprehension test

Cont. on the following page(s)

BODY REGION AND PATHOLOGY	TEST
(regions are listed from cephalad to caudal)	
Torn rotator cuff	Drop-arm test
	Supraspinatus test
Elbow	
Ligamentous instability	Ligamentous instability tests (for medial and lateral collateral ligaments)
Neurovascular compression	Elbow flexion test (for cubital tunnel syndrome)
Tendonitis	Golfer's elbow test
	Tennis elbow tests
Wrist and Hand	
Contractures	Bunnel-Littler test (for limitations at the PIP joints)
	Tight retinacular ligament test (PIP, DIP joint or collateral ligaments)
Neurovascular compression	Allen test (for vascular insufficiency to the hand)
	Froment's sign (for ulnar nerve damage)
	Phalen's test (wrist flexion test, for carpal tunnel syndrome)
	Tinel's sign (for carpal tunnel syndrome)
Rheumatoid arthritis	Intrinsic-plus test (for limitations of the intrinsic hand muscles)
Tendonitis	Finkelstein's test (for de Quervain's disease)
Low Back	
Malingering	Hoover's (sign) test (for differentiating lower limb weakness from malingering)
Nerve compression	Bowstring test (cram test or popliteal pressure sign, for the sciatic nerve)
	Brudzinski's sign (for root, meningeal, or dural irritations)

BODY REGION AND PATHOLOGY	TEST
(regions are listed from cephalad to caudal)	
	Femoral nerve traction test (for roots L2 to L4)
	Kernig's sign (Brudzinski's sign, for root, meningeal, or dural irritations)
	Naffziger test (for nerve root inflammation)
	Prone knee flexion test (also called Reverse Lasegue test for roots L2, L3)
	Sitting root test (for the sciatic nerve)
	Straight leg raising test (for the sciatic nerve)
Sacroiliac disorders	Palpation of anterior superior iliac spines (patient sitting)
	Palpation of anterior superior iliac spines (patient standing)
	Palpation of iliac crests (patient sitting)
	Palpation of iliac crests (patient standing)
	Palpation of posterior superior iliac spines (patient sitting)
	Palpation of posterior superior iliac spines (patient standing)
	Prone knee flexion test
	Side-lying iliac compression test
	Sitting flexion test
	Standing flexion test
	Standing Gillet test
	Supine iliac gapping test
	Supine long sitting test

Hip

Arthritis	Patrick's test
Contractures	Ober's test (for a tight iliotibial band)
Dislocation	Ortolani's test

Cont. on the following page(s)

BODY REGION AND PATHOLOGY	TEST
(regions are listed from cephalad to caudal)	
	Galeazzi's test
	Barlow's provocative test
	Trendelenburg's test (for detecting dislocation, weakness of the gluteus medius muscle, or extreme coxa vara)
Knee	
Anterior instability	Anterior drawer test (for anterior instability)
	Crossover test (for anterolateral instability)
	Hughston test (jerk sign) (for anterolateral instability; it is a modification of the MacIntosh test)
	Lachman's test (for anterior instability)
	Losee test (for anterolateral rotary instability)
	MacIntosh test (lateral pivot shift, or anterolateral rotary instability)
	Slocum ALRI test (for anterolateral rotary instability)
	Slocum test (for anterolateral rotary instability; it is a modification of the MacIntosh test)
Effusion	Brush or stroke test (for slight effusions)
	Patellar tap test
	Fluctuation test (for significant effusions)
Lateral instability	Adduction (varus) stress test
Medial instability	Abduction (valgus) stress test
Meniscus and tibiofemoral joint lesions	Apley grinding test (for meniscal or ligamentous lesions)

BODY REGION AND PATHOLOGY	TEST
(regions are listed from cephalad to caudal)	
	Bounce home test (for meniscal lesions)
	Helfet test (for meniscal lesions)
	Hughston Plica test (for abnormal suprapatellar plica, which can mimic a torn meniscus)
	McMurray test (for meniscal lesions)
	O'Donoghue's test (for meniscal lesions or capsular irritation)
	Wilson test (for osteochondritis dissecans)
Patellar lesions	Apprehension test (for a dislocating patella)
	Clarke's sign (for chondromalacia of the patella)
	Perkin's test (for patellar tenderness)
	Waldron test (for chondromalacia of the patella)
Posterior instability	External rotation recurvatum test (for posterolateral rotary instability)
	Hughston posterolateral drawer test (for posterolateral rotary instability)
	Hughston posteromedial drawer test (for posteromedial rotary instability)
	Jakob test (for posterolateral rotary instability)
	Posterior drawer test (for posterior instability)
	Posterior sag sign (gravity drawer test, for posterior instability)

Cont. on the following page(s)

BODY REGION AND PATHOLOGY	TEST
(regions are listed from cephalad to caudal)	
Foot and Ankle	
Achilles tendon	Thompson test (for Achilles tendon rupture)
Deep vein thrombosis	Homans' sign (for deep vein thrombosis of the leg)
Ligamentous instability	Anterior drawer test (for anterior ankle instability)
	Kleiger test (for medial instability)
	Talar tilt (for the calcaneofibular ligament)

References

1. Magee, DJ: Orthopedic Physical Assessment. WB Saunders, Philadelphia, 1987.
2. D'Ambrosia, RD: Musculoskeletal Disorders: Regional Examination and Differential Diagnosis. JB Lippincott, Philadelphia, 1977.

COMMONLY USED ORTHOPAEDIC TESTS

Common orthopaedic tests described here are listed by body region with the most cephalad regions listed first. Within body regions, the tests are listed in alphabetical order.

Cervical spine

brachial plexus tension test: A test designed to detect nerve root compression. The patient lies supine and slowly abducts and externally rotates the arm just to the point of pain. The forearm is then supinated and flexed, with the examiner supporting the shoulder and forearm. The test is positive if the patient's symptoms are reproduced or increased.

distraction test: A test designed to identify nerve root compression. The examiner places one hand under the patient's chin and the other under the occiput. The head is slowly lifted (distraction), and the test is considered positive if the radiating pain is decreased.

foraminal compression test: A test designed to identify nerve root compression. The patient laterally flexes her or his head. The examiner carefully presses down (compression) on the head. The test is positive if pain radiates into the arm toward the flexed side.

L'hermitte's sign: A test designed to identify dural irritation. The patient is in the long leg sitting position. While keeping the patient's knees extended, the examiner flexes the patient's head and hips simultaneously. The test is positive if there is a sharp pain down the spine and into the upper or lower extremities.

shoulder abduction test: A test designed to identify extradural compression, such as a herniated disk, epidural vein compression, or nerve root compression most commonly at C5 or C6. The patient is in a sitting or lying position. The patient's arm is abducted actively or passively so that the hand or forearm of the patient rests on the patient's head. The test is positive if there is a decrease in symptoms.

shoulder depression test: A test designed to detect nerve root compression or dural adhesions to the nerve or joint capsule. The examiner flexes the patient's head to one side while applying downward pressure on the opposite shoulder. The test is positive if pain is increased.

Valsalva test: A test designed to detect a space-occupying lesion in the cervical spine, such as a herniated disk or an osteophyte. The examiner instructs the patient to take a deep breath and hold the breath, as if the patient is having a bowel movement. The test is positive if symptoms are reproduced or increased.

vertebral artery test: A test designed to detect compression of the vertebral artery. The patient is in a supine position. The examiner places the patient's head into a position of extension, lateral flexion, and rotation and holds that position for 30 seconds. Each side is tested separately. The test is positive if the patient reports having a feeling of dizziness or nausea, or if nystagmus is observed.

Shoulder

Adson maneuver: A test designed to determine the presence of thoracic outlet syndrome. The patient turns his or her head toward the shoulder on the side being tested. The examiner externally rotates and extends the shoulder while the patient extends her or his head. The test is positive if the radial pulse disappears while the patient holds a deep breath.

Allen maneuver: A test designed to identify the presence of thoracic outlet syndrome. With the patient seated, the examiner flexes the patient's elbow to 90° while the patient's shoulder is abducted 90° and externally rotated. The examiner then palpates the radial pulse while the patient rotates his or her head away from the test side. The test is positive if the pulse disappears.

apprehension test for anterior shoulder dislocation: A test designed to determine whether a patient has a history of anterior dislocations. With the patient supine, the examiner slowly abducts and externally rotates the patient's arm. The test is positive if the patient becomes apprehensive and resists further motion.

apprehension test for posterior shoulder dislocation: A test designed to determine whether a patient has a history of posterior dislocations. With the patient supine, the examiner slowly flexes the patient's arm to 90° and the patient's elbow to 90°. The examiner then internally rotates the patient's arm. A posterior force is then applied to the patient's elbow. The test is positive if the patient becomes apprehensive and resists further motion.

biceps test: See Speed's test.

costoclavicular syndrome test: A test designed to determine the presence of thoracic outlet syndrome. The patient is asked to adduct her or his scapula while the examiner extends the patient's shoulder. For a positive test, symptoms should be reproduced with a decreased radial pulse to confirm the diagnosis.

drop-arm test: A test designed to determine the presence of a torn rotator cuff. With the patient seated, the examiner abducts the patient's shoulder to 90°. The test is positive if the patient is unable to lower the arm slowly to his or her side in the same arc of movement or has severe pain when attempting to do so.

Halstead maneuver: A test designed to determine the presence of thoracic outlet syndrome. With the patient seated, the examiner palpates the radial pulse and applies a downward force on the arm. The patient extends his or her neck and rotates her or his head toward the opposite side of the limb being tested. The test is positive if the pulse disappears following this maneuver.

hyperabduction syndrome test: A test designed to determine the presence of thoracic outlet syndrome. The patient abducts his or her arm above her or his head. Compression of the neurovascular bundle under the coracoid process and under the pectoralis minor muscle reproduces symptoms and results in a diminished radial pulse.

impingement sign: A test designed to identify inflammation of tissues within the subacromial space. The patient's upper extremity is forcibly flexed forward by the examiner. This manuever is thought to decrease the space between the head of the humerus and acromion process. The test is positive if the patient reports pain.

Ludington's test: A test designed for determining whether there has been a rupture of the long head of the biceps tendon. The patient is seated and clasps both hands on top of his or her head, supporting the weight of the upper limbs. The patient then alternately contracts and relaxes the biceps muscles. The test is positive if the examiner cannot palpate the long head of the biceps tendon of the affected arm during the contractions.

Speed's test (biceps test): A test designed to determine whether bicipital tendonitis is present. With the forearm supinated and elbow fully extended, the patient tries to flex the arm against resistance applied by the examiner. The test is positive if the patient reports increased pain in the area of the bicipital groove.

suprascapular nerve entrapment test: A test designed to identify entrapment of the suprascapular nerve in the suprascapular notch. Patients report pain when horizontally adducting their arm across their chest. The pain is poorly localized to the posterior aspect of the shoulder.

supraspinatus test: A test designed to identify a tear in the supraspinatus tendon. The seated patient's upper limbs are positioned horizontally at 30° anterior to the frontal plane and internally rotated. The examiner applies a downward force on the patient's limbs. The test is positive if pain and weakness are present on the involved side.

transverse humeral ligament test: A test designed to identify a torn transverse humeral ligament. The examiner abducts and internally rotates the patient's shoulder. The examiner then palpates the bicipital groove while externally rotating the patient's shoulder. The test is positive if the biceps tendon can be felt to "snap" in and out of the groove with shoulder external rotation.

Yergason's test: A test designed to identify tendonitis of the long head of the biceps. The seated patient's arm is positioned at his or her side with the elbow flexed to 90°. Supination of the forearm against resistance produces pain in the biceps tendon in the area of the bicipital groove.

Elbow

elbow flexion test: A test designed to identify cubital tunnel syndrome. The patient is asked to hold his or her elbow fully flexed for 5 minutes. The test is positive if tingling or paresthesias are felt in the ulnar nerve distribution of the forearm and hand.

golfer's elbow test: A test designed to identify the presence of inflammation in the area of the medial epicondyle. The patient flexes the elbow and wrist, supinates the forearm, and then extends the elbow.

The test is positive if the patient complains of pain over the medial epicondyle.

ligamentous instability tests: Tests designed to assess the integrity of the lateral and medial collateral ligaments of the elbow. The patient's arm is held by the examiner so that the examiner is supporting the elbow and wrist. The examiner tests the lateral collateral ligament by applying an adduction or varus force to the distal forearm with the patient's elbow held in 20° to 30° of flexion. The medial collateral ligament is similarly tested by the application of an abduction or valgus force at the distal forearm. The test is positive if pain or altered mobility is present.

tennis elbow tests: The following tests are designed to test for the presence of inflammation in the area of the lateral epicondyle.

1. The patient flexes the elbow to approximately 45° and fully supinates the forearm while making a fist. The patient is then asked to pronate the forearm and radially deviate and extend the wrist while the examiner resists these motions. For a positive test, pain is elicited in the area of the lateral epicondyle.
2. The examiner pronates the patient's arm, fully extends the elbow, and fully flexes the wrist. For a positive test, pain is elicited in the area of the lateral epicondyle.

Wrist and Hand

Allen test: A test designed to determine the patency of the vascular communication in the hand. The examiner first palpates and occludes the radial and ulnar arteries. The patient is then asked to open and close his or her fingers rapidly from three to five times to cause the palmar skin to blanch. Pressure is then released from either the radial or ulnar artery, and the rapidity with which the hand regains color is noted. The test is repeated with release of the other artery. A positive Allen's test indicates that there is a diminished or absent communication between the superficial ulnar arch and the deep radial arch.

Bunnel-Littler test: A test designed to identify intrinsic muscle or joint contractures at the proximal interphalangeal (PIP) joints. The examiner flexes the PIP joint maximally while maintaining the MCP joint in slight extension. The test is positive for a joint capsule contracture if the PIP joint cannot be flexed. The test is positive for intrinsic muscle contracture if the MCP is slightly flexed and the PIP flexes fully.

Finkelstein's test: A test designed to determine the presence of tenosynovitis of the abductor pollicis longus and extensor pollicis brevis tendons. The test is commonly used to determine the presence of de Quervain's disease. The patient makes a fist while holding the thumb inside the fingers. The patient then attempts to deviate ulnarly the first metacarpal and extend the proximal joint of the thumb. If the patient experiences pain, this is recorded as a positive test.

Froment's sign: A test designed for determining the presence of adductor pollicis weakness from ulnar nerve paralysis. The patient attempts to grasp a piece of paper between the tips of the thumb and the radial side of the index finger. The test is positive if the terminal phalanx of the patient's thumb flexes as the examiner attempts to pull the paper from the patient's grasp.

intrinsic-plus test: A test designed to identify shortening of the intrinsic muscles of the hand. This test is useful and specific when examining the hand of the patient with rheumatoid arthritis, particularly in the early stages prior to any destruction or deformity of the hand. In this test, the metacarpophalangeal joint of the finger being tested is hyperextended. The middle and distal joints flex slightly due to the passive action of tissues. The examiner then further attempts to flex passively the proximal interphalangeal joint of the finger. Any severe restriction to this movement is considered a positive sign.

Phalen's (wrist flexion) test: A test designed to determine the presence of carpal tunnel syndrome. The patient's wrists are maximally flexed by the examiner, who maintains this position by holding the patient's wrists together for 1 minute. The test is positive if paresthesias are present in the thumb, index finger, and the middle and lateral half of the ring finger.

tight retinacular ligament test: A test designed to determine the presence of shortened retinacular ligaments or a tight DIP joint capsule. The examiner holds the patient's proximal interphalangeal (PIP) joint in a fully extended position while attempting to flex the DIP joint. If the distal interphalangeal (DIP) joint does not flex, the test is positive for either a contracted collateral ligament or joint capsule. The test is positive for tight retinacular (collateral) ligaments and a normal joint capsule if, when the PIP joint is flexed, the DIP joint flexes easily.

Tinel's sign: A test designed to detect carpal tunnel syndrome. The examiner taps over the carpal tunnel of the wrist. The test is positive if the patient reports paresthesia distal to the wrist.

wrist flexion test: See Phalen's test.

Low Back (also see sacroiliac joint tests)

bowstring test (cram test or popliteal pressure sign): A test designed to identify the presence of sciatic nerve compression. A straight leg raising test is first carried out by the examiner. The leg is raised to the point where the patient reports pain. The knee is slightly flexed to reduce the symptoms. Digital pressure is then applied to the popliteal fossa. The test is positive if pain is increased.

Brudzinski's sign: See Kernig's sign.

cram test: The same as the bowstring test (see bowstring test).

femoral nerve traction test: A test designed to identify nerve root compression of the midlumbar area (L2, L3, and L4). The patient lies on the unaffected side with the unaffected limb flexed slightly for support. The examiner grasps the "affected" limb and extends the knee while gently extending the hip approximately 15°, being sure not to extend the back. The patient's knee is then flexed, further stretching the femoral nerve. The test is positive if pain radiates down the anterior thigh.

Hoover's sign test: A test designed to discriminate lower limb weakness from possible malingering. The patient relaxes in a supine position while the examiner places one hand under each heel. The patient is then asked to do a straight leg raise (knee extended). The test is positive if the patient is unable to lift the leg and there is no downward pressure from the opposite leg.

Kernig's sign: A test designed to identify meningeal irritation, nerve root involvement, or dural irritation. The patient lies in the supine position with hands cupped behind the head. The patient flexes his or her head onto the chest (Brudzinski's sign) and raises the lower extremity with knee extended (Kernig's sign). The test is positive if radiating pain is elicited.

Naffziger test: A test designed to detect a space occupying lesion in the spine. The patient lies supine while the examiner gently compresses the jugular veins for approximately 10 seconds. The patient is then asked to cough. The test is positive if coughing produces pain in the lower back.

popliteal pressure sign: See bowstring test.

prone knee flexion test (also called reverse Lasegue test: A test designed to identify L2 or L3 nerve root lesions. The patient lies prone while the examiner passively flexes the knee so that the patient's heel touches the patient's buttocks. The test is positive if unilateral symptoms are elicited or increased in the lumbar area or anterior thigh. Pain in the anterior thigh may indicate a tight quadriceps muscle.

sitting root test: A test designed to identify compression of the sciatic nerve. The patient is seated with neck flexed. The knee is actively extended while the hip remains flexed. The test is positive if pain increases.

straight leg raising test: A test designed to identify sciatic nerve root compression. With the patient supine, the examiner raises the patient's extended leg while watching the patient's reaction. The examiner stops when the patient complains of back or leg pain (and not hamstring tightness). The examiner may also dorsiflex the ankle to further increase the traction on the sciatic nerve. Back pain suggests a central herniation, and leg pain suggests a lateral disk protrusion. The test is repeated for both sides.

Sacroiliac Joint

Gillet test:

palpation of anterior superior iliac spines (patient sitting): A test designed to identify the presence of asymmetry of the sacroiliac joints that may be associated with subluxation or other pain-producing causes. The patient sits erect on a flat surface. The examiner, who is standing or squatting in front of the patient, places his or her thumbs on the inferior margins of the anterior superior iliac spines (ASIS). The examiner then moves the thumbs upward so that they are stopped by the bony prominence of the ASIS. The test is positive if one ASIS is higher than the other.

palpation of anterior superior iliac spines (patient standing): A test designed to identify the presence of asymmetry of the sacroiliac joints that may be associated with subluxation or other pain-producing causes. The patient stands with feet 12 inches apart. The examiner, standing or squatting in front of the patient, places her or his thumbs on the inferior margins of the anterior superior iliac spines (ASIS). The examiner then moves the thumbs upward so that they are stopped by the bony prominence of the ASIS. The test is positive if one ASIS is higher than the other.

palpation of iliac crests (patient sitting): A test designed to identify the presence of asymmetry of the sacroiliac joints that may be associated with subluxation or other pain-producing causes. The patient sits erect on a flat surface. The examiner, who is standing or squatting behind the patient, places the radial borders of his or her hands on the patient's waist. The hands are then moved gently downward to move aside soft tissues before the examiner's movement is stopped by the iliac crests. The test is positive if one crest is higher than the other.

palpation of iliac crests (patient standing): A test designed to identify the presence of asymmetry of the sacroiliac joints that may be associated with subluxation or other pain-producing causes. The patient stands with feet 12 inches apart. The examiner, who is standing or squatting behind the patient, places the radial borders of her or his hands on the patient's waist. The hands are then moved gently downward to move aside soft tissues before the examiner's movement is stopped by the iliac crests. The test is positive if one crest is higher than the other.

palpation of posterior superior iliac spines (patient sitting): A test designed to identify the presence of asymmetry of the sacroiliac joints that may be associated with subluxation or other pain-producing causes. The patient sits erect on a flat surface. The examiner, who is standing or squatting behind the patient, places his or her thumbs on the inferior margin of the posterior superior iliac spines (PSIS). The examiner then moves her or his thumbs upward so that they are stopped by the bony prominence of the posterior superior iliac spines (PSIS). The test is positive if one PSIS is higher than the other.

palpation of posterior superior iliac spines (patient standing): A test designed to identify the presence of asymmetry of the sacroiliac joints that may be associated with subluxation or other pain-producing causes. The patient stands with feet 12 inches apart. The examiner, who is standing or squatting behind the patient, places her or his thumbs on the inferior margin of the posterior superior iliac spines (PSIS). The examiner then moves his or her thumbs upward so that they are stopped by the bony prominence of the posterior superior iliac spines (PSIS). The test is positive if one PSIS is higher than the other.

prone knee flexion test: A test designed to identify the presence of rotation of the innominate bones relative to the sacroiliac joint. The patient, who should be wearing shoes, lies prone with arms at sides and the cervical spine in a neutral position. The examiner stands at the patient's feet and grasps the heels of the patient's shoes. The examiner places his or her index fingers just posterior to the lateral malleoli and holds the feet in a neutral position relative to pronation and supination. The examiner then flexes the patient's knees to 90° of flexion. A change in the relative position of the patient's heels is said to indicate innominate rotation. An apparent increase in leg length is said to indicate a posterior innominate rotation on the same side. An apparent decrease in leg length is said to indicate an anterior innominate rotation on the same side.

side-lying iliac compression test: A test designed to identify the presence of sacroiliac joint dysfunction. The patient lies on his or her side. The examiner stands above the patient and, with elbows fully extended, interlocks her or his palms and places them over the most cephalad margin of the iliac crest. The examiner then exerts a downward and cephalad directed force on the crest. The test is positive if the patient's painful symptoms in the sacroiliac, gluteal, or crural regions are reproduced.

sitting flexion test: A test designed to identify the presence of sacroiliac joint dysfunction. The patient sits erect on a flat surface, with feet flat on the floor and knees flexed to 90°. The hips are sufficiently abducted that the patient can bend forward between them. The examiner, who is kneeling or squatting behind the patient, places his or her thumbs on the inferior margin of the posterior superior iliac spines (PSIS). The patient bends forward as far as possible, reaching the hands toward the floor. A positive test occurs when one PSIS moves more in a cranial direction than does the other. The side with the greater movement is said to have articular restriction.

standing flexion test: A test designed to identify the presence of sacroiliac joint dysfunction. The patient stands with feet 12 inches apart. The examiner, who is standing or squatting behind the patient, places his or her thumbs on the inferior margin of the posterior superior iliac spines (PSIS). The patient then bends forward while keeping the knees straight. A positive test occurs when one PSIS moves more in a cranial direction than does the other. The side with the greater movement is said to have articular restriction. Because hamstring tightness may also cause these findings the test is not considered positive until hamstring tightness has been ruled out.

standing Gillet test: A test designed to identify the presence of sacroiliac joint dysfunction. The patient stands with feet 12 inches apart. The examiner, who is standing behind the patient, places one thumb directly under one posterior superior iliac spine (PSIS) and the other thumb on the ipsilateral tubercle of S2 (which is on the sacrum at the level of the PSIS). The patient flexes the hip and knee on the side being palpated so that she or he is standing on one leg. A positive test is one in which the PSIS does not dip downward as the extreme of hip flexion is reached. The test is repeated on the contralateral side.

supine iliac gapping test: A test designed to identify sacroiliac joint dysfunction. The patient lies supine. The examiner crosses his or her arms, placing the palms of her or his hands on the patient's anterior superior iliac spines. The examiner then presses down and laterally to strain the sacroiliac ligaments. A positive test occurs when the patient reports pain in the gluteal or posterior crural areas. If pain is felt in the lumbar region, the test is repeated after using more support for the lumbar spine.

supine long sitting test: A test designed to identify the presence of rotation of the innominate bones relative to the sacroiliac joint. The patient lies supine. The examiner places her or his thumbs on the inferior borders of the medial malleoli. The patient then sits up, being careful to do so in a symmetrical, non-twisting fashion. Changes in the relative positions of the medial malleoli are noted. If one leg appears to lengthen when the patient sits up, that is interpreted as indicating a posterior innominate rotation on that side. If one leg appears to shorten when the patient sits up, that is interpreted as indicating an anterior innominate rotation on that side.

Hip

Barlow's provocative test: See Ortolani's test. A test designed to identify hip instability in infants. The test is performed after the Ortolani test has been conducted. With the infant in the same position used for Ortolani's test, the examiner stabilizes the pelvis between the symphysis and sacrum with one hand. With the thumb of the other hand, the examiner attempts to dislocate the hip by gentle but firm posterior pressure.

Galeazzi's test: A test designed to detect unilateral congenital dislocations of the hip in children. The child is positioned supine with the hips flexed to 90° and the knees fully flexed. The test is positive if one knee is positioned higher than the other.

Ober's test: A test designed to determine the presence of a shortened (tight) iliotibial band. With the patient lying on one side, the lower limb closest to the table is flexed. The other lower limb, which is being tested, is abducted and extended. The knee of that limb is flexed to 90° and is then allowed to drop to the table. If the limb does not, this indicates that the iliotibial band is shortened (tight).

Ortolani's test: A test designed to identify a congenital hip dislocation in infants. The infant is positioned supine with the hips flexed 90° and the knees fully flexed. The examiner grasps the legs so that the examiner's thumbs are placed on the infant's medial thighs and the examiner's fingers are placed on the infant's lateral thighs. The thighs are gently abducted, and the examiner applies a gentle force to the greater trochanters with the fingers of each hand. Resistance will be felt at about 30° of abduction and, if there is a dislocation, a click will be felt as the dislocation is reduced (see the related Barlow's provocative test).

Patrick's test: A test designed to identify arthritis of the hip. With the patient lying supine, the knee is flexed and the hip is flexed, abducted, and externally rotated until the lateral malleolus rests on the opposite knee just above the patella. In this position the knee on the side being tested is gently forced downward; if pain is produced, the test is positive for the presence of osteoarthritis of the hip.

Trendelenburg's test: A test designed to identify the presence of an unstable hip. The patient stands on the leg to be tested. The test is positive if the non-weight-bearing side does not rise as the patient stands on one lower extremity. A positive test may be caused by a hip dislocation, weakness of the hip abductors, or coxa vara.

Knee

abduction (valgus stress) test: A test designed to identify medial instability of the knee. The examiner applies a valgus stress to the patient's knee while the patient's ankle is stabilized in slight lateral rotation. The test is first conducted with the knee fully extended and then repeated with the knee at 20° of flexion. Excessive movement of the tibia away from the femur indicates a positive test. Positive findings with the knee fully extended indicate a major disruption of the knee ligaments. A positive test with the knee flexed is indicative of damage to the medial collateral ligament.

adduction (varus stress) test: A test designed to identify lateral instability of the knee. The examiner applies a varus stress to the patient's knee while the ankle is stabilized. The test is done with the patient's knee in full extension and then with the knee in 20° to 30° of flexion. A positive test with the knee extended suggests a major disruption of the knee ligaments, whereas a positive test with the knee flexed is indicative of damage to the lateral collateral ligament.

ALRI test: See Slocum ALRI test.

anterior drawer (sign) test: A test designed to detect anterior instability of the knee. The patient lies supine with the knee flexed 90°. The examiner sits across the forefoot of the patient's flexed lower limb. With the patient's foot in neutral rotation, the examiner pulls forward on the proximal part of the calf. Both lower limbs are tested. The test is positive if there is excessive anterior movement of the tibia with respect to the femur.

Apley grinding test: A test designed to detect meniscal lesions. The patient lies prone with the knees flexed 90°. The examiner applies a compressive force through the foot and rotates the tibia back and forth while palpating the joint line with the other hand feeling for crepitation. The test is positive if the patient reports pain or the examiner feels crepitation. This test is then repeated by applying a distractive force to the leg, and if pain is elicited it is indicative of a ligamentous injury rather than a meniscal injury.

apprehension test: A test designed to identify dislocation of the patella. The patient lies supine with the knee resting at 30° flexion. The examiner carefully and slowly displaces the patella laterally. If the patient looks apprehensive and tries to contract the quadriceps muscle to bring the patella back to neutral, the test is positive.

bounce home test: A test designed to identify meniscal lesions. The patient lies supine, and the heel of the patient's foot is cupped by the examiner. The patient's knee is completely flexed and then allowed to extend passively. If extension is not complete or has a rubbery end-feel ("springy block"), the test is positive.

brush or stroke (wipe) test: This test is designed to identify a mild effusion in the knee. Starting below the joint line on the medial side of the patella, the examiner strokes proximally with the palm and fingers as far as the suprapatellar pouch. With the opposite hand, the examiner strokes down the lateral side of the patella. The test is positive if a wave of fluid appears as a slight bulge at the medial distal border of the patella.

Clarke's sign: A test designed to identify the presence of chondromalacia of the patella. The patient lies relaxed with knees extended as the examiner presses down slightly proximal to the base of the patella with the web of the hand. The patient is then asked to contract the quadriceps muscle as the examiner applies more force. The test is positive if the patient cannot complete the contraction without pain.

crossover test: A test designed to identify anterolateral instability of the knee. With the patient standing and the uninvolved leg crossed in front of the test leg, the examiner secures the foot of the test leg by carefully stepping on it. The patient rotates the upper torso away from the injured leg approximately 90°. In this position the patient is asked to contract the quadriceps muscles. If this action produces a feeling of "giving way" in the knee, the test is positive.

drawer sign test: See anterior drawer test and posterior drawer test.

external rotation recurvatum test: A test designed to identify posterolateral rotary instability of the knee. There are two methods for this test. Both are conducted with the patient in a supine position:
1. The examiner elevates the patient's legs by grasping the patient's great toes. The test is positive if the tibial tubercle is observed to rotate laterally while the knee goes into recurvatum.
2. The examiner flexes the knee to 30° or 40°. The knee is then slowly extended while the examiner's other hand holds the posterolateral aspect of the knee to palpate for movement. The test is positive if hyperextension and excessive lateral rotation occur in the injured limb.

fluctuation test: A test designed to identify significant knee effusion. The knee is placed in a position of 15° flexion. The examiner then places the palm of one hand over the suprapatellar pouch and the other hand anterior to the joint, with the thumb and index finger adjacent to the patellar margins. The examiner tries to feel and assess the shifting or fluctuation of synovial fluid while alternatively pressing down with one hand and then the other.

gravity drawer test: See posterior sag sign.

Helfet test: A test designed to identify meniscal lesions. The "screw home" mechanism is observed during full extension. With a torn meniscus blocking the joint, the tibial tubercle remains slightly medial in relation to the midline of the patella, and the final limit of external rotation is prevented.

Hughston plica test: A test designed to identify an abnormal suprapatellar plica. The patient lies supine, and the examiner flexes the knee and medially rotates the tibia with one arm and hand while with the other hand the patella is displaced slightly medially with the fingers over the course of the plica. The test is positive if a "pop" is elicited at the plica while the knee is flexed and extended by the examiner.

Hughston posterolateral drawer test: A test designed to identify the presence of posterolateral rotary knee instability. The procedure is similar to the Hughston posteromedial test except the patient's foot is slightly laterally rotated. The test is positive if the tibia rotates posteriorly on the lateral side an excessive amount when the examiner pushes the tibia posteriorly.

Hughston posteromedial drawer test: A test designed to identify posteromedial rotary instability of the knee. The patient lies in a supine position with the knee flexed to 90°. The examiner fixes the foot in slight medial rotation by sitting on the foot. The examiner pushes the tibia posteriorly. The test is positive if the tibia moves or rotates posteriorly on the medial aspect an excessive amount.

Hughston test (jerk sign): A test designed to identify the presence of anterolateral rotary instability of the knee. The test is a modification of the MacIntosh test for anterolateral instability. The patient lies supine with the knee flexed to 90°. The extremity is grasped at the foot with one hand while the examiner's other hand rests over the proximal, lateral aspect of the leg just distal to the knee. A valgus stress is applied to the knee and the tibia is internally rotated while the knee is slowly moved into extension. The test is positive if, when the knee is gradually extended, at 30° to 40° of flexion the lateral tibial plateau suddenly subluxes forward and does so with a jerking sensation. The knee will spontaneously reduce if the leg is further extended.

Jakob test (reverse pivot shift): A test designed to identify posterolateral rotary instability of the knee. This test can be performed with the patient either standing or supine

1. In the standing position, the patient leans against a wall with the involved extremity toward the examiner. The examiner's hands are placed above and below the test knee, and a valgus stress is applied while the patient flexes the knee. The test is positive if there is a jerk in the knee or the tibia shifts posteriorly and the knee gives way.
2. The patient lies supine. The examiner supports the patient's knee posteriorly with one hand and the heel with the other hand. The patient's foot is then laterally rotated.

jerk sign: See Hughston test.

Lachman's test: A test designed to identify injury to the anterior cruciate ligament. The patient lies supine with the examiner stabilizing the distal femur with one hand and grasping the proximal tibia with the other hand. With the knee held in slight flexion, the tibia is moved forward on the femur. A positive test is indicated by a soft end-feel and excessive observable movement of the tibia.

lateral pivot shift: See MacIntosh test.

Losee test: A test designed to identify anterolateral rotary instability of the knee. With the patient supine and relaxed, the examiner cradles the patient's foot so that the knee is flexed to 30° and the leg is externally rotated and braced against the examiner's abdomen. With the patient's hamstrings relaxed, the examiner extends the knee while the examiner's right thumb pushes the fibula anteriorly and a valgus stress is applied to the knee. The knee is allowed to rotate internally during extension. The test is positive if the lateral tibial plateau subluxes anteriorly just before full extension.

MacIntosh test (lateral pivot shift): A test designed to identify anterolateral rotary instability. The examiner grasps the leg with one hand and places the other hand over the lateral, proximal aspect of the leg. With the knee in extension, a valgus stress is applied and the leg internally rotated as the knee is flexed. At about 30° to 40° of flexion, a sudden jump is noted as the lateral tibial plateau, which has subluxed anteriorly in relation to the femoral condyle, suddenly reduces.

McMurray test: A test designed to identify meniscal lesions. The patient lies supine while the examiner grasps the foot with one hand and palpates the joint line with the other. The knee is fully flexed and the tibia rotated back and forth and then held alternately in internal and external rotation as the knee is extended. A click or crepitation may be felt over the joint line with a posterior meniscal lesion, as the knee is extended.

O'Donoghue's test: A test designed to detect meniscal injuries or capsular irritation. The patient lies supine, and the examiner flexes the knee to 90°, rotates it medially and laterally twice, and then fully flexes and rotates it again. The test is positive if pain increases on rotation.

patellar tap test: A test designed to identify significant joint effusion. The knee is flexed or extended to discomfort, and the examiner taps the surface of the patella. The test is positive if a floating of the patella is felt.

Perkin's test: A test for patellar tenderness. With the knee supported in full extension, the borders of the medial and lateral facets are palpated while the patella is displaced medially and laterally. With chondromalacia, this maneuver reveals varying degrees of tenderness.

plica test: See Hughston plica test.

posterior drawer test: A test designed to identify posterior instability of the knee. The patient lies supine with the knee flexed to 90° as the foot is held in a neutral position by the examiner sitting on it. The examiner's hands grasp the leg around the proximal tibia and attempt to move the tibia backward on the femur. The test is positive if there is excessive posterior movement of the tibia on the femur.

posterior sag sign (gravity drawer test): A test designed to identify posterior instability of the knee. The patient lies supine with the knees flexed to 90° and the feet supported. The test is positive if the tibia sags back on the femur.

posterolateral drawer sign: See Hughston posterolateral drawer test.

posteromedial drawer sign: See Hughston posteromedial drawer test.

reverse pivot shift: See Jakob test.

Slocum test: A test designed to identify anterolateral instability of the knee. The patient is positioned supine with the knee flexed to 90° and the hip flexed to 45°. The examiner sits on the patient's forefoot, which is internally rotated 30°. The examiner grasps the tibia and applies an anteriorly directed force to the tibia. The test is positive if tibial movement occurs primarily on the lateral side. The test can also be used to identify anteromedial rotary instability. This version of the test is performed with the foot laterally rotated 15°; it is positive if tibial movement primarily occurs on the medial side.

Slocum ALRI test: A test designed to identify anterolateral rotary instability. The patient is lying on the side of the uninvolved leg, which is positioned with the hips and knees flexed 45°. The foot of the test leg rests on the table in medial rotation with the knee in extension. The examiner applies a valgus stress to the knee while flexing the knee. The test is positive if the subluxation of the knee is reduced between 25° and 45°.

stroke test: See brush test.

valgus stress test: See abduction test.

varus stress test: See adduction test.

Waldron test: A test designed to identify chondromalacia of the patella. The patient does several slow deep knee bends while the examiner palpates the patella. The test is positive if pain and crepitus are present during the range of movement.

Wilson test: A test designed to identify osteochondritis dissecans. The patient is seated with the leg in the dependent position. The patient extends the knee with the tibia medially rotated until the pain increases. The test is repeated with the tibia laterally rotated during extension. The test is positive if the pain does not occur when the tibia is laterally rotated.

wipe test: See brush test.

Foot and Ankle

Achilles tendon test: See Thompson test.

anterior drawer sign: A test designed to identify anterior ankle instability. The patient lies supine and the examiner stabilizes the distal tibia and fibula with one hand while the examiner's other hand holds the foot in 20 degrees of plantar flexion. The test is positive if, while drawing the talus forward in the ankle mortise, there is straight anterior translation which exceeds that of the uninvolved side.

Homans' sign: A test designed to detect deep vein thrombosis in the lower part of the leg. The ankle is passively dorsiflexed, and any sudden increase of pain in the calf or popliteal space is noted.

Kleiger test: A test for detecting lesions of the deltoid ligament. The patient is seated with the knees flexed to 90°. The examiner holds the foot and attempts to abduct the forefoot. The test is positive if the patient complains of pain medially and laterally. The talus may be felt to displace slightly from the medial malleolus.

Talar tilt: A test designed to identify lesions of the calcaneofibular ligament. The patient is supine or lying on one side with the knee flexed to 90°. With the foot in a neutral position, the talus is tilted medially. The test is positive if the amount of adduction on the involved side is excessive.

Thompson test: A test designed to detect ruptures of the Achilles tendon. The patient is placed in a prone position or on the knees with the feet extended over the edge of the bed. The middle third of the calf muscle is squeezed by the examiner. If a normal plantar flexion response is not elicited, an Achilles tendon rupture is suspected.

References

1. Magee, DJ: Orthopedic Physical Assessment. WB Saunders, Philadelphia, 1987.
2. D'Ambrosia, RD: Musculoskeletal Disorders: Regional Examination and Differential Diagnosis. JB Lippincott, Philadelphia, 1977. Ed. 3, McRae, R: Clinical Orthopedic Examination. Churchill Livingstone, New York, 1976.

CYRIAX TERMS

End-feel

end-feel: The type of resistance felt by an examiner at the end-range of a passive range-of-motion test.

bone to bone: The abrupt halt to the movement that is felt when two hard surfaces meet, for example, at the extreme of passive extension of the normal elbow.

capsular: The feeling of immediate stoppage of movement with some give. The type of end-feel felt at the end of the range of normal shoulder extension or hip extension.

empty: The end-feel felt when the patient complains of considerable pain during passive movement but the examiner perceives no increase in resistance to joint movement.

spasm: The feeling of muscle "spasm" coming actively into play. It is said to indicate the presence of acute or subacute arthritis.

springy block: A rebound is seen and felt at the end of the range. It is said to occur with displacement of an intra-articular structure, for example, when a torn meniscus in the knee engages between the tibia and femur and prevents the last few degrees of extension.

tissue approximation: The end-feel felt when a limb segment cannot be moved further because the soft tissues surrounding the joint cannot be compressed any further. It is the sensation felt at the end-range of elbow or knee flexion.

Selective Tissue Tension Tests of Cyriax

Following are terms developed by Cyriax that relate to the method he says can be used to identify the source of the patient's pain complaints. In his system the diagnosis depends on asking the patient to move or on the application of forces. In either case, patients report what they feel. Equal importance is placed on determining which movements are painful and/or limited and which movements are full range and/or pain-free.

active range of movements: These assess the patient's ability and willingness to perform the movements requested, the range of active movements available, and the patient's ability to produce the muscle forces required for active movement. These movements are also used to determine the region of the body from which the symptoms are originating and to determine which movements and muscles to examine in detail.

painful arc: The excursion (arc) near the mid-range in which pain is felt during an active movement test. The pain disappears as this position is passed in either direction. The pain may reappear at the end-range. According to Cyriax, a painful arc implies that a structure is pinched between two bony surfaces.

passive range of movements: These assess the ability of the "inert" (noncontractile, according to Cyriax) tissues to allow motion at a joint. The patient states whether pain is provoked. Each motion possible for the joint being tested must be examined to distinguish between capsular and noncapsular patterns of movement restrictions. Any discrepancy between the range of movement obtained actively and passively is noted.

resisted movements: These are resisted isometric contractions with the limb segment near the mid-range. These movements assess the tension-producing capabilities of specific muscle groups and whether the patient's pain is originating from these muscle groups.

Reference

1. Cyriax, J: Textbook of Orthopaedic Medicine, ed 7. Bailliere Tindall, London, 1978.

Significance of Diagnostic Movements in Selective Tissue Tension Tests According to Cyriax

TESTS	RESULTS OF TESTS	CONCLUSION ACCORDING TO CYRIAX
Active and passive movements	Pain is felt in one direction during the passive movement and in the opposite direction during the active movement	A contractile structure is at fault
Passive movements	Excessive range of motion is found	Capsular or ligamentous laxity
Active and passive movements, resisted movements	Pain is felt at the end-range of active and passive movements; resisted movements are pain-free	An "inert" noncontractile structure is at fault
Resisted movements	Pain is not felt; strength is normal	No lesion
Resisted movements	Pain is felt; strength is normal	A minor lesion of muscle or tendon
Resisted movements	Pain is felt; strength is decreased	A serious lesion of the muscle or tendon
Resisted movements	Pain is not felt; strength is decreased	A complete rupture of the muscle or tendon may be present
Resisted movements	Pain is felt after a number of repetitions	Intermittent claudication may be present
Resisted movements	Pain is felt with all resisted movements	Emotional hypersensitivity or an organic cause of pain

CAPSULAR PATTERNS OF THE JOINTS AS DESCRIBED BY CYRIAX

capsular pattern: A limitation of movement or a pattern of pain at a joint that occurs in a predictable pattern. According to Cyriax, these patterns are due to lesions in either the joint capsule or the synovial membrane. Limitations of motion at a joint that do not fall into these predictable patterns are said to exhibit noncapsular patterns. Causes of noncapsular patterns are said to be ligamentous adhesions, internal derangements, and extra-articular lesions.

acromioclavicular joint: Pain only at the extremes of range.

ankle joint: If the calf muscles are of adequate length, there will be a greater limitation of plantar flexion than of dorsiflexion.

cervical spine (facet joints): Lateral flexion and rotation are equally limited, flexion is full range and painful, and extension is limited.

elbow: Greater limitation in flexion than in extension.

facet joints: See specific body region—cervical spine, lumbar spine, or thoracic spine.

finger joints: Greater limitation in flexion than in extension.

glenohumeral joint: Greatest limitation in external rotation, followed by abduction, with less limitation in internal rotation.

hip joint: Equal limitations in flexion, abduction, and medial rotation, with a slight loss in extension. There is little or no loss in lateral rotation.

knee joint: Greater limitation in flexion than in extension.

lumbar spine (facet joints): The capsular pattern for the joints of the lumbar spine cannot be determined because of the difficulty of assessing the amount of motion in these joints.

metatarsophalangeal joint (first): Greater limitation in extension than in flexion.

metatarsophalangeal joints (second through fifth): Variable.

midtarsal joint: Equal limitations in dorsiflexion, plantar flexion, adduction, and medial rotation.

radioulnar joint (distal): Full range of motion with pain at both extremes of rotation.

sacrococcygeal joints: Pain is produced when forces are applied to these joints.

sacroiliac joint: Pain is produced when forces are applied to these joints.

sternoclavicular joint: Pain only at the extremes of range.

symphysis pubis: Pain is produced when forces are applied to this joint.

talocalcaneal joint: Limitation in varus.

thoracic spine (facet joints): The capsular pattern for the joints of the thoracic spine cannot be determined because of the difficulty of assessing the amount of motion in these joints.

thumb joints: Greater limitation in flexion than in extension.

trapeziometacarpal joint: Limitations in abduction and in extension with full flexion.

wrist: Equal limitation in flexion and extension.

KALTENBORN TERMS

Grading System for Classifying Joint Motion

Hypomobility $\begin{cases} 0 = \text{No movement (ankylosis)} \\ 1 = \text{Considerable decrease in movement} \\ 2 = \text{Slight decrease in movement} \end{cases}$

Normal $\begin{bmatrix} 3 = \text{Normal} \end{bmatrix}$

Hypermobility $\begin{cases} 4 = \text{Slight increase in movement} \\ 5 = \text{Considerable increase in movement} \\ 6 = \text{Complete instability} \end{cases}$

convex-concave rule: The rule is used to guide therapists as to which direction they should move limb segments when examining joints with limitations in range of motion. When a therapist moves a convex joint surface on a concave joint surface, the convex joint surface is moved in a direction opposite the range-of-motion limitation. Conversely, when a therapist moves a concave joint surface on a convex joint surface, the concave joint surface is moved in the same direction as the range-of-motion limitation.

End-feel

end-feel: The type of resistance felt by an examiner at the end-range of a passive range-of-motion test.

firm end-feel: Results from capsular or ligamentous stretching. An example is the resistance felt by the examiner at the end-range of external rotation of the glenohumeral joint.

hard end-feel: Occurs when bone meets bone. An example is the resistance felt by the examiner at the end-range of extension of the elbow.

soft end-feel: Due to soft tissue approximation or soft tissue stretching. An example is the resistance felt by the examiner at the end-range of knee flexion.

Reference

1. Kaltenborn, FM: Mobilization of the Extremity Joints: Examination and Basic Treatment Techniques. Olaf Norlis Bokhandel, Oslo, 1980.

MacCONNAILL TERMS

arthrokinematics: The study of movements within joints.

osteokinematics: The study of the movement of bony segments around a joint axis.

roll: The movement that occurs when equidistant points on a convex surface come into contact with equidistant points on the concave surface. Roll also occurs when equidistant points on a concave surface come into contact with equidistant points on the convex surface.

slide: The movement that occurs when the same point on the convex surface comes into contact with new points on the concave surface. Slide also occurs when the same point on the concave surface comes into contact with new points on the convex surface.

spin: Rotation of a convex joint surface about a longitudinal axis on a concave joint surface. Spin also occurs when a concave surface rotates about a longitudinal axis on the convex surface.

Reference

1. Warwick, R and Williams, PL: Gray's Anatomy, ed 35. WB Saunders, Philadelphia, 1973.

MAITLAND TERMS

comparable sign: Any form of joint movement testing that causes the patient to report symptoms comparable to those associated with the patient's chief complaint.

mobilization: Passive movement test performed by an examiner in such a way that the patient can prevent the movement if he or she so chooses. Two main types of movement are

> Passive oscillatory movements that are done at a rate of two or three per second. They are of small or large amplitude and are applied anywhere in a range of movement.

> Sustained stretching that is performed with small-amplitude oscillations at the end of the range of motion.

manipulation: Manipulation is a sudden movement or thrust, of small amplitude, performed at a speed that makes the patient unable to prevent the motion. Manipulation under anesthesia (MUA) is a procedure performed with the patient under anesthesia that is used to stretch a joint to restore a full range of movement by breaking adhesions. The procedure does not consist of a sudden, forceful thrust that is performed when the patient is awake (see first definition) but is done as a steady and controlled stretch.

GRADES OF MOVEMENT ACCORDING TO MAITLAND

grade I: Small-amplitude movements performed at the beginning of the range.

grade II: Large-amplitude movements that do not reach the limit of the range. If the movement is performed near the beginning of the range, it is a II−; if taken deeply into the range, yet still not reaching the limit, it is a II+.

grade III: Large-amplitude movements performed up to the limit of the range. If the movement is applied forcefully at the limit of the range, it is a III+; if applied gently at the limit of the range, it is a III−.

grade IV: Small-amplitude movements performed at the limit of the range. Depending on the vigor of the motion, the grades can be a IV− or IV+.

Reference

1. Maitland, GD: Peripheral Manipulation, ed 2. Butterworths, Boston, 1977.

CRITERIA FOR CLASSIFICATION INTO THE SYNDROMES DESCRIBED BY McKENZIE

The following describes the common findings associated with each syndrome. Information usually obtained during the history is listed first; followed by the information obtained during the physical examination (which consists of the examination, tests for movement loss, and the use of test movements).

Postural Syndrome

- *History*
- Patients are usually 30 years of age or younger.
- Patients frequently have sedentary occupations.
- Pain is always intermittent and produced when the patient stays in one position (especially sitting and forward bending) for a prolonged period of time.
- Pain ceases with movement and activity.

- *Physical Examination*
- Deformity of the lumbar spine is not present (i.e., there is no lateral shift, or reduced, or accentuated lumbar lordosis during standing).
- All test movements are pain free.
- No loss of motion will be noted during the test movements.
- Poor sitting and standing posture is often the only positive finding.

Dysfunction Syndrome

- *History*
- Patients are likely to be over 30 years of age.
- Pain is felt at the end-range of some movements, and may interfere with the performance of certain simple tasks.
- Rapid changes in symptoms do not occur.
- Patients complain in the early stages of low back stiffness that occurs in the morning and which decreases as the day progresses.
- Patients with a longstanding history of a dysfunction syndrome are likely to have reduced flexion and extension, and are likely to have stiffness that persists throughout the day.
- Patients often feel better when active and moving about than when they are at rest.
- Pain is intermittent and occurs only when the patient's back is placed in a position near the patient's limitation of motion.
- Pain is sometimes triggered by activity that the patient is not used to.

- *Physical Examination*
- The posture is poor.
- Deformities (i.e., a lateral shift, reduced, or accentuated lumbar lordosis during standing) are not typically seen except in elderly patients.
- A loss of movement is present.
- A loss of function may occur.
- Pain is easily reproduced with some test movements.

- Pain is elicited as soon as the end-range of limited movements is reached, but the pain subsides when the patient returns to his normal standing position.
- Patients who have an adherent nerve root will have peripheralization with flexion in standing but flexion while lying supine will not cause peripheralization.
- Patients who have an adherent nerve root will laterally deviate during flexion toward the painful side.

DERANGEMENT SYNDROMES

History for All Derangement Syndromes

- Patients are likely to be between 20 and 55 years of age and are usually male.
- Derangements may arise from a single severe strain, a less severe strain applied more frequently, or a sustained flexion strain. A sustained flexion strain is the most common cause of derangement.
- Derangement syndrome patients often have constant pain that varies in intensity, while postural and dysfunction syndrome patients always have intermittent pain.
- Pain is usually worse when the patient assumes certain positions.
- Pain is often increased when patients are in the sitting position.
- Patients often have difficulty finding a comfortable sleeping position.
- Patients have a loss of movement that is almost always asymmetrical.
- During the assessment of sagittal plane movements (flexion and extension) the patient's trunk often deviates to one side.
- Patients often have a history of recurring episodes of low back pain.

History and Physical Examination for Derangement One

- Central or symmetrical low back pain is present.
- Buttock and thigh pain is only rarely present.
- Spinal extension is limited but the lumbar lordosis is normal and there is no other lumbar postural deformity.

History and Physical Examination for Derangement Two

- Central or symmetrical low back pain is present.
- Buttock and/or thigh pain may be present.
- Extension is limited.
- The reduced lumbar lordosis deformity is present while standing.
- Extension of the lumbar spine is painful.
- Following painful extension of the lumbar spine returning to a flexed position will result in relief from pain.

History and Physical Examination for Derangement Three

- Unilateral or asymmetrical low back pain is present.
- Buttock and/or thigh pain may be present.
- No deformity (i.e., a lateral shift, reduced, or accentuated lumbar lordosis) is present.

History and Physical Examination for Derangement Four

- Unilateral or asymmetrical low back pain is present.
- Buttock and/or thigh pain may be present.
- A lateral shift deformity is present while standing.

History and Physical Examination for Derangement Five

- Unilateral or asymmetrial low back pain is present.
- Buttock and/or thigh pain may be present.
- Intermittent or constant pain extends below the knee.
- No deformity (i.e., a lateral shift, reduced or accentuated lumbar lordosis) is present.

History and Physical Examination for Derangement Six

- Unilateral or asymmetrical low back pain is present.
- Buttock and/or thigh pain may be present.
- Pain will usually be constant and extend below the knee.
- A lateral shift and a reduced lumbar lordosis deformity is present.
- Neurologic deficit is often present.

History and Physical Examination for Derangement Seven

- Symmetrical or asymmetrical low back pain is present.
- Buttock and/or thigh pain may be present.
- An accentuated lumbar lordosis is present.
- The patient's lumbar spine will remain lordotic even during flexion motions (e.g., during motion testing).
- Patients describe a sudden onset of pain and may say they were easily able to touch their toes the day before the onset of pain.

Reference

1. McKenzie, RA: The Lumbar Spine: Mechanical Diagnosis and Therapy. Spinal Publications. Waikenae, New Zealand, 1981.

Systems Used to Measure Curves

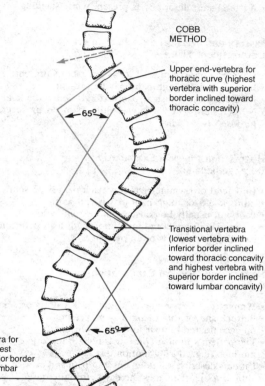

COBB
METHOD

Upper end-vertebra for
thoracic curve (highest
vertebra with superior
border inclined toward
thoracic concavity)

←65°

Transitional vertebra
(lowest vertebra with
inferior border inclined
toward thoracic concavity
and highest vertebra with
superior border inclined
toward lumbar concavity)

←65°

Lower end-vertebra for
lumbar curve (lowest
vertebra with inferior border
inclined toward lumbar
concavity)

Cobb Method. A line is drawn perpendicular to the upper margin of the vertebra that inclines most toward the concavity. A line is also drawn on the inferior border of the lower vertebra with the greatest angulation toward the concavity. The angle formed by these intersecting lines is the measure of the curvature. The apical vertebra is also usually noted.

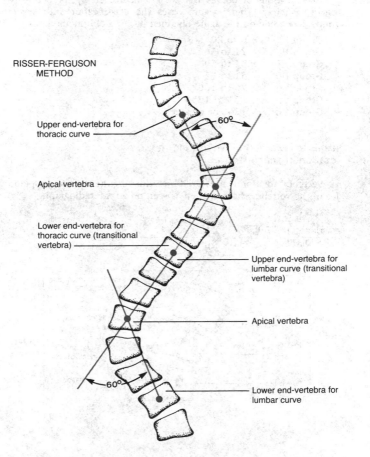

RISSER-FERGUSON
METHOD

Upper end-vertebra for
thoracic curve

60°

Apical vertebra

Lower end-vertebra for
thoracic curve (transitional
vertebra)

Upper end-vertebra for
lumbar curve (transitional
vertebra)

Apical vertebra

60°

Lower end-vertebra for
lumbar curve

Risser-Ferguson Method. The midpoints of the proximal, distal, and apical vertebra of the curvature are identified. The proximal vertebra is the highest vertebra whose superior surface tilts to the concavity of the curve. The distal vertebra is the lowest vertebra whose inferior surface tilts to the concavity of the curve. The apical vertebra is between the proximal and distal vertebrae and is parallel to the horizontal or transverse plane of the body. The angle formed by the two lines that intersect the apex from the proximal and distal midpoints is the measure of the curvature. This method is still used but is no longer accepted internationally.

Classification of Scoliotic Curves

Classifications of curves has been standardized by the Scoliosis Research Society. Their system bases the classification into seven groups depending on the angle obtained by the Cobb method.

Group I: 0 to 20°
Group II: 21 to 30°
Group III: 31 to 50°
Group IV: 51 to 75°
Group V: 76 to 100°
Group VI: 101 to 125°
Group VIII: 126° or greater

Nash-Moe Method of Measuring the Rotation of the Vertebrae

Vertebral rotation is measured by estimating the amount the pedicles of the vertebrae have rotated as seen on an A-P radiograph.

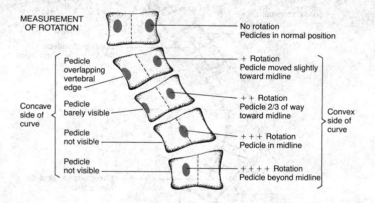

MEASUREMENT OF ROTATION

No rotation
Pedicles in normal position

Pedicle overlapping vertebral edge

+ Rotation
Pedicle moved slightly toward midline

Concave side of curve

Pedicle barely visible

+ + Rotation
Pedicle 2/3 of way toward midline

Convex side of curve

Pedicle not visible

+ + + Rotation
Pedicle in midline

Pedicle not visible

+ + + + Rotation
Pedicle beyond midline

CLASSIFICATION OF EPIPHYSEAL PLATE INJURIES

TYPE OF INJURY	DESCRIPTION AND PROGNOSIS
Type I	Complete separation of the epiphysis from the metaphysis without fracture of the bone. Type I injuries are usually caused by shear forces and are most common in newborns (birth injuries) and young children. Closed reduction is not difficult, and the prognosis is excellent, provided the blood supply to the epiphysis is intact.

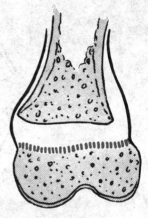

TYPE OF INJURY	DESCRIPTION AND PROGNOSIS
Type II	The line of separation extends a variable distance along the epiphyseal plate and then out through the metaphysis to produce a triangular fragment. Type II injuries are the most common type of epiphyseal fracture and occur as a result of shearing and bending forces. These injuries tend to occur in the older child. Closed reduction is relatively easy to maintain. The prognosis for growth is excellent, providing blood supply to plate is intact.

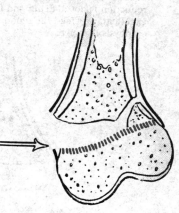

Type III

Intra-articular fracture extending from the joint surface to the deep zone of the epiphyseal plate and then along the plate to the periphery. Type III injuries are uncommon. They are caused by an intra-articular shearing force and are usually limited to the distal epiphysis. Open reduction is usually necessary. The prognosis for growth is good, provided the blood supply to the separated portion of the epiphysis has not been disrupted.

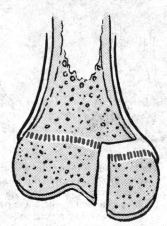

TYPE OF INJURY	DESCRIPTION AND PROGNOSIS

Type IV

An intra-articular fracture extending from the joint surface through the epiphysis, across the entire thickness of the plate, and through a portion of the metaphysis. Type IV injuries are commonly seen as fractures of the lateral condyle of the humerus. Except for undisplaced fractures, open reduction and internal skeletal fixation are necessary. Perfect reduction is necessary for a favorable prognosis of restored bone growth.

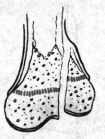 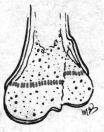

Type V

An uncommon injury that results from a severe crushing force applied through the epiphysis to one area of the plate. Type V injuries are most common in the ankle or the knee, resulting from a severe abduction or adduction injury to the joint. Weight bearing must be avoided for 3 weeks in the hope of preventing the almost inevitable premature cessation of growth. Prognosis for bone growth is usually poor.

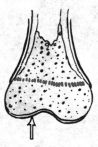 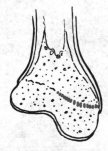

TYPE OF INJURY	DESCRIPTION AND PROGNOSIS
Type VI	A rare injury resulting from damage to the periosteum or perichondral ring. Type VI injuries can be caused by direct blows or deep lacerations from sharp objects. Because a local bony bridge tends to form across the growth plate, the prognosis for subsequent growth is poor.

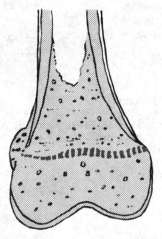

References

1. Rang, M: The Growth Plate and Its Disorders. Williams & Wilkins Baltimore, 1969.
2. Salters, RB: Textbook of Disorders and Injuries of the Musculoskeletal System, ed 2. Williams & Wilkins, Baltimore, 1983.

Contribution of the Epiphyses to Bone Growth

BONE	PROXIMAL END (%)	DISTAL END (%)
Femur	30	70
Fibula	60	40
Humerus	80	20
Radius	25	75
Tibia	55	45
Ulna	20	80

Reference

1. Rang, M: The Growth Plate and Its Disorders. Williams & Wilkins, Baltimore, 1969.

CRITERIA FOR THE CLASSIFICATION OF RHEUMATOID ARTHRITIS

> **The 1987 Revised Criteria for Classification of Rheumatoid Arthritis (traditional format)***

CRITERION	DEFINITION
1. Morning stiffness	Morning stiffness in and around the joints lasting at least 1 hour before maximal improvement.
2. Arthritis of three or more joint areas	At least three joint areas have simultaneously had soft-tissue swelling or fluid (not bony overgrowth alone) observed by a physician. The 14 possible joint areas are right or left PIP, MCP, wrist, elbow, knee, ankle, and MTP joints.
3. Arthritis of hand joints	At least one joint area swollen as above in a wrist, MCP, or PIP.
4. Symmetric arthritis	Simultaneous involvement of the same joint areas (as in 2) on both sides of the body (bilateral involvement of PIPs, MCPs, or MTPs is acceptable without absolute symmetry).
5. Rheumatoid nodules	Subcutaneous nodules, over bony prominences, or extensor surfaces, or in juxtaarticular regions, observed by a physician.
6. Serum rheumatoid factor	Demonstration of abnormal amounts of serum "rheumatoid factor" by any method that has been positive in less than 5% of normal control subjects.
7. Radiologic changes	Radiologic changes typical of rheumatoid arthritis on PA hand and wrist roentgenograms, which

Cont. on the following page(s)

CRITERION   DEFINITION

must include erosions or unequivocal bony decalcification localized to or most marked adjacent to the involved joints (osteoarthritis changes alone do not qualify).

For classification purposes, a patient shall be said to have rheumatoid arthritis if he/she has satisfied at least four of the above seven criteria. Criteria 1–4 must have been present for at least 6 weeks. Patients with two clinical diagnoses are not excluded. Designation as "classic," "definite," or "probable" rheumatoid arthritis is *not* to be made.

---

*Legend: PIPs = proximal interphalangeal joints, MCPs = metacarpophalangeal joints, MTP = metatarsophalangeal joints, PA = posteroanterior.

Diagnostic Criteria for Rheumatoid Arthritis (1958)

1. Morning stiffness.

2. Pain on motion or tenderness in at least one joint (observed by a physician).

3. Swelling (soft tissue thickening or fluid, not bony overgrowth alone) in at least one joint (observed by a physician).

4. Swelling of at least one other joint (observed by a physician).

5. Symmetric joint swelling (observed by a physician) with simultaneous involvement of the same joint on both sides of the body (bilateral involvement of PIP, MCP, or MTP joints is acceptable without absolute symmetry). Terminal phalangeal joint involvement will not fulfill this criterion.

6. Subcutaneous nodules (observed by a physician) over bony prominences, on extensor surfaces, or in juxtaarticular regions.

7. Roentgenographic changes typical of rheumatoid arthritis (which must include at least bony decalcification localized to or most marked adjacent to the involved joints and not just degenerative changes). Degenerative changes do not exclude patients from any group classified as having rheumatoid arthritis.

8. Positive agglutinin test — demonstration of the "rheumatoid factor" by any method that, in two laboratories, has been positive in not over 5% of normal controls, or positive streptococcal agglutinin test.

9. Poor mucin precipitate from synovial fluid (with shreds and cloudy solution). (An inflammatory synovial effusion with 2000 or more white cells/mm^3, without crystals can be substituted for this criterion.)

10. Characteristic histologic changes in synovium with three or more of the following: marked villous hypertrophy; proliferation of superficial synovial cells often with palisading; marked infiltration of chronic inflammatory cells (lymphocytes or plasma cells predominating) with tendency to form "lymphoid follicles"; deposition of compact fibrin either on surface or interstitially; foci of necrosis.

11. Characteristic histologic changes in nodules showing granulomatous foci with central zones of cell necrosis, surrounded by a palisade of proliferated mononuclear cells and peripheral fibrosis and chronic inflammatory cell infiltration.

A. *Classic rheumatoid arthritis* requires seven of the above criteria. In criteria 1–5 the joint signs or symptoms must be continuous for at least 6 weeks.

B. *Definite rheumatoid arthritis* requires five of the above criteria. In criteria 1–5 the joint signs or symptoms must be continuous for at least 6 weeks.

C. *Probable rheumatoid arthritis* requires three of the above criteria. In criteria 1–5 the joint signs or symptoms must be continuous for at least 6 weeks.

D. *Possible rheumatoid arthritis* (not used).

E. *Exclusions*

1. Typical rash of SLE
2. High concentrations of LE cells
3. Histologic evidence of periarteritis nodosa
4. Polymyositis and dermatomyositis
5. Scleroderma
6. Rheumatic fever
7. Gouty arthritis
8. Tophi
9. Acute infectious arthritis
10. Tuberculous arthritis
11. Reiter's syndrome
12. Shoulder-hand syndrome
13. Hypertrophic pulmonary osteoarthropathy
14. Neuropathic arthropathy
15. Ochronosis
16. Sarcoidosis
17. Multiple myeloma
18. Erythema nodosum
19. Leukemia or lymphoma
20. Agammaglobulinemia

Relative Performance of Old and New Criteria Sets for Rheumatoid Arthritis

	SENSITIVITY	SPECIFICITY	NUMBER MISCLASSIFIED
Old ARA Criteria			
Mucin clot, synovial biopsy, and nodule biopsy excluded. At least 5 out of 8 criteria must be present	92%	85%	61
Old New York Criteria			
At least 2 out of 4 criteria must be present	98%	76%	69
At least 3 out of 4 criteria must be present	81%	94%	64
New RA Criteria			
At least 4 out of 7 criteria must be present	91.2%*	89.3%	51
New Classification Tree Criteria	93.5%†	89.3%	45

*Early disease onset (<1 year–sensitivity 80.9%, specificity 88.2%)
†Early disease onset (<1 year–sensitivity 85%, specificity 90%)
‡From the Bulletin on the Rheumatic Diseases, 1989, with permission of the Arthritis Foundation.

References

1. Ropes, MW, Bennett, GA, Cobb, S, et al: 1958 Revision of diagnostic criteria for rheumatoid arthritis. Bull Rheum Dis 9:175–176, 1958
2. Blumberg, B, Bunim, JJ, Calkins, E, et al: ARA nomenclature and classification of arthritis and rheumatism (tentative). Arthritis Rheum 7:93–97, 1964.
3. Arnett, FC: Revised Criteria For Classification of Rheumatoid Arthritis. Bull Rheum Dis 38:1–6, 1989.

RHEUMATOID ARTHRITIS

Classification of Functional Capacity in Patients with Rheumatoid Arthritis*

CLASS   FUNCTIONAL CAPACITY

Class I: Complete functional capacity with ability to carry on all usual duties without handicaps

Class II: Functional capacity adequate to conduct normal activities despite handicap of discomfort or limited mobility of one or more joints

Class III: Functional capacity adequate to perform only few or none of the duties of usual occupation or of self-care

Class IV: Largely or wholly incapacitated, with patient bedridden or confined to wheelchair, permitting little or no self-care

---

*From Arnett, FC, Edworthy, S, Block, DA et al: The 1987 revised ARA criteria for rheumatic arthritis. Arthritis & Rheum 30:517, 1987.

Classification of (Stages) Progression of Rheumatoid Arthritis*

Stage I, Early

†1. No destructive changes on roentgenographic examination

2. Roentgenologic evidence of osteoporosis may be present

Stage II, Moderate

†1. Roentgenologic evidence of osteoporosis, with or without slight subchondral bone destruction; slight cartilage destruction may be present

†2. No joint deformities, although limitation of joint mobility may be present

3. Adjacent muscle atrophy

4. Extra-articular soft tissue lesions, such as nodules and tenosynovitis may be present

Stage III, Severe

†1. Roentgenologic evidence of cartilage and bone destruction, in addition to osteoporosis

†2. Joint deformity, such as subluxation, ulnar deviation, or hyperextension, without fibrous or bony ankylosis.

3. Extensive muscle atrophy

4. Extra-articular soft tissue lesions, such as nodules and tenosynovitis, may be present

Stage IV, Terminal

†1. Fibrous or bony ankylosis

2. Criteria of stage III

---

*From Primer on the Rheumatic Diseases, ed 9. Arthritis Foundation, Atlanta, 1988. Used by permission off the Arthritis Foundation.

†The criteria prefaced by daggers are those that must be present to permit classification of a patient in any particular stage or grade.

CRITERIA FOR THE DIAGNOSIS OF JUVENILE RHEUMATOID ARTHRITIS

I. General

The JRA Criteria Subcommittee in 1982 again reviewed the 1977 Criteria (1) and recommended that *juvenile rheumatoid arthritis* be the name for the principal form of chronic arthritic disease in children and that this general class should be classified into three onset subtypes: systemic, polyarticular, and pauciarticular. The onset subtypes may be further subclassified into subsets as indicated below. The following classification enumerates the requirements for the diagnosis of JRA and the three clinical onset subtypes and lists subsets of each subtype that may be useful in further classification.

II. General criteria for the diagnosis of juvenile rheumatoid arthritis:

A. Persistent arthritis of at least six weeks duration in one or more joints

B. Exclusion of other causes of arthritis (see list of exclusions)

III. JRA onset subtypes

The onset subtype is determined by manifestations during the first six months of disease and remains the principal classification, although manifestations more closely resembling another subtype may appear later.

A. Systemic onset JRA: This subtype is defined as JRA with persistent intermittent fever (daily intermittent temperatures to 103°F or more) with or without rheumatoid rash or other organ involvement. Typical fever and rash will be considered probable systemic onset JRA if not associated with arthritis. Before a definite diagnosis can be made, arthritis, as defined, must be present.

B. Pauciarticular onset JRA: This subtype is defined as JRA with arthritis in four or fewer joints during the first six months of disease. Patients with systemic onset JRA are excluded from this onset subtype.

C. Polyarticular JRA: This subtype is defined as JRA with arthritis in five or more joints during the first six months of disease. Patients with systemic JRA onset are excluded from this subtype.

D. The onset subtypes may include the following subsets:
1. Systemic onset (SO)
   a. Polyarthritis
   b. Oligoarthritis
2. Oligoarthritis (OO) (Pauciarticular onset)
   a. Antinuclear antibody (ANA) positive-chronic uveitis
   b. Rheumatoid factor (RF) positive
   c. Seronegative, B27 positive
   d. Not otherwise classified
3. Polyarthritis (PO)
   a. RF positivity
   b. Not otherwise classified

IV. Exclusions
   A. Other rheumatic diseases
      1. Rheumatic fever
      2. Systemic lupus erythematosus
      3. Ankylosing spondylitis
      4. Polymyositis and dermatomyositis
      5. Vasculitic syndromes
      6. Scleroderma
      7. Psoriatic arthritis
      8. Reiter's syndrome
      9. Sjögren's syndrome
      10. Mixed connective tissue disease
      11. Behçet's syndrome
   B. Infectious arthritis
   C. Inflammatory bowel disease
   D. Neoplastic diseases including leukemia
   E. Nonrheumatic conditions of bones and joints
   F. Hematologic diseases
   G. Psychogenic arthralgia
   H. Miscellaneous
      1. Sarcoidosis
      2. Hypertrophic osteoarthropathy
      3. Villonodular synovitis
      4. Chronic active hepatitis
      5. Familial Mediterranean fever
V. Other proposed terminology

Juvenile chronic arthritis (JCA) and juvenile arthritis (JA) are new diagnostic terms currently in use in some places for the arthritides of childhood. The diagnoses of JCA and JA are not equivalent to each other, nor to the older diagnosis of juvenile rheumatoid arthritis or Still's disease. Hence reports of studies of JCA or JA cannot be directly compared with one another nor to reports of JRA or Still's disease. Juvenile chronic arthritis is described in more detail in a report of the European Conference on the Rheumatic Diseases of Children (2) and juvenile arthritis in the report of the Ross Conference (3).

1. JRA Criteria Subcommittee of the Diagnostic and Therapeutic Criteria Committee of the American Rheumatism Association: Current proposed revisions of the JRA criteria. Arthritis Rheum 20(suppl)195–199, 1977
2. Ansell BW: Chronic arthritis in childhood. Ann Rheum Dis 37:107–120, 1978
3. Fink CW: Keynote address: Arthritis in childhood, Report of the 80th Ross Conference in Pediatric Research. Columbus, Ross Laboratories, 1979, pp 1–2
From the Primer on Rheumatic Diseases, ed 9, Arthritis Foundation, Atlanta, 1988, with permission.

Nonsteroidal Anti-Inflammatory Drugs Used for Arthritis*		
CLASS AND DRUG	USUAL SUPPLY	USUAL DAILY DOSE
Salicylates and Related Drugs		
Aspirin or buffered aspirin†	250–325-mg tabs	3–6 g
Ascriptin	325 mg aspirin and 150 mg Maalox	3–6 g
Choline magnesium trisalicylate (Trilisate†)	500-mg tabs	2–6 g
Enteric-coated aspirin (Ecotrin†)	325-mg tabs	2–6 g
Diflunisal (Dolobid†)	250-, 500-mg tabs	500–1000 mg
Choline salicylate (Arthropan†)	Liquid	1–1½ tsp q.i.d.
Salicylsalicylic acid (Disalcid†)	500, 750 mg	3000 mg
Indoles (and Related Drugs)		
Indomethacin (Indocin†)	25-, 50-, 75-mg (timed-release) capsules	75–200 mg
Sulindac (Clinoril†)	150-, 200-mg tabs	300–400 mg
Tolmetin (Tolectin†)	200-mg tabs	600–2000 mg
Propionic Acids		
Ibuprofen (Motrin†)	200-, 300-, 400-, 600-, 800-mg tabs	1.4–3.2 g
Fenoprofen (Nalfon†)	300-, 600-mg capsules	1–3 g

CLASS AND DRUG	USUAL SUPPLY	USUAL DAILY DOSE
Propionic Acids continued		
Naproxen (Naprosyn,† Anaprox†)	250-, 375-, 500-mg tabs	0.75 – 1 g
Oxicams		
Piroxicam (Feldene†)	10-, 20-mg capsules	20 mg
Anthranilic Acids		
Meclofenamate (Meclomen†)	50-, 100-mg capsules	1.5 – 2 g
Pyrazoles		
Phenylbutazone (Butazolidine†)	50, 100 mg	300 – 400 mg
Oxyphenbutazone (Tandearil†)	50, 100 mg	300 – 400 mg

*Modified from Simon, LS, Mills, LS, and Mills, JA: Drug therapy: Nonsteroidal anti-inflammatory drugs (two parts). N Engl J Med 302:1179, 1237, 1980.

*From Goldenberg, DL and Cohen, AS: Drugs in the Rheumatic Diseases. Grune & Stratton, Orlando, 1986.

†Trade name.

TRIGGER POINTS

Many treatment techniques require the location of trigger points. Travell first described these points when she stated that the "trigger area is simply derived from the fact that if you do something at one place, which we call the trigger, then something else happens in another place, which we call the reference or the target. It implies that some relationship exists between two different topographical areas" (from Reference 1).

The diagrams that follow are based on Travell's publications. The trigger points are said to be hypersensitive areas. In response to pressure, needling, extreme heat or cold, or stretch, these areas give rise to pain referred elsewhere.

Trigger Points of the Head and Neck

Sternomastoid

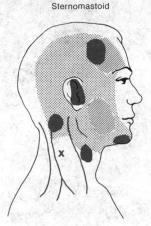

Temporalis

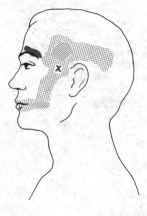

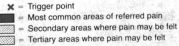

✗ = Trigger point
■ = Most common areas of referred pain
▨ = Secondary areas where pain may be felt
▧ = Tertiary areas where pain may be felt

Trigger Points of the Head and Neck (continued)

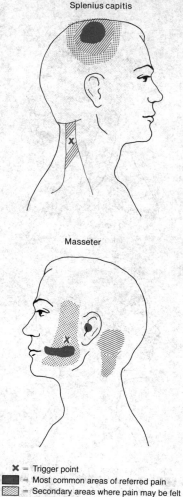

Splenius capitis

Masseter

✘ = Trigger point
■ = Most common areas of referred pain
▨ = Secondary areas where pain may be felt
▦ = Tertiary areas where pain may be felt

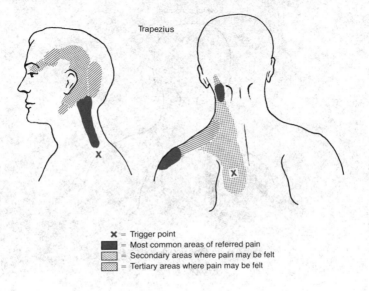

Trapezius

✘ = Trigger point

███ = Most common areas of referred pain

▨ = Secondary areas where pain may be felt

▦ = Tertiary areas where pain may be felt

Trigger Points of the Head and Neck (continued)

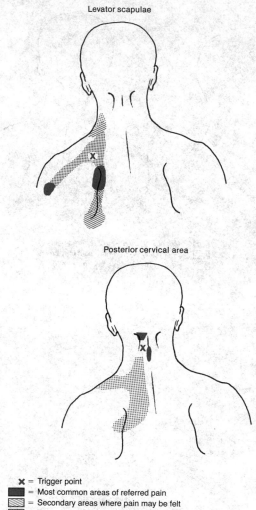

Levator scapulae

Posterior cervical area

✕ = Trigger point

█ = Most common areas of referred pain

▨ = Secondary areas where pain may be felt

▧ = Tertiary areas where pain may be felt

Trigger Points of the Hand

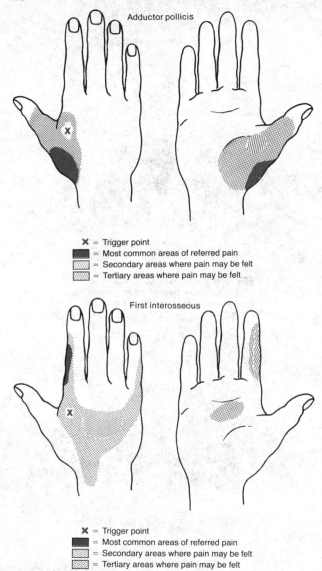

Adductor pollicis

✕ = Trigger point
◼ = Most common areas of referred pain
▨ = Secondary areas where pain may be felt
▦ = Tertiary areas where pain may be felt

First interosseous

✕ = Trigger point
◼ = Most common areas of referred pain
▨ = Secondary areas where pain may be felt
▦ = Tertiary areas where pain may be felt

Sternal area

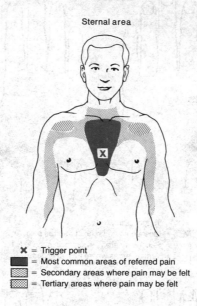

✗ = Trigger point

= Most common areas of referred pain

= Secondary areas where pain may be felt

= Tertiary areas where pain may be felt

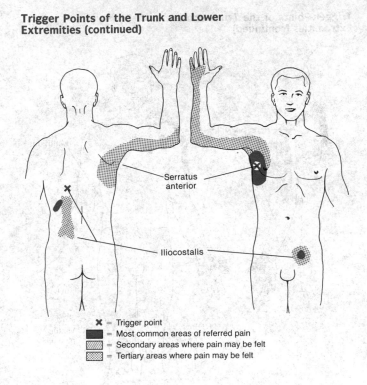

Serratus anterior

Iliocostalis

✖ = Trigger point
= Most common areas of referred pain
= Secondary areas where pain may be felt
= Tertiary areas where pain may be felt

Trigger Points of the Trunk and Lower Extremities (continued)

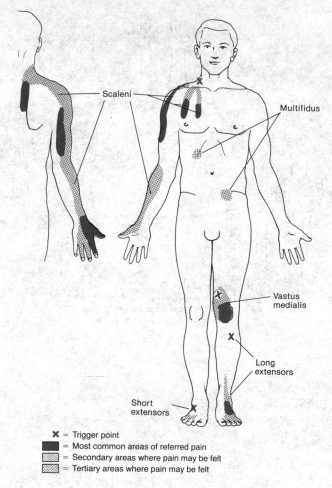

Scaleni

Multifidus

Vastus medialis

Long extensors

Short extensors

✖ = Trigger point

■ = Most common areas of referred pain

▨ = Secondary areas where pain may be felt

▨ = Tertiary areas where pain may be felt

Trigger Points of the Trunk and Lower Extremities (continued)

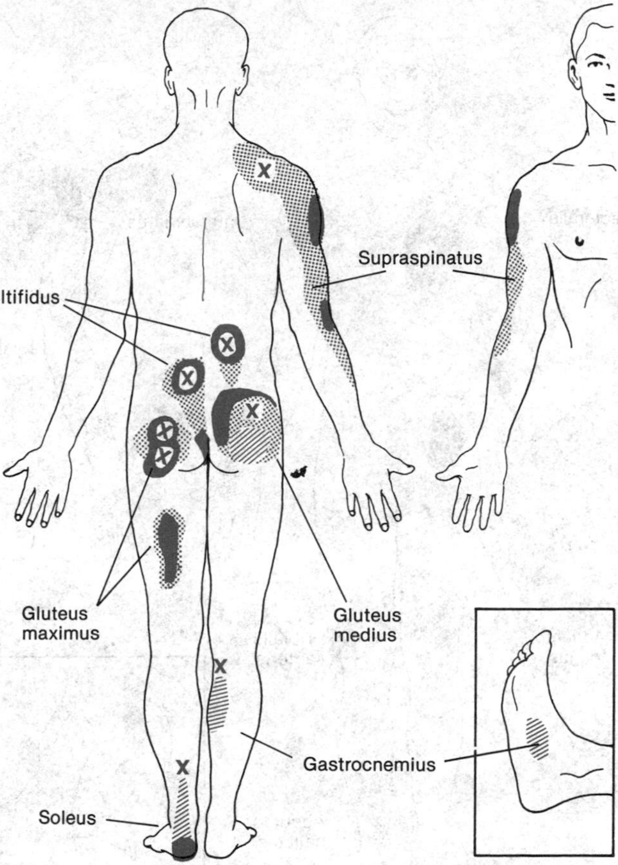

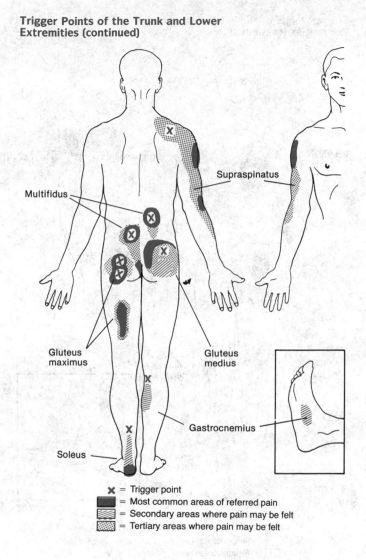

Supraspinatus
Multifidus
Gluteus maximus
Gluteus medius
Gastrocnemius
Soleus

✖ = Trigger point
■ = Most common areas of referred pain
▨ = Secondary areas where pain may be felt
░ = Tertiary areas where pain may be felt

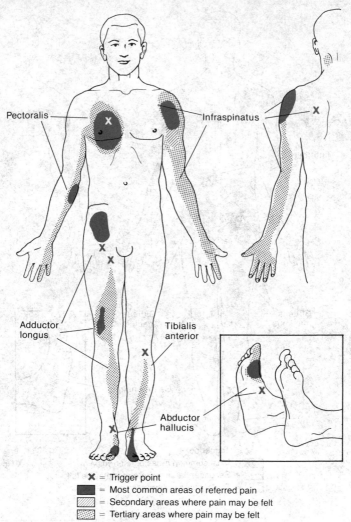

Pectoralis

Infraspinatus

Adductor
longus

Tibialis
anterior

Abductor
hallucis

✗ = Trigger point

■ = Most common areas of referred pain

▨ = Secondary areas where pain may be felt

▨ = Tertiary areas where pain may be felt

Trigger Points of the Trunk and Lower Extremities (continued)

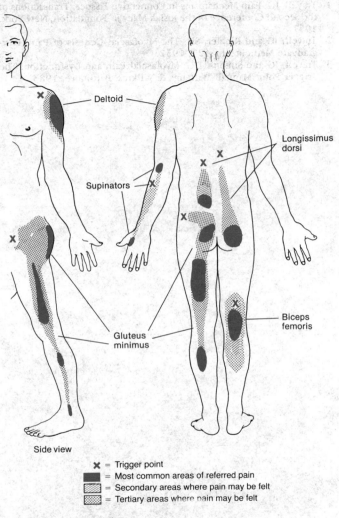

Side view

✕ = Trigger point

■ = Most common areas of referred pain

▨ = Secondary areas where pain may be felt

▧ = Tertiary areas where pain may be felt

References

1. Travell, JG: Pain Mechanisms in Connective Tissues, Transactions of the Second Conference of the Josiah Macy Jr. Foundation, New York, 1951.
2. Travell, JG and Rinzler, SH: The Myofascial Genesis of Pain. Postgraduate Medicine 11:425, 1952.
3. Travell, JG and Simons, DG: Myofascial Pain and Dysfunction: The Trigger Point Manual. Williams & Wilkins, Baltimore, 1983.

Neuroanatomy, Neurology, and Neurologic Therapy

THE BRAIN

Lateral Surface: Anatomical Features and Brodmann's Numbers

Anatomical Features

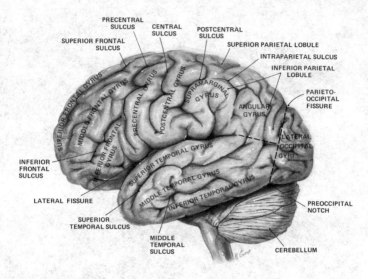

Illustrations appearing on pages 184 to 189, 191 to 209, and 229 are from Manter and Gatz's *Essentials of Clinical Neuroanatomy and Neurophysiology* by Sid Gilman, M.D., and Sarah Winans Newman, Ph.D. Artwork by Margaret Croup Brudon.

Brodmann's Numbers

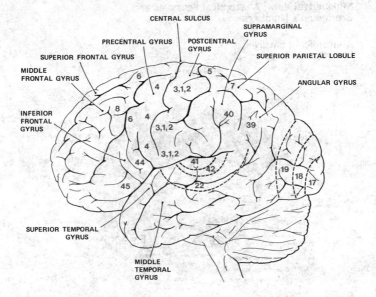

THE BRAIN

Midsagittal View: Anatomical Features and Brodmann's Numbers

Anatomical Features

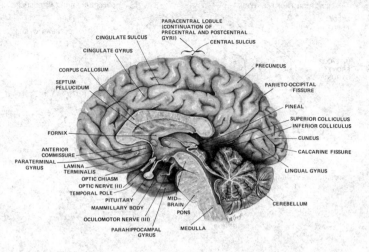

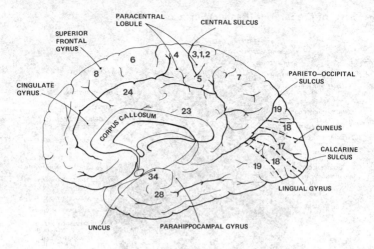

THE BRAIN

View of the Inferior (Basilar) Surface

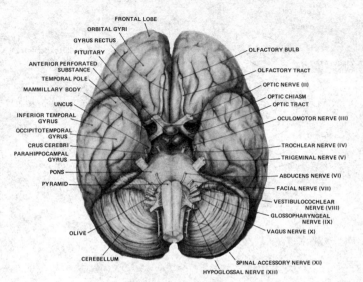

FRONTAL LOBE
ORBITAL GYRI
GYRUS RECTUS
PITUITARY
ANTERIOR PERFORATED SUBSTANCE
TEMPORAL POLE
MAMMILLARY BODY
UNCUS
INFERIOR TEMPORAL GYRUS
OCCIPITOTEMPORAL GYRUS
CRUS CEREBRI
PARAHIPPOCAMPAL GYRUS
PONS
PYRAMID
OLIVE
CEREBELLUM

OLFACTORY BULB
OLFACTORY TRACT
OPTIC NERVE (II)
OPTIC CHIASM
OPTIC TRACT
OCULOMOTOR NERVE (III)
TROCHLEAR NERVE (IV)
TRIGEMINAL NERVE (V)
ABDUCENS NERVE (VI)
FACIAL NERVE (VII)
VESTIBULOCOCHLEAR NERVE (VIII)
GLOSSOPHARYNGEAL NERVE (IX)
VAGUS NERVE (X)
SPINAL ACCESSORY NERVE (XI)
HYPOGLOSSAL NERVE (XII)

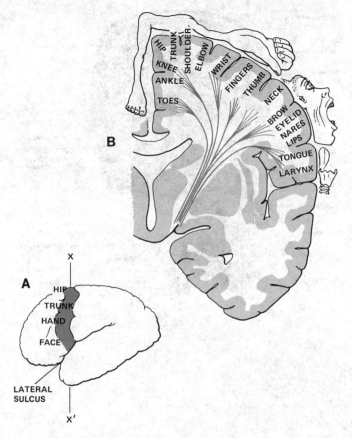

Figure A shows the somatotopical representation of the motor cortex. Illustrated is a left cortex. Figure B shows the somatotopical organization of cortical neurons in a section taken along plane x-x' in Figure A.

BLOOD SUPPLY TO THE BRAIN

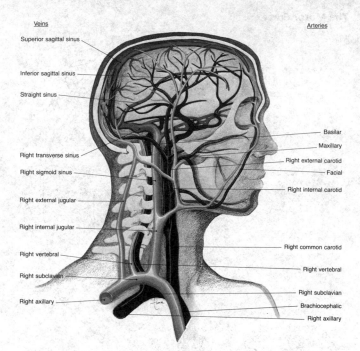

Veins

Superior sagittal sinus

Inferior sagittal sinus

Straight sinus

Right transverse sinus

Right sigmoid sinus

Right external jugular

Right internal jugular

Right vertebral

Right subclavian

Right axillary

Arteries

Basilar

Maxillary

Right external carotid

Facial

Right internal carotid

Right common carotid

Right vertebral

Right subclavian

Brachiocephalic

Right axillary

BLOOD SUPPLY TO THE BRAIN

Brain Stem: Ventral surface of the brain stem. Cross-sections are at the levels indicated in figure A by letters B, C, and D. Some territories served by arteries overlap.

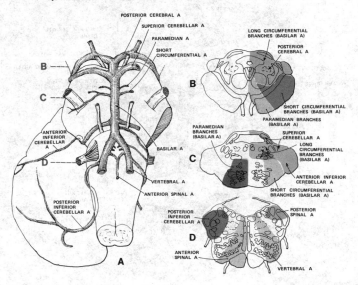

Circle of Willis

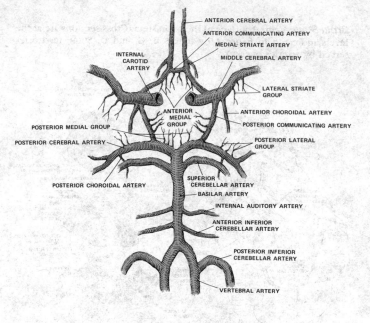

ANTERIOR CEREBRAL ARTERY
ANTERIOR COMMUNICATING ARTERY
MEDIAL STRIATE ARTERY
MIDDLE CEREBRAL ARTERY
INTERNAL CAROTID ARTERY
LATERAL STRIATE GROUP
ANTERIOR MEDIAL GROUP
ANTERIOR CHOROIDAL ARTERY
POSTERIOR COMMUNICATING ARTERY
POSTERIOR MEDIAL GROUP
POSTERIOR CEREBRAL ARTERY
POSTERIOR LATERAL GROUP
POSTERIOR CHOROIDAL ARTERY
SUPERIOR CEREBELLAR ARTERY
BASILAR ARTERY
INTERNAL AUDITORY ARTERY
ANTERIOR INFERIOR CEREBELLAR ARTERY
POSTERIOR INFERIOR CEREBELLAR ARTERY
VERTEBRAL ARTERY

BLOOD SUPPLY TO THE BRAIN

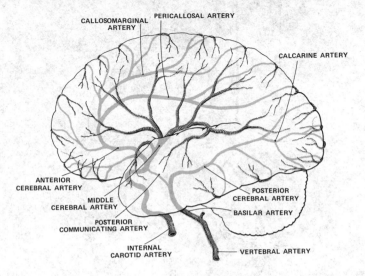

CALLOSOMARGINAL ARTERY

PERICALLOSAL ARTERY

CALCARINE ARTERY

ANTERIOR CEREBRAL ARTERY

MIDDLE CEREBRAL ARTERY

POSTERIOR COMMUNICATING ARTERY

INTERNAL CAROTID ARTERY

POSTERIOR CEREBRAL ARTERY

BASILAR ARTERY

VERTEBRAL ARTERY

Cerebral Circulation: Lateral view of a left hemisphere. The anterior and posterior cerebral arteries are normally not visible from a lateral view. Here they are shown as they are positioned on the medial surface of the hemisphere.

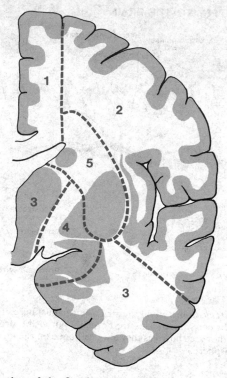

Frontal Section of the Cerebrum: Section at the level of the central sulcus. The areas of distribution are (1) the anterior cerebral artery including the callosomarginal and pericallosal arteries; (2) the middle cerebral artery; (3) the posterior cerebral artery to the diencephalon and occipital lobe; (4) the medial striate arteries to the internal capsule, globus pallidus, and amygdala; and (5) the lateral striate arteries to the caudate nucleus, putamen, and internal capsule.

THE BRAIN STEM AND DIENCEPHALON

Ventral Surface

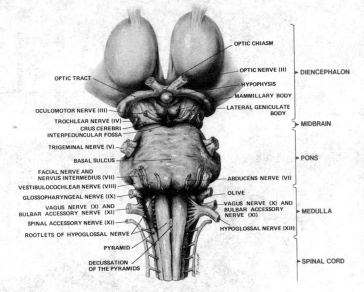

OPTIC CHIASM

OPTIC NERVE (II)

HYPOPHYSIS

MAMMILLARY BODY

LATERAL GENICULATE BODY

OPTIC TRACT

OCULOMOTOR NERVE (III)

TROCHLEAR NERVE (IV)

CRUS CEREBRI

INTERPEDUNCULAR FOSSA

TRIGEMINAL NERVE (V)

BASAL SULCUS

FACIAL NERVE AND NERVUS INTERMEDIUS (VII)

VESTIBULOCOCHLEAR NERVE (VIII)

GLOSSOPHARYNGEAL NERVE (IX)

VAGUS NERVE (X) AND BULBAR ACCESSORY NERVE (XI)

SPINAL ACCESSORY NERVE (XI)

ROOTLETS OF HYPOGLOSSAL NERVE

PYRAMID

DECUSSATION OF THE PYRAMIDS

ABDUCENS NERVE (VI)

OLIVE

VAGUS NERVE (X) AND BULBAR ACCESSORY NERVE (XI)

HYPOGLOSSAL NERVE (XII)

DIENCEPHALON

MIDBRAIN

PONS

MEDULLA

SPINAL CORD

Dorsal Surface

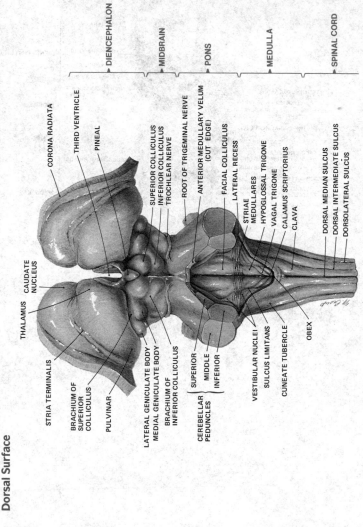

DIENCEPHALON
MIDBRAIN
PONS
MEDULLA
SPINAL CORD

CORONA RADIATA
THIRD VENTRICLE
PINEAL
SUPERIOR COLLICULUS
INFERIOR COLLICULUS
TROCHLEAR NERVE
ROOT OF TRIGEMINAL NERVE
ANTERIOR MEDULLARY VELUM (CUT EDGE)
FACIAL COLLICULUS
LATERAL RECESS
STRIAE MEDULLARES
HYPOGLOSSAL TRIGONE
VAGAL TRIGONE
CALAMUS SCRIPTORIUS
CLAVA
DORSAL MEDIAN SULCUS
DORSAL INTERMEDIATE SULCUS
DORSOLATERAL SULCUS

CAUDATE NUCLEUS
THALAMUS

STRIA TERMINALIS
BRACHIUM OF SUPERIOR COLLICULUS
PULVINAR
LATERAL GENICULATE BODY
MEDIAL GENICULATE BODY
BRACHIUM OF INFERIOR COLLICULUS
CEREBELLAR PEDUNCLES { SUPERIOR MIDDLE INFERIOR
VESTIBULAR NUCLEI
SULCUS LIMITANS
CUNEATE TUBERCLE
OBEX

THE BRAIN STEM AND DIENCEPHALON

Lateral Surface

CORONA RADIATA
LENTIFORM NUCLEUS
PULVINAR
LATERAL GENICULATE BODY
MEDIAL GENICULATE BODY
SUPERIOR COLLICULUS
INFERIOR COLLICULUS
SUPERIOR
MIDDLE } CEREBELLAR PEDUNCLES
INFERIOR
GLOSSOPHARYNGEAL NERVE
VAGUS NERVE (X) AND BULBAR ACCESSORY NERVE (XI)
DORSOLATERAL SULCUS
OPTIC NERVE
HYPOPHYSIS
OCULOMOTOR NERVE
TROCHLEAR NERVE
TRIGEMINAL NERVE
ABDUCENS NERVE
FACIAL NERVE AND NERVUS INTERMEDIUS
VESTIBULOCOCHLEAR NERVE
PYRAMID
OLIVE
HYPOGLOSSAL NERVE
SPINAL ACCESSORY NERVE
VENTROLATERAL SULCUS

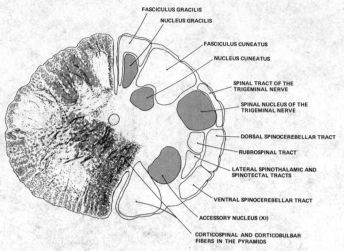

FASCICULUS GRACILIS

NUCLEUS GRACILIS

FASCICULUS CUNEATUS

NUCLEUS CUNEATUS

SPINAL TRACT OF THE TRIGEMINAL NERVE

SPINAL NUCLEUS OF THE TRIGEMINAL NERVE

DORSAL SPINOCEREBELLAR TRACT

RUBROSPINAL TRACT

LATERAL SPINOTHALAMIC AND SPINOTECTAL TRACTS

VENTRAL SPINOCEREBELLAR TRACT

ACCESSORY NUCLEUS (XI)

CORTICOSPINAL AND CORTICOBULBAR FIBERS IN THE PYRAMIDS

Lower Medulla: Section at the level of the pyramids. The left side of the illustration depicts what would be seen in a myelin-stained section, and the right side shows nuclei (colored) and tracts.

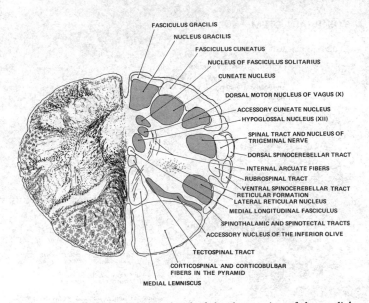

FASCICULUS GRACILIS
NUCLEUS GRACILIS
FASCICULUS CUNEATUS
NUCLEUS OF FASCICULUS SOLITARIUS
CUNEATE NUCLEUS
DORSAL MOTOR NUCLEUS OF VAGUS (X)
ACCESSORY CUNEATE NUCLEUS
HYPOGLOSSAL NUCLEUS (XII)
SPINAL TRACT AND NUCLEUS OF TRIGEMINAL NERVE
DORSAL SPINOCEREBELLAR TRACT
INTERNAL ARCUATE FIBERS
RUBROSPINAL TRACT
VENTRAL SPINOCEREBELLAR TRACT
RETICULAR FORMATION
LATERAL RETICULAR NUCLEUS
MEDIAL LONGITUDINAL FASCICULUS
SPINOTHALAMIC AND SPINOTECTAL TRACTS
ACCESSORY NUCLEUS OF THE INFERIOR OLIVE
TECTOSPINAL TRACT
CORTICOSPINAL AND CORTICOBULBAR FIBERS IN THE PYRAMID
MEDIAL LEMNISCUS

Lower medulla: Section at the level of the decussation of the medial lemniscus. The left side of the illustration depicts what would be seen in a myelin-stained section, and the right side shows nuclei (colored) and tracts.

THE BRAIN STEM

Cross-Sectional Views

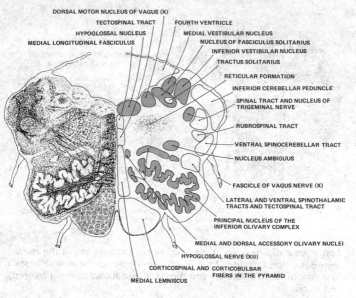

DORSAL MOTOR NUCLEUS OF VAGUS (X)
TECTOSPINAL TRACT
HYPOGLOSSAL NUCLEUS
MEDIAL LONGITUDINAL FASCICULUS
FOURTH VENTRICLE
MEDIAL VESTIBULAR NUCLEUS
NUCLEUS OF FASCICULUS SOLITARIUS
INFERIOR VESTIBULAR NUCLEUS
TRACTUS SOLITARIUS
RETICULAR FORMATION
INFERIOR CEREBELLAR PEDUNCLE
SPINAL TRACT AND NUCLEUS OF TRIGEMINAL NERVE
RUBROSPINAL TRACT
VENTRAL SPINOCEREBELLAR TRACT
NUCLEUS AMBIGUUS
FASCICLE OF VAGUS NERVE (X)
LATERAL AND VENTRAL SPINOTHALAMIC TRACTS AND TECTOSPINAL TRACT
PRINCIPAL NUCLEUS OF THE INFERIOR OLIVARY COMPLEX
MEDIAL AND DORSAL ACCESSORY OLIVARY NUCLEI
HYPOGLOSSAL NERVE (XII)
CORTICOSPINAL AND CORTICOBULBAR FIBERS IN THE PYRAMID
MEDIAL LEMNISCUS

Upper Medulla: The left side of the illustration depicts what would be seen in a myelin-stained section, and the right side shows nuclei (colored) and tracts.

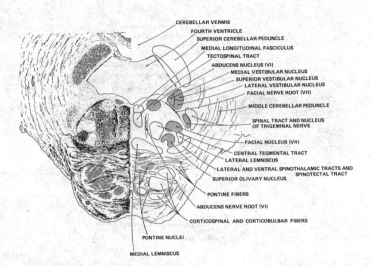

CEREBELLAR VERMIS
FOURTH VENTRICLE
SUPERIOR CEREBELLAR PEDUNCLE
MEDIAL LONGITUDINAL FASCICULUS
TECTOSPINAL TRACT
ABDUCENS NUCLEUS (VI)
MEDIAL VESTIBULAR NUCLEUS
SUPERIOR VESTIBULAR NUCLEUS
LATERAL VESTIBULAR NUCLEUS
FACIAL NERVE ROOT (VII)

MIDDLE CEREBELLAR PEDUNCLE

SPINAL TRACT AND NUCLEUS
OF TRIGEMINAL NERVE

FACIAL NUCLEUS (VII)
CENTRAL TEGMENTAL TRACT
LATERAL LEMNISCUS
LATERAL AND VENTRAL SPINOTHALAMIC TRACTS AND
SPINOTECTAL TRACT
SUPERIOR OLIVARY NUCLEUS

PONTINE FIBERS

ABDUCENS NERVE ROOT (VI)

CORTICOSPINAL AND CORTICOBULBAR FIBERS

PONTINE NUCLEI

MEDIAL LEMNISCUS

Pons: Section at the level of the nuclei of the abducens and facial nerves. The left side of the illustration depicts what would be seen in a myelin-stained section, and the right side shows nuclei (colored) and tracts.

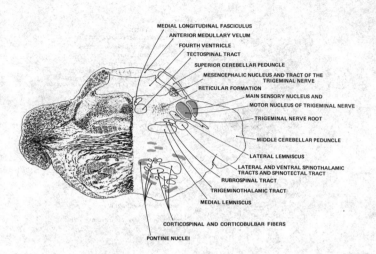

MEDIAL LONGITUDINAL FASCICULUS
ANTERIOR MEDULLARY VELUM
FOURTH VENTRICLE
TECTOSPINAL TRACT
SUPERIOR CEREBELLAR PEDUNCLE
MESENCEPHALIC NUCLEUS AND TRACT OF THE TRIGEMINAL NERVE
RETICULAR FORMATION
MAIN SENSORY NUCLEUS AND
MOTOR NUCLEUS OF TRIGEMINAL NERVE
TRIGEMINAL NERVE ROOT
MIDDLE CEREBELLAR PEDUNCLE
LATERAL LEMNISCUS
LATERAL AND VENTRAL SPINOTHALAMIC TRACTS AND SPINOTECTAL TRACT
RUBROSPINAL TRACT
TRIGEMINOTHALAMIC TRACT
MEDIAL LEMNISCUS
CORTICOSPINAL AND CORTICOBULBAR FIBERS
PONTINE NUCLEI

Pons: Section at the level of the main sensory and motor nuclei of the trigeminal nerve. The left side of the illustration depicts what would be seen in a myelin-stained section, and the right side shows nuclei (colored) and tracts.

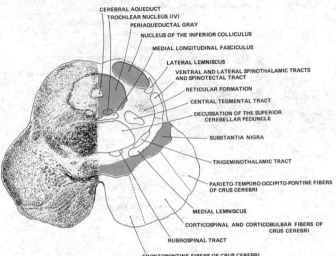

CEREBRAL AQUEDUCT
TROCHLEAR NUCLEUS (IV)
PERIAQUEDUCTAL GRAY
NUCLEUS OF THE INFERIOR COLLICULUS
MEDIAL LONGITUDINAL FASCICULUS
LATERAL LEMNISCUS
VENTRAL AND LATERAL SPINOTHALAMIC TRACTS AND SPINOTECTAL TRACT
RETICULAR FORMATION
CENTRAL TEGMENTAL TRACT
DECUSSATION OF THE SUPERIOR CEREBELLAR PEDUNCLE
SUBSTANTIA NIGRA
TRIGEMINOTHALAMIC TRACT
PARIETO-TEMPORO-OCCIPITO-PONTINE FIBERS OF CRUS CEREBRI
MEDIAL LEMNISCUS
CORTICOSPINAL AND CORTICOBULBAR FIBERS OF CRUS CEREBRI
RUBROSPINAL TRACT
FRONTOPONTINE FIBERS OF CRUS CEREBRI

Lower Midbrain: Section at the level of the inferior colliculus. The left side of the illustration depicts what would be seen in a myelin-stained section, and the right side shows nuclei (colored) and tracts.

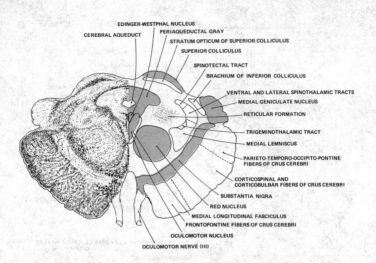

Upper Midbrain: Section at the level of the superior colliculus and the red nucleus. The left side of the illustration depicts what would be seen in a myelin-stained section, and the right side shows nuclei (colored) and tracts.

CROSS-SECTIONAL VIEWS OF THE SPINAL CORD

Cervical, Thoracic, and Lumbar Sections

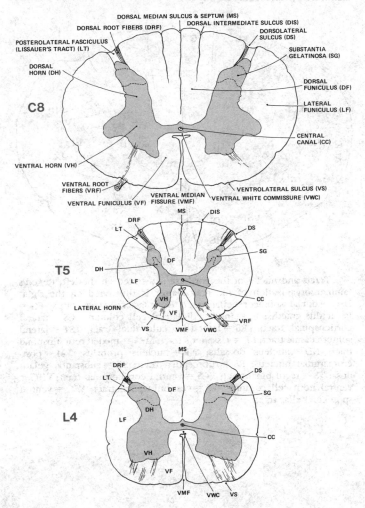

C8

DORSAL MEDIAN SULCUS & SEPTUM (MS)
DORSAL ROOT FIBERS (DRF)
DORSAL INTERMEDIATE SULCUS (DIS)
DORSOLATERAL SULCUS (DS)
POSTEROLATERAL FASCICULUS (LISSAUER'S TRACT) (LT)
SUBSTANTIA GELATINOSA (SG)
DORSAL HORN (DH)
DORSAL FUNICULUS (DF)
LATERAL FUNICULUS (LF)
CENTRAL CANAL (CC)
VENTRAL HORN (VH)
VENTRAL ROOT FIBERS (VRF)
VENTRAL FUNICULUS (VF)
VENTRAL MEDIAN FISSURE (VMF)
VENTRAL WHITE COMMISSURE (VWC)
VENTROLATERAL SULCUS (VS)

T5

MS
DIS
DRF
LT
DS
SG
DH
DF
LF
VH
CC
LATERAL HORN
VF
VS
VMF
VWC
VRF

L4

MS
DRF
DS
LT
DF
SG
DH
LF
VH
CC
VF
VMF
VWC
VS

CROSS-SECTIONAL OF THE SPINAL CORD: TRACTS AND LAMINA OF REXED

Section Approximately at C8–T1

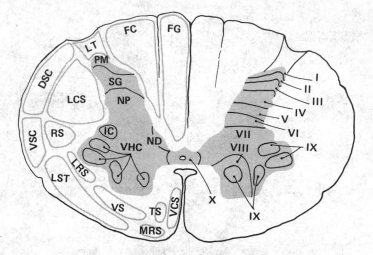

Tracts and nuclei of the cord are illustrated on the left; Rexed's laminar organization of the gray matter is illustrated on the right. DSC = dorsal spinocerebellar tract; FC = fasciculus cuneatus; FG = fasciculus gracilis; IC = intermediolateral cell column; LCS = lateral corticospinal tract; LRS = lateral reticulospinal tract; LST = lateral spinothalamic tract; LT = Lissauer's tract; MRS = medial reticulospinal tract; ND = nucleus dorsalis; NP = nucleus proprius; PM = posteromarginal nucleus; RS = rubrospinal tract; SG = substantia gelatinosa; TS = tectospinal tract; VCS = ventral corticospinal tract; VHC = ventral horn cell columns; VS = vestibulospinal tract; VSC = ventral spinocerebellar tract.

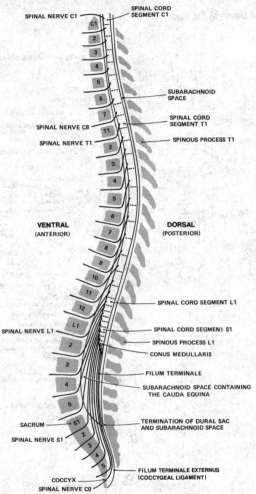

The figure shows the relationships between the spinal cord, spinal roots, vertebral segments, and the dural sac. The dural sac, the filum terminale internus, and the filum terminale externus (coccygeal ligament) are shown in color.

CUTANEOUS INNERVATION: DERMATOMES AND PERIPHERAL NERVE DISTRIBUTIONS

View of Ventral Surface

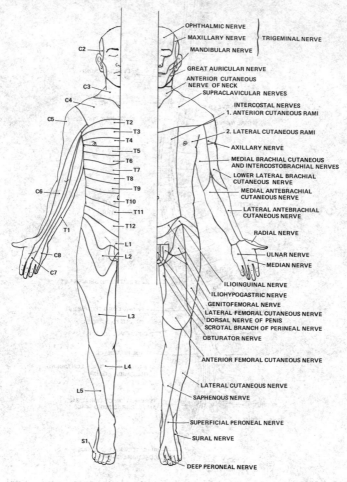

Cutaneous innervation of the front of the body. Dermatomes are on the left, and peripheral nerves are on the right.

CUTANEOUS INNERVATION: DERMATOMES AND PERIPHERAL NERVE DISTRIBUTIONS

View of Dorsal Surface

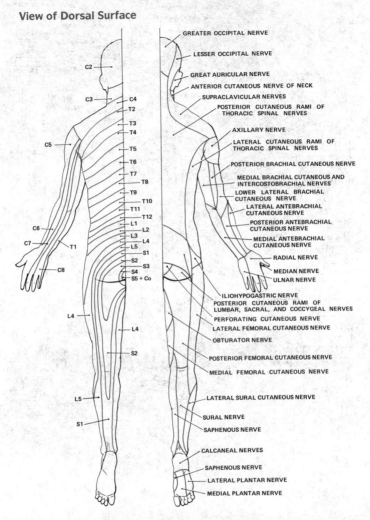

Cutaneous innervation of the back of the body. Dermatomes are on the left, and peripheral nerves are on the right.

THE AUTONOMIC NERVOUS SYSTEM

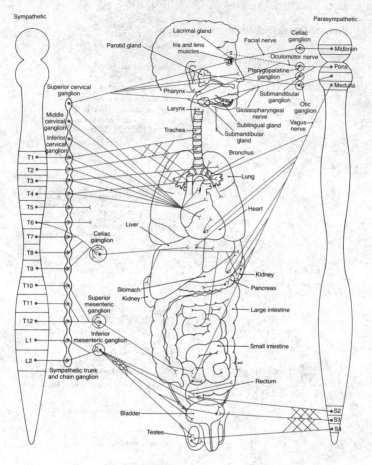

CIRCULATION OF THE CEREBROSPINAL FLUID

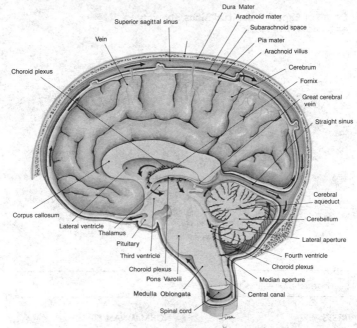

Superior sagittal sinus

Dura Mater

Arachnoid mater

Subarachnoid space

Pia mater

Arachnoid villus

Vein

Cerebrum

Fornix

Choroid plexus

Great cerebral vein

Straight sinus

Cerebral aqueduct

Cerebellum

Corpus callosum

Lateral aperture

Lateral ventricle

Fourth ventricle

Thalamus

Choroid plexus

Pituitary

Median aperture

Third ventricle

Central canal

Choroid plexus

Pons Varolii

Medulla Oblongata

Spinal cord

CIRCULATION OF THE CEREBROSPINAL FLUID

Detail of Superior Sagittal Sinus Showing Arachnoid Granulation

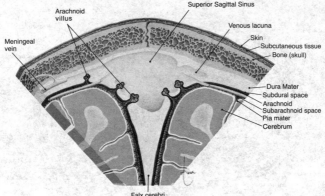

Normal CSF Values in Adults	
TESTS	**NORMAL VALUES**
Volume	90 – 150 ml
Pressure	Newborn: 30 – 80 mm H_2O Children: 50 – 100 mm Adults: 75 – 150 mm
Total cell count	Infants: 0 – 20/cu mm Adults: 0 – 5/cu mm (all cells are lymphocytes)
Specific gravity	1.006 – 1.008
Osmolality	280 – 290 mOsm/kg
Glucose	45 – 85 mg/dl
Protein	15 – 45 mg/dl (lumbar) 15 – 25 mg/dl (cisternal) 5 – 15 mg/dl (ventricular)

TESTS	NORMAL VALUES
Lactic acid	24 mg/dl
Glutamine	90 – 150 ml
Colloidal gold	0 (none)
A/G ratio (albumin to globulin)	8 : 1
Chloride	118 – 132 mEq/liter
Urea nitrogen	6 – 16 mg/dl
Creatinine	0.5 – 1.2 mg/dl
Cholesterol	0.2 – 0.6 mg/dl
Uric acid	0.5 – 4.5 mg/dl
Bilirubin	0 (none)
LDH	1/10 that of serum
pH	7.30 – 7.40
Chloride	118 – 132 mEq/Liter
Sodium	144 – 154 mEq/Liter
Potassium	2.0 – 3.5 mEq/Liter
CO_2 content	25 – 30 mEq/Liter (m mol)
PCO_2	42 – 53 mm Hg
PO_2	40 – 44 mm Hg
Calcium	2.1 – 2.7 mEq/Liter
Magnesium	2.4 – 3.1 mEq/Liter

Reference

1. Fischbach, F: A Manual of Laboratory Diagnostic Tests, ed 2. JB Lippincott, Philadelphia, 1984.

Normal and Pathological Findings in Cerebrospinal Fluid

CONDITION	APPEARANCE	PRESSURE (mm water)	CELLS (per Ml)	PROTEIN
Normal				
Lumbar	Clear and colorless	70–200	0–5	15–45 mg/dl
Ventricular	Clear and colorless	70–190	0–5	5–15 mg/dl
Pathological State				
Traumatic tap	Bloody; supernatant fluid yellow	Normal	Red blood cells	4 mg/dl rise per 5000 red cells
Cerebral, ventricular, or subarachnoid hemorrhage	Bloody; supernatant fluid yellow	Slightly increased	Red blood cells	4 mg/dl rise per 5000 red cells
Meningitis (acute purulent)	Clear, cloudy, milky, or xantho-chromic; occasional clot formation	Greatly increased (250–700)	Polymorphonuclear leukocytes (over 1000)	Increased

Acute tuberculosis	Opalescent to turbid; faint fibrin web or pellicle formation	Moderately increased (200–450)	10–500 (lymphocytes)	Increased
Acute syphilis	Clear to turbid; fibrin clots	Moderately increased (200–350)	100–1000 (mostly lymphocytes)	Slightly increased
Syphilis (meningovascular parenchymatous)	Clear and colorless	Normal	Normal or increased	Slightly increased
Brain tumor	Usually clear and colorless	Increased	Normal or increased	Increased
Brain abscess	Clear and colorless	Greatly increased	Polymorphonuclear leukocytes normal or increased	Increased
Subdural hematoma	Yellow, clear, or colorless	Usually increased	Normal	Normal or slightly increased
Encephalitis	Clear and colorless	Normal	Normal or increased (mostly lymphocytes)	Normal or slightly increased

Cont. on the following page(s)

Normal and Pathological Findings in Cerebrospinal Fluid *Continued*				
CONDITION	APPEARANCE	PRESSURE (mm water)	CELLS (per Ml)	PROTEIN
Uremia	Clear and colorless	Slightly increased	Normal	Normal or slightly increased
Lead encephalopathy	Clear or slightly cloudy	Increased	Lymphocytes	Normal or slightly increased
Arterial hypertension	Clear	Normal or increased	Normal	Normal or slightly increased
Epilepsy (idiopathic)	Normal fluid	Normal	Normal	Normal
Multiple sclerosis	Normal fluid	Normal or low	Normal or increased	Normal or increased (increased gamma globulin)

Condition	Appearance			
Poliomyelitis, acute	Opalescent; may be faintly yellow; delicate fibrin webs	Slightly increased	Slightly increased	Slightly increased (for a few weeks)
Spinal cord tumor (with partial block)	Clear and colorless	Normal	Normal	Slightly increased
Spinal cord tumor (with complete block)	Yellow	Normal or low	Slightly increased	Marked rise (200–600 mg/dl)
Diabetic coma	Clear and colorless (glucose elevated)	Decreased	Normal	Normal or slightly increased
Acute alcoholic coma	Clear and colorless	Slightly increased	May be slightly increased	Normal

CLASSIFICATION OF THE CRANIAL NERVES

Definitions

Afferent Components
GSA (general somatic afferents): Innervate receptors for touch, pain, or temperature sensibility of the skin; innervate sensory organs of muscle, joint, and tendon.

SSA (special somatic afferents): Innervate specialized receptors of ectodermal origin, specifically those for vision and vestibular and auditory sensibility.

GVA (general visceral afferents): Innervate touch, pain, or temperature receptors that are related to mucous or serous membranes, hollow organs, or glands; innervate chemoreceptors and baroreceptors.

SVA (special visceral afferents): Innervate specialized receptors found in the cranial region that are associated with visceral activity, specifically those for taste and smell.

Efferent Components
GSE (general somatic efferents): Motoneurons that innervate skeletal muscle that was not derived from the branchial arch mesoderm.

SVE (specialized visceral efferents): Motoneurons that innervate skeletal muscle that was derived from the embryonic branchial arch mesoderm, including muscles of the jaw, facial expression, pharynx, and larynx.

GVE (general visceral efferents): Motoneurons that are part of the autonomic nervous system and innervate smooth muscle, cardiac muscle, and glands.

Reference

1. Gilman, S and Newman, SW: Manter and Gatz's Essentials of Clinical Neuroanatomy and Neurophysiology, ed 7. FA Davis, Philadelphia, 1987.

CRANIAL NERVE
NUMBER NAME

COMPONENTS

I.	Olfactory	SVA
II.	Optic	SSA
III.	Oculomotor	GSE, GVE
IV.	Trochlear	GSA, GSE
V.	Trigeminal	GSA, SVE
VI.	Abducens	GSA, GSE
VII.	Facial	GSA, GVA, GVE, SVA, SVE
VIII.	Vestibulocochlear	SSA
IX.	Glossopharyngeal	GSA, GVA, GVE, SVA, SVE
X.	Vagus	GSA, GVA, SVA, SVE, GVE
XI.	Accessory	GSA, SVE
XII.	Hypoglossal	GSA, GSE

OVERVIEW OF CRANIAL NERVE INNERVATION

Sensory Innervation

MODALITY	NUMBER	CLASSIFICATION
Olfaction	I	SVA
Vision	II	SSA
Taste	VII, IX, X	SVA
Hearing and vestibular organs	VIII	SSA
Skin overlying face and scalp to vertex	V	GSA
Majority of mucosal membranes	V	GSA
Remainder of mucosal membranes	VII, IX, X	GVA

Motor Innervation

STRUCTURE	NUMBER	CLASSIFICATION
Muscles within orbit	III, IV, and VI	GSE
Muscles of the tongue	XII	GSE
Muscles of mastication, tensor tympani, tensor palati (tensor veli palatini), anterior belly of digastric, mylohyoid	V	Mandibular division, SVE
Muscles of facial expression and the stapedius, stylohyoid, posterior belly of digastric	VII	SVE
Mucosal and glandular secretions including lacrimal, mucous glands, nose, palate, oral cavity; submandibular and sublingual glands	VII	GVE
Parotid gland	IX	GVE

SYMPATHETIC AND PARASYMPATHETIC COMPONENTS OF THE CRANIAL NERVES

Sympathetic Components

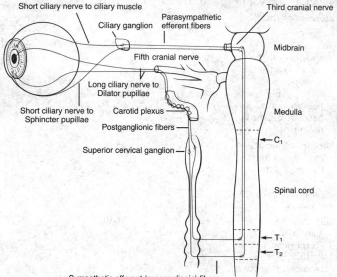

Cell bodies for the sympathetic nerve supply to the head are located in the superior cervical ganglion. Postganglionic fibers reach visceral targets such as the smooth muscle of blood vessels or the dilator pupillae by ascending with the internal carotid artery or any of its branches.

Parasympathetic Distribution to the Head

CRANIAL NERVE	GANGLION	INNERVATES	COURSE
Oculomotor	Ciliary	Sphincter pupillae and the ciliary muscles	Short ciliary nerves to the sphincter pupillae (for pupillary constriction) and to the ciliary muscle (for increased lens convexity)
Facial	Pterygopalatine	Lacrimal gland and mucosa	Via lacrimal nerve and gland and glands of nose and palate
Facial	Submandibular	Submandibular and sublingual glands and mucosa	Via chorda tympani and submaxillary ganglion and on to the submandibular and sublingual salivary glands
Glossopharyngeal	Otic	Parotid gland	Lesser petrosal nerve through the otic ganglion to the parotid gland

Reference

1. Clemente, CD, (ed): Gray's Anatomy, ed 30. Lea & Febiger, Philadelphia, 1985.

CRANIAL NERVE	DISTRIBUTION	FUNCTION
Olfactory	Olfactory mucosa	Smell
Optic	Retina	Vision
Oculomotor	Superior division: rectus superior (superior rectus) and levator palpebra	Eye movements
	Inferior division: rectus inferior (inferior rectus) and rectus medialis (medial rectus) muscles; obliquus inferior (inferior oblique) muscle and parasympathetic accommodation fibers to the ciliary ganglion and on to the sphincter pupillae and ciliary muscles	Eye movements
Trochlear	Obliquus superior (superior oblique) muscle	Eye movements
Trigeminal	Ophthalmic nerve: eyeball and face	Sensation of the face, scalp, eyeball, and tongue (not for taste)
	Maxillary nerve: upper jaw and face	

CRANIAL NERVE	DISTRIBUTION	FUNCTION
	Mandibular nerve: muscles of mastication and to lower part of face and anterior two thirds of tongue	
Abducens	Rectus lateralis (lateral rectus) muscle	Eye movements
Facial	Muscles of face and scalp	Facial expression
	Anterior two thirds of the tongue	Taste
	Submandibular, sublingual, and lacrimal glands	Secretion (saliva and tears) lingual and lacrimal glands
	external auditory meatus	Pain and temperature of the external auditory meatus
Vestibulocochlear	Cochlear nerve	Hearing
	Vestibular nerve	To semicircular canals, utricle, and saccule
Glossopharyngeal	Tympanic	Sensory to middle ear
	Lesser petrosal nerve	Innervates parotid gland (via the otic ganglion)
	Carotid	Chemoreceptors and baroreceptors
	Pharyngeal	Mucosal membranes of the pharynx

"Cont. on the following page(s)"

CRANIAL NERVE	DISTRIBUTION	FUNCTION
	Muscular	Innervates stylopharyngeus muscle
	Tonsillar	Sensation to the tonsils
	Lingual	General sensation and taste to the posterior one third of the tongue and papillae
Vagus	Meningeal	Dura mater and posterior fossa of the skull
	Auricular	Sensation around the external acoustic meatus
	Pharyngeal	Motor nerves of the pharynx
	Superior laryngeal	Sensory to the muscles and mucous membranes of the larynx
	Recurrent laryngeal (left and right)	Motor innervation to the muscles of the larynx, sensation to lower larynx, and branches to esophagus and trachea

CRANIAL NERVE	DISTRIBUTION	FUNCTION
	Cardiac	Joins cardiac plexus
Vagus (con't.)	Pulmonary	Lung
	Esophageal	Esophagus and posterior pericardium
	Gastric	Stomach
	Celiac	Contributes to celiac plexus
	Hepatic	Liver
Accessory	Cranial with vagus and larynx	Muscles of pharynx and soft palate
	Spinal motor innervation to sternomastoid and trapezius	Neck movements
Hypoglossal	All muscles of the tongue except the palatoglossus	Movement of the tongue

CRANIAL NERVE TESTING

Nerve Examination and Types of Deficits

I.	Olfactory	The patient is asked to identify familiar odors (tobacco, garlic, coffee) with eyes closed.
II.	Optic	**field testing:** One eye is covered as patient looks at the examiner's nose; staring at the peripheral extent of each quadrant, the examiner moves a finger in front of the patient toward the center of vision; patient states when she or he first sees the finger, thus revealing any gross deficits. **retinal lesion:** Blind spot in affected eye. **optic nerve lesion:** Partial or complete blindness. **complete lesion of optic tract or of one lateral geniculate body:** Blindness in opposite halves of both visual fields. **temporal lobe abnormality:** Blindness in upper quadrant of both visual fields on the side opposite lesion. **parietal lobe lesion:** Contralateral blindness in lower quadrants of both eyes. **occipital lobe lesion:** Contralateral blindness in corresponding half of each visual field.
III.	Oculomotor	Test for an inability to elevate, depress, and adduct affected eye.
IV.	Trochlear	Test for an inability to depress and adduct the affected eye.
V.	Trigeminal	Test sensations in all areas of the face bilaterally and look for inability to sense specific stimuli or for differences in threshold in response to the same stimulus bilaterally; examine corneal reflex by determining if patient blinks in response to light touch of cotton to cornea; palpate masseter and temporalis muscles in response to command to close jaw; test jaw reflex by striking the middle of chin with a reflex hammer with patient's mouth slightly open; normally there is a sudden, slight jaw closing.
VI.	Abducens	Test for an inability to abduct the affected eye.

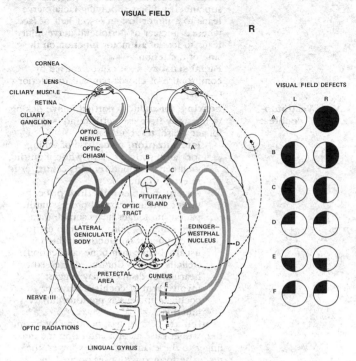

VISUAL FIELD

L   R

CORNEA
LENS
CILIARY MUSCLE
RETINA
CILIARY GANGLION
OPTIC NERVE
OPTIC CHIASM
PITUITARY GLAND
OPTIC TRACT
LATERAL GENICULATE BODY
EDINGER—WESTPHAL NUCLEUS
PRETECTAL AREA
CUNEUS
NERVE III
OPTIC RADIATIONS
LINGUAL GYRUS

VISUAL FIELD DEFECTS

L   R
A
B
C
D
E
F

The visual pathways. Lesions along the pathway from the eye to the visual cortex (lesions A through F) result in deficits in the visual fields, which are shown as black areas on the corresponding visual field diagrams. The pathway through the pretectum and nerve III, which mediates reflex constriction of the pupil in response to light, is also shown.

VII. Facial — Patient imitates examiner's facial expressions; maintenance of eye closure as examiner attempts to manually open eye; sensation tested by having patient identify taste of stimuli (sugar, salt, and so on) placed on one half of anterior tongue and with sips of water at a neutral temperature between stimuli.

facial muscle motor loss: Involvement of supranuclear fibers supplying facial nerve leads to a motor loss in lower half of face, whereas nuclear or peripheral nerve injury leads to loss of all motor function on the side of the lesion.

Facial sensory loss: can be caused by compromise of chorda tympani to anterior tongue.

VIII. **Vestibulo-cochlear**

hearing: for auditory portion, move ticking watch away from ear until sound is no longer heard; test both ears.

lateralization: place base of tuning fork atop patient's skull while inquiring whether the sound remains central or is referred to one side.

air and bone conduction: place tuning fork on mastoid process until patient no longer hears sound; then hold vibrating portion next to ear to determine air conduction (which is usually better than bone conduction). Deficits such as tinnitus, decreased hearing, or deafness may suggest involvement of cochlear nerve or cochlear nucleus at pontomedullary junction.

vestibular: Test for past-pointing by having the patient raise an arm and bring the index finger to the examiner's index finger; the test is performed with eyes opened and closed; with vestibular disorders the patient misses the examiner's finger by pointing to one side or the other; the patient may also have difficulty in performing the finger-to-nose test; nystagmus may also be present; caloric testing (infiltrating one ear with cold water at 18° to 20° C) should demonstrate vertigo, past-pointing, and nystagmus, whereas a patient with a defective vestibular system will not necessarily show such changes.

IX. **Glosso-pharyngeal**

See tests listed under the vagus nerve.

X. **Vagus**

Touch side of pharynx with applicator stick to elicit gag reflex and note rise in uvula when its mucous membrane is stroked (the glossopharyngeal nerve supplies the sensory portion of this reflex); patient's ability to swallow and to speak clearly without hoarseness as well as to demonstrate symmetrical vocal cord movements and soft palate movement suggest an intact vagus nerve to pharynx, larynx, and soft palate.

| XI. | Accessory | Shoulder shrug against resistance (upper trapezius), resistance to lateral neck flexion with rotation (sternomastoid). |
| XII. | Hypoglossal | Patient protrudes tongue while examiner checks for lateral deviation, atrophy, or tremor. |

Reference

1. Chusid, JG: Correlative Neuroanatomy and Functional Neurology, ed 19. Lange Medical Publications, Los Altos CA, 1985.

Adduction

Rectus medialis
(medial rectus)

Rectus superioris
(superior rectus)

Rectus inferior
(inferior rectus)

Medial Rotation

Obliquus superior
(superior
oblique)

Rectus superior
(superior rectus)

Depression

Obliquus superior
(superior
oblique)

Rectus inferior
(inferior rectus)

Abduction

Obliquus inferior
(inferior
oblique)

Obliquus superior
(superior
oblique)

Rectus lateralis
(lateral rectus)

Lateral Rotation

Obliquus inferior
(inferior
oblique)

Rectus inferior
(inferior rectus)

Elevation

Rectus lateralis
(lateral rectus)

Rectus superior
(superior rectus)

Obliquus inferior
(inferior
oblique)

BY MUSCLE

Muscle	Innervation	Function
Rectus superior (superior rectus)	Oculomotor (III)	Elevation, adduction, medial rotation
Obliquus superior (superior oblique)	Trochlear (IV)	Depression, abduction, medial rotation
Rectus inferior (inferior rectus)	Oculomotor (III)	Depression, adduction, lateral rotation
Obliquus inferior (inferior oblique)	Oculomotor (III)	Elevation, abduction, lateral rotation
Rectus medialis (medial rectus)	Oculomotor (III)	Adduction
Rectus lateralis (lateral rectus)	Abducens (VI)	Abduction

Reference

1. Anderson, JE: Grant's Atlas of Anatomy, ed 8. Williams & Wilkins, Baltimore, 1983.

Clinical Tests for Function of Extraocular Muscles	

MUSCLE	MOVEMENT OF EYE REQUESTED
Rectus lateralis (lateral rectus)	Outward (abduction)
Rectus medialis (medial rectus)	Inward (adduction)
Rectus superioris (superior rectus)	Elevation and adduction
Rectus inferioris (inferior rectus)	Depression and adduction
Obliquus Superioris (superior oblique)	Depression and adduction
Obliquus Inferioris (inferior oblique)	Elevation and adduction

THE EYE AND THE ORBIT

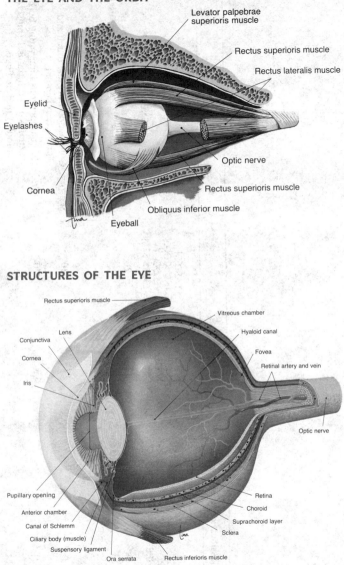

Levator palpebrae superioris muscle

Rectus superioris muscle

Rectus lateralis muscle

Eyelid

Eyelashes

Optic nerve

Cornea

Rectus superioris muscle

Obliquus inferior muscle

Eyeball

STRUCTURES OF THE EYE

Rectus superioris muscle

Vitreous chamber

Lens

Hyaloid canal

Conjunctiva

Fovea

Cornea

Retinal artery and vein

Iris

Optic nerve

Pupillary opening

Retina

Anterior chamber

Choroid

Canal of Schlemm

Suprachoroid layer

Ciliary body (muscle)

Sclera

Suspensory ligament

Ora serrata

Rectus inferioris muscle

Classification of Nerve Fibers

SENSORY AND MOTOR FIBERS	SENSORY FIBERS	LARGEST FIBER DIAMETER (MICROMETERS)	FASTEST CONDUCTION VELOCITY (METERS/SEC)	GENERAL COMMENTS
A-α	Ia	22	120	Motor: The large alpha motoneurons of lamina IX, innervating extrafusal muscle fibers
				Sensory: The primary afferents of muscle spindles
A-α	Ib	22	120	Sensory: Golgi tendon organs, touch and pressure receptors
A-β	II	13	70	Motor: The motoneurons innervating both extrafusal and intrafusal (muscle spindle) muscle fibers

Fiber Type				
A-γ		8	40	Sensory: The secondary afferents of muscle spindles, touch and pressure receptors, and pacinian corpuscles (vibratory sensors)
				Motor: The small gamma motoneurons of lamina IX, innervating intrafusal fibers (muscle spindles)
A-δ	III	5	15	Sensory: Small, lightly myelinated fibers; touch, pressure, pain, and temperature
B		3	14	Motor: Small, lightly myelinated preganglionic autonomic fibers
C	IV	1	2	Motor: All postganglionic autonomic fibers (all are unmyelinated)
				Sensory: Unmyelinated pain and temperature fibers

Reference

1. Gilman, S and Newman, SW: Manter and Gatz's Essentials of Clinical Neuroanatomy and Neurophysiology, ed 7. FA Davis, Philadelphia, 1987.

ANATOMICAL CLASSIFICATION OF PERIPHERAL NEUROPATHIES

Symmetrical Generalized Neuropathies (Polyneuropathies)

DISTAL AXONOPATHIES

Toxic: drugs, industrial and environmental chemicals
Metabolic: uremia, diabetes, porphyria, endocrine
Deficiencies: thiamine, pyridoxine
Genetic: HMSN II (hereditary motor sensory neuropathy type II)
Malignancy associated: oat-cell carcinoma, multiple myeloma

MYELINOPATHIES

Toxic: diphtheria, buckthorn
Immunologic: acute inflammatory polyneuropathy (Guillain-Barré), chronic inflammatory polyneuropathy
Genetic: Refsum's disease, metachromatic leukodystrophy

NEURONOPATHIES

Somatic Motor

Undetermined: amyotrophic lateral sclerosis
Genetic: hereditary motor neuropathies

Somatic Sensory

Infectious: herpes zoster neuronitis
Malignancy associated: sensory neuropathy syndrome
Toxic: pyridoxine sensory neuropathy
Undetermined: subacute sensory neuropathy syndrome

Autonomic

Genetic: hereditary dysautonomia (HSN IV: hereditary sensory neuropathy type IV)

Ischemia: polyarteritis, diabetes, rheumatoid arthritis

Infiltration: leukemia, lymphoma, granuloma, schwannoma, amyloid

Physical injuries: severance, focal crush, compression, stretch and traction, entrapment

Immunologic: brachial and lumbar plexopathy

Reference

1. Schaumberg, HH, Spencer, PS, and Thomas, PK: Disorders of Peripheral Nerves. FA Davis, Philadelphia, 1986.

ANATOMICAL CLASSIFICATIONS OF ACUTE NERVE INJURIES

Terms Used to Describe Acute Nerve Injuries: Lesions and Clinical Features
(see figures for illustrations of each lesion type)

SUGGESTED NOMENCLATURE	PREVIOUS NOMENCLATURE	ANATOMIC LESION	COMMON CLINICAL FEATURES
Class 1	Neuropraxia Transient	Conduction block Ischemia	A rapidly reversible loss of nerve function occurs
	Delayed reversible	Demyelination	Dysfunction of the nerve persists for a few weeks
Class 2	Axonotmesis	Axonal interruption	Total loss of function occurs in the nerve until there is regeneration of the damaged

Class 3	Neurotmesis			
	Partial	Nerve fiber interruption Damage to Schwann cell tube and endoneural connective tissue	axon; Wallerian degeneration occurs distal to the site of the lesion; regenerating axons are guided back to their terminations via the intact Schwann cell tubes and other endoneural connective tissue	Reinnervation may be incomplete because of a failure of the regenerating axon to find its proper terminus
	Complete	Total nerve severance	Reinnervation will not occur unless the nerve is surgically repaired; neuroma formation and aberrant regeneration are common	

Reference

1. Schaumberg, HH, Spencer, PS, and Thomas, PK: Disorders of Peripheral Nerves. FA Davis, Philadelphia, 1986.

Class 1 (Neurapraxia) Nerve Injury

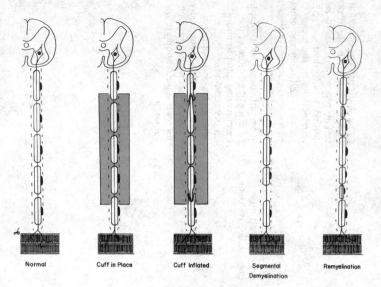

Normal   Cuff in Place   Cuff Inflated   Segmental Demyelination   Remyelination

CLASS I — ACUTE NERVE INJURY
(e.g. Compression)

Class 1 (neurapraxia) nerve injury associated with compression by a cuff. Axon movement at both edges of the cuff causes intussusception of the attached myelin across the node of Ranvier into the adjacent paranode. Affected paranodes demyelinate. Remyelination begins following cuff removal and conduction eventually resumes. Conduction is normal in the nerve above and below the cuff since the axon has not been damaged.

Class 2 (Axonotmesis) Nerve Injury

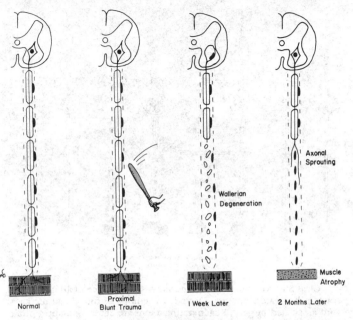

Normal · **Proximal Blunt Trauma** · **I Week Later** (Wallerian Degeneration) · **2 Months Later** (Axonal Sprouting, Muscle Atrophy)

CLASS 2 NERVE INJURY

Class 2 nerve injury (axonotmesis) from a crush injury to a limb. Axonal disruption occurs at the site of injury. Wallerian degeneration takes place throughout the axon distal to the injury with loss of axon, myelin, and nerve conduction. Preservation of Schwann cell tubes and other endoneurial connective tissue ensures that regenerating axons have the opportunity to reach their previous terminals and, hopefully, re-establish functional connections.

Class 3 (Neurotmesis) Nerve Injury

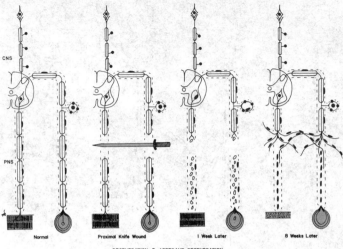

DEGENERATION & ABBERANT REGENERATION
IN (CLASS 3) NERVE INJURY

Class 3 nerve injury (neurotmesis) with severance of all neural and connective tissue elements. There is little hope of functional recovery without skilled surgery. Regenerating axons are entering inappropriate Schwann cell tubes (aberrant regeneration).

PERIPHERAL NERVE ENTRAPMENT SYNDROMES

(listed alphabetically under upper and lower extremity syndromes)

Upper Extremity Syndromes

anterior interosseous nerve syndrome: The anterior interosseus nerve is compromised at or near its site of origin from the median nerve. Entrapment may occur as a result of thrombosis of the vessels that accompany the nerve, an accessory head of the flexor pollicis longus, an enlarged bicipital bursa, a tendinous origin of the deep head of the pronator muscle, or from either forearm fracture undergoing open reduction or supracondylar fractures in children. This syndrome is characterized by pain or discomfort in the volar aspect of the proximal forearm area with eventual weakness or paralysis of the pronator quadratus and flexor pollicis longus, and the flexor digitorum profundus slips to the index and middle finger.

carpal tunnel syndrome: Compression of the median nerve as it passes through the tunnel formed by the concavity in the two rows of carpal bones and the flexor retinaculum. The causes may be inflammatory, as in tenosynovitis of the flexor tendons or rheumatoid arthritis, hormonal dysfunction, or bony deformity secondary to fracture, acromegaly, or congenital stenosis. The syndrome presents as pain and paresthesias, usually worse at night, involving the digits supplied by the median nerve. There may be weakness and atrophy of the abductor pollicis brevis, the opponens pollicis, and the first and second lumbricales.

cubital tunnel syndrome: Entrapment of the ulnar nerve at the cubital tunnel, which is formed by the ulnar groove between the medial epicondyle of the humerus and the olecranon. This syndrome can be caused by ganglion formation, arthritis, an old fracture of the lateral humeral epicondyle, and dislocation of the ulnar nerve when the elbow is flexed. Sensory involvement is localized over the ulnar aspect of the hand on both the palmar and dorsal aspects. The motor weakness is manifested in the forearm by the flexor carpi ulnaris and in the hand by the adductor pollicis, and the flexor digitorum profundus, lumbricales, and interosseus muscles (fourth and fifth digits). These weaknesses result in a radial deviation on wrist flexion and a mild clawing of the fourth and fifth fingers.

flexor carpi ulnaris syndrome: Entrapment of the ulnar nerve as it passes under the arcuate ligament between the two heads of the flexor carpi ulnaris muscle. The symptoms are similar to those described for cubital tunnel syndrome.

posterior interosseous nerve entrapment: The posterior interosseous nerve, a branch of the radial nerve, may be entrapped as it passes through the two heads of the supinator muscle via an aponeurotic arch (arcade of Frohse). Most cases of this syndrome are found to be secondary to either thickening or narrowing of the arcade of Frohse. Predisposing factors are diabetes mellitus, leprosy, periarteritis nodosa, and heavy metal poisoning. The complete syndrome presents as pain or discomfort over the proximal or lateral aspect of the forearm. The patient radially deviates on dorsiflexion of the wrist and the fingers and thumb cannot be extended at the MCP joints.

pronator teres syndrome: Occurs when the median nerve is entrapped as it passes between the two heads of the pronator teres. Symptoms are pain or discomfort over the volar proximal third of the forearm, which is aggravated when the forearm is overly pronated and the wrist flexed. Paresthesias may be present in the radial three half digits. Muscle weakness is highly variable. The flexor carpi radialis, the flexor digitorum superficialis, and the median lumbricales are often weak. The most common causes of this syndrome are:

1. Narrowing of the space between the two heads of the pronator
2. Direct trauma of the volar upper third of the forearm
3. Repetitive motion of the limb (forearm pronation with finger flexion)
4. An anatomical variation
5. Chronic external compression of the upper forearm

spiral groove syndrome: Entrapment or direct trauma to the radial nerve at the spiral groove of the humerus between the medial and lateral heads of the triceps. This syndrome usually occurs as a complication of humeral fractures or direct pressure on the nerve (Saturday Night palsy). Fully manifested, its symptoms are a drop wrist with a flexed metacarpophalangeal joint and an adducted thumb. All muscles innervated by the radial nerve may be paralyzed, except for the triceps.

supracondylar process syndrome: The median nerve, accompanied by the brachial or ulnar artery, may become entrapped beneath the ligament of Struthers. This ligament originates from a bony process above the medial condyle and runs to the medial epicondyle of the elbow (it is present in about 1 percent of limbs). The patient presents with pronator teres weakness, and the radial or ulnar pulse may decrease or vanish when the arm is fully extended and supinated.

Ulnar (Guyon's) tunnel syndrome: Entrapment of the ulnar nerve as it travels through the ulnar tunnel from the forearm into the hand. This tunnel is formed by the pisohamate ligament at the wrist. Entrapment occurs usually as a result of a space-occupying lesion within the tunnel such as with rheumatoid arthritis or from the formation of ganglions. The symptoms are pain over the palmar aspect of the ulnar side of the hand and the fifth digit and the ulnar aspect of the fourth digit. Motor function shows the typical "preacher" or "benediction" hand. Atrophy of the hypothenar and interosseus muscles (especially the first dorsal interossei) may become very noticeable.

Lower Extremity Syndromes

anterior compartment syndrome: Compression of the anterior tibial artery and veins and the deep branch of the peroneal nerve, as a result of increased pressure within the confines of the anterior compartment. Blood supply to the muscles within this osteofascial compartment is compromised. This syndrome may result from anterior tibial tendonitis associated with running long distances, a direct blow to the anterior aspect of the leg, or an overly tight cast to the leg. Early symptoms are intense pain in the anterior aspect of the leg with signs of vascular depletion in the foot. Muscular loss appears as an inability to dorsiflex the ankle, the toes, and the big toe. There is hypesthesia or anesthesia in the dorsal aspect of the first web space.

common peroneal nerve syndrome: Injury or entrapment of the common peroneal nerve at the fibular head and neck, as it winds around the fibula head. Some of the most common causes of this syndrome are excessive pressure from poorly applied casts or bandages, excessive pressure in bedridden patients allowed to remain in external rotation, fracture of the neck of the fibula, severe acute genu varum, and direct trauma to the nerve. In patients with a fully developed syndrome, the patient's foot appears in full plantar flexion and slight inversion as a result of weakness or paralysis in all the muscles of the anterior and lateral compartment of the leg. The patient has a steppage gait.

meralgia paraesthetica: Compression of the lateral femoral cutaneous nerve as it passes into the thigh under the inguinal ligament just medial to the anterior superior iliac spine. It is brought on by trauma, postural abnormalities, occupations requiring long periods of hip flexion, obesity, and wearing of a tight belt or truss. The patient usually complains of discomfort or pain in the lateral aspect of the thigh.

piriformis syndrome: Entrapment of the sciatic nerve as it emerges from the pelvis through the greater sciatic foramen, passing between the piriformis muscle above and the obturator internus below. The common causes of this syndrome are sustained piriformis muscle contraction and fibrotic muscle changes secondary to direct trauma, as in posterior dislocation of the hip joint. The patient has motor and sensory changes involving the posterior aspect of the thigh and the entire leg and foot. Muscle weakness of the hamstrings, gluteus maximus, ankle dorsiflexors, plantar flexors, and the intrinsics of the foot can result in a gluteus maximus lurch as well as difficulty in walking on toes or heels.

popliteal fossa entrapment: Compression of the tibial nerve as it passes through the popliteal fossa. It is usually caused by a Baker's cyst. Enlarged cysts may also compress the common peroneal and sural nerves. Other causes are proliferation of the synovial tissue in patients with rheumatoid arthritis. The patient presents with incomplete flexion of the knee joint and pain behind the knee or in the calf muscles when the foot is dorsiflexed. The gastrocnemius, tibialis posterior, flexor hallucis longus, flexor digitorum longus, and the intrinsic muscles of the foot (except for extensor digitorum brevis) are weak or paralyzed. The entire plantar surface of the foot is hypesthetic or anesthetic.

tarsal tunnel syndrome: Compression of the posterior tibial nerve or its branches as it passes under the flexor retinaculum behind the medial malleolus of the ankle joint. The most common causes of this syndrome are tenosynovitis of the flexor hallucis longus, flexor digitorum longus, or tibialis posterior caused by local trauma or systemic connective tissue diseases; venous distension or engorgement within the tunnel from chronic venous insufficiency or distortion of the canal from either developmental (pes planus, pes valgus); or traumatic deformities (fracture of the medial malleolus or fracture/dislocations of the calcaneus or talus). There is severe weakness of plantar flexion and edema in the back of the leg.

Reference

1. Perotto, A and Delagi, E: Peripheral nerve entrapment syndromes. In Ruskin, A (ed): Current Therapy in Physiatry, Physical Medicine and Rehabilitation. WB Saunders, Philadelphia, 1984.

CERVICAL PLEXUS

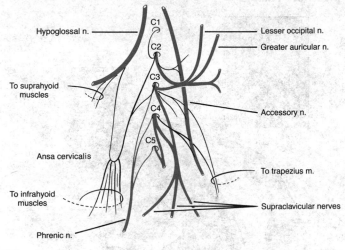

Hypoglossal n.

C1

Lesser occipital n.

C2

Greater auricular n.

To suprahoid muscles

C3

Accessory n.

C4

Ansa cervicalis

C5

To trapezius m.

To infrahyoid muscles

Supraclavicular nerves

Phrenic n.

Anatomy: The cervical plexus is formed by anterior primary rami of C1, C2, C3, and C4. The plexus lies almost entirely beneath the sternomastoid muscle.

BRACHIAL PLEXUS

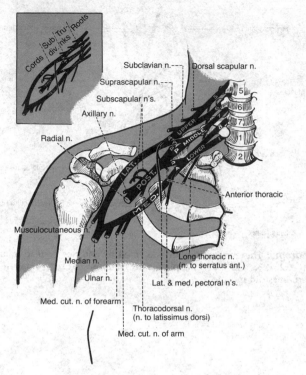

Subclavian n.
Dorsal scapular n.
Suprascapular n.
Subscapular n's.
Axillary n.
Radial n.
Anterior thoracic
Musculocutaneous n.
Median n.
Long thoracic n.
(n. to serratus ant.)
Ulnar n.
Lat. & med. pectoral n's.
Med. cut. n. of forearm
Thoracodorsal n.
(n. to latissimus dorsi)
Med. cut. n. of arm

The brachial plexus. Note that extensor muscles are innervated by posterior divisions, and anterior divisions innervate flexors. Each of the three trunks (upper, middle, and lower) has an anterior and posterior division. The posterior divisions form the posterior cord, and the anterior divisions form the lateral and medial cords.

BRACHIAL PLEXUS

Anatomy. The brachial plexus is formed by anterior primary rami of spinal segments C5, C6, C7, C8, and T1. The upper trunk is formed from the fibers of C5 and C6. The middle trunk is formed from the fibers of C7, and the lower trunk is formed from fibers of C8 and T1. The trunks divide into anterior and posterior divisions. The anterior divisions contribute to nerves that innervate flexors, and the posterior divisions contribute to nerves that innervate extensors. The anterior divisions of the middle and upper trunk form the lateral cord. The posterior divisions from all three trunks form the posterior cord. The anterior division of the lower trunk forms the medial cord. The cords are named for their relationships with the axillary artery, around which the plexus wraps.

Injuries to the Brachial Plexus

Upper Plexus Injury (Erb-Duchenne). This is the most common injury to the brachial plexus and occurs when damage is done to the roots of C5 and C6. Common mechanisms of injury are traction injuries (as occur at birth) and compression injuries. Months or years after radiation therapy for breast cancer, upper plexus damage may become apparent. Upper plexus injuries result in paralysis of the deltoid, biceps, and brachialis, brachioradialis muscles, and sometimes the supraspinatus, infraspinatus, and subscapularis muscles. If the roots are avulsed from the spinal cord, the rhomboids, serratus anterior, levator scapula, and the scalenes muscles will also be affected.

With upper plexus injuries, the arm is held limply at the patient's side, internally rotated and adducted. The elbow is extended and the forearm is pronated in what is called the *waiter's tip* position. Biceps and brachioradialis reflexes are lost. Sensation is lost in the region of the deltoid and the radial surfaces of the forearm and hand.

Lower Plexus Injury (Klumpke). This occurs when damage is done to the roots of C8 and T1. Forceful upward pull of the arm at birth may cause this pattern of damage. Compression of the lower part of the brachial plexus may occur due to space-occupying lesions (such as tumors) and is often due to the presence of a cervical rib. Lower plexus injuries result in paralysis of all the intrinsic hand muscles and weakness of the medial fingers and wrist flexors. Extensors of the forearm may also be weak.

A clawhand deformity is seen with lower plexus injuries, that is, the fourth and fifth digits are hyperextended at the MCP joints and flexed at the IP joints, the first phalanx is hyperextended, and the fifth finger remains abducted. Guttering of the hand may be seen due to atrophy of the intrinsic muscles. Sensation is lost in the region of the ulnar side of the arm, forearm, and hand. Lower plexus lesions are often accompanied by disturbances in the sympathetic nervous system (e.g., Horner's syndrome). Trophic changes in the arm may occur that can include edema and changes in the appearance of the skin and nails.

Brachial Plexus Latency Determinations From Specific Nerve Root Stimulation				
			LATENCY ACROSS PLEXUS (ms)	
PLEXUS	SITE OF STIMULATION	RECORDING SITE	RANGE	MEAN ± SD
Brachial (upper trunk and lateral cord)	C5 and C6	Biceps	4.8 – 6.2	5.3 ± 0.4
Brachial (posterior cord)	C6, C7, C8	Triceps	4.4 – 6.1	5.4 ± 0.4
Brachial (lower trunk and medial cord)	C8, T1, ulnar nerve	Abductor digiti minimi	3.7 – 5.5	4.7 ± 0.5

Adapted from Kimura's modification of MacLean

Nerve Conduction Times From Erb's Point to Muscle

MUSCLE	n*	DISTANCE (cm)	LATENCY (ms)
Biceps	19	20	4.6 ± 0.6
	15	24	4.7 ± 0.6
	14	28	5.0 ± 0.5
Deltoid	20	15.5	4.3 ± 0.5
	17	18.5	4.4 ± 0.4
Triceps	16	21.5	4.5 ± 0.4
	23	26.5	4.9 ± 0.5
	16	31.5	5.3 ± 0.5
Supraspinatus	19	8.5	2.6 ± 0.3
	16	10.5	2.7 ± 0.3
Infraspinatus	20	14	3.4 ± 0.4
	15	17	3.4 ± 0.5

*Number of subjects tested to obtain values.

From Kimura, J: Electrodiagnosis in Diseases of Nerve and Muscle: Principles and Practice. FA Davis, Philadelphia, 1989, p. 119.

LONG THORACIC NERVE, ANTERIOR THORACIC NERVE, LATERAL PECTORAL NERVE, AND THE MEDIAL PECTORAL NERVE

Course and Distribution

(muscles innervated by nerves are listed in italics)

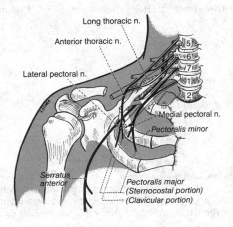

LONG THORACIC NERVE AND ANTERIOR THORACIC NERVES

Nerve

Long thoracic nerve, also called the external respiratory nerve of Bell, nerve to serratus anterior, or posterior thoracic nerve (a term that also includes the dorsal scapular nerve).

Origin: Arises from anterior primary rami of C5, C6, and C7.

Innervates

Motor
Serratus anterior muscle

Cutaneous and joint
None

Common Injuries

Traction: due to the long course of the nerve and because it is held in place by the scaleni and slips of the serratus anterior, it is prone to stretch injuries (e.g., lifting of heavy objects); prolonged compression from lying on the lateral aspect of the trunk can lead to damage.

Surgery: proximity to the axilla makes the nerve vulnerable during various form of surgery (e.g., during breast surgery).

Trauma to the base of the neck: forces exerted to the base of the neck damage the nerve because it is trapped against the lower cervical vertebrae.

Effects of Injuries
Instability of the scapula; winging of the scapula with medial rotation of the lower part of the scapula; shoulder girdle is displaced posteriorly.

Special Tests

During a wall push-up or during protraction of the scapula, look for winging of the scapula; slight winging of the scapula at rest can be noted, and this winging increases with shoulder flexion.

Nerve

Anterior thoracic nerve (gives rise to the medial pectoral nerve and the lateral pectoral nerve).

Origin

The anterior thoracic nerve arises from the proximal portion of the lateral and medial cords of the brachial plexus; the fibers that form the lateral pectoral nerve are from C5, C6, and C7; the fibers that form the medial pectoral nerve are from C8 and T1.

Innervates

Motor

Lateral pectoral nerve: superior and clavicular portions of the pectoralis major muscle. Medial pectoral nerve: pectoralis minor muscle and the inferior part of the sternocostal portion of the pectoralis major muscle.

Cutaneous and Joint

None

Common Injuries

Isolated injuries to these nerves are rare. Fibers that form the nerves may be damaged when there is a nerve root or brachial plexus injury.

Effects of Injuries

Depending on the extent of injury, weakness or paralysis of the pectoral muscles; the shoulder is held slightly posterior and may be elevated or depressed.

Special Tests

When an examiner elevates the patient's shoulders by placing his hands in the axillae, the shoulder of the affected side rises higher than that of the normal side; when the patient flexes both arms to approximately 90°, the affected arm deviates laterally.

DORSAL SCAPULAR NERVE, NERVE TO SUBCLAVIUS, AND SUPRASCAPULAR NERVE

Course and Distribution: Posterior View

(muscles innervated by nerves are listed in italics)

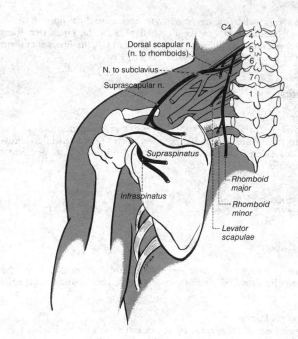

DORSAL SCAPULAR NERVE, NERVE TO SUBCLAVIUS, AND SUPRASCAPULAR NERVE

Nerve

Dorsal scapular nerve (also called posterior scapular nerve or the nerve to the rhomboids).

Origin

Arises from anterior primary rami of C5.

Innervates

Motor
Rhomboid minor and rhomboid major muscles; contributes innervation to the levator scapulae muscle, which also receives innervation from C3 and C4.

Cutaneous and Joint
None

Common Injuries

Injury to the C5 root is more common than injury to the nerve.

Effects of Injuries
Depending on the extent of injury, weakness or paralysis of the rhomboid muscles and paresis of the levator scapulae; the inferior portion of the vertebral border of the scapula wings posteriorly.

Special Tests

When the patient is asked to brace the shoulders (i.e., stand at attention with shoulders square), the scapula of the affected shoulder is obliquely positioned with the upper vertebral border lying medially and the inferior portion lying laterally; damage to the dorsal scapular nerve can be differentiated from injury to the C5 root only by EMG testing, which indicates that the lesion is isolated to the rhomboid muscles and the levator scapulae muscle.

Nerve

Nerve to subclavius (also called subclavian nerve).

Origin

Arises from the upper trunk of the brachial plexus from fibers originating at C5 and C6.

Innervates

Motor
Subclavius muscle

Cutaneous and Joint
None

Common Injuries

Isolated injury to the nerve is uncommon.

Effects of Injuries
Depending on the extent of injury, weakness or paralysis of the subclavius muscle results in slight forward displacement of the lateral end of the clavicle.

Special Tests

None

Nerve

Suprascapular nerve

Origin

Arises from the upper trunk of the brachial plexus from fibers originating at C5 and C6.

Innervates

Motor
Supraspinatus muscle and infraspinatus muscle.

Cutaneous and Joint
No cutaneous distribution; supplies posterior capsule of the gleno-humeral joint.

Common Injuries

Traction and pressure: downward displacement on the shoulder stretches the nerve and can cause injury (e.g., as occurs with Erb's palsy or due to gymnastics).

Trauma: wounds above the scapula will frequently affect the nerve.

Effects of Injuries
Atrophy of the supraspinatus muscle and infraspinatus muscle. There is difficulty initiating abduction and external rotation at the glenohumeral joint. When at rest, the arm may be kept slightly medially rotated.

Special Tests

To test for loss of function of the infraspinatus muscle, test for lateral rotation; EMG testing reveals only denervation of supraspinatus and infraspinatus muscles without any denervation to other muscles innervated by C5 and C6.

THORACODORSAL NERVE AND SUBSCAPULAR NERVES

Course and Distribution

(muscles innervated by nerves are listed in italics)

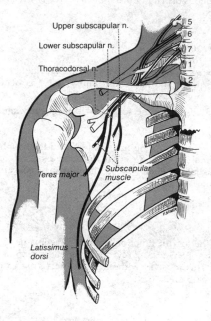

THORACODORSAL NERVE AND SUBSCAPULAR NERVES

Nerve

Thoracodorsal nerve

Origin

Arises from the posterior cord of the brachial plexus from fibers originating at C6, C7, and C8.

Innervates

Motor
Latissimus dorsi muscle

Cutaneous and Joint
None

Common Injuries

Isolated injuries to the nerve are rare; damage is associated with injuries to the posterior cord of the brachial plexus.

Effects of Injuries
Paralysis of the latissimus dorsi muscle that may result in winging of the inferior angle of the scapula and an inability to powerfully extend the arm.

Special Tests

The examiner resists shoulder extension; if the latissimus dorsi muscle is denervated, there is weakness.

Nerve

Subscapular nerves

Origin

The upper (superior) subscapular nerve and the lower (inferior) subscapular nerve arise from the posterior cord of the brachial plexus from fibers originating at C5 and C6 (the upper subscapular nerve is also called the short subscapular nerve).

Innervates

Motor
Upper subscapular nerve innervates the subscapularis muscle; lower subscapular nerve innervates the subscapularis muscle and the teres major muscle.

Cutaneous and Joint
None

Common Injuries

Isolated injuries to the nerves are rare; damage is associated with injuries to the posterior cord of the brachial plexus.

Effects of Injuries
Paralysis of the subscapularis muscle, resulting in weakness of medial rotation. Paralysis of the teres major muscle does not significantly affect function.

Special Tests

The examiner resists medial rotation; there is weakness rather than loss of motion if the nerve is damaged because other medial rotators are still innervated.

AXILLARY NERVE

Course and Distribution: Posterior View

(muscles innervated by nerves are listed in italics)

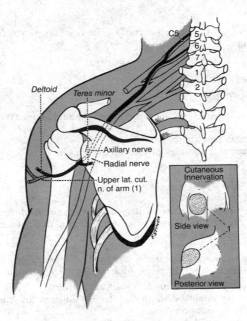

AXILLARY NERVE

Nerve

Axillary nerve (also called circumflex nerve)

Origin

Arises from the posterior cord of the brachial plexus from fibers originating at C5 and C6.

Innervates

Motor
Deltoid muscle (all three parts) and the teres minor muscle.

Cutaneous and Joint
Cutaneous in the area of the deltoid muscle.

Common Injuries

Fractures: because the axillary nerve wraps around the proximal humerus, any fracture in the region of the surgical neck of the humerus may be accompanied by an axillary nerve lesion.

Dislocations: movement of the humerus after a dislocation at the glenohumeral joint may result in an axillary nerve lesion.

Forceful hyperextension of the shoulder: with hyperextension of the shoulder (as might occur during a wrestling match), the axillary nerve may be compromised.

Inappropriate use of crutches: pressure on the axillary region due to leaning on crutches can cause a compression injury to the axillary nerve.

Other Trauma: contusions in the shoulder region or injuries to the scapula may be accompanied by axillary nerve lesions. Because the nerve passes between the coracoid process of the scapula and the humerus, compression of these structures often results in an entrapment syndrome.

Effects of Injuries
Paralysis of the deltoid muscle with resultant atrophy causes a change in the contour of the shoulder; the shoulder becomes flattened and loses its normal rounded shape. There is a decreased ability to

abduct, flex, and extend the arm at the glenohumeral joint. Paralysis of the teres minor muscle does not significantly affect function.

Special Tests

Muscle testing of the deltoid muscle, especially in the fully abducted position, reveals severe weakness. Confirmation of denervation of the teres minor muscle can be determined only through EMG because the infraspinatus muscle is also an external rotator of the arm.

MUSCULOCUTANEOUS NERVE

Course and Distribution

(muscles innervated by nerves are listed in italics)

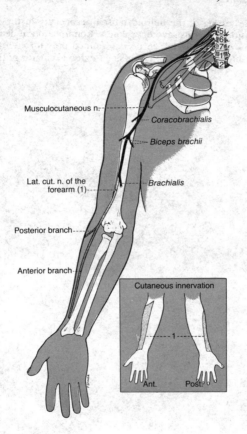

Musculocutaneous n.

Coracobrachialis

Biceps brachii

Brachialis

Lat. cut. n. of the forearm (1)

Posterior branch

Anterior branch

Cutaneous innervation

1

Ant.   Post.

MUSCULOCUTANEOUS NERVE

Nerve

Musculocutaneous nerve

Origin

Arises from the lateral cord of the brachial plexus from fibers originating at C5, C6, and C7.

Innervates

Motor
Coracobrachialis muscle, biceps brachii muscle, and most of the brachialis muscle

Cutaneous and Joint
In the forearm, the musculocutaneous nerve gives rise to the lateral cutaneous nerve of the forearm that innervates the lateral forearm; the cutaneous division is also called the lateral antebrachial cutaneous nerve.

Common Injuries

Fractures or dislocations of the humerus can lead to lesions of the musculocutaneous nerve, as can open wounds (e.g., stab wounds). The nerve can also be entrapped by the coracobrachialis muscle or injured during surgery.

Effects of Injuries
Paralysis of the biceps brachii muscle and the brachialis muscle results in weak elbow flexion. The loss of the biceps is especially noticeable when elbow flexion is attempted with the forearm supinated. Weakness in supination occurs. Paralysis of the coracobrachialis muscle does not significantly affect function.

Special Tests

Test for the biceps brachii stretch reflex; extreme weakness when the elbow flexors are muscle-tested with the forearm fully supinated; weakness when muscle-testing for supination. Although EMG testing of the biceps brachii muscle, brachialis muscle, and the coracobrachialis muscle can show denervation, to determine specific nerve damage this should be accompanied by findings of impaired nerve conduction velocities.

MUSCULOCUTANEOUS NERVE

Values for Electrodiagnostic Testing*

AGE (years)	MOTOR NERVE CONDUCTION BETWEEN ERB'S POINT AND AXILLA				ORTHODROMIC SENSORY NERVE CONDUCTION BETWEEN ERB'S POINT AND AXILLA			ORTHODROMIC SENSORY NERVE CONDUCTION BETWEEN AXILLA AND ELBOW		
	n†	RANGE OF CONDUCTION VELOCITIES (m/s)	RANGE OF AMPLITUDES (µV) AXILLA	RANGE OF AMPLITUDES (µV) ERB'S POINT	n†	RANGE OF CONDUCTION VELOCITIES (m/s)	RANGE OF AMPLITUDES (µV)	n	RANGE OF CONDUCTION VELOCITIES (m/s)	RANGE OF AMPLITUDE (µV)
15–24	14	63–78	9–32	7–27	14	59–76	3.5–30	15	61–75	17–75
25–34	6	60–75	8–30	6–26	6	57–74	3–25	8	59–73	16–72
35–44	8	58–73	8–28	6–24	7	54–71	2.5–21	8	57–71	16–69
45–54	10	55–71	7–26	6–22	10	52–69	2–18	13	55–69	15–65
55–64	9	53–68	7–24	5–21	9	49–66	2–15	10	53–67	14–62
65–74	4	50–66	6–22	5–19	4	47–64	1.5–12	6	51–65	13–59

*From Trojaborg with permission.
†Number of subjects tested to obtain values in the table.

LATERAL AND MEDIAL CUTANEOUS NERVES

Values for Electrodiagnostic Testing

NERVE	NUMBER OF PATIENTS SEEN	AGE (years) (MEAN)	DISTANCE (cm)	LATENCY ONSET (ms)	LATENCY PEAK (ms)	CONDUCTION VELOCITY (m/s)	AMPLITUDE (μV)
Lateral cutaneous nerve	30	20–84 (35)	12	1.8 ± 0.1	2.3 ± 0.1	65 ± 4	24.0 ± 7.2
Lateral cutaneous nerve	154	17–80 (45)	14		2.8 ± 0.2	62 ± 4	18.9 ± 9.9
Medial cutaneous nerve	155	17–80 (45)	14		2.7 ± 0.2	63 ± 5	11.4 ± 5.2
Medial cutaneous nerve	30	23–60 (38)	18	2.7 ± 0.2	3.3 ± 0.2	66 ± 4	15.4 ± 4.1

(Adapted from Kimura, J: Electrodiagnosis in Diseases of Nerve and Muscle: Principles and Practice, ed 2. FA Davis, Philadelphia, 1989, p. 122.)

271

Course and Distribution

(muscles innervated by nerves are listed in italics)

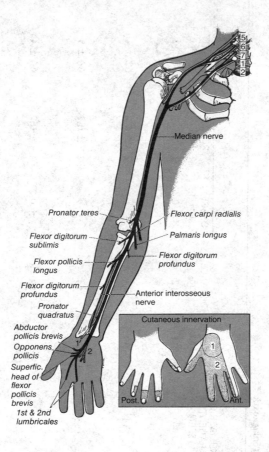

Median nerve

Pronator teres

Flexor digitorum sublimis

Flexor pollicis longus

Flexor digitorum profundus

Pronator quadratus

Abductor pollicis brevis

Opponens pollicis

Superfic. head of flexor pollicis brevis

1st & 2nd lumbricales

Flexor carpi radialis

Palmaris longus

Flexor digitorum profundus

Anterior interosseous nerve

Cutaneous innervation

Post.   Ant.

MEDIAN NERVE

Nerve

Median nerve

Origin

Portions of the medial and lateral cords of the brachial plexus join together to form the median nerve. These fibers, which originated at C6, C7, C8, and T1, pass through the anterior divisions of the upper, middle, and lower trunks of the brachial plexus. Sometimes fibers from C5 also are part of the median nerve.

Innervates

Motor

Supplies all the muscles in the anterior aspect of the forearm with the exception of the flexor carpi ulnaris muscle and the medial half of the flexor digitorum profundus muscle; the main trunk of the nerve supplies the pronator teres, flexor carpi radialis, palmaris longus, and the flexor digitorum superficialis muscles; the anterior osseous nerve (a pure motor nerve) innervates the flexor pollicis longus, the lateral half of the flexor digitorum profundus, and the pronator quadratus muscle before passing through the carpal tunnel to innervate lumbricals one and two; at the level of the distal carpal ligament, a recurrent (muscular) thenar branch is given off to innervate the abductor pollicis brevis, the lateral half of the flexor pollicis brevis, and the opponens pollicis muscle.

Cutaneous and Joint

Supplies the skin over the lateral (radial) side of the palm and the palmar and dorsal (terminal parts) aspects of the lateral three-and-a-half digits.

Common Injuries

Entrapment syndromes: the median nerve can be entrapped at many points as it courses down the arm; often entrapment of the median nerve is also accompanied by entrapment of the ulnar nerve (see ulnar nerve).

Thoracic outlet syndrome: due to either the scalenus-anticus syndrome, the presence of a cervical rib, or some other narrowing of the thoracic outlet where the median nerve can be compressed near its proximal origin.

Ligament of Struther's syndrome (supracondylar process syndrome): due to the presence of an anomalous ligament that forms a fibrous tunnel near the medial condyle of humerus, the median nerve can be compressed.

Pronator teres syndrome: the median nerve can be compressed as it passes between the deep and superficial heads of the pronator teres muscle. Trauma, fracture of the humerus, and hypertrophy of the pronator teres muscle can cause the entrapment; repetitive motion of the limb with the forearm in pronation and the fingers flexed (e.g., using a screwdriver) can also result in compression. An anomalous fibrous band connecting the pronator teres muscle to the flexor digitorum superficialis muscle can also compress the median nerve; compression may also occur if the nerve has an anomalous path that takes it behind both heads of the pronator teres muscle.

Anterior interosseous syndrome: as the median nerve gives rise to the anterior interosseous nerve (just below the level of the radial tuberosity), it can be compressed by several different anomalous structures, including fibrous sheaths, and the tendinous origin of the long flexors. Thrombosis of the vessels that are in close proximity with the nerve can cause entrapment, as can the presence of an accessory head of the flexor pollicis longus muscle. Forearm fractures and supracondylar fractures in children may also result in compression.

Carpal tunnel syndrome: as the median nerve enters the hand, it runs beneath a wide, fibrous ligamentous band which forms the *carpal tunnel*; this is a common site of median nerve compression. In women the syndrome may, in some cases, be caused by hormonal factors that occur with pregnancy or during the menstrual cycle; in addition, hypothyroidism has been thought to cause the syndrome. Inflammatory events that occur with tenosynovitis of the flexor tendons, rheumatoid arthritis, or overuse syndromes may also cause compression at the carpal tunnel. Moreover, congenital bony deformities, deformities secondary to fractures, or acromegaly may also cause the syndrome.

Digital nerve entrapment syndrome: the interdigital nerve that supplies the skin of the second and third digits and half of the fourth digit may be compressed against the edge of the deep transverse metacarpal ligament. This syndrome appears to be caused by trauma (such as phalangeal fractures), tumors, or inflammation of the MCP joints.

Trauma

In addition to causing compression syndromes, trauma may lead to direct injuries to the median nerve.

Humeral fractures: may lead to disruption of the median nerve above the elbow. This is especially true of supracondylar fractures.

Lacerations of the wrist: the superficial course of the median nerve at the wrist makes it vulnerable to damage from accidental lacerations (that occur with falls on sharp objects) or lacerations associated with suicide attempts.

Carpal bone injuries: because the median nerve courses directly over the carpal bones, trauma to these bones often results in damage to the nerve. This damage may occur with fractures or dislocations or from direct trauma at the time the carpal bone was injured.

Effects of Injuries

The deficits associated with damage to the median nerve depend on the severity of the injury and the site of the lesion. To determine specific deficits for each syndrome and type of injury, the course of the nerve must be considered and the resultant loss of motor and sensory function distal to the site determined (see the listing of peripheral nerve entrapment syndromes for descriptions of the symptoms of some of the more common syndromes). Pain is a common feature of the entrapment syndromes; however, sensory effects can also include hypesthesia, paresthesia, and even complete sensory loss.

General Motor Defects With Median Nerve Lesions

Loss of opposition of the thumb, loss of ability to make a fist, and atrophy of the thenar eminence.

Common deformities seen with median nerve lesions:

Simian (ape) hand: occurs due to denervation and resultant atrophy of muscles in the thenar eminence. Opposition is lost. As a result of the atrophy and paralysis, the hand flattens.

Benediction sign: occurs because of paralysis to the flexors of the middle and ring fingers. When a person with a median nerve injury attempts to make a fist, these fingers do not fully flex, and they remain in a position similar to that used when clergy make a benediction.

Special Tests

Depending on the severity and site of the lesion, many different tests can be used to ascertain median nerve damage. General muscle and sensory testing can be used to indicate the level of the lesion by determining which portion of the nerve is damaged.

Motor

If, as part of general paralysis or weakness of all muscles innervated by the median nerve, muscles above the elbow are affected (e.g., flexor carpi radialis muscle and other long flexors), the main portion of the nerve must be injured; if the long flexors (those muscles first innervated by the nerve) are spared but there is isolated paralysis of the flexor pollicis longus muscle, the lateral half of the flexor digitorum profundus muscle, and the pronator quadratus muscle, damage to the anterior interosseous nerve is indicated; if paralysis or paresis is isolated to the abductor pollicis brevis, lateral half of the flexor pollicis brevis, and the opponens pollicis muscles, then damage to the thenar branch is indicated.

Cutaneous and Joint

Total sensory loss of the tip of the index finger and decreased sensation on the lateral (radial) side of the palm and the lateral three-and-a-half digits over their palmar aspects indicates interruption of the nerve at a level above the lower third of the forearm; lesions distal to the origin of the palmar cutaneous branch (which arises proximal to the level of the wrist) result in preserved sensation of the more proximal portions of the dorsal surface of the hand, but loss of sensation in the most distal distribution of the median nerve (e.g., loss of sensation in the distal portion of the second and third fingers and some loss in the distal fourth finger).

Specific Tests

Adson's maneuver (test for thoracic outlet syndrome): the patient turns the head to the side of the suspected lesion, extends the neck fully, and takes and holds a deep breath while the examiner checks for a decreased radial pulse (in some patients the effect may be more noticeable if the patient turns the head away from the side of the suspected lesion); if the thoracic outlet is compromised, this maneuver further narrows the outlet and indicates whether the median nerve is likely to be compressed at this level.

Tests for compression by ligament of Struther's (supracondylar process syndrome): an examiner checks for decrease or absence of radial and/or ulnar pulses when the forearm is fully extended and supinated; the presence of weakness and EMG abnormalities of the pronator teres muscle indicates possible compression due to a ligament of Struthers (this muscle is usually not affected by the pronator teres syndrome); nerve conduction testing can also be used to determine blockage across the antecubital fossa.

Tests for pronator teres syndrome: test for a pattern of weakness in the flexor carpi radialis muscle, flexor digitorum superficialis muscle, thenar muscles, and lumbricals one and two. Nerve conduction velocity testing indicates a slowing of velocity across the elbow, and there will be a diminished evoked response (see test for ligament of Struthers). The EMG shows denervation in affected muscles. Electrodiagnostic testing for pronator teres syndrome is usually not considered positive based on findings of abnormalities in the pronator teres because this muscle is usually spared in this syndrome. Phalen's sign and testing for normal conduction latencies are used to rule out carpal tunnel syndrome (see appropriate tests).

Tests for anterior interosseous syndrome: the patient is asked to make an "OK" sign (an *O* between the thumb and index finger) using the first two digits. The shape is observed. If there is damage to the interosseous nerve, a triangle (the "pinch sign") rather than a circle will be formed. Routine nerve conduction studies of the median nerve are normal with this syndrome, but slowed conduction velocities of the anterior interosseous nerve may be discerned by recording compound muscle action potentials from the pronator quadratus muscle after stimulation of the nerve at the elbow; EMG shows denervation in the flexor pollicis longus, flexor digitorum profundus (first and second fingers), and pronator quadratus muscles.

Tests for carpal tunnel syndrome: the examiner taps the patient's wrist over the carpal tunnel; if pain is felt in the cutaneous distribution of the median nerve (Tinel's sign), carpal tunnel syndrome is likely. The examiner can use Phalen's test by forcefully flexing the patient's wrist and holding it in that position for a minute; in this way the carpal tunnel is compressed and pain in the distribution of the median nerve is felt if carpal tunnel syndrome is present. In carpal tunnel syndrome, conduction abnormalities of sensory and motor fibers are usually seen in the wrist-to-palm segment of the median nerve with the distal segment of the nerve remaining relatively normal; EMG may be normal, or, in severe cases, signs of denervation may be seen in the median nerve – innervated lumbricals.

Observable signs: look for the benediction sign or the appearance of a simian hand.

MEDIAN NERVE

Values for Electrodiagnostic Testing*

SITE OF STIMULATION	AMPLITUDE† MOTOR (mV) SENSORY (µV)	LATENCY‡ TO RECORDING SITE (ms)	DIFFERENCE BETWEEN RIGHT AND LEFT (ms)	CONDUCTION TIME BETWEEN TWO POINTS (ms)	CONDUCTION VELOCITY (m/s)
Motor fibers					
Palm	6.9 ± 3.2 (3.5)§	1.86 ± 0.28 (2.4)¶	0.19 ± 0.17 (0.5)¶	1.65 ± 0.25 (2.2)¶	48.8 ± 5.3 (38)**
Wrist	7.0 ± 3.0 (3.5)	3.49 ± 0.34 (4.2)	0.24 ± 0.22 (0.7)	3.92 ± 0.49 (4.9)	57.7 ± 4.9 (48)
Elbow	7.0 ± 2.7 (3.5)	7.39 ± 0.69 (8.8)	0.31 ± 0.24 (0.8)	2.42 ± 0.39 (3.2)	63.5 ± 6.2 (51)
Axilla	7.2 ± 2.9 (3.5)	9.81 ± 0.89 (11.6)	0.42 ± 0.33 (1.1)		

Sensory fibers Digit				
Palm	39.0 ± 16.8 (20)	1.37 ± 0.24 (1.9)	0.15 ± 0.11 (0.4)	1.37 ± 0.24 (1.9)	58.8 ± 5.8 (47)
Wrist	38.5 ± 15.6 (19)	2.84 ± 0.34 (3.5)	0.18 ± 0.14 (0.5)	1.48 ± 0.18 (1.8)	56.2 ± 5.8 (44)
Elbow	32.0 ± 15.5 (16)	6.46 ± 0.71 (7.9)	0.29 ± 0.21 (0.7)	3.61 ± 0.48 (4.6)	61.9 ± 4.2 (53)

*Mean ± standard deviation (SD) in 122 nerves from 61 patients, 11 to 74 years of age (average, 40), with no apparent disease of the peripheral nerves.

†Amplitude of the evoked response, measured from the baseline to the negative peak.

‡Latency, measured to the onset of the evoked response, with the cathode at the origin of the thenar nerve in the palm.

§Lower limits of normal, based on the distribution of the normative data.

¶Upper limits of normal, calculated as the mean + 2 SD.

**Lower limits of normal, calculated as the mean − 2 SD.

(Adapted from Kimura, J: Electrodiagnosis in Diseases of Nerve and Muscle: Principles and Practice, ed. 2. FA Davis; Philadelphia, 1989, p. 107.)

ULNAR NERVE

Course and Distribution

(muscles innervated by nerves are listed in italics)

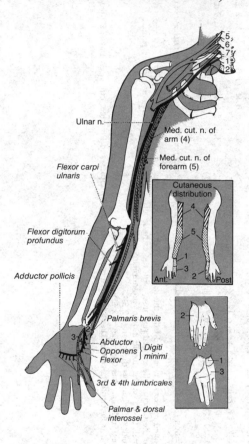

ULNAR NERVE

Nerve

Ulnar nerve

Origin

The medial cord of the brachial plexus gives rise to the ulnar nerve. Fibers originate in C8 and T1 and pass through the lower trunk of the brachial plexus and the anterior division before joining the medial cord.

Innervates

Motor
In the upper arm a branch of the ulnar nerve supplies the flexor carpi ulnaris muscle and the medial half of the flexor digitorum profundus muscle; in the hand a superficial branch is given off to supply the palmaris brevis muscle, while a deep branch innervates the hypothenar muscles, the opponens digiti minimi, abductor digiti minimi, and flexor digiti minimi muscles; after supplying innervation to the hypothenar muscles, the deep branch supplies interossei, third and fourth lumbricals, adductor pollicis muscle, and the deep head (or medial half) of the flexor pollicis brevis muscle.

Cutaneous and Joint
An articular branch is given off in the elbow region, where it innervates that joint; the dorsal branch (a pure cutaneous nerve) is given off in the forearm and continues down the forearm, winding around the ulna to supply the skin over the dorsal aspect of the hand and dorsal aspects of the medial one-and-a-half fingers (half of the fourth and all of the fifth digit); a superficial branch arises near the pisiform bone to innervate the volar aspects of the medial one and half fingers (half of the fourth and all of the fifth digit); a palmar branch also arises near the wrist to innervate the proximal hypothenar region.

Common injuries

Entrapment syndromes and mononeuropathies: the ulnar nerve can be entrapped and damaged at many points as it courses down the arm. Often entrapment of the ulnar nerve is also accompanied by entrapment of the median nerve (see median nerve).

Thoracic outlet syndrome: the ulnar nerve, like the median nerve, may be compressed at the thoracic outlet (see thoracic outlet syndrome described under the median nerve).

Inappropriate use of crutches: pressure on the axillary region, due to a patient leaning on crutches, can cause a compression injury to the ulnar nerve.

Tardy ulnar palsy and cubital tunnel syndrome: the term *tardy ulnar palsy* was once reserved for damage to the ulnar nerve secondary to trauma in the elbow region; now, however, the term is used to describe entrapment at the elbow due to traumatic and nontraumatic causes. This syndrome may occur in association with thoracic outlet syndrome (see thoracic outlet syndrome). The most common entrapment at the elbow is in the cubital tunnel, where the nerve is large and underlies the aponeurotic band between the two heads of the flexor carpi ulnaris muscle. Joint deformities, repetitive motion at the elbow, and inflammatory conditions may all cause entrapment at the tunnel, and trauma to the elbow is known to lead to ulnar nerve damage.

Anomalous anatomical features at the elbow: a ligament of Struthers, if present, may cause compression of the ulnar nerve similar to the way such a ligament affects the median nerve (see ligament of Struthers syndrome under the median nerve). The presence of an anomalous anconeus muscle (an epitrochleoanconeus muscle) can compress the ulnar nerve near the elbow; a hypertrophied flexor carpi ulnaris muscle may also press on the ulnar nerve.

Compression at Guyon's canal (ulnar tunnel): the ulnar nerve can be entrapped as it crosses from the forearm into the hand through Guyon's canal (the ulnar tunnel). The tunnel is formed by the pisohamate ligament superficially, and the base of the tunnel is formed by the pisiform and the hamate bones; space-occupying lesions within the tunnel of the type that can occur with rheumatoid arthritis and ganglia can cause damage to the ulnar nerve. Persons who engage in activities that can traumatize the hypothenar region (e.g., persons who engage in karate or who have jobs requiring them to use the hypothenar portion of their hands to press or bang) are also at risk.

Bicycle rider's syndrome: prolonged bicycle riding causes compression of the ulnar nerve in the hypothenar region; a similar compression injury may occur from pressing the hypothenar region on a crutch.

Digital nerve entrapment syndrome: the digital nerves that supply the skin of the fifth digits and half of the fourth digit may be compressed against the edge of the deep transverse metacarpal ligament; this syndrome appears to be caused by trauma (such as phalangeal fractures), tumors, or inflammation of the MCP joints.

Effects of Injuries

The deficits associated with damage to the ulnar nerve depend on the severity of the injury to the nerve and the site of the lesion; to determine specific deficits for each syndrome and type of injury, the course of the nerve must be considered and the resultant loss of motor and sensory function distal to the site determined (see the listing of peripheral nerve entrapment syndromes for descriptions of the symptoms of some of the more common syndromes). Pain is a common feature of the entrapment syndromes; however, sensory effects can also include hypesthesia, paresthesia, and even complete sensory loss.

Motor deficits at the hand: clawhand occurs with lesions to the ulnar nerve because of the unopposed action of the radial nerve–innervated extensor digitorum communis muscle in the fourth and fifth digits. The first phalanx is hyperextended and the distal two phalanges are flexed while the fifth finger remains abducted; there is an inability to abduct or adduct the fingers because of a loss of the interossei muscles; flexion at the DIP joints of the fourth and fifth digit is lost because of denervation of the medial half of the flexor digitorum profundus muscle; denervation of the adductor pollicis muscle results in weakened opposition of the thumb, and there is also a total loss of opposition by the fifth finger and an inability to abduct the little finger.

Motor deficits at the wrist: resisted palmar flexion of the wrist results in deviation of the wrist to the radial side because of denervation the flexor carpi ulnaris muscle.

Special Tests

Adson's maneuver (test for thoracic outlet syndrome): the patient turns head to the side of the suspected lesion, extends neck fully, and takes and holds a deep breath while the examiner checks for a decreased radial pulse (in some patients the effect may be more noticeable if the patient turns head away from the side of the suspected lesion). If the thoracic outlet is compromised, this maneuver further narrows the outlet and indicates whether the ulnar nerve is likely to be compressed at this level.

Tests for compression by ligament of Struthers (supracondylar process syndrome): the examiner checks for decrease or absence of radial and/or ulnar pulses when the forearm is fully extended and supinated.

Froment's sign: the patient is asked to grasp a piece of paper between thumb and index finger; because of paralysis of the adductor pollicis muscle, the patient flexes the thumb. This flexion becomes more pronounced when the examiner pulls the paper away.

Observable signs: guttering occurs between the fingers because of atrophy of the intrinsic muscles. There is flattening of the hypothenar eminence due to atrophy of the palmaris brevis muscle and the muscles of the fifth digit.

ULNAR NERVE

Values for Electrodiagnostic Testing*

SITE OF STIMULATION	AMPLITUDE†: MOTOR (mV) SENSORY (µV)	LATENCY‡ TO RECORDING SITE (ms)	DIFFERENCE BETWEEN RIGHT AND LEFT (ms)	CONDUCTION TIME BETWEEN TWO POINTS (ms)	CONDUCTION VELOCITY (m/s)
Motor Fibers					
Wrist	5.7 ± 2.0 (2.8)§	2.59 ± 0.39 (3.4)¶	0.28 ± 0.27 (0.8)¶	3.51 ± 0.51 (4.5)¶	58.7 ± 5.1 (49)**
Below elbow	5.5 ± 2.0 (2.7)	6.10 ± 0.69 (7.5)	0.29 ± 0.27 (0.8)	1.94 ± 0.37 (2.7)	61.0 ± 5.5 (50)
Above elbow	5.5 ± 1.9 (2.7)	8.04 ± 0.76 (9.6)	0.34 ± 0.28 (0.9)	1.88 ± 0.35 (2.6)	66.5 ± 6.3 (54)
Axilla	5.6 ± 2.1 (2.7)	9.90 ± 0.91 (11.7)	0.45 ± 0.39 (1.2)		

Sensory Fibers

Digit

Wrist	35.0 ± 14.7 (18)	2.54 ± 0.29 (3.1)	0.18 ± 0.13 (0.4)	2.54 ± 0.29 (3.1)	54.8 ± 5.3 (44)
Below elbow	28.8 ± 12.2 (15)	5.67 ± 0.59 (6.9)	0.26 ± 0.21 (0.5)	3.22 ± 0.42 (4.1)	64.7 ± 5.4 (53)
Above elbow	28.3 ± 11.8 (14)	7.46 ± 0.64 (8.7)	0.28 ± 0.27 (0.8)	1.79 ± 0.30 (2.4)	66.7 ± 6.4 (54)

*Mean ± standard deviation (SD) in 130 nerves from 65 patients, 13 to 74 years of age (average, 39), with no apparent disease of the peripheral nerves.

†Amplitude of the evoked response, measured from the baseline to the negative peak.

‡Latency, measured to the onset of the evoked response, with the cathode 3 cm above the distal crease in the wrist.

§Slower limits of normal, based on the distribution of the normative data.

¶Upper limits of normal, calculated as the mean + 2 SD.

**Lower limits of normal, calculated as the mean − 2 SD.

(Adapted from Kimura, J: Electrodiagnosis in Diseases of Nerve and Muscle: Principles and Practice, ed. 2. FA Davis, Philadelphia, 1989, p. 114.)

Course and Distribution

(muscle innervated by nerves are listed in italics)

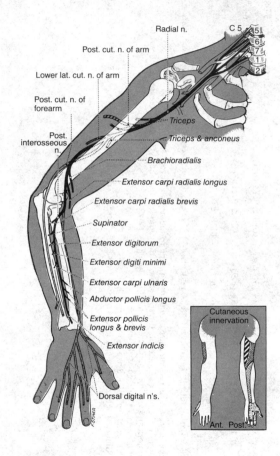

Radial n.

Post. cut. n. of arm

Lower lat. cut. n. of arm

Post. cut. n. of forearm

Post. interosseous n.

C 5

Triceps

Triceps & anconeus

Brachioradialis

Extensor carpi radialis longus

Extensor carpi radialis brevis

Supinator

Extensor digitorum

Extensor digiti minimi

Extensor carpi ulnaris

Abductor pollicis longus

Extensor pollicis longus & brevis

Extensor indicis

Dorsal digital n's.

Cutaneous innervation

Ant. Post.

RADIAL NERVE

Nerve

Radial nerve

Origin

The radial nerve arises from the posterior cord of the brachial plexus. Fibers originating in C5, C6, C7, C8, and T1 pass through the posterior divisions of the upper, middle, and lower trunks to contribute to the radial nerve.

Innervates

Motor

After traveling in the posterior compartment of the arm, the radial nerve travels in the cubital fossa anterior to the lateral epicondyle of the humerus; at this point it gives rise to lateral muscular branches that innervate the brachioradialis, and the extensor carpi radialis longus muscles; a deep branch (posterior interosseous nerve) continues on to innervate the triceps, anconeus, extensor carpi radialis brevis, supinator, extensor digitorum, extensor digiti minimi, extensor carpi ulnaris, abductor pollicis longus, extensor pollicis longus, extensor pollicis brevis, and extensor indicis muscles.

Cutaneous and Joint

After leaving the brachial plexus, the radial nerve courses deep to the axillary artery and winds around the upper arm in the spiral groove, where it gives off the posterior (antebrachial) cutaneous nerve, which innervates the medial posterior portion of the arm; a lower lateral cutaneous nerve innervates the medial portion of the arm on the anterior and posterior surfaces; the radial nerve continues on in the arm and at the level of the epicondyle gives off the superficial radial nerve (a sensory nerve), which supplies the dorsum of the hand on the radial side via dorsal digital nerves; the posterior interosseous nerve innervates joint structures of the wrist and the carpal bones

Common Injuries

Entrapment syndromes and mononeuropathies: the radial nerve is especially vulnerable to compression because of its location in the brachial plexus and its proximity to the humerus.

Saturday night palsies: pressure on the nerve at the spiral groove causes damage to the radial nerve; when a person is drunk and falls asleep with an arm against a hard object, this is called *Saturday night palsy;* the result is denervation of all muscles innervated by the radial nerve except the triceps muscle.

Inappropriate use of crutches: pressure on the nerve at the spiral groove causes damage to the radial nerve. This may occur when patients lean on their crutches.

Sequelae to fractures: during the repair of humeral fractures, newly formed callus may compress the radial nerve.

Compression at the arcade of Frohse (posterior interosseous nerve entrapment): the posterior interosseous branch of the radial nerve passes through a fibrous arch (the arcade of Frohse) at the level of the supinator muscle, and it may be compressed at this site.

Tennis elbow: compression of a branch of the radial nerve at the lateral epicondyle of the humerus may give rise to pain at the elbow. This form of tennis elbow may also involve entrapment of the deep branch of the nerve.

Trauma

Because the radial nerve runs superficially during part of its course and because it lies against the rigid spiral groove of the humerus, the nerve is very vulnerable to trauma. Shoulder dislocations, humeral fractures, and radial neck fractures can all cause damage to the radial nerve. The location of the radial nerve also makes it highly vulnerable to gunshot and stab wounds.

Effects of Injuries

The deficits associated with damage to the radial nerve depend on the severity of the injury to the nerve and the site of the lesion; to determine specific deficits for each syndrome and type of injury, the course of the nerve must be considered and the resultant loss of motor and sensory function distal to the site determined.

General motor defects with radial nerve lesions: a lesion of the radial nerve above the innervation of the triceps muscle is possible, but quite rare; most lesions to the radial nerve affect all muscles innervated by the radial nerve except the triceps. The general findings with such lesions are an inability to extend at the MCP joints, the wrist, and the thumb (tenodesis action may allow passive extension); inability to supinate unless the biceps muscle is used; weakness in palmar abduction of the thumb, although opposition is preserved; and paralysis of the brachioradialis muscle resulting in weakness of elbow flexors.

Special Tests

Palm-to-palm test (wrist drop): when separating hands that have been placed palm to palm, the hand of the affected side drops at the wrist. Wrist drop during functional activities is also an observable sign of radial nerve injury.

Impaired gripping: patients have trouble gripping objects because of their inability to extend their wrists.

RADIAL NERVE

Values for Electrodiagnostic Testing*

CONDUCTION	n†	CONDUCTION VELOCITY (m/s) OR CONDUCTION TIME (ms)	AMPLITUDE: MOTOR (mV) SENSORY (µV)	DISTANCE (cm)
Motor				
Axilla–elbow	8	69 ± 5.6	11 ± 7.0	15.7 ± 3.3
Elbow–forearm	10	62 ± 5.1	13 ± 8.2	18.1 ± 1.5
Forearm–muscle	10	2.4 ± 0.5	14 ± 8.8	6.2 ± 0.9
Sensory				
Axilla–elbow	16	71 ± 5.2	4 ± 1.4	18.0 ± 0.7
Elbow–wrist	20	69 ± 5.7	5 ± 2.6	20.0 ± 0.5
Wrist–thumb	23	58 ± 6.0	13 ± 7.5	13.8 ± 0.4

*(Adapted from Trojaborg, W and Sindrup, EH: Motor and sensory conduction in different segments of the radial nerve in normal subjects. J Neurol Neurosurg Psychiatry 32:354–359, 1969.)
†Number of subjects tested to obtain values in the table.

LUMBAR PLEXUS

The lumbar plexus is formed from the anterior primary rami of L1, L2, and L3, with a contribution from L4. There is often a contribution from T12 (the subcostal nerve). The lower part of the plexus gives off the lumbosacral trunk, which contributes to the sacral plexus.

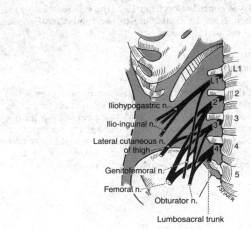

LUMBAR PLEXUS

Anatomy

The lumbar plexus lies within the psoas major muscle and is composed of the anterior primary rami of L1, L2, and L3, with a contribution from L4. A contribution from T12 (the subcostal nerve) is quite common. Fibers from L4 contribute to the lumbosacral trunk, which forms part of the sacral plexus.

Injuries to the Lumbar Plexus

True lesions of the lumbar plexus are rare because the plexus lies deep within the abdomen. Damage to the plexus is often accompanied by fatal injuries. Fractures, dislocations, and space-occupying lesions (such as tumors), however, may occasionally damage the plexus. Stereotypical patterns of damage to the lumbar plexus are essentially non-existent, although structures giving rise to the plexus may be associated with cauda equina lesions or spinal cord injuries.

Lumbar Plexus Latency Determinations from Specific Nerve Root Stimulation*

PLEXUS	SITE OF STIMULATION	RECORDING SITE	LATENCY ACROSS PLEXUS (ms)	
			RANGE	MEAN ± SD
Lumbar	L2 to L4 Femoral nerve	Vastus medialis	2.0–4.4	3.4 ± 0.6

*Adapted from MacLean, IC: Nerve root stimulation to evaluate conduction across the brachial and lumbosacral plexuses. Third Annual Continuing Education Course, American Association of Electromyography and Electrodiagnosis, September 25, 1980, Philadelphia.

ILIO-INGUINAL NERVE AND GENITOFEMORAL NERVE

Course and Distribution

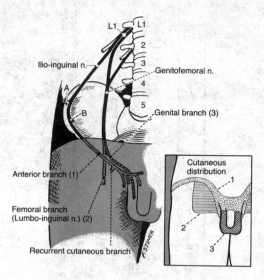

ILIO-INGUINAL AND
GENITOFEMORAL NERVES

Nerve

Ilio-inguinal nerve

Origin

The ilio-inguinal nerve is formed by fibers from L1, L2, L3, and L4. Although it is part of the lumbar plexus, it is functionally similar to thoracic nerve because it innervates a segmental region.

Innervates

Motor
The nerve gives off segmental innervation to the obliquus internus abdominis and the transversus abdominis muscles.

Cutaneous and Joint
A cutaneous branch arises in the medial portion of the inguinal canal; an anterior branch innervates the anterior abdominal wall that overlies the pubic symphysis, the base and dorsum of the penis and the upper part of the scrotum in the male or the mons pubis and the labium majus in the female, and the thigh medial to the femoral triangle; a lateral recurrent branch innervates the skin over the thigh adjacent to the inguinal ligament.

Common Injuries

The nerve is rarely damaged; however, if it is injured, the deficit is manifest in a segmental pattern of loss. Damage may occur during surgery.

Effects of Injuries
Segmental deficits are of little clinical importance; however, some patients with ilio-inguinal neuropathies report pain in the groin, especially when they stand.

Special Tests

If an examininer applies pressure just medial to the ASIS and causes pain to radiate into the crural region, there is evidence of an ilioinguinal neuropathy.

Nerve

Genitofemoral (genitocrural) nerve

Origin

Fibers from the roots of L1 and L2 unite to form the genitofemoral nerve. The nerve branches to form the lumboinguinal (femoral) branch and genital (external spermatic) branch.

Innervates

Motor
The genital (external spermatic) nerve innervates the cremasteric muscle.

Cutaneous and Joint
The genital (external spermatic) nerve innervates the skin of the inner aspect of the upper thigh and in males the scrotum and in females the labium; the lumboinguinal (femoral branch) nerve innervates the skin over the femoral triangle.

Common Injuries

Trauma to the groin may result in injury to the genitofemoral nerve; the nerve is sometimes injured during surgery or damaged by adhesions following surgery.

Effects of Injuries
With lesions pain may be felt in the inguinal region; there is a loss of sensation over the femoral triangle, and in males the cremasteric reflex is absent.

Special Tests

To test the nerve in males, the examiner strokes the inner aspect of the thigh, and the testicle elevates if the genitofemoral nerve is intact.

LATERAL CUTANEOUS NERVE OF THE THIGH AND THE OBTURATOR NERVE

Course and Distribution

(muscles innervated by nerves are listed in italics)

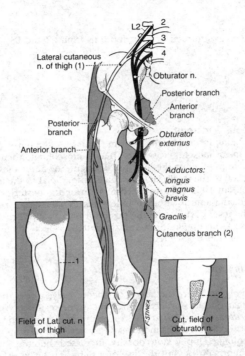

Lateral cutaneous n. of thigh (1)

L2

2

3

4

Obturator n.

Posterior branch

Anterior branch

Posterior branch

Anterior branch

Obturator externus

Adductors:
longus
magnus
brevis

Gracilis

Cutaneous branch (2)

Field of Lat. cut. n of thigh

Cut. field of obturator n.

LATERAL CUTANEOUS NERVE OF THE THIGH AND THE OBTURATOR NERVE

Nerve

Lateral cutaneous nerve of the thigh

Origin

The nerve is formed by contributions from L2 and L3.

Innervates

Motor
None

Cutaneous and Joint
After being formed by fibers from L2 and L3, the nerve penetrates the psoas major muscle, crosses the iliacus muscle, and then descends downward to pass below the inguinal ligament; the nerve moves from a position deep to the fascia lata to become superficial to the fascia lata; at a level about 10 cm below the ASIS, anterior and posterior branches are formed; the anterior branch innervates the anterior aspect of the thigh to the level of the knee; the posterior branch supplies the lateral two thirds of the upper thigh and the lateral aspect of the buttocks below the greater trochanter.

Common Injuries

In the region where the lateral cutaneous nerve passes through the inguinal ligament, it is prone to entrapment; the resultant syndrome is called *meralgia paresthetica*. The exact mechanism resulting in compression at the inguinal ligament may vary between persons, although trauma, prolonged hip flexion, obesity, increased abdominal pressures, postural abnormalities, and the use of a tight belt or corset are often implicated.

Effects of Injuries
Meralgia paresthetica results in a sensory disturbance in the lateral aspect of the thigh; patients may report burning, pain, numbness, paresthesia, or even anesthesia.

Special Tests

Sensory nerve conduction studies are used to determine if there is slowing across the suspected site of compression.

Nerve

Obturator nerve

Origin

Fibers from the anterior primary rami of L3 and L4 give rise to the obturator nerve. Sometimes there are also fibers from L2.

Innervates

Motor
The obturator passes through the psoas major muscle, emerging at the inner border of that muscle to descend posterior to the common iliac vessels; after passing through the obturator foramen, an anterior (superficial) branch and a posterior (deep) branch are given off; the anterior branch supplies the adductor longus, adductor brevis, and gracilis muscles; the posterior branch supplies the obturator externus, part of the adductor magnus, and the adductor brevis muscles.

Cutaneous and Joint
The anterior branch gives rise to a cutaneous branch that innervates the medial aspect of the thigh and the hip joint.

Common Injuries

The obturator nerve may be damaged during labor or from the pressure caused by a gravid uterus. Pelvic fractures may also result in obturator nerve damage, as may surgical procedures designed to correct obturator hernias.

Effects of Injuries
Weakness of adduction, internal rotation, and external rotation of the thigh are seen with damage to the obturator nerve. With injuries to the nerve, pain in the groin may be felt to radiate along the medial aspect of the thigh.

Special Tests

The primary symptom of obturator nerve damage is the pain that radiates along the medial thigh. The pain may be greatest in the region of the knee.

FEMORAL NERVE

Course and Distribution

(muscles innervated by nerves are listed in italics)

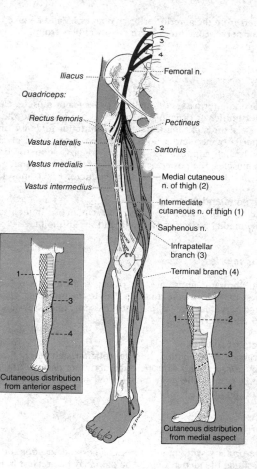

Iliacus

Quadriceps:

Rectus femoris

Vastus lateralis

Vastus medialis

Vastus intermedius

Femoral n.

Pectineus

Sartorius

Medial cutaneous n. of thigh (2)

Intermediate cutaneous n. of thigh (1)

Saphenous n.

Infrapatellar branch (3)

Terminal branch (4)

Cutaneous distribution from anterior aspect

Cutaneous distribution from medial aspect

FEMORAL NERVE

Nerve

Femoral nerve

Origin

Fibers from the anterior primary rami of L2, L3, and L4 give rise to the femoral nerve.

Innervates

Motor
The femoral nerve passes through the psoas major muscle and emerges from the lateral border before passing below the inguinal ligament and giving off a branch to innervate the iliacus muscle; after passing beneath the inguinal ligament to reach the thigh, the nerve innervates the pectineus, sartorius, and quadriceps femoris muscles.

Cutaneous and Joint
Below the inguinal ligament, the femoral nerve gives rise to sensory nerves; the anterior femoral cutaneous nerve supplies the anterior portion of the thigh while the saphenous nerve descends downward; the saphenous nerve, along with the femoral vessels, pass under the sartorius muscle (in the subsartorial canal); the saphenous nerve gives off an infrapatellar branch that supplies sensory innervation to the medial aspect of the knee; the main branch of the saphenous nerve continues down the leg to supply sensory innervation to the medial side of the leg and foot.

Common Injuries

The femoral nerve is vulnerable to compression as it passes through the pelvis; damage may be caused by tumors of the vertebrae, psoas abscesses, retroperitoneal lymphadenopathies, hematomas, and fractures of the pelvis and upper femur. Direct trauma to the nerve may occur with proximal femoral fractures or during cardiac catherization. Femoral neuropathies may also be caused by vascular compromise and secondary to diabetes. The saphenous portion of the femoral nerve may be compressed as it exits the subsartorial canal (in Hunter's canal); the compression may be due to obstructive vascular disease that causes the femoral artery to press on the nerve.

Effects of Injuries

The deficits associated with damage to the femoral nerve depend on the severity of the injury to the nerve and the site of the lesion. To determine specific deficits for each type of injury, the course of the nerve must be considered and the resultant loss of motor and sensory function distal to the site determined.

General motor deficits: If the lesion is above the innervation of the iliacus muscle, there is weakness in hip flexion. The nerve to the quadriceps muscle is the most often injured branch of the femoral nerve; loss of innervation of the quadriceps results in difficulty in walking because of an inability to keep the knee from buckling; walking down stairs is especially difficult with paralysis of the quadriceps muscle.

General sensory deficits: sensory disturbances of the anterior thigh and medial side of leg and foot occur with lesions to the sensory portions of the femoral nerve. With saphenous nerve injuries, pain is felt in the medial aspect of the knee; this pain often radiates distally to the medial side of the foot.

Special Tests

Denervation of the quadriceps muscle results in weakness often requiring the patient to use a hand to steady the thigh; there is loss of the quadriceps reflex. With painful lesions to the saphenous nerve, the pain becomes worse with exercise and especially when the patient climbs stairs.

FEMORAL NERVE

Values for Electrodiagnostic Testing*

STIMULATION POINT	RECORDING SITE	N+	AGE	ONSET LATENCY (ms)	CONDUCTION VELOCITY (m/s)
Just below inguinal ligament	14 cm from stimulus point	42	8–79	3.7 ± 0.45	70 ± 5.5 between the two recording sites
	30 cm from stimulus point	42	8–79	6.0 ± 0.60	

(Adapted from Gassel, MM: A study of femoral nerve conduction time. Arch Neurol 9:57–64, 1963.)
+Number of subjects tested to obtain values in the table.

SAPHENOUS NERVE

Values for Electrodiagnostic Testing

METHOD	AGE (years)	INGUINAL LIGAMENT–KNEE			KNEE–MEDIAL MALLEOLUS		
		n†	AMPLITUDE (µV)	CONDUCTION VELOCITY	n†	AMPLITUDE (µV)	CONDUCTION VELOCITY (m/s)
Orthodromic	17–38	33	4.2 ± 2.3	59.6 ± 2.3	10	4.8 ± 2.4	52.3 ± 2.3
Orthodromic	<40	28	5.5 ± 2.6	58.9 ± 3.2	22	2.1 ± 1.1	51.2 ± 4.7
	>40	41	5.1 ± 2.7	57.9 ± 4.0	32	1.7 ± 0.8	50.2 ± 5.0
Antidromic	20–79			Peak latency of 3.6 ± 1.4 for 14 cm	80	9.0 ± 3.4	41.7 ± 3.4
Orthodromic	18–56	71					54.8 ± 1.9

†Number of subjects tested to obtain values in the table.

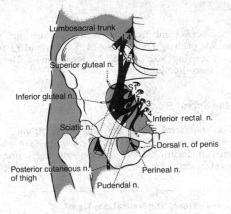

The sacral plexus is formed by the lumbosacral trunk, which comes from the lumbar plexus (L4), and the anterior primary rami of L5, S1, S2, and S3. Contributions may also come from S4.

Anatomy

The lumbosacral trunk from the lumbar plexus joins with fibers from the anterior primary rami of L4, L5, S1, S2, and S3 to form the sacral plexus. There may also be contributions from S4. The plexus lies in front of the sacroiliac joint.

Injuries to the Sacral Plexus

Injuries to the sacral plexus are quite rare, although damage to roots of the lumbar region occurs relatively frequently with disk disease. Fractures, dislocations, and space-occupying lesions (such as tumors), however, may occasionally cause damage to the plexus.

Sacral Plexus Latency Determinations from Specific Nerve Root Stimulation

PLEXUS	SITE OF STIMULATION	RECORDING SITE	LATENCY ACROSS PLEXUS (ms)	
			RANGE	MEAN ± SD
Sacral	L5 and S1 Sciatic nerve	abductor hallucis	2.5–4.9	3.9 ± 0.7

SCIATIC NERVE, TIBIAL NERVE, AND COMMON PERONEAL NERVE

Course and Distribution

(muscles innervated by nerves are listed in italics)

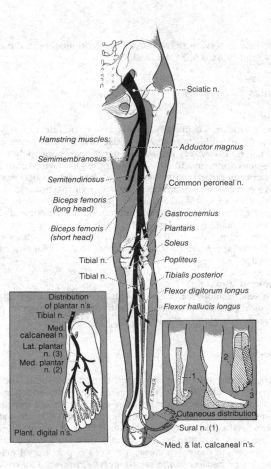

Hamstring muscles:

Semimembranosus

Semitendinosus

Biceps femoris (long head)

Biceps femoris (short head)

Tibial n.

Tibial n.

Distribution of plantar n's.
Tibial n.
Med. calcaneal n.
Lat. plantar n. (3)
Med. plantar n. (2)

Plant. digital n's.

Sciatic n.

Adductor magnus

Common peroneal n.

Gastrocnemius

Plantaris

Soleus

Popliteus

Tibialis posterior

Flexor digitorum longus

Flexor hallucis longus

F. STINER

Cutaneous distribution
Sural n. (1)
Med. & lat. calcaneal n's.

SCIATIC NERVE, TIBIAL NERVE, AND COMMON PERONEAL NERVE

Nerve

Sciatic nerve

Origin

The sciatic nerve is derived from fibers originating in the anterior primary rami of L4, L5, S1, S2, and S3.

Innervates

Motor
The sciatic nerve initially travels as one bundle but is actually made up of divisible units that give rise to the tibial nerve and the common peroneal nerve; the sciatic nerve leaves the pelvis via the greater sciatic foramen and courses under the gluteus maximus muscle to pass between the greater trochanter and the ischial tuberosity; in the thigh the nerve descends between the adductor magnus and the hamstring muscles; rami from the tibial portion of the nerve innervate the long head of the biceps femoris, semitendinosus, semimembranosus, and adductor magnus muscles; in the thigh rami of the peroneal portion innervate the short head of the biceps femoris muscle; above the popliteal fossa the nerve divides, giving rise to the tibial and common peroneal nerves.

Cutaneous and Joint
The sciatic nerve has no direct cutaneous innervation; the tibial and peroneal nerves, which are derived from the sciatic nerve, provide cutaneous innervation to the lateral leg and foot.

Common Injuries

Intramuscular injections improperly given may injure the sciatic nerve in the buttock region. Fractures of the pelvis and femur may result in damage to the sciatic nerve. Wounds (stab and gunshot) are common causes of damage to the sciatic nerve, and it is often affected by tumors originating in the genitourinary tract or rectum. Compression of the nerve may also be due to pressure from a gravid uterus or from an abscess in the pelvic floor. A Baker's popliteal cyst may compress the lower portion of the sciatic nerve. Prolonged squatting can cause damage to the sciatic nerve due to pressure on the nerve as it passes between ischial tuberosity and the greater trochanter or as it passes between the adductor magnus and the hamstring muscles.

Piriformis syndrome may occur when the nerve is compressed between the piriformis and the obturator internus muscles as it exits the pelvis in the greater sciatic foramen; sustained contractions of the piriformis muscle and fibrotic changes in the piriformis muscle secondary to trauma have been implicated in causing piriformis syndrome.

Effects of Injuries

The deficits associated with damage to the sciatic nerve will depend on the severity of the injury to the nerve and the site of the lesion; to determine specific deficits for each type of injury, the course of the nerve must be considered and the resultant loss of motor and sensory function distal to the site determined. Lesions to the sciatic nerve are always accompanied by loss of function of the common peroneal nerve, the tibial nerve, or both.

General motor deficits: with loss of the sciatic nerve, there is loss of voluntary flexion at the knee due to denervation of the hamstring muscles. Paralysis of all the muscles of the leg and foot leads to a steppage gait and an inability to run; foot drop is noticeable. With piriformis syndrome, there can be weakness of the hamstrings and all the muscles innervated by the peroneal and tibial nerve derivates.

General sensory deficits: with lesions of the sciatic nerve, there is a loss of sensation on the lateral side of the leg and the foot; with piriformis syndrome, pain and/or diminished sensation may be felt on the posterior aspect of the leg and the plantar surface of the foot.

Special Tests

Loss of the Achilles reflex and the plantar reflex is seen with lesions of the sciatic nerve; there is an inability to stand on the toes or heels. If the nerve is damaged, placing the sciatic nerve on stretch by straight leg raising may evoke Lasègue's sign (pain along the distribution of the sciatic nerve). With sciatic nerve damage, joint position sense is lost for the foot and toes.

Nerve

Tibial nerve

Origin

The tibial nerve arises from the sciatic nerve above the level of the popliteal fossa. It contains fibers from the anterior primary rami of L4, L5, S1, S2, and S3.

Innervates

Motor

The tibial nerve passes through the popliteal fossa and down the back of the leg and gives off branches that innervate both heads of the gastrocnemius, plantaris, soleus, popliteus, and the tibialis posterior muscles; the portion of nerve below the popliteal fossa was called the *posterior tibial nerve* but is now considered part of the tibial nerve; below the popliteal fossa, the tibial nerve innervates the flexor digitorum longus and flexor hallucis longus muscles; after the tibial nerve passes the level of the heel, it divides into two terminal branches—the medial plantar nerve and the lateral plantar nerve.

The medial plantar nerve innervates the flexor digitorum brevis, abductor hallucis, flexor hallucis brevis, and the first lumbrical muscles, and the lateral plantar nerve, which innervates the quadratus plantae, abductor digiti minimi, flexor digiti minimi brevis, opponens digiti minimi, the plantar and dorsal interossei, and the second, third, and fourth lumbrical muscles.

Cutaneous and Joint

In the region of the popliteal fossa, the sural nerve, a cutaneous division of the tibial nerve, branches off and descends down the lateral leg; the sural nerve supplies innervation to the posterolateral leg and gives rise to the lateral calcaneal nerve at the level of the heel; the lateral calcaneal nerve innervates the posterolateral heel area; as the tibial nerve reaches the heel, it gives rise to the medial calcaneal nerve, which innervates the posteromedial heel area.

After the tibial nerve passes the level of the heel, it divides into two branches—the medial plantar nerve and the lateral plantar nerve; digital nerves from the medial plantar nerve innervate the medial plantar surface of the foot and the plantar surfaces of the medial three-and-a-half digits; digital nerves from the lateral plantar nerve innervate the lateral portion of the plantar surface of the foot and the plantar surfaces of the lateral one-and-a-half toes.

Common Injuries

Damage to the sciatic nerve usually involves portions that form the tibial nerve. Isolated damage to the tibial nerve is usually due to an injury in or below the popliteal space; this region is particularly vulnerable to trauma. The tibial nerve is often compressed by the flexor retinaculum (the tarsal tunnel) as it passes behind and beneath the medial malleolus; this is called *tarsal tunnel syndrome* and is thought to occur as a result of trauma, tenosynovitis, or venous stasis of the posterior tibial vein.

The digital branches of the medial and lateral plantar nerves may be compressed under the metatarsal heads, giving rise to Morton's neuroma, a painful condition of the foot. Symptoms similar to those seen with Morton's neuroma are caused by other mechanical problems, such as irritation by ligaments placed on stretch due to the wearing of high-heeled shoes; hallux valgus, rheumatoid arthritis, congenital malformations, or trauma may also cause pain.

Effects of Injuries

The deficits associated with damage to the tibial nerve will depend on the severity of the injury to the nerve and the site of the lesion; to determine specific deficits for each type of injury, the course of the nerve must be considered and the resultant loss of motor and sensory function distal to the site determined. With damage to the tibial nerve, there is an inability to plantar flex, adduct, and invert the foot and an inability to flex, abduct, and adduct the toes; patients are unable to stand on their toes and find walking fatiguing and even painful.

Tarsal tunnel syndrome results in pain and/or sensory loss on the plantar surface of the foot. This pain may be most severe after prolonged walking or standing; pain may be restricted to the area of the medial foot and the great toe.

Special Tests

With lesions of the tibial nerve, the Achilles reflex is lost. To test for tarsal tunnel syndrome, the examiner taps the medial malleolus just above the margin of the flexor retinaculum; paresthesias felt in the foot are indicative of tarsal tunnel syndrome.

TIBIAL NERVE

Values for Electrodiagnostic Testing*

SITE OF STIMU-LATION	AMPLITUDE† (mV)	LATENCY† TO RECORDING SITE (ms)	DIFFERENCE BETWEEN TWO SIDES (ms)	CONDUCTION TIME BETWEEN TWO POINTS (ms)	CONDUCTION VELOCITY (m/s)
Ankle	5.8 ± 1.9 (2.9)§	3.96 ± 1.00 (6.0)¶	0.66 ± 0.57 (1.8)¶		
Knee	5.1 ± 2.2 (2.5)	12.05 ± 1.53 (15.1)	0.79 ± 0.61 (2.0)	8.09 ± 1.09 (10.3)¶	48.5 ± 3.6 (41)**

*Mean ± standard deviation (SD) in 118 nerves from 59 patients, 11 to 78 years of age (average, 39), with no apparent disease of the peripheral nerves.

†Amplitude of the evoked response, measured from the baseline to the negative peak.

‡Latency, measured to the onset of the evoked response, with a standard distance of 10 cm between the cathode and the recording electrode.

§Lower limits of normal, based on the distribution of the normative data.

¶Upper limits of normal, calculated as the mean + 2 SD.

**Lower limits of normal, calculated as the mean − 2 SD.

Latency Comparison Between Two Nerves in the Same Limb*			
SITE OF STIMULATION	PERONEAL NERVE (ms)	TIBIAL NERVE (ms)	DIFFERENCE (ms)
Ankle	3.89 ± 0.87 (5.6)†	4.12 ± 1.06 (6.2)†	0.77 ± 0.65 (2.1)†
Knee	12.46 ± 1.38 (15.2)	12.13 ± 1.48 (15.1)	0.88 ± 0.71 (2.3)

*Mean ± standard deviation (SD) in 104 nerves from 52 patients, 17 to 86 years of age (average, 41), with no apparent disease of the peripheral nerve.

†Upper limits of normal, calculated as the mean + 2 SD.

313

SURAL NERVE

Values for Electrodiagnostic Testing

STIMULATION POINT	RECORDING SITE	n*	AGE (years)	AMPLITUDE (μV)	LATENCY (ms)	CONDUCTION VELOCITY (m/s)
Foot	High ankle	40	13–41	6.3 (1.9–17)		44.0 ± 4.7
Lower third of leg	Lateral malleolus	38	1–15	23.1 ± 4.4	1.46 ± 0.43	52.1 ± 5.1
		62	Over 15	23.7 ± 3.8	2.27 ± 0.43 (Peak)	46.2 ± 3.3
15 cm above lateral malleolus	Dorsal aspect of foot	71	15–30			51.2 ± 4.5
			40–65			48.3 ± 5.3

14 cm above lateral malleolus	Lateral malleolus	101	13–66	3.50 ± 0.25 (Peak)		40.1
Lower third of leg	Lateral malleolus	80	20–79	3.7 ± 0.3 (Peak)	18.9 ± 6.7	41.0 ± 2.5
Distal 10 cm	Lateral malleolus	102				33.9 ± 3.25
Middle 10 cm		102				51.0 ± 3.8
Proximal 10 cm		102				51.6 ± 3.8
14 cm above lateral malleolus	Lateral malleolus	52	10–40	2.7 ± 0.3 (Onset)	20.9 ± 8.0	52.5 ± 5.6
			41–84	2.8 ± 0.3 (Onset)	17.2 ± 6.7	51.1 ± 5.9

*Number of subjects tested to obtain values in the table.

(Adapted from Kimura, J: Electrodiagnosis in Diseases of Nerve and Muscle: Principles and Practice, ed. 2. FA Davis, Philadelphia, 1989, p. 131).

Nerve

Common peroneal (lateral popliteal) nerve

Origin

The common peroneal nerve arises from the sciatic nerve above the level of the popliteal fossa. It contains fibers from the anterior primary rami of L4, L5, S1, and S2.

Innervates

Motor

The common peroneal nerve arises from the sciatic nerve at the upper part of the popliteal fossa, descends along the posterior border of the biceps femoris muscle, and courses around the head of the fibula to the anterior compartment of the leg; below the head of the fibula, it divides to form the deep peroneal nerve, which innervates the tibialis anterior, extensor digitorum longus, extensor hallucis longus, peroneus tertius, and extensor digitorum brevis muscles, and the superficial peroneal nerve, which innervates the peroneus longus and the peroneus brevis muscles.

Cutaneous and Joint

At the level of the popliteal fossa, the common peroneal nerve gives off the superior and inferior articular branches that innervate the knee joint; the lateral cutaneous nerve exits the common peroneal above the head of the fibula (see figure on page 322 with superficial peroneal nerve); this branch innervates the lateral upper leg; branches of the superficial peroneal nerve innervate the anterior portion of the leg, with the exception of the space between the great toe and the first toe, which is innervated by the deep peroneal nerve; the deep peroneal nerve also supplies the ankle joint, the inferior tibiofibular joint, and the joints of the toes.

Common Injuries

Damage to the sciatic nerve usually involves portions that form the common peroneal nerve. Because of the superficial course of the common peroneal nerve as it crosses by the head of the fibula, the nerve is more likely to be damaged than are either of its major branches. As a result of the firm attachment of the nerve to the fibular head, there is an additional predisposing factor to injury because the nerve cannot easily move when compressed.

Habitual sitting in a cross-legged position or prolonged squatting may compress the common peroneal nerve at the neck of the fibula; the nerve may also be injured at this site when people are sleeping or while they are anesthetized. Improper application of elastic bandages and plaster casts can damage the nerve near the fibula. People who are bedridden and allowed to maintain their legs in excessive external rotation are also prone to compression injuries of the common peroneal nerve.

Effects of Injuries

Complete lesions to the common peroneal nerve result in paralysis of the muscles of the anterior and lateral compartments of the leg; the subject cannot dorsiflex or evert the foot. Patients exhibit a steppage gait (e.g., to compensate for lack of dorsiflexion they use excessive hip flexion), and at heel strike the lateral border of the foot contacts the ground before the heel. Foot-drop deformities commonly develop in patients who have lesions of the common peroneal nerve; sensation is lost in the lateral portion of the leg and in the dorsum of the foot with this lesion. Pain is a rare component of common peroneal injuries; when pain is present, it is quite mild.

Special Tests

Lesions to the common peroneal nerve can be differentiated from spinal root and sciatic nerve lesions because the Achilles reflex is preserved with the common peroneal nerve lesion and there is also normal inversion of the foot. Lesions of the common peroneal nerve are relatively apparent because of the pattern of motor loss and the foot-drop that is not accompanied by symptoms of sciatic nerve damage.

PERONEAL NERVE

Values for Electrodiagnostic Testing*

SITE OF STIMULATION	AMPLITUDE† (mV)	LATENCY‡ TO RECORDING SITE (ms)	DIFFERENCE BETWEEN RIGHT AND LEFT (ms)	CONDUCTION TIME BETWEEN TWO POINTS (ms)	CONDUCTION VELOCITY (m/s)
Ankle	5.1 ± 2.3 (2.5)§	3.77 ± 0.86 (5.5)¶	0.62 ± 0.61 (1.8)¶		
Below knee	5.1 ± 2.0 (2.5)	10.79 ± 1.06 (12.9)	0.65 ± 0.65 (2.0)	7.01 ± 0.89 (8.8)¶	48.3 ± 3.9 (40)**
Above knee	5.1 ± 1.9 (2.5)	12.51 ± 1.17 (14.9)	0.65 ± 0.60 (1.9)	1.72 ± 0.40 (2.5)	52.0 ± 6.2 (40)

*Mean ± standard deviation (SD) in 120 nerves from 60 patients, 16 to 86 years of age (average, 41), with no apparent disease of the peripheral nerves.

†Amplitude of the evoked response, measured from the baseline to the negative peak.

‡Latency, measured to the onset of the evoked response, with a standard distance of 7 cm between the cathode and the recording electrode.

§Lower limits of normal, based on the distribution of the normative data.

¶Upper limits of normal, calculated as the mean + 2 SD.

**Lower limits of normal, calculated as the mean − 2 SD.

(Adapted from Kimura, J: Electrodiagnosis in Diseases of Nerve and Muscle: Principles and Practice, ed. 2. FA Davis, Philadelphia, 1989.)

DEEP PERONEAL NERVE

Course and Distribution

(muscles innervated by nerves are listed in italics)

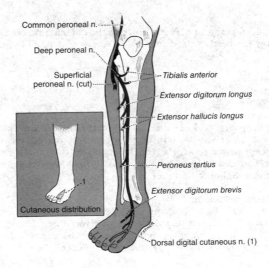

Common peroneal n.

Deep peroneal n.

Superficial peroneal n. (cut)

Tibialis anterior

Extensor digitorum longus

Extensor hallucis longus

Peroneus tertius

Extensor digitorum brevis

Cutaneous distribution

Dorsal digital cutaneous n. (1)

DEEP PERONEAL NERVE

Nerve

Deep peroneal nerve

Origin

The deep peroneal nerve arises from the common peroneal nerve just below the head of the fibula. The fibers originated in L4, L5, and S1.

Innervates

Motor
The deep peroneal nerve arises below the neck of the fibula and then courses anteriorly down the leg along the interosseous membrane; as the nerve passes down the leg, it innervates the tibialis anterior, extensor digitorum longus, extensor hallucis longus, peroneus tertius, and extensor digitorum muscles.

Cutaneous and Joint
At the level of the foot, the deep peroneal nerve gives rise to a dorsal cutaneous branch that innervates the space between the great toe and the first toe; the deep peroneal nerve also supples the ankle joint, the inferior tibiofibular joint, and the joints of the toes

Common Injuries

Isolated injuries to the deep peroneal nerve are less likely than are injuries to the common peroneal nerve. With complete common peroneal nerve lesions, there is loss of innervation to all structures innervated by the deep peroneal nerve (see common peroneal nerve); lesions of the deep peroneal nerve, however, can occur in the region of the fibular neck. Increased pressure in the anterior compartment of the leg can lead to anterior compartment syndrome, where the vascular supply to muscles of the anterior leg is compromised and there is impairment of the deep peroneal nerve.

Effects of Injuries
After injury to the deep peroneal nerve, the patient cannot dorsiflex the foot. Patients exhibit a steppage gait (i.e., to compensate for lack of dorsiflexion, they use excessive hip flexion), and at heel strike the lateral border of the foot contacts the ground before the heel. Foot-drop deformities commonly develop in these patients.

Special Tests

Lesions to the deep peroneal nerve can be differentiated from root and sciatic nerve lesions because the Achilles reflex is preserved with the deep peroneal nerve lesions, and there is also normal inversion of the foot. Lesions of the deep peroneal nerve are relatively apparent because of the pattern of motor loss and the foot-drop that is not accompanied by symptoms of sciatic nerve damage. Lesions of the deep peroneal nerve can be differentiated from those of the common peroneal nerve because the cutaneous area supplied by the superficial peroneal nerve (the anterior leg) is not affected, but the space between the big toe and the first toe may lose sensation.

SUPERFICIAL PERONEAL NERVE

Course and Distribution

(muscles innervated by nerves are listed in italics)

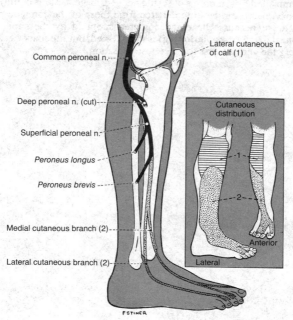

SUPERFICIAL PERONEAL NERVE

Nerve

Superficial peroneal nerve

Origin

The superficial peroneal nerve is formed by the continuation of the common peroneal nerve in the lateral crural compartment after the deep peroneal nerve has branched off below the level of the fibular neck. The fibers originated in the L4, L5, and S1 roots.

Innervates

Motor
As the superficial peroneal nerve passes down the leg, it innervates the peroneus longus and the peroneus brevis muscles.

Cutaneous and Joint
Above the ankle, medial and lateral cutaneous branches arise from the superficial peroneal nerve; these branches innervate the anterior portion of the leg and foot with the exception of the space between the great toe and the first toe, which is innervated by the deep peroneal nerve.

Common Injuries

Isolated injuries to the superficial peroneal nerve are very rare and are much less likely than injuries to the common peroneal nerve. With complete common peroneal nerve lesions, there is loss of innervation to all structures innervated by the superficial perofneal nerve (see common peroneal nerve).

Effects of Injuries
With complete lesions of the superficial peroneal nerve, there is an inability to evert the foot. Dorsiflexion is preserved but is always accompanied by inversion. Sensory loss is most notable on the medial part of the dorsum of the foot.

Special Tests

The loss of eversion, preservation of inversion and dorsiflexion, and the pattern of sensory loss on the dorsum of the foot are indicative of the rare isolated lesion to the superficial peroneal nerve.

SUPERFICIAL PERONEAL NERVE

Values for Electrodiagnostic Testing*

STIMULATION POINT	RECORDING SITE	n†	AGE (years)	AMPLITUDE (µV)	LATENCY (ms)	CONDUCTION VELOCITY (m/s)	
5 cm above, 2 cm medial to lateral malleolus	Dorsum of foot	50	1–15	13.0 ± 4.6	1.22 ± 0.40	53.1 ± 5.3	(Distal segment)
		50	Over 15	13.9 ± 4.0	(Peak) 2.24 ± 0.49	47.3 ± 3.4	(Distal segment)

					(Peak)		(Proximal segment)
Anterior edge of fibula, 12 cm above the active electrode	Medial border of lateral malleolus	50	3–60	20.5 ± 6.1	2.9 ± 0.3	65.7 ± 3.7	
					(Peak)		(Proximal segment)
Anterolateral aspect of leg, 14 cm above the active electrode	Medial border of lateral malleolus	80		18.3	2.8 ± 0.3	51.2 ± 5.7	
				(Onset)			

*Data from Di Benedetto, Jabre and Izzo et al. Kimura ZE

†Number of subjects tested to obtain values in the table.

REFLEX TESTING

Muscle Stretch Reflexes (listed in cephalad to caudal order)

REFLEX	STIMULUS	RESPONSE	SEGMENTAL LEVEL AND NERVE
Jaw (maxillary)	Tap mandible in half-open position	Closure of jaw	Pons (trigeminal nerve)
Biceps	Tap biceps tendon	Contraction of biceps	C5 and C6 (musculocutaneous nerve)
Brachioradialis (periosteoradial)	Styloid process of radius (insertion of brachioradialis)	Flexion of elbow and pronation of forearm	C5 and C6 (musculocutaneous nerve)

Triceps	Tap triceps tendon	Extension of elbow	C6 to C8 (radial nerve)
Wrist extension	Tap wrist extensor tendons	Extension of wrist	C7 and C8 (radial nerve)
Wrist flexion	Tap wrist flexor tendons	Flexion of wrist	C6 to C8 (median nerve)
Patellar	Tap patellar tendon	Extension of leg at knee	L2 to L4 (femoral nerve)
Tendocalcaneus	Tap Achilles tendon	Plantar flexion at ankle	S1 and S2 (tibial nerve)

References

1. Mancall, EL: Alpers and Mancall's Essentials of the Neurologic Examination, ed 2. FA Davis, Philadelphia, 1981.
2. Chusid, JG: Correlative Neuroanatomy and Functional Neurology. Lange Medical Publishers, Los Altos, CA, 1985.

Grading of Muscle Stretch (DTR) Reflexes

0	Areflexia
+	Hyporeflexia
1 to 3	Average
3+ to 4+	Hyperreflexia

Major Superficial Reflexes (listed in cephalad to caudal order)

REFLEX	STIMULUS	RESPONSE	SEGMENTAL LEVEL
Corneal (conjunctival)	Touching cornea with hair or cotton wisp	Contraction of orbicularis oculi (closing the eye)	Pons (afferent: trigeminal nerve; efferent: facial nerve)
Nasal (sneeze)	Lightly touch nasal mucosa with cotton wisp	Sneezing	Pons and medulla (afferent: trigeminal nerve; efferent: trigeminal nerve, facial, glossopharyngeal, and vagus nerves)
Pharyngeal (gag)	Touching posterior wall of pharynx	Contraction of pharynx	Medulla (afferent: glossopharyngeal nerve; efferent: vagus nerve)
Palatal (uvular)	Touching soft palate	Elevation of palate	Medulla (afferent: glossopharyngeal nerve; efferent: vagus)
Scapular (interscapular)	Stroking skin between scapulae	Contraction of scapular muscles	C5 to T1
Epigastric	Stroking downward from the nipples	Dimpling of epigastrium ipsilaterally	T7 to T9

Abdominal	Stroking beneath costal margins and above the inguinal ligament	Contraction of the abdominal muscles in the stimulated quadrant	T8 to T12 (depending on the quadrant stimulated)
Cremasteric	Stroking medial surface of upper thigh	Ipsilateral elevation of testicle	L1 and L2 (afferent: femoral nerve; efferent: genitofemoral)
Gluteal	Stroking skin of buttock	Contraction of glutei	L4 and L5 (superior gluteal nerve)
Bulbocavernosus	Pinching dorsum of glans of the penis	Contraction of the bulbous urethra	S3 and S4 (afferent: pudendal nerve; efferent: pelvic autonomic)
Superficial anal	Pricking perineum	Contraction of rectal sphincters	S5 and coccygeal (pudendal nerves)
Plantar	Stroke sole of foot	Plantar flexion of toes (children may also retract foot)	S1 and S2 (tibial nerve)

References

1. Mancall, EL: Alpers and Mancall's Essentials of the Neurologic Examination, ed 2. FA Davis, Philadelphia, 1981.
2. Chusid, JG: Correlative Neuroanatomy and Functional Neurology. Lange Medical Publishers, Los Altos, CA 1985.

Major Visceral Reflexes (listed in cephaled to caudal order)

REFLEX	STIMULUS	RESPONSE	SEGMENTAL LEVEL
Light reflex	Examiner projects light on the retina	Constriction of pupil	Mesencephalon
Consensual light	Examiner projects light into the eye opposite the one being evaluated	Constriction of the pupil in the eye not receiving the light	Commissural pathways in the pretectal area are tested, as are the same pathways used in the light reflex
Accommodation	Examiner asks the patient to look at a nearby object	Eyes should converge with constriction of the pupils	Occipital cortex (if light reflexes exist) and mesencephalon (afferent: optic nerve; efferent: oculomotor)
Ciliospinal reflex	Examiner applies a painful stimulus to patient's neck (pinching)	Dilation of pupil	T1 and T2 for sympathetic portion (efferent) and whatever area is used for sensory
Blink reflex (of Descartes)	Unexpected movement of object near and toward eyes	Closure of the eyes	Mesencephalon and occipital cortex (afferent: optic nerve; efferent: facial nerve)

| Oculocardiac | Examiner applies pressure on eye | Slowing of heart rate | Medulla (afferent: trigeminal nerve; efferent: vagus nerve) |
| Carotid sinus reflex | Examiner applies pressure over carotid sinus | Slowing of heart rate and fall in blood pressure | Medulla (afferent: glossopharyngeal nerve; efferent: vagus nerve) |

Reference

1. Chusid, JG: Correlative Neuroanatomy and Functional Neurology. Lange Medical Publishers, Los Altos, CA, 1985.

MAJOR PATHOLOGICAL REFLEXES

Reflexes That Indicate Pathology Affecting Corticospinal Systems

These reflexes can often be seen in normal infants who are younger than seven months of age.

Major Pathological Reflexes: Upper Extremity (in alphabetical order)

NAME	STIMULUS	RESPONSE
Bechterew's sign	Patient alternately flexes and relaxes the forearm	If the sign is positive, the arm falls back into the extended position in a slow, jerky fashion
Chaddock wrist sign	Examiner strokes the ulnar side of forearm (pressure on tendon of palmaris longus)	Flexion of wrist with extension and possible fanning of fingers
Clonus	Rapid extension of the wrist by the examiner	Rapid reciprocal flexion and extension
Extension-adduction (Dagnini reflex)	Examiner percusses the dorsum of hand on radial side	Slight adduction and extension of wrist
Finger flexion (Trömner's reflex)	The examiner taps the palmar surface or tips of the middle three fingers	Flexion of the fingers
Forced grasping	Examiner strokes the patient's palm in a radial direction	Grasp reaction
Gordon's sign	Examiner compresses the region of pisiform bone	Extension of flexed fingers
Hoffmann's sign	Examiner snaps the nail of the middle finger	Flexion of fingers and thumb

Sign	Maneuver	Response
Kleist hooking sign	Pressure by examiner against the flexor surface of the finger tips	Flexion of fingers
Klippel and Weil thumb sign	The patient's flexed fingers are rapidly extended by the examiner	Flexion and adduction of the thumb
Leri's sign	Examiner forcefully flexes the wrist and fingers	Absence of elbow flexion
Mayer's sign	Examiner forcefully flexes the proximal phalanges of the supinated hand	Absence of adduction and opposition of the thumb
Mendel-Bechterew reflex of the hand	Examiner percusses the dorsal aspect of the carpals and metacarpals on the radial side	Flexion of the fingers
Palm-chin reflex (Marinesco-Radiovici)	Examiner stimulates of thenar eminence	Contraction of muscles of chin and elevation of the corner of the mouth
Rossolimo's sign of the hand	Examiner percusses the palmar aspect of the metacarpophalangeal joint	Flexion of the fingers
Souque's sign	Patient attempts to raise paretic arm	Fingers adduct and extend
Sterling's sign	Resisted adduction of nonparetic arm	Adduction of paretic arm
Strümpell's pronation sign	Patient flexes the forearm	The hand touches the shoulder (normally the palm should touch the shoulder)
Thumb-adductor reflex (Babinski of the hand or Marie Foix of the hand)	Examiner strokes the hypothenar region	Adduction and flexion of thumb, sometimes flexion of adjacent fingers with extension of the little finger

Major Pathological Reflexes: Lower Extremity (in alphabetical order)		
NAME	STIMULUS	RESPONSE
Babinski's sign	Examiner strokes the outer edge of sole of foot	Extension of the great toe, flexion of small toes, and spreading of small toes
Bechterew-Mendel reflex	Tapping on the lateral surface of the dorsum of the foot	Flexion of the toes
Chaddock toe sign	Examiner strokes the lateral aspect of the dorsum of the foot and lateral malleolus	Response similar to that seen with Babinski's sign (extension of great toe, flexion of small toes, and spreading of small toes)
Clonus	Examiner rapidly dorsiflexes the ankle	Continued and prolonged reciprocal plantar flexion and dorsiflexion of the ankle
Crossed extension	With the subject supine and both legs flexed at the hip, examiner stimulates the sole of the foot	Extension of the contralateral extremity
Extensor thrust	Examiner vigorously dorsiflexes the foot of a leg that has been flexed at the hip	Extension of that entire lower extremity
Gonda's sign	Examiner strongly flexes a toe and then rapidly releases it into extension (with a snap)	Extension of the big toe

Gordon's leg sign	Examiner squeezes the calf	Response similar to that seen with Babinski's sign (extension of great toe, flexion of small toes, and spreading of small toes)
Grasset-Gaussel phenomenon	The supine patient is asked to raise each leg and then both legs; if the paretic leg is raised, the examiner then passively raises the nonparetic leg	A positive sign is when both legs cannot be raised together and the paretic limb falls back down if it is raised when the examiner lifts the nonparetic limb
Hirschberg's sign	Examiner strokes the medial border of foot	Adduction and internal rotation (inversion) of foot
Hoover's sign	Examiner places palms under the heels of the supine patient and the patient is asked to press downward; the patient is then also asked to lift the nonparetic limb while the examiner resists the movement	If there is true hemiplegia (nonhysterical), there will be no pressure felt under the heel of the paretic limb when the patient is asked to press down and no increased pressure when the patient is asked to move the nonparetic limb
Huntington's sign	Patient coughs or strains	The paretic limb will flex at the hip and there will be extension at the knee
Marie-Foix	Examiner forcefully flexes the patient's toes	There is flexion at the hip and knee
Néri's sign	The supine patient attempts alternate straight leg raising	Flexion at the knee on the paretic limb

Cont. on the following page(s)

Major Pathological Reflexes: Lower Extremity (in alphabetical order) *Continued*

NAME	STIMULUS	RESPONSE
Oppenheim's reflex	Examiner strokes downward on the medial aspect of leg	Response similar to that seen with Babinski's sign (extension of great toe, flexion of small toes, and spreading of small toes)
Patellar clonus (trepidation sign)	With the leg fully extended and relaxed, a downward movement of the patella is caused by the examiner	Rapid up-and-down movements of the patella
Ramiste's sign	The supine patient attempts either hip adduction or abduction of the nonparetic limb	The paretic limb moves in the same way as the nonparetic limb (the effect is more dramatic if resistance is added to the nonparetic limb)
Rossolimo's sign	Examiner taps on balls of the patient's foot	Flexion of toes
Schäffer's reflex	Examiner squeezes the patient's Achilles tendon	Response similar to that seen with Babinski's sign (extension of great toe, flexion of small toes, and spreading of small toes)
Stransky's sign	Patient abducts the small toe	Extension of the great toe
Strümpell's tibialis anterior sign	Patient flexes the hip	Dorsiflexion and adduction of the foot (the effect is more dramatic if resistance is added to the hip flexion)

Additional Pathological Reflexes (in alphabetical order)		
NAME	STIMULUS	RESPONSE
Babinski's platysma sign	Examiner resists neck flexion or mouth opening	Normally the platysma on the nonparetic side contracts while the platysma on the paretic side does not contract
Glabella (McCarthy's reflex)	Examiner taps the glabella	Contraction of orbicularis oculi
Snout reflex	Examiner taps middle of upper lip	Movement of upper lips

References

1. Mancall, EL: Alpers and Mancall's Essentials of the Neurologic Examination, ed 2. FA Davis, Philadelphia, 1981.
2. Chusid, JG: Correlative Neuroanatomy and Functional Neurology. Lange Medical Publishers, Los Altos, CA, 1985.

CLINICAL ELECTRODIAGNOSIS

Electrodes

The two types of electrodes used for clinical electromyography are *surface* (or skin) electrodes and *percutaneous* (or indwelling) electrodes. The segment of the electrode that makes direct electrical contact with the tissue is referred to as the *detection surface*. Detection surfaces are used either singularly (*monopolar*) or in pairs (*bipolar*).

Surface Electrodes

Surface electrodes are applied to the overlying skin and can be used to record the global activity of evoked muscle and nerve action potentials and to stimulate peripheral nerves in nerve conduction tests. Recording electrodes can either be *passive*, wherein the detection surface senses the current on the skin through its skin-electrode interface, or *active*, wherein the input impedance of the electrode is greatly increased, rendering it less sensitive to the impedance of the electrode-skin interface. The chief advantage of surface electrodes is convenience, whereas the disadvantages are that they can only be used effectively with superficial muscles and they cannot be easily used to detect signals selectively from small muscles.

Percutaneous Electrodes

For clinical purposes, the most commonly used percutaneous electrodes are needle electrodes, which are used to record from a single motor unit or just a few motor units. A wide variety of needle electrodes is available; however, the most common is the concentric electrode. The monopolar configuration of the concentric electrode contains one insulated wire in the cannula with the tip of the wire bared to act as a detection surface. The bipolar configuration of the concentric electrode contains a second wire in the cannula that provides a second detection surface. The main advantages of the needle electrode are its small pickup area (high selectivity) and the convenience with which new muscle territories can be explored by repositioning the needle.

Needle Electrode Configurations

Schematic illustration of standard or coaxial bipolar (*a*), concentric bipolar (*b*), monopolar (*c*), and single fiber needles (*d* and *e*). Dimensions vary, but the diameters of the outside cannulas shown resemble 26-gauge hypodermic needles (460 µm) for *a, d,* and *e,* a 23-gauge needle (640 µm) for *b,* and a 28-gauge needle (360 µm) for *c.* The exposed tip areas measure 150 by 300 µm with spacing between wires of 200 µm center to center for *b,* 0.14 sq mm for *c,* and 25 µm in diameter for *d* and *e.* A flat-skin electrode completes the circuit with unipolar electrodes shown in *c* and *d.*

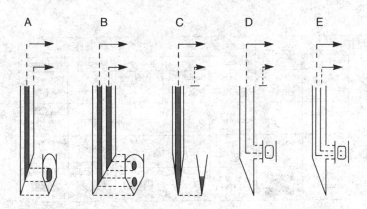

A   B   C   D   E

Clinical Electromyography:
Typical EMG Pattern

The figure shows the typical patterns of EMG activity of various diseases and lesions. *Insertional activity* is the electrical activity recorded when the needle is inserted or moved within the muscle. *Spontaneous activity* is the electrical activity recorded after the cessation of insertional activity in resting muscle. The *motor unit potential* is the compound electrical wave formed by the depolarization of the muscle fibers belonging to a motor unit. The size and shape of the potential are of diagnostic significance. The *interference pattern* is the electrical activity recorded from a muscle during maximal voluntary effort.

LESION / EMG steps	NORMAL	NEUROGENIC LESION		MYOGENIC LESION		
		Motoneuron	CNS	Myopathy	Myotonia	Polymyositis
1 Insertional activity	Normal	Increased	Normal	Normal	Myotonic discharge	Increased
2 Spontaneous activity	—	Fibrillation Positive wave	—	—		Fibrillation Positive wave
3 Motor unit potential	0.5–1.0 mV 5–10 ms	Large unit Limited recruitment	Normal	Small unit Early recruitment	Myotonic discharge	Small unit Early recruitment
4 Interference pattern	Full	Reduced Fast firing rate	Reduced Slow firing rate	Full amplitude Low	Full amplitude Low	Full amplitude Low

Reference

1. Kimura, J: Electrodiagnosis in Diseases of Nerve and Muscle: Principles and Practice, ed 2. FA Davis, Philadelphia, 1989.

AAEE GLOSSARY OF TERMS IN CLINICAL ELECTROMYOGRAPHY

*A wave: A compound action potential evoked consistently from a muscle by submaximal electric stimuli to the nerve and frequently abolished by supramaximal stimuli. The amplitude of the A wave is similar to that of the F wave, but the latency is more constant. The A wave usually occurs before the F wave, but may occur afterwards. The A wave is due to normal or pathologic axonal branching.

absolute refractory period: See *refractory period.*

accommodation: True accommodation in neuronal physiology is a rise in the threshold transmembrane depolarization required to initiate a spike when depolarization is slow or a subthreshold depolarization is maintained. In the older literature, accommodation described the observation that the final intensity of current applied in a slowly rising fashion to stimulate a nerve was greater than the intensity of a pulse of current required to stimulate the same nerve. The latter may largely be an artifact of the nerve sheath and bears little relation to true accommodation as measured intracellularly.

accommodation curve: See *strength-duration curve.*

action current: The electric currents associated with an *action potential.*

action potential (AP): The brief regenerative electric potential that propagates along a single axon or muscle fiber membrane. The action potential is an all-or-none phenomenon; whenever the stimulus is at or above threshold, the action potential generated has a constant size and configuration. See also *compound action potential, motor unit action potential.*

active electrode: Synonymous with *exploring electrode.* See *recording electrode.*

adaptation: A decline in the frequency of the spike discharge as typically recorded from sensory axons in response to a maintained stimulus.

AEPs: See *auditory evoked potentials.*

afterdischarge: The continuation of an impulse train in a neuron, axon, or muscle fiber following the termination of an applied stimulus. The number of extra impulses and their periodicity in the train may vary depending on the circumstances.

afterpotential: The membrane potential between the end of the spike and the time when the membrane potential is restored to its resting value. The membrane during this period may be depolarized or hyperpolarized.

amplitude: With reference to an *action potential,* the maximum voltage difference between two points, usually baseline to peak or peak to peak. By convention, the amplitude of the *compound muscle action potential* is measured from the baseline to the most negative peak. In contrast, the amplitude of a *compound sensory nerve action potential, motor unit potential, fibrillation potential, positive sharp wave, fasciculation potential*, and most other *action potentials* is measured from the most positive peak to the most negative peak.

anodal block: A local block of nerve conduction caused by *hyperpolarization* of the nerve cell membrane by an electric stimulus. See *stimulating electrode*.

anode: The positive terminal of a source of electric current.

antidromic: Propagation of an impulse in the direction opposite to physiologic conduction; e.g., conduction along motor nerve fibers away from the muscle and conduction along sensory fibers away from the spinal cord. Contrast with *orthodromic*.

AP: See *action potential*.

artifact (also artefact): A voltage change generated by a biologic or nonbiologic source other than the ones of interest. The *stimulus artifact* is the potential recorded at the time the stimulus is applied and includes the *electric* or *shock artifact*, which represents cutaneous spread of stimulating current to the recording electrode. The stimulus and shock artifacts usually precede the activity of interest. A *movement artifact* refers to a change in the recorded activity caused by movement of the recording electrodes.

auditory evoked potentials (AEPs): Electric waveforms of biologic origin elicited in response to sound stimuli. AEPs are classified by their latency as short-latency brainstem AEPs (BAEPs) with a latency of up to 10 ms, middle-latency AEPs with a latency of 10 – 50 ms, and long-latency AEPs with a latency of over 50 ms. See *brainstem auditory evoked potentials*.

axon reflex: Use of term discouraged as it is incorrect. No reflex is considered to be involved. See preferred term, *A wave*.

axon response: See preferred term, *A wave*.

axon wave: See *A wave*.

axonotmesis: Nerve injury characterized by disruption of the axon and myelin sheath, but with preservation of the supporting connective tissue, resulting in axonal degeneration distal to the injury site.

backfiring: Discharge of an antidromically activated motor neuron.

BAEPs: See *brainstem auditory evoked potentials*.

BAERs: Abbreviation for *brainstem auditory evoked responses*. See preferred term, *brainstem auditory evoked potentials*.

baseline: The potential recorded from a biologic system while the system is at rest.

benign fasciculation: Use of term discouraged to describe a firing pattern of fasciculation potentials. The term has been used to describe a clinical syndrome and/or the presence of fasciculations in nonprogressive neuromuscular disorders. See *fasciculation potential*.

BERs: Abbreviation for *brainstem auditory evoked responses*. See preferred term, *brainstem auditory evoked potentials*.

bifilar needle recording electrode: *Recording electrode* that measures variations in voltage between the bare tips of two insulated wires cemented side by side in a steel cannula. The bare tips of the electrodes are flush with the level of the cannula. The latter may be grounded.

biphasic action potential: An *action potential* with two phases.

biphasic end-plate activity: See *endplate activity (biphasic)*.

bipolar needle recording electrode: See preferred term, *bifilar needle recording electrode*.

bipolar stimulating electrode: See *stimulating electrode*.

bizarre high-frequency discharge: See preferred term, *complex repetitive discharge*.

bizarre repetitive discharge: See preferred term, *complex repetitive discharge*.

bizarre repetitive potential: See preferred term, *complex repetitive discharge*.

blink reflex: See *blink responses*.

blink response: Strictly defined, one of the *blink responses*. See *blink responses*.

blink responses: *Compound muscle action potentials* evoked from orbicularis oculi muscles as a result of brief electric or mechanical stimuli to the cutaneous area innervated by the supraorbital (or less commonly, the infraorbital) branch of the trigeminal nerve. Typically, there is an early compound muscle action potential (*R1 wave*) ipsilateral to the stimulation site with a latency of about 10 ms and a bilateral late compound muscle action potential (*R2 wave*) with a latency of approximately 30 ms. Generally, only the *R2 wave* is associated with a visible twitch of the orbicularis oculi. The configuration, amplitude, duration, and latency of the two components, along with the sites of recording and the sites of stimulation, should be specified. *R1* and *R2 waves* are probably oligosynaptic and polysynaptic brainstem reflexes, respectively, together called the *blink reflex*, with the afferent arc provided by the sensory branches of the trigeminal nerve and the efferent arc provided by the facial nerve motor fibers.

brainstem auditory evoked potentials (BAEPs): Electric waveforms of biologic origin elicited in response to sound stimuli. The normal BAEP consists of a sequence of up to seven waves, named I to VII, which occur during the first 10 ms after the onset of the stimulus and have positive polarity at the vertex of the head.

brainstem auditory evoked responses (BAERs, BERs): See preferred term, *brainstem auditory evoked potentials*.

BSAPs: Abbreviation for brief, small, abundant potentials. Use of term is discouraged. It is used to describe a recruitment pattern of brief-duration, small-amplitude, overly abundant motor unit action potentials. Quantitative measurements of motor unit potential duration, amplitude, numbers of phases, and recruitment frequency are to be preferred to qualitative descriptions such as this. See *motor unit action potential*.

BSAPPs: Abbreviation for brief, small abundant, polyphasic potentials. Use of term is discouraged. It is used to describe a recruitment pattern of brief-duration, small-amplitude, overly abundant, polyphasic motor unit action potentials. Quantitative measurements of motor unit potential duration, amplitude, numbers of phases, and recruitment frequency are to be preferred to qualitative descriptions such as this. See *motor unit action potential*.

cathode: The negative terminal of a source of electric current.

central electromyography (central EMG): Use of electromyographic recording techniques to study reflexes and the control of movement by the spinal cord and brain.

chronaxie (also chronaxy): See *strength-duration curve*.

clinical electromyography: Synonymous with *electroneuromyography*. Used to refer to all electrodiagnostic studies of human peripheral nerves and muscle. See also *electromyography* and *nerve conduction studies*.

coaxial needle electrode: See synonym, *concentric needle electrode*.

collision: When used with reference to nerve conduction studies, the interaction of two action potentials propagated toward each other from opposite directions on the same nerve fiber so that the refractory periods of the two potentials prevent propagation past each other.

complex action potential: See preferred term, *serrated action potential*.

complex motor unit action potential: A *motor unit action potential* that is polyphasic or serrated. See preferred terms, *polyphasic action potential or serrated action potential*.

complex repetitive discharge: Polyphasic or serrated action potentials that may begin spontaneously or after a needle movement. They have a uniform frequency, shape, and amplitude, with abrupt onset, cessation, or change in configuration. Amplitude ranges from 100 μV to 1 mV and frequency of discharge from 5 to 100 Hz. This term is preferred to *bizarre high-frequency discharge, bizarre repetitive discharge, bizarre repetitive potential, near constant frequency trains, pseudomyotonic discharge,* and *synchronized fibrillation*.

compound action potential: See *compound mixed nerve action potential, compound motor nerve action potential, compound nerve action potential, compound sensory nerve action potential,* and *compound muscle action potential*.

compound mixed nerve action potential (compound mixed NPA): A compound nerve action potential is considered to have been evoked from afferent and efferent fibers if the recording electrodes detect activity on a mixed nerve with the electric stimulus applied to a segment of the nerve that contains both afferent and efferent fibers. The amplitude, latency, duration, and phases should be noted.

compound motor nerve action potential (compound motor NAP): A compound nerve action potential is considered to have been evoked from efferent fibers to a muscle if the recording electrodes detect activity only in a motor nerve or a motor branch of a mixed nerve, or if the electric stimulus is applied only to such a nerve or a ventral root. The amplitude, latency, duration, and phases should be noted. See *compound nerve action potential.*

compound muscle action potential (CMAP): The summation of nearly synchronous muscle fiber action potentials recorded from a muscle commonly produced by stimulation of the nerve supplying the muscle either directly or indirectly. Baseline-to-peak amplitude, duration, and latency of the negative phase should be noted, along with details of the method of stimulation and recording. Use of specific named potentials is recommended, e.g., *M wave, F wave, H wave, T wave, A wave* and *R1 wave* or *R2 wave (blink responses).*

compound nerve action potential (compound NAP): The summation of nearly synchronous nerve fiber action potentials recorded from a nerve trunk, commonly produced by stimulation of the nerve directly or indirectly. Details of the method of stimulation and recording should be specified, together with the fiber type (sensory, motor, or mixed).

compound sensory nerve action potential (compound SNAP): A compound nerve action potential is considered to have been evoked from afferent fibers if the recording electrodes detect activity only in a sensory nerve or in a sensory branch of a mixed nerve, or if the electric stimulus is applied to a sensory nerve or a dorsal nerve root, or an adequate stimulus is applied synchronously to sensory receptors. The amplitude, latency, duration, and configuration should be noted. Generally, the amplitude is measured as the maximum peak-to-peak voltage, the latency as either the *latency* to the initial deflection or the *peak latency* to the negative peak, and the duration as the interval from the first deflection of the waveform from the baseline to its final return to the baseline. The compound sensory nerve action potential has been referred to as the *sensory response* or *sensory potential.*

concentric needle electrode: *Recording electrode* that measures an electric potential difference between the bare tip of an insulated wire, usually stainless steel, silver, or platinum, and the bare shaft of a steel cannula through which it is inserted. The bare tip of the central wire (*exploring electrode*) is flush with the level of the cannula (*reference electrode*).

conditioning stimulus: See *paired stimuli.*

conduction block: Failure of an action potential to be conducted past a particular point in the nervous system whereas conduction is possible below the point of the block. Conduction block is documented by demonstration of a reduction in the area of an evoked potential greater than that normally seen with electric stimulation at two different points on a nerve trunk; anatomic variations of nerve pathways and technical factors related to nerve stimulation must be excluded as the cause of the reduction in area.

conduction distance: See *conduction velocity.*

conduction time: See *conduction velocity.*

conduction velocity (CV): Speed of propagation of an *action potential* along a nerve or muscle fiber. The nerve fibers studied (motor, sensory, autonomic, or mixed) should be specified. For a nerve trunk, the maximum conduction velocity is calculated from the *latency* of the evoked potential (muscle or nerve) at maximal or supramaximal intensity of stimulation at two different points. The distance between the two points (*conduction distance*) is divided by the difference between the corresponding latencies (*conduction time*). The calculated velocity represents the conduction velocity of the fastest fibers and is expressed as meters per second (m/s). As commonly used, the term *conduction velocity* refers to the maximum conduction velocity. By specialized techniques, the conduction velocity of other fibers can be determined as well and should be specified, e.g., minimum conduction velocity.

contraction: A voluntary or involuntary reversible muscle shortening that may or may not be accompanied by *action potentials* from muscle. This term is to be contrasted with the term *contracture*, which refers to a condition of fixed muscle shortening.

contraction fasciculation: Rhythmic, visible twitching of a muscle with weak voluntary or postural contraction. The phenomenon occurs in neuromuscular disorders in which the motor unit territory is enlarged and the tissue covering the muscle is thin.

contracture: The term is used to refer to immobility of a joint due to fixed muscle shortening. Contrast *contraction*. The term has also been used to refer to an electrically silent, involuntary state of maintained muscle contraction, as seen in phosphorylase deficiency, for which the preferred term is *muscle cramp.*

coupled discharge: See preferred term, *satellite potential.*

cps (also c/s): See *cycles per second.*

cramp discharge: Involuntary repetitive firing of *motor unit action potentials* at a high frequency (up to 150 Hz) in a large area of muscles, usually associated with painful muscle contraction. Both the discharge frequency and the number of *motor unit action potentials* firing increase gradually during development and both subside gradually with cessation. See *muscle cramp*.

c/s (also cps): See *cycles per second*.

CV: See *conduction velocity*.

cycles per second: Unit of frequency. (cps or c/s). See also *hertz* (Hz).

decremental response: See preferred term, *decrementing response*.

decrementing response: A reproducible decline in the amplitude and/or area of the *M wave* of successive responses to *repetitive nerve stimulation*. The rate of stimulation and the total number of stimuli should be specified. Decrementing responses with disorders of neuromuscular transmission are most reliably seen with slow rates (2 – 5 Hz) of nerve stimulation. A decrementing response with repetitive nerve stimulation commonly occurs in disorders of neuromuscular transmission but can also be seen in some neuropathies, myopathies, and motor neuron disease. An artifact resembling a decrementing response can result from movement of the stimulating or recording electrodes during repetitive nerve stimulation. Contrast with *incrementing response*.

delay: As originally used in clinical electromyography, delay referred to the time between the beginning of the horizontal sweep of the oscilloscope and the onset of an applied stimulus. The term is also used to refer to an information storage device (delay line) used to display events occurring before a trigger signal.

denervation potential: The term has been used to describe a *fibrillation potential*. The use of this term is discouraged because fibrillation potentials may occur in settings where transient muscle membrane instability occurs in the absence of denervation, e.g., hyperkalemia periodic paralysis. See preferred term, *fibrillation potential*.

depolarization: See *polarization*.

depolarization block: Failure of an excitable cell to respond to a stimulus because of depolarization of the cell membrane.

discharge: Refers to the firing of one or more excitable elements (neurons, axons, or muscle fibers) and as conventionally applied refers to the all-or-none potentials only. Synonymous with *action potential*.

discharge frequency: The rate of repetition of potentials. When potentials occur in groups, the rate of recurrence of the group and the rate of repetition of the individual components in the groups should be specified. See also *firing rate*.

discrete activity: See *interference pattern*.

distal latency: See *motor latency* and *sensory latency*.

double discharge: Two action potentials (*motor unit action potential, fibrillation potential*) of the same form and nearly the same amplitude, occurring consistently in the same relationship to one another at intervals of 2 to 20 ms. Contrast with *paired discharge*.

doublet: Synonymous with *double discharge*.

duration: The time during which something exists or acts. (1) The total duration of individual potential *waveforms* is defined as the interval from the beginning of the first deflection from the baseline to its final return to the baseline, unless otherwise specified. For example, the duration of the *M wave* may refer to the interval from the deflection of the first negative phase from the baseline to its return to the baseline. (2) The duration of a single electric stimulus refers to the interval of the applied current or voltage. (3) The duration of recurring stimuli or action potentials refers to the interval from the beginning to the end of the series.

earth electrode: Synonymous with *ground electrode*.

EDX: See *electrodiagnosis*.

electric artifact: See *artifact*.

electric inactivity: Absence of identifiable electric activity in a structure or organ under investigation. See preferred term, *electric silence*.

electric silence: The absence of measurable electric activity due to biologic or nonbiologic sources. The sensitivity and signal-to-noise level of the recording system should be specified.

electrode: A conducting device used to record an electric potential (*recording electrode*) or to apply an electric current (*stimulating electrode*). In addition to the *ground electrode* used in clinical recordings, two electrodes are always required either to record an electric potential or to apply an electric current. Depending on the relative size and location of the electrodes, however, the stimulating or recording condition may be referred to as *monopolar* or *unipolar*. See *ground electrode, recording electrode,* and *stimulating electrode*. Also see specific needle electrode configurations: *monopolar, unipolar, concentric, bifilar recording, bipolar stimulating, multilead, single fiber,* and *macro-EMG needle electrodes*.

electrodiagnosis (EDX): The recording and analysis of responses of nerves and muscles to electric stimulation and the identification of patterns of insertion, spontaneous, involuntary and voluntary action potentials in muscle and nerve tissue. See also *electromyography, electroneurography, electroneuromyography,* and *evoked potential studies*.

electrodiagnostic medicine: A specific area of medical practice in which a physician uses information from the clinical history, observations from the physical examination, and the techniques of *electrodiagnosis* to diagnose and treat neuromuscular disorders. See *electrodiagnosis*.

electromyelography: The recording and study of electric activity from the spinal cord and/or from the cauda equina.

electromyogram: The record obtained by *electromyography*.

electromyograph: Equipment used to activate, record, process, and display nerve and muscle action potentials for the purpose of evaluating nerve and muscle function.

electromyography (EMG): Strictly defined, the recording and study of insertion, spontaneous, and voluntary electric activity of muscle. It is commonly used to refer to nerve conduction studies as well. See also *clinical electromyography* and *electroneuromyography*.

electroneurography (ENG): The recording and study of the action potentials of peripheral nerves. Synonymous with *nerve conduction studies*.

electroneuromyography (ENMG): The combined studies of *electromyography* and *electroneurography*. Synonymous with *clinical electromyography*.

EMG: See *electromyography*.

end-plate activity: Spontaneous electric activity recorded with a needle electrode close to muscle end-plates. May be either of two forms:

1. *Monophasic:* Low-amplitude (10–20 μV), short-duration (0.5–1 ms), monophasic (negative) potentials that occur in a dense, steady pattern and are restricted to a localized area of the muscle. Because of the multitude of different potentials occurring, the exact frequency, although appearing to be high, cannot be defined. These nonpropagated potentials are probably miniature end-plate potentials recorded extracellularly. This form of end-plate activity has been referred to as *endplate noise* or *sea shell sound* (*sea shell noise* or *roar*).

2. *Biphasic:* Moderate-amplitude (100–300 μV), short-duration (2–4 ms), biphasic (negative-positive) spike potentials that occur irregularly in short bursts with a high frequency (50–100 Hz), restricted to a localized area within the muscle. These propagated potentials are generated by muscle fibers excited by activity in nerve terminals. These potentials have been referred to as *biphasic spike potentials, end-plate spikes,* and, incorrectly, *nerve potentials*.

end-plate noise: See *end-plate activity (monophasic)*.

end-plate potential (EPP): The graded nonpropagated membrane potential induced in the postsynaptic membrane of the muscle fiber by the action of acetylcholine released in response to an action potential in the presynaptic axon terminal.

end-plate spike: See *end-plate activity (biphasic)*.

end-plate zone: The region in a muscle where the neuromuscular junctions of the skeletal muscle fibers are concentrated.

ENG: See *electroneurography*.

ENMG: See *electroneuromyography*.

EPP: See *end-plate potential*.

EPSP: See *excitatory postsynaptic potential*.

evoked compound muscle action potential: See *compound muscle action potential.*

evoked potential: Electric waveform elicited by and temporally related to a stimulus, most commonly an electric stimulus delivered to a sensory receptor or nerve, or applied directly to a discrete area of the brain, spinal cord, or muscle. See *auditory evoked potential, brainstem auditory evoked potential, spinal evoked potential, somatosensory evoked potential, visual evoked potential, compound muscle action potential,* and *compound sensory nerve action potential.*

evoked potential studies: Recording and analysis of electric waveforms of biologic origin elicited in response to electric or physiologic stimuli. Generally used to refer to studies of waveforms generated in the peripheral and central nervous system, whereas *nerve conduction studies* refers to studies of waveforms generated in the peripheral nervous system. There are two systems for naming complex waveforms in which multiple components can be distinguished. In the first system, the different components are labeled PI or NI for the initial positive and negative potentials, respectively, and PII, NII, PIII, NIII, and so on, for subsequent positive and negative potentials. In the second system, the components are specified by polarity and average peak latency in normal subjects to the nearest millisecond. The first nomenclature principle has been used in an abbreviated form to identify the seven positive components (I–VII) of the normal *brainstem auditory evoked potential.* The second nomenclature principle has been used to identify the positive and negative components of *visual evoked potentials* ($\overline{N75}$, P100) and *somatosensory evoked potentials* (P9, P11, P13, P14, N20, P23). Regardless of the nomenclature system, it is possible under standardized conditions to establish normal ranges of amplitude, duration, and latency of the individual components of these *evoked potentials.* The difficulty with the second system is that the latencies of components of evoked potentials depend upon the length of the pathways in the neural tissues. Thus the components of an SEP recorded in a child have different average latencies from the same components of an SEP recorded in an adult. Despite this problem, there is no better system available for naming these components at this time. See *auditory evoked potentials, brainstem auditory evoked potentials, visual evoked potentials, somatosensory evoked potentials.*

evoked response: Tautology. Use of term discouraged. See preferred term, *evoked potential.*

excitability: Capacity to be activated by or react to a stimulus.

excitatory postsynaptic potential (EPSP): A local, graded depolarization of a neuron in response to activation by a nerve terminal of a synapse. Contrast with *inhibitory postsynaptic potential.*

exploring electrode: Synonymous with *active electrode.* See *recording electrode.*

F reflex: See preferred term, *F wave.*

F response: Synonymous with *F wave.* See preferred term, *F wave.*

F wave: A *compound action potential* evoked intermittently from a muscle by a supramaximal electric stimulus to the nerve. Compared with the maximal amplitude *M wave* of the same muscle, the F wave has a smaller amplitude (1–5% of the *M wave*), variable configuration and a longer, more variable latency. The F wave can be found in many muscles of the upper and lower extremities, and the latency is longer with more distal sites of stimulation. The F wave is due to antidromic activation of motor neurons. It was named by Magladery and McDougal in 1950. Compare to the *H wave* and the *A wave.*

facilitation: Improvement of neuromuscular transmission that results in the activation of previously inactive muscle fibers. Facilitation may be identified in several ways:

1. *Incrementing response:* A reproducible increase in the amplitude associated with an increase in the area of successive electric responses (*M waves*) during *repetitive nerve stimulation.*
2. *Postactivation* or *posttetanic facilitation:* Nerve stimulation studies performed within a few seconds after a brief period (2–15 s) of nerve stimulation producing *tetanus* or after a strong voluntary contraction may show changes in the configuration of the *M wave*(s) compared to the results of identical studies of the rested neuromuscular junction as follows:
   a. *Repair of the decrement:* A diminution of the decrementing response seen with slow rates (2–5 Hz) of *repetitive nerve stimulation.*
   b. *Increment after exercise:* An increase in the amplitude associated with an increase in the area of the M wave elicited by a single supramaximal stimulus. *Facilitation* should be distinguished from pseudofacilitation. *Pseudofacilitation* occurs in normal subjects with *repetitive nerve stimulation* at high (20–50 Hz) rates or after strong volitional contraction, and probably reflects a reduction in the temporal dispersion of the summation of a constant number of muscle fiber action potentials. *Pseudofacilitation* produces a response characterized by an increase in the amplitude of the successive M waves with a corresponding decrease in the duration of the M wave, resulting in no change in the area of the negative phase of the successive M waves.

far-field potential: Electric activity of biologic origin generated at a considerable distance from the recording electrodes. Use of the terms *near-field potential* and *far-field potential* is discouraged because all potentials in clinical neurophysiology are recorded at some distance from the generator and there is no consistent distinction between the two terms.

fasciculation: The random, spontaneous twitching of a group of muscle fibers or a motor unit. This twitch may produce movement of the overlying skin (limb), mucous membrane (tongue), or digits. The electric activity associated with the spontaneous contraction is called the *fasciculation potential*. See also *myokymia*. Historically the term *fibrillation* has been used to describe fine twitching of muscle fibers visible through the skin or mucous membrane, but this usage is no longer acceptable.

fasciculation potential: The electric potential often associated with a visible *fasciculation* which has the configuration of a *motor unit action potential* but which occurs spontaneously. Most commonly these potentials occur sporadically and are termed "single fasciculation potentials." Occasionally, the potentials occur as a grouped discharge and are termed a "brief repetitive discharge." The occurrence of repetitive firing of adjacent fasciculation potentials, when numerous, may produce an undulating movement of muscle (see *myokymia*). Use of the terms *benign fasciculation* and *malignant fasciculation* is discouraged. Instead, the configuration of the potentials, peak-to-peak amplitude, duration, number of phases, and stability of configuration, in addition to frequency of occurrence, should be specified.

fatigue: Generally, a state of depressed responsiveness resulting from protracted activity and requiring an appreciable recovery time. Muscle fatigue is a reduction in the force of contraction of muscle fibers and follows repeated voluntary contraction or direct electric stimulation of the muscle.

fiber density: (1) Anatomically, fiber density is a measure of the number of muscle or nerve fibers per unit area. (2) In *single fiber electromyography*, the fiber density is the mean number of *muscle fiber action potentials* fulfilling amplitude and rise time criteria belonging to one motor unit within the recording area of the *single fiber needle electrode* encountered during a systematic search in the weakly, voluntarily contracted muscle. See also *single fiber electromyography, single fiber needle electrode*.

fibrillation: The spontaneous contractions of individual muscle fibers that are not visible through the skin. This term has been used loosely in electromyography for the preferred term, *fibrillation potential*.

fibrillation potential: The electric activity associated with a spontaneously contracting (fibrillating) muscle fiber. It is the action potential of a single muscle fiber. The action potentials may occur spontaneously or after movement of the needle electrode. The potentials usually fire at a constant rate, although a small proportion fire irregularly. Classically, the potentials are biphasic spikes of short duration (usually less than 5 ms) with an initial positive phase and a peak-to-peak amplitude of less than 1 mV. When recorded with concentric or monopolar needle electrodes, the firing rate has a wide range (1–50 Hz) and often decreases just before cessation of an individual discharge. A high-pitched regular sound is associated with the discharge of fibrillation potentials and has been described in the old literature as "rain on a tin roof." In addition to this classic form of fibrillation potentials, *positive* *sharp waves* may also be recorded from fibrillating muscle fibers when the potential arises from an area immediately adjacent to the needle electrode.

firing pattern: Qualitative and quantitative descriptions of the sequence of discharge of potential waveforms recorded from muscle or nerve.

firing rate: Frequency of repetition of a potential. The relationship of the frequency to the occurrence of other potentials and the force of muscle contraction may be described. See also *discharge frequency*.

frequency: Number of complete cycles of a repetitive waveform in one second. Measured in *hertz* (Hz) or *cycles per second* (cps or c/s).

frequency analysis: Determination of the range of frequencies composing a potential waveform, with a measurement of the absolute or relative amplitude of each component frequency.

full interference pattern: See *interference pattern*.

functional refractory period: See *refractory period*.

G1, G2: Synonymous with *Grid 1, Grid 2,* and newer terms, *Input Terminal 1, Input Terminal 2.* See *recording electrode*.

"giant" motor unit action potential: Use of term discouraged. It refers to a *motor unit action potential* with a peak-to-peak amplitude and duration much greater than the range recorded in corresponding muscles in normal subjects of similar age. Quantitative measurements of amplitude and duration are preferable.

Grid 1: Synonymous with *G1, Input Terminal 1,* or *active* or *exploring electrode.* See *recording electrode*.

Grid 2: Synonymous with *G2, Input Terminal 2,* or *reference electrode.* See *recording electrode*.

ground electrode: An electrode connected to the patient and to a large conducting body (such as the earth) used as a common return for an electric circuit and as an arbitrary zero potential reference point.

grouped discharge: The term has been used historically to describe three phenomena: (1) irregular, voluntary grouping of *motor unit action potentials* as seen in a tremulous muscular contraction, (2) involuntary grouping of *motor unit action potentials* as seen in *myokymia*, (3) general term to describe repeated firing of *motor unit action potentials*. See preferred term, *repetitive discharge*.

H reflex: Abbreviation or Hoffmann reflex. See *H wave*.

H response: See preferred term *H wave*.

H wave: A compound muscle action potential having a consistent latency evoked regularly, when present, from a muscle by an electric stimulus to the nerve. It is regularly found only in a limited group of physiologic extensors, particularly the calf muscles. The H wave is most easily obtained with the cathode positioned proximal to the anode. Compared with the maximum amplitude *M wave* of the same muscle, the H wave has a smaller amplitude, a longer latency, and a lower optimal stimulus intensity. The latency is longer with more distal sites of stimulation. A stimulus intensity sufficient to elicit a maximal amplitude M wave reduces or abolishes the H wave. The H wave is thought to be due to a spinal reflex, the Hoffmann reflex, with electric stimulation of afferent fibers in the mixed nerve to the muscle and activation of motor neurons to the muscle through a monosynaptic connection in the spinal cord. The reflex and wave are named in honor of Hoffmann's description (1918). Compare the *F wave*.

habituation: Decrease in size of a reflex motor response to an afferent stimulus when the latter is repeated, especially at regular and recurring short intervals.

hertz: (Hz) Unit of frequency equal to *cycles per second*.

Hoffmann reflex: See *H wave*.

hyperpolarization: See *polarization*.

Hz: See *hertz*.

increased insertion activity: See *insertion activity*.

increment after exercise: See *facilitation*.

incremental response: See preferred term, *incrementing response*.

incrementing response: A reproducible increase in amplitude and/or area of successive responses (M wave) to *repetitive nerve stimulation*. The rate of stimulation and the number of stimuli should be specified. An incrementing response is commonly seen in two situations. First, in normal subjects the configuration of the M wave may change with repetitive nerve stimulation so that the amplitude progressively increases as the duration decreases, but the area of the M wave remains the same. This phenomenon is termed *pseudofacilitation*. Second, in disorders of neuromuscular transmission, the configuration of the M wave may change with repetitive nerve stimulation so that the amplitude progressively increases as the duration remains the same or increases, and the area of the M wave increases. This phenomenon is termed *facilitation*. Contrast with *decrementing response*.

indifferent electrode: Synonymous with *reference electrode*. Use of term discouraged. See *recording electrode*.

inhibitory postsynaptic potential (IPSP): A local graded hyperpolarization of a neuron in response to activation at a synapse by a nerve terminal. Contrast with *excitatory postsynaptic potential*.

injury potential: The potential difference between a normal region of the surface of a nerve or muscle and a region that has been injured; also called a "demarcation potential." The injury potential approximates the potential across the membrane because the injured surface is almost at the potential of the inside of the cell.

Input Terminal 1: The input terminal of the differential amplifier at which negativity, relative to the other input terminal, produces an upward deflection on the graphic display. Synonymous with *active* or *exploring electrode* (or older term, *Grid 1*). See *recording electrode*.

Input Terminal 2: The input terminal of the differential amplifer at which negativity, relative to the other input terminal, produces a downward deflection on the graphic display. Synonymous with *reference electrode* (or older term, *Grid 2*). See *recording electrode*.

insertion activity: Electric activity caused by insertion or movement of a needle electrode. The amount of the activity may be described as normal, reduced, increased (prolonged), with a description of the waveform and repetitive rate.

interdischarge interval: Time between consecutive discharges of the same potential. Measurements should be made between the corresponding points on each waveform.

interference: Unwanted electric activity arising outside the system being studied.

interference pattern: Electric activity recorded from a muscle with a needle electrode during maximal voluntary effort. A *full interference pattern* implies that no individual *motor unit action potentials* can be clearly identified. A *reduced interference pattern (intermediate interference pattern)* is one in which some of the individual MUAPs may be identified while other individual MUAPs cannot be identified because of overlap. The term *discrete activity* is used to describe the electric activity recorded when each of several different MUAPs can be identified. The term *single unit pattern* is used to describe a single MUAP, firing at a rapid rate (should be specified) during maximum voluntary effort. The force of contraction associated with the interference pattern should be specified. See also *recruitment pattern*.

intermediate interference pattern: See *interference pattern*.

International 10–20 System: A system of electrode placement on the scalp in which electrodes are placed either 10% or 20% of the total distance between the nasion and inion in the sagittal plane, and between right and left preauricular points in the coronal plane.

interpeak interval: Difference between the peak latencies of two components of a waveform.

interpotential interval: Time between two different potentials. Measurement should be made between the corresponding parts on each waveform.

involuntary activity: *Motor unit potentials* that are not under voluntary control. The condition under which they occur would be described, for example, spontaneous or reflex potentials and, if elicited by a stimulus, the nature of the stimulus. Contrast with *spontaneous activity*.

IPSP: See *inhibitory postsynaptic potential*.

irregular potential: See preferred term, *serrated action potential*.

iterative discharge: See preferred term, *repetitive discharge*.

jitter: Synonymous with "single fiber electromyographic jitter." Jitter is the variability with consecutive discharges of the *interpotential interval* between two muscle fiber action potentials belonging to the same motor unit. It is usually expressed quantitatively as the mean value of the difference between the interpotential intervals of successive discharges (the mean consecutive difference, MCD). Under certain conditions, jitter is expressed as the mean value of the difference between interpotential intervals arranged in the order of decreasing interdischarge intervals (the mean sorted difference, MSD).

Jolly test: A technique described by Jolly (1895), who applied an electric current to excite a motor nerve while recording the force of muscle contraction. Harvey and Masland (1941) refined the technique by recording the M wave evoked by repetitive, supramaximal nerve stimulation to detect a defect of neuromuscular transmission. use of the term is discouraged. See preferred term, *repetitive nerve stimulation*.

late component (of a motor unit action potential): See preferred term, *satellite potential*.

late response: A general term used to describe an evoked potential having a longer latency than the *M wave*. See *A wave, F wave, H wave, T wave*.

latency: Interval between the onset of a stimulus and the onset of a response. Thus the term *onset latency* is a tautology and should not be used. The *peak latency* is the interval between the onset of a stimulus and a specified peak of the evoked potential.

latency of activation: The time required for an electric stimulus to depolarize a nerve fiber (or bundle of fibers as in a nerve trunk) beyond threshold and to initiate a regenerative action potential in the fiber(s). This time is usually on the order of 0.1 ms or less. An equivalent term now rarely used in the literature is the "utilization time."

latent period: See synonym, *latency*.

linked potential: See preferred term, *satellite potential*.

long-latency SEP: That portion of a *somatosensory evoked potential* normally occurring at a time greater than 100 ms after stimulation of a nerve in the upper extremity at the wrist or the lower extremity at the knee or ankle.

M response: See synonym, *M wave*.

M wave: A *compound action potential* evoked from a muscle by a single electric stimulus to its motor nerve. By convention, the M wave elicited by supramaximal stimulation is used for motor nerve conduction studies. Ideally, the recording electrodes should be placed so that the initial deflection of the evoked potential is negative. The *latency*, commonly called the *motor latency*, is the latency (ms) to the onset of the first phase (positive or negative) of the M wave. The amplitude (MV) is the baseline-to-peak amplitude of the first negative phase, unless otherwise specified. The *duration* (ms) refers to the duration of the first negative phase, unless otherwise specified. Normally, the configuration of the M wave (usually biphasic) is quite stable with repeated stimuli at slow rates (1–5 Hz). See *repetitive nerve stimulation*.

macro motor unit action potential (macro MUAP): The average electric activity of that part of an anatomic motor unit that is within the recording range of a *macro-EMG electrode*. The potential is characterized by its consistent appearance when the small recording surface of the macro-EMG electrode is positioned to record action potentials from one muscle fiber. The following parameters can be specified quantitatively: (1) maximal peak-to-peak amplitude, (2) area contained under the waveform, (3) number of phases.

macro MUAP: See *macro motor unit action potential*.

macroelectromyography (macro-EMG): General term referring to the technique and conditions that approximate recording of all *muscle fiber action potentials* arising from the same motor unit.

macro-EMG: See *macroelectromyography*.

macro-EMG needle electrode: A modified *single fiber electromyography* electrode insulated to within 15 mm from the tip and with a small recording surface (25 μm in diameter) 7.5 mm from the tip.

malignant fasciculation: Use of term discouraged to describe a firing pattern of fasciculation potentials. Historically, the term was used to describe large, polyphasic fasciculation potentials firing at a slow rate. This pattern has been seen in progressive motor neuron disease, but the relationship is not exclusive. See *fasciculation potential*.

maximal stimulus: See *stimulus*.

maximum conduction velocity: See *conduction velocity*.

MCD: Abbreviation for mean consecutive difference. See *jitter*.

mean consecutive difference (MCD): See *jitter*.

membrane instability: Tendency of a cell membrane to depolarize spontaneously, with mechanical irritation, or after voluntary activation.

MEPP: Miniature end-plate potential.

microneurography: The technique of recording peripheral nerve action potentials in man by means of intraneural electrodes.

midlatency SEP: That portion of the waveforms of a *somatosensory evoked potential* normally occurring within 25–100 ms after stimulation of a nerve in the upper extremity at the wrist, within 40–100 ms after stimulation of a nerve in the lower extremity at the knee, and within 50–100 ms after stimulation of a nerve in the lower extremity at the ankle.

miniature end-plate potential (MEPP): The postsynaptic muscle fiber potentials produced through the spontaneous release of individual quanta of acetylcholine from the presynaptic axon terminals. As recorded with conventional concentric needle electrodes inserted in the end-plate zone, such potentials are characteristically monophasic, negative, or relatively short duration (less than 5 ms) and generally less than 20 μV in amplitude.

MNCV: Abbreviation for *motor nerve conduction velocity*. See *conduction velocity*.

monophasic action potential: See *action potential* with one phase.

monophasic end-plate activity: See *end-plate activity (monophasic)*.

monoplar needle recording electrode: A solid wire, usually stainless steel, usually coated, except at its tip, with an insulating material. Variations in voltage between the tip of the needle (active or exploring electrode) positioned in a muscle and a conductive plate on the skin surface or a bare needle in subcutaneous tissue (reference electrode) are measured. By convention, this recording condition is referred to as a monopolar needle electrode recording. It should be emphasized, however, that potential differences are always recorded between two electrodes.

motor latency: Interval between the onset of a stimulus and the onset of the resultant *compound muscle action·potential (M wave)*. The term may be qualified, as "proximal motor latency" or "distal motor latency," depending on the relative position of the stimulus.

motor nerve conduction velocity (MNCV): See *conduction velocity*.

motor point: The point over a muscle where a contraction of a muscle may be elicited by a minimal-intensity, short-duration electric stimulus. The motor point corresponds anatomically to the location of the terminal portion of the motor nerve fibers (end-plate zone).

motor response: (1) The compound muscle action potential (*M wave*) recorded over a muscle with stimulation of the nerve to the muscle, (2) the muscle twitch or contraction elicited by stimulation of the nerve to a muscle, (3) the muscle twitch elicited by the muscle stretch reflex.

motor unit: The anatomic unit of an anterior horn cell, its axon, the neuromuscular junctions, and all of the muscle fibers innervated by the axon.

motor unit action potential (MUAP): Action potential reflecting the electric activity of a single anatomic motor unit. It is the compound action potential of those muscle fibers within the recording range of an electrode. With voluntary muscle contraction, the action potential is characterized by its consistent appearance with, and relationship to, the force of contraction. The following parameters should be specified, quantitatively if possible, after the recording electrode is placed so as to minimize the *rise time* (which by convention should be less than 0.5 ms):
1. Configuration
   a. *Amplitude*, peak-to-peak (μV or mV).

    b. *Duration*, total (ms).

    c. Number of *phases* (monophasic, biphasic, triphasic, tetraphasic, polyphasic).

    d. Sign of each *phase* (negative, positive).

    e. Number of *turns*.

    f. Variation of shape, if any, with consecutive discharges.

    g. Presence of *satellite* (linked) *potentials*, if any.

2. *Recruitment* characteristics

    a. Threshold of activation (first recruited, low threshold, high threshold).

    b. *Onset frequency* (Hz).

    c. *Recruitment frequency* (Hz) or *recruitment interval* (ms) of individual potentials.

Descriptive terms implying diagnostic significance are not recommended, e.g., "myopathic," "neuropathic," "regeneration," "nascent," "giant," BSAP, and BSAPP. See *polyphasic action potential, serrated action potential*.

motor unit fraction: See *scanning EMG*.

motor unit potential (MUP): See synonym, *motor unit action potential*.

motor unit territory: The area in a muscle over which the muscle fibers belonging to an individual motor unit are distributed.

movement artifact: See *artifact*.

MSD: Abbreviation for mean sorted difference. See *jitter*.

MUAP: See *motor unit action potential*.

multielectrode: See *multilead electrode*.

multilead electrode: Three or more insulated wires inserted through a common metal cannula with their bared tips at an aperture in the cannula and flush with the outer circumference of the cannula. The arrangement of the bare tips relative to the axis of the cannula and the distance between each tip should be specified.

multiple discharge: Four or more *motor unit action potentials* of the same form and nearly the same amplitude occurring consistently in the same relationship to one another and generated by this same axon or muscle fiber. See *double* and *triple discharge*.

multiplet: See *multiple discharge*.

MUP: Abbreviation for *motor unit potential*. See preferred term, *motor unit action potential*.

muscle action potential: Term commonly used to refer to a *compound muscle action potential*.

muscle cramp: Most commonly, an involuntary, painful muscle *contraction* associated with electric activity (See *cramp discharge*). Muscle cramps may be accompanied by other types of *repetitive discharges*, and in some metabolic myopathies (McArdle's disease) the painful, contracted muscles may show *electric silence*.

muscle fiber action potential: Action potential recorded from a single muscle fiber.

muscle fiber conduction velocity: The speed of propagation of a single *muscle fiber action potential*, usually expressed as meters per second. The muscle fiber conduction velocity is usually less than most nerve conduction velocities, varies with the rate of discharge of the muscle fiber, and requires special techniques for measurement.

muscle stretch reflex: Activation of a muscle follows stretch of the muscle, for example, by percussion of a muscle tendon.

myoedema: Focal muscle contraction produced by muscle percussion and not associated with propagated electric activity; may be seen in hypothyroidism (myxedema) and chronic malnutrition.

myokymia: Continuous quivering or undulating movement of surface and overlying skin and mucous membrane associated with spontaneous, repetitive discharge of *motor unit potentials*. See *myokymic discharge, fasciculation,* and *fasciculation potential*.

myokymic discharge: *Motor unit action potentials* that fire repetitively and may be associated with clinical myokymia. Two firing patterns have been described. Commonly, the discharge is a brief, repetitive firing of single units for a short period (up to a few seconds) at a uniform rate (2 – 60 Hz) followed by a short period (up to a few seconds) of silence, with repetition of the same sequence for a particular potential. Less commonly, the potential recurs continuously at a fairly uniform firing rate (1 – 5 Hz). Myokymic discharges are a subclass of *grouped discharges* and *repetitive discharges*.

myopathic motor unit potential: Use of term discouraged. It has been used to refer to low-amplitude, short-duration, polyphasic *motor unit action potentials*. The term incorrectly implies specific diagnostic significance of a motor unit potential configuration. See *motor unit action potential*.

myopathic recruitment: Use of term discouraged. It has been used to describe an increase in the number of and firing rate of *motor unit action potentials* compared with normal for the strength of muscle contraction.

myotonia: The clinical observation of delayed relaxation of muscle after voluntary contraction or percussion. The delayed relaxation may be electrically silent, or accompanied by propagated electric activity, such as *myotonic discharge, complex repetitive discharge,* or *neuromyotonid discharge*.

myotonic discharge: Repetitive discharge at rates of 20 – 80 Hz are of two types: (1) biphasic (positive-negative) spike potentials less than 5 ms in duration resembling *fibrillation potentials*. (2) positive waves of 5 – 20 ms in duration resembling *positive sharp waves*. Both potential forms are recorded after needle insertion, after voluntary muscle contraction or after muscle percussion, and are due to independent, repetitive discharges of single muscle fibers. The amplitude and frequency of the potentials must both wax and wane to be identified as myotonic discharges. This change produces a characteristic musical sound in the audio display of the electromyograph due to the corresponding change in pitch, which has been likened to the sound of a dive bomber. Contrast with *waning discharge.*

myotonic potential: See preferred term, *myotonic discharge.*

NAP: Abbreviation for nerve action potential. See *compound nerve action potential.*

nascent motor unit potential: From the Latin "nascens," to be born. Use of term is discouraged as it incorrectly implies diagnostic significance of a motor unit potential configuration. Term has been used to refer to very-low-amplitude, long-duration, highly polyphasic motor unit potentials observed during early states of reinnervation of muscle. See *motor unit action potential.*

NCS: See *nerve conduction studies.*

NCV: Abbreviation for *nerve conduction velocity.* See *conduction velocity.*

near constant frequency trains: See preferred term, *complex repetitive discharge.*

near-field potential: Electric activity of biologic origin generated near the recording electrodes. Use of the terms *near-field potential* and *far-field potential* is discouraged because all potentials in clinical neurophysiology are recorded at some distance from the generator and there is no consistent distinction between the two terms.

needle electrode: An electrode for recording or stimulating, shaped like a needle. See specific electrodes: *bifilar (bipolar) needle recording electrode, concentric needle electrode, macro-EMG needle electrode, monopolar needle recording electrode, multilead electrode, single fiber needle electrode,* and *stimulating electrode.*

nerve action potential (NAP): Strictly defined, refers to an action potential recorded from a single nerve fiber. The term is commonly used to refer to the compound nerve action potential. See *compound nerve action potential.*

nerve conduction studies (NCS): Synonymous with *electroneurography.* Recording and analysis of electric *waveforms* of biologic origin elicited in response to electric or physiologic *stimuli.* Generally *nerve conduction studies* refers to studies of waveforms generated in the peripheral nervous system, whereas *evoked potential studies* refers to studies of waveforms generated in both the peripheral and central nervous system. The waveforms recorded in *nerve conduction studies* are *compound sensory nerve action potentials.* The *compound sensory nerve action potentials* are generally referred to as *sensory nerve action potentials.* The *compound muscle action potentials* are generally referred to by letters that have historical origins: *M wave, F wave, H wave, T wave, A wave, R1 wave,* and *R2 wave.* It is possible under standardized conditions to establish normal ranges of amplitude, duration, and latencies of these *evoked potentials* and to calculate the maximum conduction velocity of sensory and motor nerves.

nerve conduction velocity (NCV): Loosely used to refer to the maximum nerve conduction velocity. See *conduction velocity*.

nerve fiber action potential: Action potential recorded from a single nerve fiber.

nerve potential: Equivalent to *nerve action potential*. Also commonly, but inaccurately, used to refer to the biphasic form of *end-plate activity*. The latter use is incorrect because muscle fibers, not nerve fibers, are the source of these potentials.

nerve trunk action potential: See preferred term, *compound nerve action potential*

neurapraxia: Failure of nerve conduction, usually reversible, due to metabolic or microstructural abnormalities without disruption of the axon. See preferred electrodiagnostic term, *conduction block*.

neuromyotonia: Clinical syndrome of continuous muscle fiber activity manifested as continuous muscle rippling and stiffness. The accompanying electric activity may be intermittent or continuous. Terms used to describe related clinical syndromes are continuous muscle fiber activity, Isaac syndrome, Isaac-Merton syndrome, quantal squander syndrome, generalized myokymia, pseudomyotonia, normocalcemic tetany, and neurotonia.

neuromyotonic discharge: Bursts of *motor unit action potentials* which originate in the motor axons firing at high rates (150–300 Hz) for a few seconds, and which often start and stop abruptly. The amplitude of the response typically wanes. Discharges may occur spontaneously or be initiated by needle movement, voluntary effort and ischemia, or percussion of a nerve. These discharges should be distinguished from *myotonic discharges* and *complex repetitive discharges*.

neuropathic motor unit potential: Use of term discouraged. It was used to refer to abnormally high-amplitude, long-duration, polyphasic *motor unit action potentials*. The term incorrectly implies a specific diagnostic significance of a motor unit potential configuration. See *motor unit action potential*.

neuropathic recruitment: Use of term discouraged. It has been used to describe a recruitment pattern with a decreased number of *motor unit action potentials* firing at a rapid rate. See preferred terms, *reduced interference pattern, discrete activity, single unit pattern*.

neurotmesis: Partial or complete severance of a nerve, with disruption of the axons, their myelin sheaths, and the supporting connective tissue, resulting in degeneration of the axons distal to the injury site.

noise: Strictly defined, potentials produced by electrodes, cables, amplifier, or storage media and unrelated to the potentials of biologic origin. The term has been used loosely to refer to one form of *end-plate activity*.

onset frequency: The lowest stable frequency of firing for a single *motor unit action potential* that can be voluntarily maintained by a subject.

onset latency: Tautology. See *latency*.

order of activation: The sequence of appearance of different *motor unit action potentials* with increasing strength of voluntary contraction. See *recruitment*.

orthodromic: Propagation of an impulse in the direction the same as physiologic conduction, for instance, conduction along motor nerve fibers towards the muscle and conduction along sensory nerve fibers towards the spinal cord. Contrast with *antidromic*.

paired discharge: Two action potentials occurring consistently in the same relationship with each other. Contrast with *double discharge*.

paired response: Use of term discouraged. See preferred term, *paired discharge*.

paired stimuli: Two consecutive stimuli. The time interval between the two stimuli and the intensity of each stimulus should be specified. The first stimulus is called the *conditioning stimulus* and the second stimulus is the *test stimulus*. The *conditioning stimulus* may modify the tissue excitability, which can then be evaluated by the response to the *test stimulus*.

parasite potential: See preferred term, *satellite potential*.

peak latency: Interval between the onset of a stimulus and a specified peak of the evoked potential.

phase: That portion of a *wave* between the departure from, and the return to, the *baseline*.

polarization: As used in neurophysiology, the presence of an electric potential difference across an excitable cell membrane. The potential across the membrane of a cell when it is not excited by an input or spontaneously active is termed the *resting potential*; it is at a stationary nonequilibrium state with regard to the electric potential difference across the membrane. *Depolarization* describes a reduction in the magnitude of the polarization toward the zero potential while *hyperpolarization* refers to an increase in the magnitude of the polarization relative to the resting potential. *Repolarization* describes an increase in polarization from the depolarized state toward, but not above, the normal resting potential.

polyphasic action potential: An *action potential* having five or more phases. See *phase*. Contrast with *serrated action potential*.

positive sharp wave: A biphasic, positive-negative *action potential* initiated by needle movement and recurring in a uniform, regular pattern at a rate of 1–50 Hz; the discharge frequency may decrease slightly just before cessation of discharge. The initial positive deflection is rapid (<1 ms), its duration is usually less than 5 ms, and the amplitude is up to 1 mV. The negative phase is of low amplitude, with a duration of 10–100 ms. A sequence of positive sharp waves is commonly referred to as a *train of positive sharp waves*. Positive sharp waves can be recorded from the damaged area of fibrillating muscle fibers. Its configuration may result from the position of the needle electrode which is felt to be adjacent to the depolarized segment of a muscle fiber injured by the electrode. Note that the positive sharp waveform is not specific for muscle fiber damage. *Motor unit action potentials* and potentials in *myotonic discharges* may have the configuration of positive sharp waves.

positive wave: Loosely defined, the term refers to a positive sharp wave. See *positive sharp wave*.

postactivation depression: A descriptive term indicating a reduction in the amplitude associated with a reduction in the area of the M wave(s) in response to a single *stimulus* or *train of stimuli* which occurs a few minutes after a brief (30–60 s), strong voluntary contraction or a period of *repetitive nerve stimulation* that produces *tetanus*. *Postactivation exhaustion* refers to the cellular mechanisms responsible for the observed phenomenon of *postactivation depression*.

postactivation exhaustion: A reduction in the safety factor (margin) of neuromuscular transmission after sustained activity of the neuromuscular junction. The changes in the configuration of the M wave due to *postactivation exhaustion* are referred to as *postactivation depression*.

postactivation facilitation: See *facilitation*.

postactivation potentiation: Refers to the increase in the force of contraction (mechanical response) after *tetanus* or strong voluntary contraction. Contrast *postactivation facilitation*.

posttetanic facilitation: See *facilitation*.

posttetanic potentiation: The incrementing mechanical response of muscle during and after *repetitive nerve stimulation* without a change in the amplitude of the action potential. In spinal cord physiology, the term has been used to describe enhancement of excitability or reflex outflow of the central nervous system following a long period of high-frequency stimulation. This phenomenon has been described in the mammalian spinal cord, where it lasts minutes or even hours.

potential: A physical variable created by differences in charges, measurable in volts, that exists between two points. Most biologically produced potentials arise from the difference in charge between two sides of a cell membrane. See *polarization*.

potentiation: Physiologically, the enhancement of a response. Some authors use the term *potentiation* to describe the incrementing mechanical response of muscle elicited by *repetitive nerve stimulation*, that is, *posttetanic potentiation*, and the term *facilitation* to describe the incrementing electric response elicited by *repetitive nerve stimulation*, that is, *postactivation facilitation*.

prolonged insertion activity: See *insertion activity*.

propagation velocity of a muscle fiber: The speed of transmission of a muscle fiber action potential.

proximal latency: See *motor latency* and *sensory latency*.

pseudofacilitation: See *facilitation*.

pseudomyotonic discharge: Use of term discouraged. It has been used to refer to different phenomena, including (1) *complex repetitive discharges*, and (2) *repetitive discharges* that do not wax or wane in both frequency and amplitude, and end abruptly. These latter discharges may be seen in disorders such as polymyositis in addition to disorders with *myotonic discharges*. See preferred term, *waning discharge*.

pseudopolyphasic action potential: Use of term discouraged. See preferred term, *serrated action potential*.

R1, R2 waves: See *blink responses*.

recording electrode: Device used to record electric potential difference. All electric recordings require two *electrodes*. The recording electrode close to the source of the activity to be recorded is called the *active* or *exploring electrode*, and the other recording electrode is called the *reference electrode*. Active electrode is synonymous with *Input Terminal 1* (or older terms *Grid 1* and *G1*) and the reference electrode with *Input Terminal 2* (or older terms *Grid 2* and *G2*).

In some recordings, it is not certain which electrode is closer to the source of the biologic activity, that is, recording with a *bifilar (bipolar) needle recording electrode*. In this situation, it is convenient to refer to one electrode as Input Electrode 1 and the other electrode as Input Electrode 2.

By present convention, a potential difference that is negative at the active electrode (Input Terminal 1) relative to the reference electrode (Input Terminal 2) causes an upward deflection on the oscilloscope screen. The term "monopolar recording" is not recommended, because all recording requires two electrodes; however, it is commonly used to describe the use of an intramuscular needle exploring electrode in combination with a surface disk or subcutaneous needle reference electrode. A similar combination of needle electrodes has been used to record nerve activity and also has been referred to as "monopolar recording."

recruitment: The successive activation of the same and additional motor units with increasing strength of voluntary muscle contraction. See *motor unit action potential*.

recruitment frequency: Firing rate of a *motor unit action potential (MUAP)* when a different MUAP first appears with gradually increasing strength of voluntary muscle contraction. This parameter is essential to assessment of *recruitment pattern*.

recruitment interval: The *interdischarge interval* between two consecutive discharges of a *motor unit action potential (MUAP)* when a different MUAP first appears with gradually increasing strength of voluntary muscle contraction. The reciprocal of the recruitment interval is the *recruitment frequency*.

recruitment pattern: A qualitative and/or quantitative description of the sequence of appearance of *motor unit action potentials* with increasing strength of voluntary muscle contraction. The *recruitment frequency* and *recruitment interval* are two quantitative measures commonly used. See *interference pattern* for qualitative terms commonly used.

reduced insertion activity: See *insertion activity*.

reduced interference pattern: See *interference pattern*.

reference electrode: See *recording electrode*.

reflex: A stereotyped *motor response* elicited by a sensory *stimulus*.

refractory period: The *absolute refractory period* is the period following an *action potential* during which no stimulus, however strong, evokes a further response. the *relative refractory period* is the period following an *action potential* during which a stimulus must be abnormally large to evoke a second response. The *functional refractory period* is the period following an *action potential* during which a second *action potential* cannot yet excite the given region.

regeneration motor unit potential: Use of term discouraged. See *motor unit action potential*.

relative refractory period: See *refractory period*.

repair of the decrement: See *facilitation*.

repetitive discharge: General term for the recurrence of an *action potential* with the same or nearly the same form. The term may refer to recurring potentials recorded in muscle at rest, during voluntary contraction, or in response to single nerve stimulus. See *double discharge, triple discharge, multiple discharge, myokymic discharge, myotonic discharge, complex repetitive discharge*.

repetitive nerve stimulation: The technique of repeated supramaximal stimulations of a nerve while recording M waves from muscles innervated by the nerve. The number of stimuli and the frequency of stimulation should be specified. Activation procedures performed prior to the test should be specified, for example, sustained voluntary contraction or contraction induced by nerve stimulation. If the test was performed after an activation procedure, the time elapsed after the activation procedure was completed should also be specified. The technique is commonly used to assess the integrity of neuromuscular transmission. For a description of specific patterns of responses, see the terms *incrementing response, decrementing response, facilitation,* and *postactivation depression*.

repolarization: See *polarization*.

residual latency: Refers to the calculated time difference between the measured distal latency of a motor nerve and the expected distal latency, calculated by dividing the distance between the stimulus cathode and the active recording electrode by the maximum conduction velocity measured in a more proximal segment of a nerve. The residual latency is due in part to neuromuscular transmission time and to slowing of conduction in terminal axons due to decreasing diameter and the presence of unmyelinated segments.

response: Used to describe an activity elicited by a *stimulus*.

resting membrane potential: Voltage across the membrane of an excitable cell at rest. See *polarization*.

rheobase: See *strength-duration curve*.

rise time: The interval from the onset of a change of a potential to its peak. The method of measurement should be specified.

satellite potential: A small action potential separated from the main MUAP by an isoelectric interval and firing in a time-locked relationship to the main *action potential*. These potentials usually follow, but may precede, the main action potential. Also called *late component, parasite potential, linked potential,* and *coupled discharge* (less preferred terms).

scanning EMG: A technique by which an electromyographic electrode is advanced in defined steps through muscle while a separate *SFEMG* electrode is used to trigger both the oscilloscope sweep and the advancement device. This recording technique provides temporal and spatial information about the motor unit. Distinct maxima in the recorded activity are considered to be generated by muscle fibers innervated by a common branch of the axon. These groups of fibers form a *motor unit fraction*.

sea shell sound (sea shell roar or noise): Use of term discouraged. See *end-plate activity, monophasic*.

sensory delay: See preferred terms, *sensory latency* and *sensory peak latency*.

sensory latency: Interval between the onset of a stimulus and the onset of the *compound sensory nerve action potential*. This term has been loosely used to refer to the *sensory peak latency*. The term may be qualified as "proximal sensory latency" or "distal sensory latency," depending on the relative position of the stimulus.

sensory nerve action potential (SNAP): See *compound sensory nerve action potential*.

sensory nerve conduction velocity: See *conduction velocity*.

sensory peak latency: Interval between the onset of a *stimulus* and the peak of the negative phase of the *compound sensory nerve action* *potential*. Note that the term *latency* refers to the interval between the onset of a stimulus and the onset of a response.

sensory potential: Used to refer to the compound sensory nerve action potential. See *compound sensory nerve action potential*.

sensory response: Used to refer to a sensory evoked potential, for example, *compound sensory nerve action potential*.

SEP: See *somatosensory evoked potential*.

serrated action potential: An action potential waveform with several changes in direction (*turns*) which do not cross the baseline. This term is preferred to the terms *complex action potential* and *pseudopolyphasic action potential*. See also *turn* and *polyphasic action potential*.

SFEMG: See *single fiber electromyography*.

shock artifact: See *artifact*.

short-latency somatosensory evoked potential (SSEP): That portion of the waveforms of a *somatosensory evoked potential* normally occurring within 25 ms after stimulation of the median nerve in the upper extremity at the wrist, 40 ms after stimulation of the common peroneal nerve in the lower extremity at the knee, and 50 ms after stimulation of the posterior tibial nerve in the lower extremity at the ankle.

> **Median nerve SSEPs:** Normal short-latency response components to median nerve stimulation are designated $P\overline{9}$, $P\overline{11}$, $P\overline{13}$, $P\overline{14}$, $N\overline{20}$, and $P\overline{23}$ in records taken between scalp and noncephalic reference electrodes, and $N\overline{9}$, $N\overline{11}$, $N\overline{13}$, and $N\overline{14}$ in cervical spine-scalp derivation. It should be emphasized that potentials having opposite polarity but similar latency in spine-scalp and scalp-noncephalic reference derivations do not necessarily have identical generator sources.

> **Common peroneal nerve SSEPs:** Normal short-latency response components to common peroneal stimulation are designated $P\overline{27}$ and $N\overline{35}$ in records taken between scalp and noncephalic reference electrodes, and L3 and T12 from a cervical spine-scalp derivation.

> **Posterior tibial nerve SSEPs:** Normal short-latency response components to posterior tibial nerve stimulation are designated as the PF potential in the popliteal fossa, $P\overline{37}$ and $N\overline{45}$ waves in records taken between scalp and noncephalic reference electrode, and L3 and T12 potentials from a cervical spine-scalp derivation.

silent period: A pause in the electric activity of a muscle such as that seen after rapid unloading of a muscle.

single fiber electromyography (SFEMG): General term referring to the technique and conditions that permit recording of a single *muscle fiber action potential*. See *single fiber needle electrode* and *jitter*.

single fiber EMG: See *single fiber electromyography*.

single fiber needle electrode: A needle *electrode* with a small recording surface (usually 25 μm in diameter) permitting the recording of single muscle fiber action potentials between the active recording surface and the cannula. See *single fiber electromyography*.

single unit pattern: See *interference pattern*.

SNAP: Abbreviation for *sensory nerve action potential*. See *compound sensory nerve action potential*.

somatosensory evoked potentials (SEPs): Electric waveforms of biologic origin elicited by electric stimulation or physiologic activation of peripheral sensory fibers, for example, the median nerve, common peroneal nerve, or posterior tibial nerve. The normal SEP is a complex waveform with several components that are specified by polarity and average peak latency. The polarity and latency of individual components depend upon (1) subject variables, such as age, sex, (2) stimulus characteristics, such as intensity, rate of stimulation, and (3) recording parameters, such as amplifier time constants, electrode placement, electrode combinations. See *short-latency somatosensory evoked potentials*.

spike: (1) In cellular neurophysiology, a short-lived (usually in the range of 1–3 ms), all-or-none change in membrane potential that arises when a graded response passes a threshold. (2) The electric record of a nerve impulse or similar event in muscle or elsewhere. (3) In clinical EEG recordings, a wave with duration less than 80 ms (usually 15–80 ms).

spinal evoked potential: Electric waveforms of biologic origin recorded over the sacral, lumbar, thoracic, or cervical spine in response to electric stimulation or physiologic activation of peripheral sensory fibers. See preferred term, *somatosensory evoked potential*.

spontaneous activity: Electric activity recorded from muscle or nerve at rest after insertion activity has subsided and when there is no voluntary contraction or external stimulus. Compare with *involuntary activity*.

SSEP: See *short-latency somatosensory evoked potential*.

staircase phenomenon: The progressive increase in the force of a muscle contraction observed in response to continued low rates of direct or indirect muscle stimulation.

stigmatic electrode: Of historic interest. Used by Sherrington for *active* or *exploring electrode*.

stimulating electrode: Device used to apply electric current. All electric stimulation requires two electrodes; the negative terminal is termed the *cathode* and the positive terminal, the *anode*. By convention, the stimulating electrodes are called "bipolar" if they are encased or attached together. Stimulating electrodes are called "monopolar" if they are not encased or attached together. Electric stimulation for *nerve conduction studies* generally requires application of the cathode to produce depolarization of the nerve trunk fibers. If the anode is inadvertently placed between the cathode and the recording electrodes, a focal block of nerve conduction (*anodal block*) may occur and cause a technically unsatisfactory study.

stimulus: Any external agent, state, or change that is capable of influencing the activity of a cell, tissue, or organism. In clinical *nerve conduction studies*, an electric stimulus is generally applied to a nerve or muscle. The electric stimulus may be described in absolute terms or with respect to the evoked potential of the nerve or muscle. In absolute terms, the electric stimulus is defined by a duration (ms), a waveform (square, exponential, linear, etc.) and a strength or intensity measured in voltage (V) or current (mA). With respect to the evoked potential, the stimulus may be graded as subthreshold, threshold, submaximal, maximal, or supramaximal. A *threshold stimulus* is that stimulus just sufficient to produce a detectable response. Stimuli less than the threshold stimulus are termed *subthreshold*. The *maximal stimulus* is the stimulus intensity after which a further increase in the stimulus intensity causes no increase in the amplitude of the evoked potential. Stimuli of intensity below this level but above threshold are *submaximal*. Stimuli of intensity greater than the maximal stimulus are termed *supramaximal*. Ordinarily, supramaximal stimuli are used for nerve conduction studies. By convention, an electric stimulus of approximately 20 percent greater voltage/current than required for the maximal stimulus may be used for supramaximal stimulation. The frequency, number, and duration of a series of stimuli should be specified.

stimulus artifact: See *artifact*.

strength-duration curve: Graphic presentation of the relationship between the intensity (Y axis) and various durations (X axis) of the threshold electric stimulus for a muscle with the stimulating cathode positioned over the *motor point*. The *rheobase* is the intensity of an electric current of infinite duration necessary to produce a minimal visible twitch of a muscle when applied to the motor point. In clinical practice, a duration of 300 ms is used to determine the rheobase. The *chronaxie* is the time required for an electric current twice the *rheobase* to elicit the first visible muscle twitch.

submaximal stimulus: See *stimulus*.

subthreshold stimulus: See *stimulus*.

supramaximal stimulus: See *stimulus*.

surface electrode: Conducting device for stimulating or recording placed on a skin surface. The material (metal, fabric), configuration (disk, ring), size, and separation should be specified. See *electrode* (*ground, recording, stimulating*).

synchronized fibrillation: See preferred term, *complex repetitive discharge*.

T wave: A compound action potential evoked from a muscle by rapid stretch of its tendon, as part of the muscle stretch reflex.

temporal dispersion: Relative desynchronization of components of a compound action potential due to different rates of conduction of each synchronously evoked component from the stimulation point to the recording electrode.

terminal latency: Synonymous with preferred term, *distal latency*. See *motor latency*, and *sensory latency*.

test stimulus: See *paired stimuli*.

tetanic contraction: The contraction produced in a muscle through repetitive maximal direct or indirect stimulation at a sufficiently high frequency to produce a smooth summation of successive maximum twitches. The term may also be applied to maximum voluntary contractions in which the firing frequencies of most or all of the component motor units are sufficiently high that successive twitches of individual motor units fuse smoothly. Their tensions all combine to produce a steady, smooth maximum contraction of the whole muscle.

tetanus: The continuous contraction of muscle caused by repetitive stimulation or discharge of nerve or muscle. Contrast *tetany*.

tetany: A clinical syndrome manifested by muscle twitching, cramps, and carpal and pedal spasm. These clinical signs are manifestations of peripheral and central nervous system nerve irritability from several causes. In these conditions, *repetitive discharges (double discharge, triple discharge, multiple discharge)* occur frequently with voluntary activation of *motor unit action potentials* or may appear as *spontaneous activity* and are enhanced by systemic alkalosis or local ischemia.

tetraphasic action potential: *Action potential* with four phases.

threshold: The level at which a clear and abrupt transition occurs from one state to another. The term is generally used to refer to the voltage level at which an *action potential* is initiated in a single axon or a group of axons. It is also operationally defined as the intensity that produced a response in about 50 percent of equivalent trials.

threshold stimulus: See *stimulus*.

train of positive sharp waves: See *positive sharp wave*.

train of stimuli: A group of stimuli. The duration of the group or the number of stimuli and the frequency of the stimuli should be specified.

triphasic action potential: *Action potential* with three phases.

triple discharge: Three *motor unit action potentials* of the same form and nearly the same amplitude, occurring consistently in the same relationship to one another and generated by this same axon or muscle fiber. The interval between the second and the third action potential often exceeds that between the first two, and both are usually in the range of 2–20 ms.

triplet: See *triple discharge*.

turn: Point of change in direction in the waveform and the magnitude of the voltage change following the turning point. It is not necessary that the voltage change passes through the baseline. The minimal excursion required to constitute a change should be specified.

unipolar needle electrode: See synonym, *monopolar needle recording electrode*.

utilization time: See preferred term, *latency of activation*.

VEPs: See *visual evoked potentials*.

VERs: Abbreviation for *visual evoked responses*. See *visual evoked potentials*.

visual evoked potentials (VEPs): Electric waveforms of biologic origin are recorded over the cerebrum and elicited by light stimuli. VEPs are classified by stimulus rate as transient or steady state VEPs, and can be further divided by presentation mode. The normal transient VEP to checkerboard pattern reversal or shift has a major positive occipital peak at about 100 ms (P100), often preceded by a negative peak (N75). The precise range of normal values for the latency and amplitude of P100 depends on several factors: (1) subject variables, such as age, sex, and visual acuity, (2) stimulus characteristics, such as type of stimulator, full-field or half-field stimulation, check size, contrast, and luminescence, and (3) recording parameters, such as placement and combination of recording electrodes.

visual evoked responses (VERs): See *visual evoked potentials*.

volitional activity: See *voluntary activity*.

voltage: Potential difference between two recording sites.

volume conduction: Spread of current from a potential source through a conducting medium, such as the body tissues.

voluntary activity: In electromyography, the electric activity recorded from a muscle with consciously controlled muscle contraction. The effort made to contract the muscle should be specified relative to that of a corresponding normal muscle, for example, minimal, moderate, or maximal. If the recording remains isoelectric during the attempted contraction of the muscle and artifacts have been excluded, it can be concluded that there is no voluntary activity.

waning discharge: General term referring to a *repetitive discharge* that gradually decreases in frequency or amplitude before cessation. Contrast with *myotonic discharge*.

wave: An undulating line constituting a graphic representation of a change, for instance, a changing electric potential difference. See *A wave, F wave, H wave,* and *M wave*.

waveform: The shape of a *wave*. The term is often used synonymously with wave.

ELECTROENCEPHALOGRAPHS*

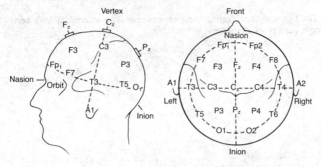

L.F.

L.P.

L.O.

R.F.

R.P.

R.O.

*From: Mancall, EL: Alpers and Mancall's Essentials of the Neurologic Examination, ed 2. FA Davis, Philadelphia, 1982.

The upper figure shows the placement of EEG electrodes and the names used for each electrode. The lower figure shows a normal EEG with a normal 8 to 10 per sec rhythm. In the lower figure *L* represents left and *R* right; *F* means the recording was from the frontal lobe, and *P* represents parietal and *O,* occipital.

EEG Patterns

The figure on the right shows representative patterns of EEG activity for a variety of disorders.

NORMAL AND ABNORMAL ELECTROENCEPHALOGRAM WAVE PATTERNS

Frontal-Motor

Parietal-Occipital

NORMAL ADULT
10/sec. activity in occipital area

PETIT MAL SEIZURE
Synchronous 3/sec. spikes and waves

50μv.
1 sec.

GRAND MAL SEIZURE
High-voltage spikes, generalized

Right Temporal

Left Temporal

TEMPORAL LOBE EPILEPSY
Right temporal spike focus

Right Frontal

Left Frontal

BRAIN TUMOR
Left frontal slow wave focus

Right Frontal

ENCEPHALITIS
Diffuse slowing

CLASSIFICATION OF EPILEPTIC SEIZURES

Categories of Epilepsy and Seizures
(in alphabetical order)

grand mal (tonic-clonic) seizure: A common type of seizure with sudden onset of unconsciousness, tonic contraction of muscles, loss of postural control, and a cry caused by the respiratory muscles causing a forced expiration. This is followed by generalized contraction of the muscles of the extremities. The seizure is often preceded by an aura. Two to five minutes after consciousness has been lost and contractions have subsided, consciousness is gradually regained. Fecal and urinary incontinence may occur, as well as biting of the tongue. There is postictal amnesia for the time of the seizure. Complete functional recovery from the seizure may take several days.

Jacksonian (focal) epilepsy: With this type of epilepsy, there is a localized seizure with spasms confined to one part of the body or one group of muscles. The spasm may spread to involve adjacent areas of the body.

petit mal (absence) seizures: Seizures in which there is a sudden brief cessation of activity (this may last a few seconds or a few minutes). During the seizure, postural maintenance is not lost, and there are no convulsive muscle contractions. Seizures may occur very frequently (as many as a hundred times a day).

psychomotor (temporal lobe) epilepsy: Seizures that are not grand mal, petit mal, or Jacksonian. Psychomotor seizures are characterized by automatisms. The seizure often begins with an aura. The seizure progresses to include motor symptoms that are often associated with emotional or behavioral states. The movements are stereotypical and nonpurposeful (e.g., lip smacking, leg kicking, picking at clothing, chewing). The movements will be similar during subsequent seizures. With temporal lobe lesions, cognitive and emotional functions are often altered. Hallucinations may occur, as well as sexual arousal and a feeling of déjà vu. The person may feel violent, depressed, or fearful. Postictally there is amnesia for the time of the seizure, with some drowsiness and confusion.

status epilepticus: A state in which there are prolonged seizures with short periods of recovery between attacks. When these seizures are tonic-clonic, they may be life-threatening.

References

1. Strub, RL and Black, FW: Neurobehavioral Disorders: A Clinical Approach. FA Davis, Philadelphia, 1988.
2. Appel, S ed: Current Neurology, Vol. 4. John Wiley & Sons, New York, 1982.

I. Partial or focal seizures (seizures beginning locally)
  A. Simple partial seizures (usually without impairment of consciousness)
    1. With motor symptoms
      a. Focal motor
      b. Jacksonian (seizures due to focal irritation of a portion of the motor cortex; motor involvement starts in areas associated with the damaged region of the cortex and may spread to other areas)
      c. Versive
      d. Postural
      e. Somatic inhibitory
      f. Aphasic
      g. Phonatory (vocalization and arrest of speech)
    2. With special sensory or somatosensory symptoms
      a. Somatosensory
      b. Visual
      c. Auditory
      d. Olfactory
      e. Gustatory
      f. Vertiginous
    3. With autonomic symptoms
    4. Compound forms (includes psychic symptoms)
  B. Complex partial (psychomotor or temporal lobe) seizures (usually with impairment of consciousness)
    1. With only impaired consciousness
    2. With cognitive symptoms
      a. With dysmnesic disturbance (impairment of memory)
      b. With ideational disturbances
    3. With affective symptoms
    4. With psychosensory symptoms
      a. illusions
      b. hallucinations
    5. With psychomotor symptoms (automatisms)
    6. Compound forms
  C. Partial seizures secondarily generalized
II. Generalized seizures (bilaterally symmetrical without local onset)
  A. Absences (petit mal)
    1. Simple absences with impairment of consciousness only
    2. Complex absences with other associated phenomena
      a. With mild clonic components (myoclonic)
      b. With increase of postural tone (retropulsive)
      c. With diminution or abolition of postural tone (atonic)
      d. With automatisms
      e. With automatic phenomena (e.g., enuresis)
      f. Mixed forms

B. Bilateral massive epileptic myoclonus (myoclonic jerks)
C. Infantile spasms
D. Clonic seizures
E. Tonic seizures
F. Tonic-clonic seizures (grand mal seizures)
G. Atonic seizures
    1. Very brief in duration (drop attacks)
    2. Longer in duration (including atonic absences)
III. Unilateral or predominantly unilateral seizures
IV. Unclassified epileptic seizures (seizures that cannot be classified due to a lack of data)

Drugs Used to Treat Epileptic Seizures*

CHEMICAL CLASS	POSSIBLE MECHANISM OF ACTION
Hydantoins Ethotoin Mephenytoin Phenacemide Phenytoin	Stabilizes neuronal membrane by impairing movement of sodium across the membrane
Barbiturates Phenobarbital Methabarbital Methobarbital Primidone	Potentiate inhibitory effects of GABA: directly affect fluidity/organization of pre- and postsynaptic membrane
Succinimides Ethosuximide Methsuximide Phensuximide	Increase glucose transport and utilization in central neurons
Valproic Acid	May indirectly increase central glucose production and utilization by increasing systemic gluconeogenic (ketone) precursors; higher doses increase central GABA concentrations
Carbamazepine	Stabilize neuronal membrane in a manner similar to hydantoin drugs
Benzodiazepines Clonazepam Chlorazepate	Potentiate inhibitory effects of GABA

*Adapted from Ciccone, C: Pharmacology in Rehabilitation, FA Davis, Philadelphia, 1990.

COMA

Glasgow Coma Scale

The Glasgow coma scale is used to reflect changes in a patient's consciousness. The scale can be used to quantify the degree of coma. Three indicators of consciousness are used: the stimulus needed to elicit eye opening, the type of verbal response, and the type of motor response. A score of 7 or less means that the patient is in coma, whereas a score of 9 or greater excludes the diagnosis of coma.

Glasgow Coma Scale*

EYE OPENING	POINTS	BEST VERBAL RESPONSE	POINTS	BEST MOTOR RESPONSE	POINTS
				Obey Commands	6
				Do not classify a grasp reflex or a change in posture as a response	
		Oriented	5	*Localized*	5
		Patient knows who and where he is, and the year, season, and month		Moves a limb to attempt to remove stimulus	
Spontaneous	4	*Confused*	4	*Flexor: Normal*	
Indicates arousal mechanisms in brain stem are active		Responses to questions indicate varying degrees of confusion and disorientation		Entire shoulder or arm is flexed in response to painful stimuli	
To Sound	3	*Inappropriate*	3		
Eyes open to any sound stimulus		Speech is intelligible but sustained			
To Pain	2				
Apply stimulus to limbs, not to face					
Never	1				

conversation is not possible

Incomprehensible   2

Unintelligible sounds such as moans and groans are made

None   1

Flexion: Abnormal   3

Slow stereotyped assumption of decorticate rigidity posture in response to painful stimuli

Extension   2

Abnormal with adduction and internal rotation of the shoulder and pronation of the forearm

None   1

Be certain that a lack of response is not due to a spinal cord injury

---

*This scale, originally described in 1974 and further discussed in 1979 by Teasdale and his associates, is widely used in assessing head injury patients, both at the time of the injury and as the patient is followed. The score is recorded every 2 to 3 days.

Diagnostic Features of Coma-Like States*

DIAGNOSIS	LEVEL OF CONSCIOUSNESS	VOLUNTARY MOVEMENT	SPEECH	EYE RESPONSES	LIMB TONE	REFLEXES
Akinetic mute (apathetic—midbrain)	Lethargy	Little and infrequent; but when sufficiently stimulated, can move *all* extremities purposefully	With stimulation, can produce normal, short phrases	Open when stimulated; usually good eye contact	Usually normal; sometimes slight increase	Can be normal. Occasionally asymmetrical with pathologic reflexes
Akinetic mute (coma—vigil—septal)	Wakeful, with occasional outbursts. Some patients are somnolent	Little but purposeful; arms usually move much better than legs	Little; can occasionally produce normal phrases. Also, can have outbursts of unintelligible utterances	Open during much of the day in most patients. Eye contact variable	Often increased in legs	Frequently have increased leg reflexes. Babinski signs, snout, grasp often present
Apallic state (decorticate)	Awake; no meaningful interaction with environment	No or little purposeful movement; mostly reflex or mass movements	None or occasional grunting	Open, searching, but no real eye contact	Increased in all extremities. Extremities often in flexion	Increased in all extremities with pathologic reflexes

Persistent vegetative state	Awake; no or little interaction with environment	Usually little or none, depending upon areas of brain damaged. Mostly primitive postural reflexes	None or occasional grunts or groans. Some patients produce a few words	Open, searching, but no real eye contact	Variable, usually increased. Extremities often in flexion	Variable, usually increased with pathologic reflexes
Locked-in syndrome	Awake and alert; able to communicate meaningfully with examiners by eye movement	None or slight, except for eye movement	None	Open, with normal following and good eye contact. Some patients have restricted lateral gaze	Increased	Increased in all extremities

*From: Strub, RL and Black, FW: The Mental Status Examination in Neurology, ed 2, FA Davis, Philadelphia, 1986.

References

1. Teasdale, G and Jennett, B: Assessment of coma and impaired consciousness: A practical scale. Lancet 2:81, 1974.
2. Teasdale, G, et al: Adding up the Glasgow coma score. ACTA Neurochir (Suppl) 28:13, 1979.
3. Strub, RL and Black, FW: The Mental Status Examination in Neurology, ed 2. FA Davis, Philadelphia, 1986.

HYDROCEPHALUS

Classification of Chronic Hydrocephalus

Chronic hydrocephalus may produce dementia or mental retardation. The syndrome of acute hydrocephalus is a neurologic emergency and does not manifest itself as a dementia.

Nonobstructive (Ex Vacuo or Compensatory) Hydrocephalus

Due to degeneration or destruction of cerebral tissue with secondary increase in ventricular size. There is an increase in the volume of the cerebrospinal fluid (CSF) as a compensation for cerebral atrophy due to primary CNS disease. Nonobstructive hydrocephalus is seen with the following disorders:

1. Alzheimer's disease
2. Pick's disease
3. Multiple cerebral infarctions
4. Huntington's disease

Reference

1. Samuels, MA: Manual of Neurologic Therapeutics, ed 2.

Obstructive Hydrocephalus

Obstructive hydrocephalus is classified according to the site of the CSF blockage.
1. Communicating (normal pressure, low pressure, tension): blockage is outside of the ventricular system; there is free communication between the ventricles and the subarachnoid space. Communicating hydrocephalus is seen with the following disorders:
   a. Postsubarachnoid hemorrhage
   b. Postmeningitis
   c. Idiopathic
2. Noncommunicating (internal): Blockage is within the ventricular system so that there is no flow between the ventricular system and the subarachnoid space. Noncommunicating hydrocephalus is seen with the following conditions:
   a. Aqueductal stenosis
   b. Masses compressing the fourth ventricle (e.g., cerebellar tumors)
   c. Malformation at the foramen magnum (e.g., Arnold-Chiari malformation and Dandy-Walker malformation)

SHUNTING PROCEDURES
FOR HYDROCEPHALUS

Intracranial Shunts

In selected cases of noncommunicating hydrocephalus, an intracranial shunt may be used to divert cerebrospinal fluid (CSF) from the obstructed segment of the ventricular system to the subarachnoid space beyond the block. This procedure is usually reserved for cases in which the ventricular obstruction is not amenable to direct operation (e.g., pineal tumor) and in which the subarachnoid space is competent.

Features
1. Reestablishes a normal route for CSF flow and absorption
2. Performed with a minimal number of mechanical devices
3. Rarely requires revision to accommodate somatic growth

Procedures
1. **Third ventriculostomy shunt:** Establishment of a permanent fistula between the third ventricle and the basilar cistern. The most common technique employs the subfrontal approach.
2. **Ventriculocisternostomy** (Torkildsen) **shunt:** Diverting CSF from one lateral ventricle to the cisterna magna by means of a rubber tube or catheter. It is technically simpler than the third ventriculostomy shunt and can be used in cases in which the third ventricle is not grossly dilated or when the ventricle is directly involved by tumor.

Extracranial Shunts

These shunts divert CSF to the bloodstream or the body cavity. This procedure is the preferred method of treating most cases of communicating hydrocephalus that are not amenable to direct operations or intracranial shunts. Repeated revisions are usually required to accommodate somatic growth, and procedures are often associated with mechanical obstruction or infections.

Features: The majority of shunting devices consist of three integrated components:
1. Ventricular catheter
2. Connecting flush pump
3. Distal catheter

Procedures
1. **Ventriculoperitoneal shunt:** Diversion of CSF from one lateral ventricle to the peritoneal cavity. Considered safer and simpler than ventriculoatrial shunt and usually performed as the initial shunting procedure, particularly when somatic growth is a factor.

2. **Ventriculoatrial shunt:** Diversion of CSF from one lateral ventricle to the right atrium of the heart by means of a valve-regulated shunt. A catheter is introduced to the atrium via the facial or jugular vein. This procedure is considered to be the procedure of choice for patients with hydrocephalus not amenable to direct operation or intracranial shunting in whom somatic growth is complete.

3. **Direct cardiac shunt:** Direct implantation of ventricular shunt to the right atrium of the heart. It is a newly developed procedure that allows for somatic growth and holds promise as a single-stage operation.

4. Miscellaneous procedures:

   a. **Ventriculopleural shunt:** Useful alternative shunt in older children, particularly when objective proof of a functioning shunt is required and when atrial and peritoneal routes are unavailable.

   b. **Lumbar subarachnoid-peritoneal shunt:** Procedure of choice in patients with pseudotumor cerebri requiring prolonged CSF drainage. Scoliosis can be a late complication.

   c. **Lumbar subarachnoid-ureteral shunt:** Requires removal of one kidney and is indicated only for cases of communicating hydrocephalus as a last resort.

Reference

1. Milhorat, TH: *Pediatric Neurosurgery* (Contemporary Neurology Series 16) FA Davis, Philadelphia, 1978.

INNERVATION OF THE URINARY BLADDER AND RECTUM

Peripheral Nervous System for Voluntary Control

pudendal nerve (S2,S3,S4): Supplies the voluntary muscles of the external anal and urethral sphincters, which provide a means for voluntary control over these orifices. Sensory fibers to the mucosa of the anal canal and to the urethra are also supplied.

Autonomic Nervous System

sympathetic fibers: Reach the rectum by both the inferior mesenteric and the inferior hypogastric plexuses, and the urinary bladder through the inferior hypogastric plexus. Preganglionic fibers originate from the upper lumbar area. The afferents associated with the sympathetic system are associated with painful sensations (e.g., overdistension) from the bladder and rectum. The sympathetic efferents cause contraction of the internal anal and vesical sphincters, with relaxation of the muscular walls of these organs.

parasympathetic fibers: Reach the rectum and urinary bladder from the inferior hypogastric plexus. Preganglionic fibers enter this plexus by the pelvic splanchnic nerves. The afferents associated with the parasympathetic system carry information regarding normal sensations of bladder and rectal distension. The parasympathetic efferents supply the urinary bladder and the rectal muscle for micturition and defecation.

References

1. Clemente, CD, ed: Gray's Anatomy, ed 30. Lea & Febiger, Philadelphia, 1985.
2. Gilman, S and Newman, SW: Manter and Gatz's Essentials of Clinical Neuroanatomy and Neurophysiology, ed 7. FA Davis, Philadelphia, 1987.

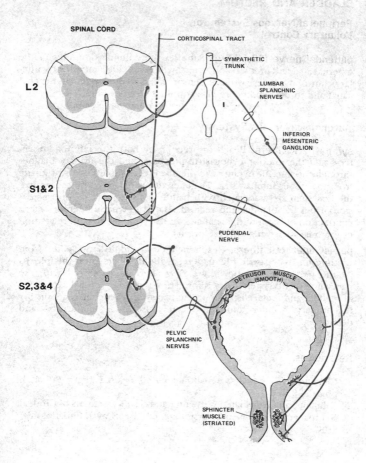

Autonomic innervation of the urinary bladder and associated somatic innervation of the sphincter.

*From: Gilman, S and Newman, SW: Manter and Gatz's Essentials of Clinical Neuroanatomy and Neurophysiology, ed 7. FA Davis, Philadelphia, 1987.

THE NEUROGENIC BLADDER

Classification of Neurogenic Bladders

The term *neurogenic bladder* refers to many disorders and does not connote a specific diagnosis or single etiology. The following classification system is followed by a simpler description of functional bladder types.

Sensorimotor Neuron Lesion

1. Lesions above the conus medullaris spinal reflex center (commonly called *upper motor neuron lesions*)
   a. Complete
   b. Incomplete
2. Lower motor neuron lesions (below the conus medullaris)
   a. Complete
   b. Incomplete
3. Mixed lesions
   a. Complete
   b. Incomplete

Sensory Neuron Lesions

1. Complete
2. Incomplete

Motor Neuron Lesions

1. Complete
2. Incomplete

Functional Bladder Types

atonic bladder (also called the flaccid, denervated, afferent or hypotonic bladder): These types of bladders are caused by lesions to the parasympathetic pathways to and from the bladder, which result in loss of the afferent or the efferent limb of the reflex arc from the detrusor muscle. These bladders may also be the result of destruction to the last few segments of the spinal cord (S3) in the conus medullaris (as in fractures of the spine at the thoracolumbar junction). Cystometrograms are flat, and there is retention with overflow. Abdominal straining may empty the bladder more. Cystograms may differ slightly according to the lesion site. The external sphincter is usually tonically active for the denervated bladder, whereas for lesions of the sacral portion of the cord, the external sphincter is usually flaccid.

spastic bladder (also called the reflex or efferent neurogenic bladder): Caused by lesions of the higher pathways to and from the cortex, with preservation of the spinal sacral segments and their innervation. This type of bladder is commonly associated with disorders of the pyramidal tracts, as in gunshot wounds, multiple sclerosis, whiplash injuries, or transverse myelitis. The cystometrogram is "jumpy," showing many uninhibited contractions without the patient feeling the need to void. Bladder capacity is reduced, and the residual urine further decreases the true capacity. Incontinence, dribbling, and residual urine are often present with this type of bladder, even with training and medication.

References

1. Chusid, J: Correlative Neuroanatomy and Functional Neurology, ed 19. Lange Medical Publications, Los Altos CA, 1985.
2. Gilman, S and Newman, SW (eds): Manter and Gatz's Essentials of Clinical Neuroanatomy and Neurophysiology, ed 7. FA Davis, Philadelphia, 1987.
3. John Blandy, Lecture Notes on Urology, Blackford Scientific, Publications, Oxford, 1976.

CYSTOMETROGRAMS

Cystometry is a urodynamic study used to assess bladder function. The resultant cystometrograph (CMG) reflects the contractility of the detrusor muscle and the bladder's ability to respond to changes in volume. The bladder's responsiveness to stretch is also evaluated. The patient's report of fullness, desire to void, and reports of pain are noted on the CMG.

The CMG is performed by introducing a catheter into the bladder of the recumbent patient in order to completely empty the bladder. Sterile water (at 37°C) or carbon dioxide is then introduced into the bladder as pressure is recorded by use of a manometer. Patients report any sensations of fullness and indicate when they feel the need to void. Patients are then instructed to void; during voiding, patients are asked to cease voiding.

During a normal cystometrogram, pressure within the bladder remains below 20 cm H_2O until the urge to void occurs between 350 and 500 cc. At that point, pressure rises to 60 to 80 cm H_2O. Uninhibited bladder contractions are absent during bladder filling. Bladder capacity is 350 to 600 cc with no residual urine.

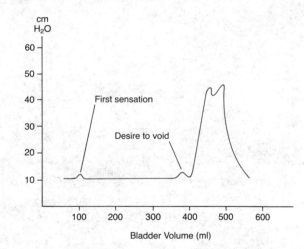

NORMAL CYSTOMETROGRAM

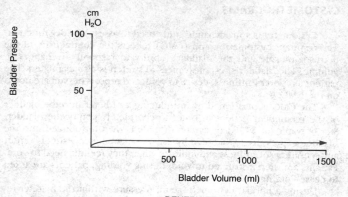

DENERVATED BLADDER

The denervated bladder resulting from injury to the parasympathetic pathways.

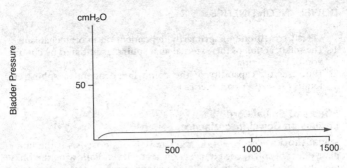

The destruction of the spinal reflex center for the bladder will result in the same condition as will injury of the parasympathetic pathways.

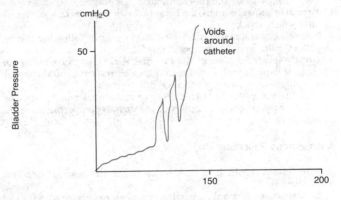

Cortical inhibition cut off by an "upper motor neuron" lesion.

References

1. Chusid, JG: Correlative Neuroanatomy and Functional Neurology, ed 19. Lange Medical Publications, Los Altos CA, 1985.
2. Blandy, J: Lecture Notes on Urology. Blackford Scientific Publications, Oxford, 1976.
3. Kottke, F, Stillwell, GK, and Lehman, J: Krusen's Handbook of Physical Medicine and Rehabilitation, ed 3. WB Saunders, Philadelphia, 1982.

BOWEL INCONTINENCE

Fecal continence is primarily dependent on two mechanisms:
1. The reflex action of the external anal sphincter initiated by contraction of the rectum
2. The reservoir capability of the colon independent of sphincteric action (*reservoir continence*)

Effects of Spinal Cord
Lesions on Bowel Incontinence

spinal shock: Fecal retention and paralysis of peristalsis is the immediate effect of spinal cord transection at any level. Following the phase of spinal shock, one of the following conditions may occur, depending on the type of lesion.

Automatic Reflex Activity

For lesions above the thoracolumbar junction:
1. Peristalsis, bowel sounds, anal and bulbocavernosus reflexes return after spinal shock.
2. Intermittent automatic reflex defecation occurs following the return of reflex activity and peristalsis.
3. Greatly increased tone of the external anal sphincter (during the stage of hyperreflexia) results in increased resistance to the expulsive function of sigmoid and rectum.

For lesions above T6, hyperreflexive abdominal muscles may interfere with the propulsive activity of the various compartments of the intestinal tract.

Autonomous Function

For lesions resulting in destruction of the lumbosacral or spinal roots, there is:
1. Lower motor neuron type paralysis (flaccid, denervation) with loss of normal response of sigmoid and rectum to distension
2. Loss of tone (reflexes) of the external sphincter
3. Impaired function of the levator ani
4. Progressive accumulation of feces leading to impaction and fecal incontinence. The patient is usually dependent on digital evacuation aided by increased intra-abdominal pressure, suppositories, and enemas.

Reference

1. Guttmann, L: Spinal Cord Injuries Comprehensive Management and Research, ed 2. Blackwell Scientific Publications, London, 1976.

CLASSIFICATION OF CEREBRAL PALSY

There are many different classifications of cerebral palsy. Confusion and incompatability between terminology can result. The most widely used system of classification is based on clinical presentation and was adopted by the American Academy for Cerebral Palsy (now the American Academy of Cerebral Palsy and Developmental Medicine). The system is based on the topographic distribution of muscle tone (reflex disorders) and movement disorders. This particular classification system is useful clinically because it describes cerebral palsy in terms of the motor deficit and distribution. An important limitation of this classification system is that it does not take into consideration developmental changes that commonly occur in the child with cerebral palsy.

The following classification begins with a description of the physiologic (motor) disorder followed by specific subtypes of cerebral palsy that include topology.

spasticity: Characterized by increased muscle tone (hyper-reflexia), stereotyped and limited movements, pathological stretch reflexes with clonus, persistence of primitive and tonic reflexes, and poor development of postural reflex mechanisms.

spastic hemiplegia: One side of the entire body is affected, the upper extremity more than the lower extremity. It is often associated with strabismus, oral motor dysfunction, somatosensory dysfunction, and perceptual learning disorders. Seizures often develop with maturity.

spastic triplegia: Involves the extremities, usually both legs and one arm. It may represent incomplete quadriplegia.

spastic quadriplegia (tetraplegia): Often related to birth asphyxia in term infants or grade 3 and 4 intraventricular bleeds in immature infants. There is involvement of all four extremities as well as head, neck, and trunk. It often presents first with hypotonia. In severe disorders, the child's posture and movement are dominated by either flexion or extension tone. Ability to move against gravity is very slight. It is associated with problems with vision, hearing, seizures, mental retardation, and oral-motor abilities.

spastic diplegia: Terminology seldom used. It is most frequently related to problems of prematurity. The total body is affected (bilateral paralysis); there is greater involvement in trunk and lower extremities than upper extremities and face. One side often is more involved than the other (double hemiplegia). Associated problems occur with speech, oral-motor function, and esotropia (crossed eyes).

athetosis (dyskinetic syndrome): Characterized by an abnormal amount and type of involuntary motion with varying amounts of tension, normal reflexes, asymmetrical involvement. Abnormal movements are exaggerated by voluntary movement, postural adjustments, and changes in emotion or speech. Often it is associated with impaired speech and poor respiratory and oral-motor control; it is related to erythroblastosis and birth asphyxia. (Note: not all of the following classification of athetosis have been adopted by the American Academy of Cerebral Palsy; they are included for completeness.)

rotary athetoid: Common type that involves muscles that function as rotators; rotary motion usually slow. Feet describe circular motion, hands pronate and supinate, and shoulders internally and externally rotate. There are varying degrees of muscle tension.

tremor (tremorlike) athetoid: Common type that involves irregular and uneven involuntary contraction and relaxation involving flexors and extensors, abductors and adductors. Rotary motion is not seen.

dystonic athetoid: Extremities, head, neck, and trunk assume distorted positions. There is increased muscle tone. Different abnormal positions may be assumed over time.

choreoathetoid: Involuntary, unpredictable, small movements of the distal parts of the extremities.

tension athetoid: A state of increased muscle tension blocking involuntary athetoid movements. Tension is not constant. Tension must be the dominant characteristic for this classification to be applicable; it is normally a temporary classification.

nontension athetoid: Involuntary movements without increased muscle tone. It is a temporary classification identifying a treatment phenomena and is frequently seen as an initial symptom of cerebral palsy in small babies.

flailing athetoid: A rare type of athetosis. Arms and legs are thrown violently from shoulder and hip, but there is little involvement of hands, wrists, fingers, or knees.

ataxia (ataxic cerebral palsy): Associated with developmental deficits of the cerebellum, it is characterized by disturbance in the sense of balance and equilibrium, dyssynergias, and low postural tone. There is bilateral distribution affecting trunk and legs more than arms and hands, as well as a widespread stance and gait. Spastic diplegia and athetosis are often concomitant. Ataxia often follows initial stage of hypotonia. Associated problems include nystagmus, poor eye tracking, delayed and poorly articulated speech, astereognosis, and poor depth perception.

hypotonia (flaccid cerebral palsy): Often a transient stage in the evolution of athetosis or spasticity, it is characterized by decreased muscle tone, real or apparent weakness, and increased range of movement. A child typically assumes "froglike" position when placed supine and uses hands to support trunk during sitting.

mixed types: Any cerebral palsy child that does not fit characterizations described. This label is used most commonly to indicate spastic diplegia mixed with athetosis.

References

1. Campbell, SK: Pediatric Neurologic Physical Therapy. Churchill Livingstone, New York, 1984.
2. Thompson, GH, Rubin, IL, and Bilenker, RM: Comprehensive Management of Cerebral Palsy. Grune & Stratton, New York, 1982.

TYPES OF SPINA BIFIDA

A normal spine with an intact spinal cord is seen on the left. Illustrations of types of spina bifida (midline closure defects) are to the right. Although defects may occur anywhere along the vertebral column, they are most common in the lumbar and lumbosacral regions.

Spina bifida occulta is a failure of the vertebral lamina to develop and is usually asymptomatic; however, it may be associated with other birth defects. Spina bifida with meningocele is a midline defect with herniation of the meninges. Depending on the severity of the herniation and associated problems, there may or may not be any neural defect. Spina bifida with meningomyelocele is a midline defect with herniation of neural tissue. In addition to neural deficits, this condition may be life-threatening due to complications such as infection (meningitis) and hydrocephalus.

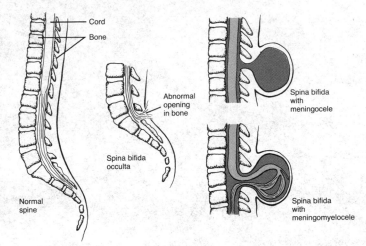

Reference

1. Lovell, WW and Winter, RB (eds): Pediatric Orthopaedics, ed 2, Vol 1. JB Lippincott, Philadelphia, 1986.

MUSCULAR DYSTROPHY

Classification of Muscular Dystrophies

The following classification of muscular dystrophies is based on genetic criteria and distribution of muscle degeneration. Each category is followed by a list of characteristic features.

Duchenne Muscular Dystrophy (Pseudohypertrophic Muscular Dystrophy)

- Inherited as an X-linked recessive gene (passed to boys by their relatively unaffected mothers).
- Diagnosis rarely made before 3 years.
- Characterized by slow motor development and late onset of sitting, walking, and running.
- Waddling lordotic gait, difficulty in climbing stairs, and hypertrophy of calf muscles are typical.
- Deltoid, brachioradialis, and tongue may also be hypertrophied.
- Moderately severe form demonstrates Gowers' sign.
- Moderate to slight mental retardation is common (IQ is 85 on average).
- Majority develop cardiomyopathy; death occurs in 75 percent of patients before 20 years of age.

Becker Muscular Dystrophy (Slowly Progressive Muscular Dystrophy)

- X-linked recessive dystrophy resembling Duchenne's variety but less severe, with later onset, and survival is prolonged until middle adult life.
- Proximal weakness of upper and lower extremities and pseudohypertrophy.
- Initially develops difficulty in gait, climbing stairs, and rising from the floor.
- Patient eventually develops contractures and skeletal deformities, but these are less conspicuous than with Duchenne's variety; early myocardial disease may develop.
- Mental retardation is less common than in Duchenne's variety.

Facioscapulohumeral Dystrophy (of Landouzy-Déjérine)

- Inherited as an autosomal dominant trait; affects both sexes equally.

- Rather benign and slowly progressive weakness of the face, shoulder, and upper arm.
- Onset is typically toward the end of the first decade or beginning of second.
- Less classical forms of this dystrophy type include infantile facioscapulohumeral dystrophy, facioscapulohumeral dystrophy with late exacerbation, and a form that is concurrent with Coats' syndrome.

Limb-Girdle Dystrophy

- Probably includes a group of disorders with progressive weakness of the hip and shoulder muscles.
- There is variety in the inheritance, age of onset, progression of the illness, and distribution and severity of weakness.
- Patients may eventually be confined to a wheelchair, but skeletal deformities are not frequent.
- Death may occur from cardiopulmonary complications and terminal pneumonia.

Humeroperoneal Muscular Dystrophy (Emery-Dreifuss Disease)

- X-linked recessive disorder.
- Present during first decade of life; tendency to walk on toes and the development of elbow contractures are among the first manifestations.
- Wasting and weakness of scapulohumeroperoneal distribution that is very slowly progressive.
- May develop cardiac conduction abnormalities that are threatening to life.

Scapuloperoneal Dystrophy

- May be a variety of facioscapulohumeral dystrophy.
- Often inherited as autosomal dominant, but an x-linked recessive pattern has also been described.
- Peroneal and anterior tibial muscle groups are involved early, followed by shoulder muscle weakness; patients may also have facial weakness.

Hereditary Distal Myopathy

- Common in Sweden but less frequent elsewhere.
- Inheritance is autosomal dominant with onset between 40 and 60 years of age.

- Clumsiness in the hands and then slowly progresses and involves the feet and anterior compartment muscles of the leg.
- Typically it does not progress to total incapacity.

Ocular Myopathies

- Three types: ocular dystrophy, oculopharyngeal dystrophy, and oculocraniosomatic neuromuscular disease.
- Controversy exists as to whether these ocular diseases are true myopathies.

Functional Stages of Duchenne Muscular Dystrophy

STAGE	DESCRIPTION
I	Walks and climbs stairs without assistance
II	Walks and climbs stairs with the aid of railings
III	Walks and climbs stairs slowly with the aid of railings (greater than 25 seconds for eight standard steps)
IV	Walks unassisted and rises from chair but cannot climb stairs
V	Walks unassisted but cannot rise from chair or climb stairs
VI	Walks only with assistance or walks independently with long-leg braces
VII	Walks in long-leg braces but requires assistance for balance
VIII	Stands in long-leg braces but unable to walk, even with assistance
IX	In a wheelchair or bed

References

1. Brooke, MH: A Clinician's View of Neuromuscular Diseases, ed 2. Williams & Wilkins, Baltimore, 1986.
2. Molnar, GE (ed): Pediatric Rehabilitation. Williams & Wilkins, Baltimore, 1979.

COMMUNICATION DISORDERS

Aphasia

Aphasia is a disturbance to language caused by focal or diffuse damage to the language areas of the brain. Aphasia results in linguistic errors in word choice, comprehension, or syntax rather than problems of articulation or pronunciation. The term *aphasia* encompasses a variety of syndromes that are described below.

Types of Aphasia

anomic aphasia: Nominal or amnesia aphasia; characterized by difficulty in naming objects and by word-finding problems. Reading, writing, and comprehension are usually unimpaired. A variety of lesions in the dominant hemisphere can result in anomia. The most severe forms usually involve the second and third temporal gyri and the parietotemporal area.

Broca's aphasia: Expressive aphasia; characterized by severe difficulty in verbal expression and mild difficulty in understanding complex syntax. Comprehension of both spoken and written language is excellent; verbal output is telegraphic or agrammatic. Patients are also impaired in object naming and in writing abilities. Most patients with Broca's aphasia are right hemiplegics with large, deep lesions affecting the inferior frontal lobe (this includes Broca's area 44). Language recovery is slow, with fluency and grammatical complexity often permanently impaired.

conduction aphasia: Characterized by deficits in the repetition of spoken language, halting speech with word-finding pauses, and literal paraphasia (letter or whole-word substitutions). Comprehension and reading are not usually impaired, but there may be errors in object naming and writing. Lesions causing this type of aphasia are usually in the areas of the supramarginal gyrus and arcuate fasciculus or the insula and auditory cortex.

crossed aphasia: A transient aphasia that often occurs in right-handed patients with a right-hemisphere lesion and no history of left-hemisphere damage or familial left-handedness. Patients are often agrammatic with decreased comprehension. Naming abilities are preserved. Reading and writing are rarely impaired.

global aphasia: The most common and severe form of aphasia, it is characterized by spontaneous speech that is either absent or reduced to a few stereotyped words or sounds. Comprehension is reduced or absent. Repetition, reading, and writing are impaired to the same level as spontaneous speech. Lesions are usually large, involving the entire perisylvian area of the frontal, temporal, and parietal lobes. An occlusion of the internal carotid area or the middle cerebral artery at its origin is the most common cause. Prognosis for the recovery of speech is poor.

subcortical (thalamic) aphasia: Aphasia associated with vascular lesions of the thalamus, putamen, caudate, or internal capsule. Patients are dysarthric and have mild anomia and comprehension deficits.

transcortical aphasia: The linguistic opposite of conduction aphasia. Patients with transcortical motor aphasia are able to repeat, comprehend, and read well but have restricted spontaneous speech. Patients with transcortical sensory aphasia can repeat words but do not comprehend the meaning of the words. Spontaneous speech and naming are fluent but paraphasic (letter or whole-word substitutions). Some patients have combined motor and sensory transcortical aphasia. Patients with the complete syndrome can only repeat and tend to echo what they hear (echolalia). Lesions are extensive.

Wernicke's aphasia: The linguistic opposite of Broca's aphasia, characterized by fluent, effortless, well-articulated speech that is frequently out of context and containing many paraphasias (letter or whole-word substitutions). There are severe disturbances of auditory comprehension resulting in inappropriate responses to questions. Reading, writing, and repetition of words are also impaired, and naming is paraphasic. Patients are often mistakenly thought to have psychotic illnesses. The lesion is in the posterior language area (area 1) and usually includes the superior temporal gyrus (area 22), where auditory comprehension is processed.

Agraphia

A syndrome in which writing ability is disturbed by an acquired brain lesion. Agraphia is not an abnormality in writing mechanics. With the exception of patients with pure word deafness, all aphasia patients have some degree of agraphia. Lesions in the posterior language area (where the message is translated into visual symbols) or the frontal language area (for motor processing) cause agraphia. There are rare instances in which isolated pure agraphia has been seen.

Aprosody

A syndrome in which the melodic qualities of language are disturbed by an acquired brain lesion. A dramatic change is heard in the intonation patterns of expressive language that results in a monotonal delivery of speech. Perisylvian lesions and anterior lesions can result in aprosody. Patients with a posterior lesion cannot comprehend the prosodic qualities of language but can express themselves with proper intonation.

Dysarthria (Articulation Disturbances)

These are speech disorders that result from loss of control of the muscles of articulation. This disturbance may be due to a variety of diseases. Among the structures that can be implicated in lesions causing dysarthria are the cortical motor area, basal ganglia, corticobulbar tract, motoneurons of the ninth, tenth, and twelfth cranial nerves, and the muscles used for articulation.

Reference

1. Goodglass, H and Kaplan, E: Assessment of Aphasia and Related Disorders. Lea & Febiger, Philadelphia, 1972.

TESTS OF LANGUAGE PERFORMANCE

Comprehensive Aphasia Batteries

Aphasia Language Performance Scales: A 30-minute test of communicative ability designed to determine whether a patient is suitable for speech therapy.

Boston Diagnostic Aphasia Examination: Assesses all areas of language in a systematic fashion. The test is used for describing aphasic disorders, planning treatment, and research.

Communication Abilities In Daily Living: A test for functional communication ability in aphasic adults, primarily used by speech therapists to identify which aspects of communication should be treated.

Multilingual Aphasia Examination: A research-derived examination that evaluates the major components of speech and language. Subtests can be administered independently.

Neurosensory Center Comprehensive Examination for Aphasia: Assesses 20 different components of language and includes tests for tactile and visual functioning. It is oriented to neurolinguistic research.

Porch Index of Communicative Ability (PICA): A psychometrically oriented test battery used to quantify verbal, gestural, and graphic language abilities, as well as a variety of other communicative functions. It is most frequently used by speech pathologists to establish baseline levels, predict possible recovery, and to measure treatment outcome or spontaneous recovery.

Western Aphasia Battery: An adaptation and standardization of the Boston Diagnostic Aphasia Examination, it assesses a number of functions related to communication, such as arithmetic, praxis, constructional ability, and Raven's Matrices. This relatively new test has not been fully evaluated for clinical and research applications.

Tests of Language Abilities

Boston Naming Test: A test of single-word expressive vocabulary or naming ability that is the reciprocal of the Peabody Picture Vocabulary Test – Revised (PPVT-R). It requires the patient to name a 60-item series of pictured objects ordered in increasing difficulty. If the patient is unable to name an item, the examiner first provides a categorical cue and then a phonemic cue. Provisional norms are provided for children, normal adults, and aphasic adults.

Peabody Picture Vocabulary Test – Revised (PPVT-R): A recently revised and standardized test of single-word vocabulary comprehension. It contains two equivalent sets of stimuli plates that contain four pictures. There are also two associated lists of 175 words that are ordered in ascending difficulty. The patient must indicate which of each set of four pictures is most like the word provided by the examiner. Norms are provided for subjects between 2 ½ and 41 years of age.

Sentence Repetition Tests: The Spreen-Benton Sentence Repetition Test and the Sentence Repetition Test are the two most widely used sentence repetition tests. Both tests evaluate the patient's ability to repeat immediately a series of sentences of increasing length and semantic complexity. Normative data are available for normal and neurologically impaired adults.

Token Tests: Simple-to-administer tests of language comprehension. Plastic tokens are manipulated by the patient in response to a series of hierarchically ordered verbal commands. Comprehension is therefore tested at several levels of difficulty. It is useful in the assessment of the aphasic patient, as well as patients with comprehension deficits secondary to dementia or other neurologic conditions.

verbal fluency tests: Verbal fluency—the ability to produce spontaneous speech fluently without undue word-finding difficulty—is typically evaluated by tabulating the number of words the patient produces within a restricted category and time limit (usually 60 s). Two easily and commonly administered tests are the Animal Naming Test and Controlled Oral Word Association Test. There are normative data for both tests.

References

1. Lezak, MD: Neuropsychological Assessment. Oxford University Press, New York, 1983.
2. Kertesz, A: Aphasia and Related Disorders: Taxonomy, Localization, and Recovery. Grune & Stratton, New York, 1979.

CLINICAL PROBLEM	EXAMPLES OF FUNCTIONAL DEFICITS
Lesion: Left Hemisphere	
Aphasias	Lacks functional speech
Ideomotor and ideational apraxias	Cannot plan and execute serial steps in performances
Number alexia	Cannot recognize symbols to do simple computations
Right-left discrimination	Unable to distinguish right from left on self or reverse on others
Slow in organization and performance	Cannot remember what he or she intended to do next
Lesion: Right Hemisphere	
Visuospatial	Cannot orient self to changes in environment while going from one treatment area to another
Left unilateral neglect of self	Generally unaware of objects to left and propels wheelchair into them
Body Image	Distorted awareness and impression of self
Dressing apraxia	Applies sweater to right side, but unable to do left-side application
Constructional apraxia	Unable to transpose two-dimensional instructions into three-dimensional structure, as per "do-it-yourself" kits
Illusions of shortening of time	Patient arrives extremely early for appointments
Number concepts — spatial type	Unable to align columns and rows of digits
Rapid organization and performance	Errors from haste; may cause accidents
Depth of language skills	May mention task related to prestroke occupation, but cannot go into details of it

PARKINSON'S SYNDROME

Drugs Used in the Treatment of Parkinson's Syndrome*

DRUG	DOSAGE	PRECAUTIONS AND REMARKS
Anticholinergic Drugs		
Trihexyphenidyl (Artane)	1–5 mg 3 times daily, starting at low dosage and slowly increasing. For oculogyric crisis use 10 mg 3 times daily.	May precipitate acute glaucoma in elderly persons and are contraindicated in patients with glaucoma. Blurred vision, dryness of mouth, vertigo, and tachycardia are early toxic symptoms; late symptoms are vomiting, dizziness, mental confusion, and hallucinations. The synthetic drugs are apt to cause more dizziness than the natural alkaloids and are somewhat less potent parasympatholytics.
Biperiden (Akineton)	2 mg 3–4 times daily	
Procyclidine (Kemadrin)	2.5–5 mg 3 times daily after meals	

Drug	Dosage	Side effects
Benztropine mesylate (Cogentin)	0.5 mg 1–2 times daily, increasing by 0.5 mg at intervals of several days to 5 mg daily or toxicity. Often most effective as single dose at bedtime.	Side effects similar to those of trihexyphenidyl (Artane).
Dopaminergic Drugs		
Levodopa (Dopar, Larodopa, etc)	250 mg 3 times daily. Increase to tolerance (4–8 g daily)	Nausea, vomiting, postural hypotension, choreiform movements
Levodopa and carbidopa (Sinemet)	3–6 tablets daily of Sinemet 25/250	Nausea, vomiting, postural hypotension, dyskinesias
Amantadine (Symmetrel)	100 mg twice daily	Jitteriness, insomnia, depression, confusion, hallucinations, livedo reticularis
Bromocriptine mesylate (Parlodel)	1.25 mg twice daily with food. Increase slowly as necessary by adding 2.5 mg daily at 2- to 4-week intervals.	Nausea, abnormal involuntary movement, hallucinations, confusion, drowsiness

*From Chusid, JG: Correlative Neuroanatomy and Functional Neurology, ed 19. Lange Medical Publications, Los Altos, CA, 1985, with permission.

Prognostic Classification of Parkinson's Disease

SCHWAB CLASSIFICATION OF PROGRESSION*			HOEHN AND YAHR CLASSIFICATION OF DISABILITY†	
GRADE	CHRONOLOGY OF DISEASE MANIFESTATIONS	COMMENTS	STAGE	CHARACTER OF DISABILITY
1	Symptoms generally remain stable for at least 5 years after diagnosis.	Diagnosis may be uncertain. Minimal therapy is required. Ability to live independently is usually not threatened.	I	Minimal or absent; unilateral if present.
2	Some evidence of progression may be observed after 5 years. Disease may remain unilateral.	With appropriate pharmacotherapy, most patients can remain independent.	II	Minimal bilateral or midline involvement. Balance not impaired.
3	Marked progression is observed after 3 to 5 years.	Partial incapacitation is likely, but most patients are still	III	Impaired righting reflexes. Unsteadiness when turning or

			rising from chair. Some activities are restricted, but patient can live independently and continue some forms of employment.
4	Disease progresses to severe tremor and rigidity after 3 to 5 years. Manifestations are usually bilateral after 8 to 10 years.	able to live independently 10 years after diagnosis.	
		Patient may remain ambulatory, but serious disability may supervene.	IV — All symptoms present and severe. Requires help with some activities of daily living.
5	Onset of disease is abrupt. Severe bilateral tremor, rigidity, and akinesia are present within a few months. Marked incapacity and motor deficiency are present within 1 year.	Outlook is for severe or total disability.	V — Confined to bed or wheelchair unless aided.

Disease may remain unilateral.

*Adapted from Schwab, RS: Progression and Prognosis in Parkinson's Disease. J Nerve Ment Dis 130:556, 1960.
†Adapted from Hoehn, MM and Yahr, MD: Parkinsonism: Onset, Progression, and Mortality. Neurology 17:433, 1967.

COGNITIVE FUNCTIONING

Ranchos Los Amigos
Cognitive Functioning Scale

I – **No response** Patient appears to be in a deep sleep and is completely unresponsive to any stimuli.

II – **Generalized Response** Patient reacts inconsistently and nonpurposefully to stimuli in a nonspecific manner. Responses are limited and often the same regardless of stimulus presented. Responses may be physiologic changes, gross body movements, and/or vocalization.

III – **Localized responses** Patient reacts specifically but inconsistently to stimuli. Responses are directly related to the type of stimulus presented. May follow simple commands in an inconsistent, delayed manner, such as closing eyes or squeezing hand.

IV – **Confused-agitated** Patient is in heightened state of activity. Behavior is bizarre and nonpurposeful relative to immediate environment. Does not discriminate among persons or objects; is unable to cooperate directly with treatment efforts. Verbalizations frequently are incoherent and/or inappropriate to the environment; confabulation may be present. Gross attention to environment is very brief; selective attention is often nonexistent. Patient lacks short-term and long-term recall.

V – **Confused-inappropriate** Patient is able to respond to simple commands fairly consistently. However, with increased complexity of commands or lack of any external structure, responses are nonpurposeful, random, or fragmented. Demonstrates gross attention to the environment but is highly distractible and lacks ability to focus attention on a specific task. With structure, may be able to converse on a social automatic level for short periods of time. Verbalization is often inappropriate and confabulatory. Memory is severely impaired; often shows inappropriate use of objects; may perform previously learned tasks with structure but is unable to learn new information.

VI – **Confused-appropriate** Patient shows goal-directed behavior but is dependent on external input or direction. Follows simple directions consistently and shows carry-over for relearned problems but appropriate to the situation; past memories show more depth and detail than recent memory.

VII – **Automatic-appropriate** Patient appears appropriate and oriented within hospital and home settings: goes through daily routine automatically, but frequently robotlike with minimal to absent confusion and has shallow recall of activities. Shows carryover for new learning but at a decreased rate. With structure is able to initiate social or recreational activities; judgment remains impaired.

VIII – **Purposeful and appropriate** Patient is able to recall and to integrate past and recent events and is aware of and responsive to environment. Shows carryover for new learning and needs no supervision once activities are learned. May continue to show a decreased ability relative to premorbid abilities, abstract reasoning, tolerance for stress, and judgment in emergencies or unusual circumstances.

(From Adult Brain Injury Service of the Rancho Los Amigos Medical Center, with permission.)

LEVEL   DESCRIPTION

Arousal
The patient has difficulty initiating attention to purposeful tasks.
The patient's behavior is purposeless, reflexive, inconsistent, and
dependent in all functional areas. They may show some visual
tracking and are usually not vocal.

2 Attention

Low Level

The patient initiates attention but has difficulty sustaining
attention. Patient is able to follow one-step commands but
inconsistently. The patient may function automatically in
overlearned behaviors. Patient does not initiate activities and may
wander if left unsupervised.

High Level

The patient's main deficit area is in sustaining and switching
attention. The patient is distractible and perseverative. He or she
may recall pieces of information but is unable to integrate
information.

3 Discrimination
Patient is able to sustain and to switch attention sufficiently to
integrate small amounts of information. Patient initiates activities
but may still show some perseveration and impulsivity. Behavior
can be partly modified by feedback. Recall over time is improved.

4 Organization

Low Level

Patient can integrate multiple pieces of information for a task but
tends to be concrete and have difficulty sequencing the task.
Patient can begin simple problem solving.

High Level

Patient can use selective attention to perceive stimuli or task
elements accurately, select a strategy, and reach a solution. Patient
continues to be concrete, has trouble generalizing and carrying
over learning from one setting to another. In stressful situations,
shows breakdown in cognitive function.

LEVEL   DESCRIPTION

5 Higher-level cognitive function
The patient is able to do complex problem solving but is limited
owing to limited flexibility, insight, social behavior, and
endurance. The patient is susceptible to breakdown of behavior
outside of a structured setting (e.g., school or work). In stressful
situations, shows preserved cognitive functions. Cognitive
processing is slow.

(From Braintree Hospital Cognitive Continuum, with permission.)

COORDINATION

Coordination Tests (in alphabetical order)*

TEST	DESCRIPTION
Alternate heel to knee; heel to toe	From a supine position, the patient is asked to touch his knee and big toe alternately with the heel of the opposite extremity.
Alternate nose to finger	The patient alternately touches the tip of his nose and the tip of the therapist's finger with the index finger. The position of the therapist's finger may be altered during testing to assess ability to change distance, direction, and force of movement.
Drawing a circle	The patient draws an imaginary circle in the air with either upper or lower extremity (a table or the floor also may be used). This also may be done using a figure-eight pattern. This test may be performed in the supine position for lower extremity assessment.
Finger to finger	Both shoulders are abducted to 90° with the elbows extended. The patient is asked to bring both hands toward the midline and approximate the index fingers from opposing hands.
Finger to nose	The shoulder is abducted to 90° with the elbow extended. The patient is asked to bring the tip of the index finger to the tip of the nose. Alterations may be made in the initial starting position to assess performance from different planes of motion.
Finger opposition	The patient touches the tip of the thumb to the tip of each finger in sequence. Speed may be gradually increased.

Finger to therapist's finger

The patient and therapist sit opposite each other. The therapist's index finger is held in front of the patient. The patient is asked to touch the tip of the index finger to the therapist's index finger. The position of the therapist's finger may be altered during testing to assess ability to change distance, direction, and force of movement.

Fixation or position holding

Upper extremity: The patient holds arms horizontally in front.
Lower extremity: The patient is asked to hold the knee in an extended position.

Heel on shin

From a supine position, patient slides the heel of one foot up and down the shin of the opposite lower extremity.

Mass grasp

An alternation is made between opening and closing fist (from finger flexion to full extension). Speed may be gradually increased.

Pointing and past pointing

The patient and therapist are opposite each other, either sitting or standing. Both patient and therapist bring shoulders to a horizontal position of 90° of flexion with elbows extended. Index fingers are touching, or the patient's finger may rest lightly on the therapist's. The patient is asked to fully flex the shoulder (fingers will be pointing toward ceiling) and then return to the horizontal position such that index fingers will again approximate. Both arms should be tested, either separately or simultaneously. A normal response consists of an accurate return to the starting position. In an abnormal response, there is typically a "past pointing," or movement beyond the target. Several variations to this test include movements in other directions such as toward 90° of shoulder abduction or toward 0° of shoulder flexion (finger will point toward floor). Following each movement, the patient is asked to return to the initial horizontal starting position.

Pronation/supination

With elbows flexed to 90° and held close to body, the patient alternately turns his palms up and down. This test also may be performed with shoulders flexed to

Cont. on the following page(s)

Coordination Tests (in alphabetical order)* *Continued*

TEST	DESCRIPTION
	90° and elbows extended. Speed may be gradually increased. The ability to reverse movements between opposing muscle groups can be assessed at many joints. Examples include active alternation between flexion and extension of the knee, ankle, elbow, fingers, and so forth.
Rebound test	The patient is positioned with the elbow flexed. The therapist applies sufficient manual resistance to produce an isometric contraction of biceps. Resistance is suddenly released. Normally, the opposing muscle group (triceps) will contract and "check" movement of the limb. Many other muscle groups can be tested for this phenomenon, such as the shoulder abductors or flexors, and elbow extensors.
Tapping (foot)	The patient is asked to "tap" the ball of one foot on the floor without raising the knee; heel maintains contact with floor.
Tapping (hand)	With the elbow flexed and the forearm pronated, the patient is asked to "tap" his hand on the knee.
Toe to examiner's finger	From a supine position, the patient is instructed to touch his great toe to the examiner's finger. The position of finger may be altered during testing to assess ability to change distance, direction, and force of movement.

*Tests should be performed first with eyes open and then with eyes closed. Abnormal responses include a gradual deviation from the "holding" position and/or a diminished quality of response with vision occluded. Unless otherwise indicated, tests are performed with the patient in a sitting position.

Tests for Common Disturbances that Affect Coordination (in alphabetical order)	

DEFICIT	SAMPLE TEST
Asthenia	Fixation or position holding (upper and lower extremity) Application of manual resistance to assess muscle strength
Bradykinesia	Walking, observation of arm swing Walking, alter speed and direction Request that a movement or gait activity be stopped abruptly Observation of functional activities
Disturbances of gait	Walk along a straight line Walk sideways, backward March in place Alter speed of ambulatory activities Walk in a circle
Disturbances of posture	Fixation or position holding (upper and lower extremity) Displace balance unexpectedly in sitting or standing Standing, alter base of support Standing, one foot directly in front of the other Standing on one foot
Dysdiadochokinesia	Finger to nose Alternate nose to finger Pronation/supination Knee flexion/extension Walking with alternations in speed
Dysmetria	Pointing and past pointing Drawing a circle or figure eight Heel on shin Placing feet on floor markers while walking
Hypotonia	Passive movement Deep tendon reflexes
Movement decomposition	Finger to nose Finger to therapist's finger Alternate heel to knee Toe to examiner's finger

Cont. on the following page(s)

DEFICIT	SAMPLE TEST
Rigidity	Passive movement Observation during functional activities Observation of resting posture(s)
Tremor (intention)	Observation during functional activities (tremor will typically increase as target is approached or when the patient attempts to hold a position) Alternate nose to finger Finger to finger Finger to therapist's finger Toe to examiner's finger
Tremor (postural)	Observation of normal standing posture
Tremor (resting)	Observation of patient at rest Observation during functional activities (tremor will diminish significantly or disappear)

BRUNNSTROM

Signe Brunnstrom described six stages of recovery for the hemiplegic patient. This classification is widely used, although some of the terms, such as spasticity, were not clearly defined. The following table describes those stages.

Brunnstrom's Stages of Hemiplegic Recovery

STAGE	MOVEMENT	SPASTICITY	EVALUATION METHOD
One	None	Absent	No voluntary movement is present; little or no resistance to passive movement
Two	Weak associated movements in synergy; little or no active finger flexion	Developing	When movement is attempted, there are associated movements in synergy (in the upper extremity seen first with flexion)
Three	All movements are in synergy; mass grasp in hand	Marked	Full upper extremity synergy; hip, knee, and ankle flexion are coupled in either sitting or standing

Cont. on the following page(s)

Brunnstrom's Stages of Hemiplegic Recovery *Continued*

STAGE	MOVEMENT	SPASTICITY	EVALUATION METHOD
Four	Some deviation from synergies; lateral prehension and semivoluntary finger extension	Decreasing	The patient in this stage can: (1) place his hand behind his back; (2) flex at the glenohumeral joint with his elbow extended; (3) pronate and supinate his forearm while the elbow is flexed to 90°; (4) sit and dorsiflex his foot while keeping the foot on the floor; (5) sit and slide his foot on the floor by flexing his knee past 90°.
Five	Almost free from synergies; palmar prehension and voluntary mass extension of digits	Further decrease from stage four	The patient in this stage can perform the tests for stage four with greater ease and: (1) abduct at the glenohumeral joint with the elbow extended; (2) flex at the shoulder joint past 90° with the elbow extended; (3) pronate and supinate the forearm with the elbow extended, especially

with abduction at the glenohumeral joint; (4) stand non-weight-bearing with the affected limb, flex the knee, and extend at the hip; (5) stand with the heel forward, knee extended, and dorsiflex the ankle.

The patient in the this stage can: perform the tests for stage five with greater ease and: (1) stand and abduct the hip; (2) sit, reciprocally contract the medial and lateral hamstring muscles, causing inversion and eversion.

Six	Free of synergy, slightly awkward; all types of prehension (grasps) can be controlled; individual finger movements present	Only during active rapid movements

Reference

1. Brunnstrom, S: Movement Therapy in Hemiplegia. Harper & Row, New York, 1970.

Brunnstrom's Classification of Synergies

The following tables present Signe Brunnstrom's descriptions of hemiplegic synergy patterns. For both the upper and lower extremities, the flexion and extension synergies are listed. Brunnstrom states that, when a person is dominated by a synergy, all of the movements in either the flexion or extension columns occur together.

Upper Extremity Synergies*		
JOINT	FLEXION	EXTENSION
Scapulothoracic	Retraction and/or elevation	Protraction
Glenohumeral	− Abduction to 90°	+ Adduction
	− External rotation	+ Internal rotation
Elbow	+ Flexion	− Extension
Radioulnar	Supination	+ Pronation
Wrist	Flexion	− Extension
Fingers	Flexion	Flexion

+ indicates a strong component of a synergy.

− indicates a weak component of a synergy.

*Although Brunnstrom states that the upper extremity flexion synergy dominates in hemiplegia, she believes that a typical posture for the patient includes the strongest component of each synergy, that is, glenohumeral internal rotation, elbow flexion, radioulnar pronation, and wrist and finger flexion with the thumb in the palm.

Lower Extremity Synergies*		

JOINT	FLEXION	EXTENSION
Hip	+ Flexion, abduction, external rotation	− Extension (limited to the neutral or 0° position), + Adduction, − Internal rotation
Knee	Flexion to 90°	+ Extension
Ankle	+ Dorsiflexion	+ Plantar flexion
Subtalar	Inversion	+ Inversion
Toes	Dorsiflexion (extension)	Plantar flexion (flexion), great toe may extend

+ indicates a strong component of a synergy.

− indicates a weak component of a synergy.

*In the lower extremity, the extensor synergy dominates.

Reference

1. Brunnstrom, S: Movement Therapy in Hemiplegia. Harper & Row, New York, 1970.

PROPRIOCEPTIVE NEUROMUSCULAR FACILITATION

PNF Terms and Techniques
(in alphabetical order)

The definitions presented are those of Knott and Voss. The definitions include a statement explaining the intent of the techniques.

approximation: Joint compression for the purpose of stimulating afferent nerve endings.

contract-relax: Occurs when a limb is passively moved to its point of limitation in the range of motion and then the patient contracts the muscles to be stretched. The therapist resists all movement from this contraction except rotation. The patient is then asked to relax, and the therapist moves the limb in the opposite direction to the motion that would have been caused by the contraction. This is a PNF relaxation technique designed to increase motion of the agonist; also see hold-relax and slow reversal-hold-relax.

hold-relax: Is similar to contract-relax, except that, when the patient contracts, no motion, not even rotation, is allowed to occur and following the isometric contraction the patient's own contraction causes movement to take place. This is a PNF relaxation technique designed to increase motion of the agonist; also see contract-relax and slow reversal-hold-relax.

manual contact: Deep, painless pressure through the therapist's contact for the purpose of stimulating muscle, tendon, and joint afferents.

maximal resistance: Resistance to stronger muscles to obtain "overflow" to weaker muscles.

reinforcement: Use of major muscle groups, or other body parts, in a coordinated fashion to bring about a desired movement pattern.

repeated contractions: An isometric contraction anywhere in the range of motion that is followed by an isotonic contraction for the purpose of facilitating the agonist and relaxing the antagonist.

rhythmic initiation: Passive motion, then assistive motion, and then resistive motion for the purpose of increasing a patient's ability to move.

rhythmic stabilization: Alternating isometric contractions of the agonist and antagonist muscles for the purpose of stimulating movement of the agonist, developing stability, and relaxing the antagonist.

slow reversal: Alternation of activity of opposing muscle groups to stimulate active motion of the agonist, relaxation of the antagonist, and coordination between agonist and antagonist patterns.

slow reversal–hold: Alternation of activity of opposing muscle groups with a pause between reversals to achieve relaxation of the antagonist and to stimulate the agonist.

slow reversal—hold—relax: The patient actively brings the extremity to the point of limitation and then reverses the direction of the motion, while the therapist resists rotation and prevents all other motions. In practice this means that, following movement into rotation, the therapist is resisting an isometric contraction of the shortened muscle. Following the isometric contraction, the patient is told to relax and then to move the limb in the direction in which it was limited. The procedure is then repeated. This is a PNF relaxation technique designed to increase motion of the agonist; also see contract-relax and hold-relax.

timing for emphasis: Maximal resistance of more powerful muscle groups to obtain "overflow" to weaker muscle groups.

traction: Force used to separate joint surfaces by manual contact. The stated purpose is to make joint motion less painful and presumably to stimulate stretch receptors.

Reference

1. Voss, DE, Ionta, MK, and Meyers, BJ: Proprioceptive Neuromuscular Facilitation, ed 3. Harper & Row, Philadelphia, 1985.

PNF Diagonals According to Knott and Voss

PNF diagonals are named according to the movement that will take place. To place a limb in the starting position for a diagonal, the limb is placed in a position so that maximum movement will take place. For example, D₁ flexion starts with the humerus internally rotated, abducted, and extended at the shoulder. The movement is then into external rotation, adduction, and flexion.

Upper Extremity Diagonals

JOINT (PROXIMAL TO DISTAL)	DIAGONAL ONE (D1)		DIAGONAL TWO (D2)	
	FLEXION	EXTENSION	FLEXION	EXTENSION
Scapulothoracic	Rotation, abduction, anterior elevation	Rotation, adduction, posterior depression	Rotation, adduction, posterior elevation	Rotation, abduction, anterior depression
Glenohumeral	External rotation, adduction, flexion	Internal rotation, abduction, extension	External rotation, abduction, flexion	Internal rotation, adduction, extension
Elbow (may be kept flexed or extended)	Flexion	Extension	Flexion	Extension
Radioulnar	Supination	Pronation	Supination	Pronation
Wrist	Flexion, radial deviation	Extension, ulnar deviation	Extension, radial deviation	Flexion, ulnar deviation

	Flexion, adduction to the radial side	Extension, abduction to the ulnar side	Extension, abduction to the radial side	Flexion, adduction to the ulnar side
Fingers				
Thumb	Flexion, abduction	Extension, abduction	Extension, adduction	Flexion, abduction

Lower Extremity Diagonals

JOINT (PROXIMAL TO DISTAL)	DIAGONAL ONE (D1)		DIAGONAL TWO (D2)	
	FLEXION	EXTENSION	FLEXION	EXTENSION
Hip	External rotation, adduction, flexion	Internal rotation, abduction, extension	Internal rotation, abduction, flexion	External rotation, adduction, extension
Knee (may be kept flexed or extended)	Flexion or extension	Extension or flexion	Flexion or extension	Extension or flexion
Ankle	Dorsiflexion	Plantar flexion	Dorsiflexion	Plantar flexion
Subtalar	Inversion	Eversion	Eversion	Inversion
Toes	Extension, abduction to the tibial side	Flexion, adduction to the fibular side	Extension, abduction to the fibular side	Flexion, adduction to the tibial side

Reference

1. Voss, DE, Ionta, MK, and Meyers, BJ: Proprioceptive Neuromuscular Facilitation, ed 3. Harper & Row, Philadelphia, 1985.

429

Functional Expectations for Spinal Cord–Injured Patients*

MOST DISTAL NERVE ROOT SEGMENTS INNERVATED AND KEY MUSCLES	AVAILABLE MOVEMENTS	FUNCTIONAL CAPABILITIES (ASSISTIVE EQUIPMENT MAY BE REQUIRED)	EQUIPMENT AND ASSISTANCE REQUIRED
C1, C2, C3 Face and neck muscles (cranial innervation)	Talking Mastication Sipping Blowing	1. Total dependence in ADL Activation of light switches, page turners, call buttons, electrical appliances, and speaker phones 2. Locomotion	Respirator dependent; may use phrenic nerve stimulator during the day Full-time attendant required Environmental control units Electric wheelchair (typical components include a high, electrically controlled reclining back, a seatbelt and trunk support); a portable respirator may be attached; microswitch or sip-and-puff controls may be used
C4 Diaphragm Trapezius	Respiration Scapular elevation	1. ADL a. Limited self-feeding	Mobile arm supports (possibly with powered elbow orthosis), powered

430

flexor hinge hand splint
Adapted eating equipment (long straws, built-up handles on utensils, plate guards, and so forth)
Plexiglas lapboard
Electric typewriter using head or mouth stick or sip-and-puff controls; another option is a rubber-tipped stick held in hand by a splint (in combination with mobile arm supports and powered splints)

b. Typing

Head or mouth stick
Environmental control unit for powered page turner
Environmental control units

c. Page turning

d. Activation of light switches, call buttons, electrical appliances, and speaker phone

2. Locomotion

Electric wheelchair with mouth, chin, breath, or sip-and-puff controls
Electric reclining back on wheelchair

3. Pressure relief

Cont. on the following page(s)

Functional Expectations for Spinal Cord–Injured Patients* *Continued*

MOST DISTAL NERVE ROOT SEGMENTS INNERVATED AND KEY MUSCLES	AVAILABLE MOVEMENTS	FUNCTIONAL CAPABILITIES (ASSISTIVE EQUIPMENT MAY BE REQUIRED)	EQUIPMENT AND ASSISTANCE REQUIRED
		4. Transfers and bed mobility	Dependent
		5. Skin inspection	Dependent
		6. Cough with glossopharangeal breathing	Dependent
		7. Recreation	Head or mouth stick
		a. Table games such as cards or checkers	Built-up playing pieces
		b. Painting and drawing	
			Full-time attendant required
C5 Biceps Brachialis Brachioradialis	Elbow flexion and supination Shoulder external rotation	1. ADL: able to accomplish all activities of a C4 quadriplegic with less adaptive equipment and more skill	Assistance is required in setting up patient with necessary equipment; patient can then accomplish activity independently
Deltoid Infraspinatus Rhomboid (major and minor) Supinator	Shoulder abduction to 90° Limited shoulder flexion	a. Self-feeding	Mobile arm supports Adapted utensils

b. Typing	Electric typewriter Hand splints Adapted typing sticks Some patients may require mobile arm supports or slings
c. Page turning	Same as above
d. Limited upper extremity dressing	Assistance required
e. Limited self-care (i.e., washing, brushing teeth, and grooming)	Hand splints Adapted equipment (wash mitt, adapted toothbrush, and so forth)
2. Locomotion	Manual wheelchair with handrim projections Electric wheelchair with joystick or adapted upper extremity controls
3. Transfer activities	Overhead swivel bar Sliding board Dependent
4. Skin inspection and pressure relief	Dependent
5. Cough with manual pressure to diaphragm	Assistance required
6. Driving	Van with hand controls Part-time attendant required

Cont. on the following page(s)

Functional Expectations for Spinal Cord–Injured Patients* *Continued*		
MOST DISTAL NERVE ROOT SEGMENTS INNERVATED AND KEY MUSCLES	AVAILABLE MOVEMENTS	FUNCTIONAL CAPABILITIES (ASSISTIVE EQUIPMENT MAY BE REQUIRED)	EQUIPMENT AND ASSISTANCE REQUIRED

MOST DISTAL NERVE ROOT SEGMENTS INNERVATED AND KEY MUSCLES	AVAILABLE MOVEMENTS	FUNCTIONAL CAPABILITIES (ASSISTIVE EQUIPMENT MAY BE REQUIRED)	EQUIPMENT AND ASSISTANCE REQUIRED
C6 Extensor carpi radialis Infraspinatus Latissimus dorsi Pectoralis major (clavicular portion) Pronator teres Serratus anterior Teres minor	Shoulder flexion, extension, internal rotation, and adduction Scapular abduction and upward rotation Forearm pronation Wrist extension (tenodesis grasp)	1. ADL a. Self-feeding b. Dressing c. Self-care d. Bed mobility 2. Locomotion 3. Transfer activities 4. Skin inspection and pressure relief	Universal cuff Intertwine utensils in fingers Adapted utensils Utilizes momentum, button hooks, zipper pulls, or other adaptations; dependent on momentum to extend limbs Cannot tie shoes Flexor hinge splint Universal cuff Adaptive equipment Independent Manual wheelchair with projection or friction surface handrims Independent with sliding board Independent

C7

Extensor pollicus longus and brevis
Extrinsic finger extensors
Flexor carpi radialis
Triceps

Elbow extension
Wrist flexion
Finger extension

5. Bowel and bladder care

6. Cough with application of pressure to abdomen

7. Driving

8. Wheelchair sports

1. ADL
   a. Self-feeding
   b. Dressing

   c. Self-care

2. Locomotion

3. Transfers

Can be independent, depending on bowel and bladder routine

Independent

Automobile with hand controls and U-shaped cuff attached to steering wheel
Usually requires assistance in getting wheelchair into car
Limited participation

Independent
Independent
Button hook may be required
Shower chair
Adapted hand shower nozzle
Adapted handles on bathroom items may be required
Manual wheelchair with friction surface handrims
Independent (usually without sliding board)

Cont. on the following page(s)

435

Functional Expectations for Spinal Cord–Injured Patients* Continued

MOST DISTAL NERVE ROOT SEGMENTS INNERVATED AND KEY MUSCLES	AVAILABLE MOVEMENTS	FUNCTIONAL CAPABILITIES (ASSISTIVE EQUIPMENT MAY BE REQUIRED)	EQUIPMENT AND ASSISTANCE REQUIRED
		4. Bowel and bladder care	Independent with appropriate equipment (digital stimulator, suppositories, raised toilet seat, urinary drainage device, and so forth)
		5. Manual cough	Independent
		6. Housekeeping	Light kitchen activities Requires wheelchair-accessible kitchen and living environment Adapted kitchen tools
		7. Driving	Automobile with hand controls Able to get wheelchair in and out of car
C8 to T1 Extrinsic finger flexors Flexor carpi ulnaris Flexor pollicis longus and brevis	Full innervation of upper extremity muscles	1. ADL	Independent in all self-care and personal hygiene Some adaptive equipment may be required (e.g., tub seat, grab bars, and so forth)

Intrinsic finger flexors	2. Locomotion	Manual wheelchair with standard handrims
	3. Housekeeping	Independent in light housekeeping and meal preparation
		Some adaptive equipment may be required (e.g., reachers)
		Requires a wheelchair-accessible living environment
	4. Driving	Automobile with hand controls
	5. Employment	Able to work in a building free of architectural barriers
T4 to T6	1. ADL	Independent in all areas
Top half of intercostals	2. Physiologic standing (not practical for functional ambulation)	Standing table
Long muscles of back (sacrospinalis and semispinalis)		Bilateral knee-ankle orthoses with spinal attachment
Improved trunk control		Some patients may be able to ambulate for short distances with assistance
Increased respiratory reserve	3. Housekeeping	Independent with routine activities
		Requires a wheelchair-accessible living environment

Cont. on the following page(s)

Functional Expectations for Spinal Cord–Injured Patients* Continued		
MOST DISTAL NERVE ROOT SEGMENTS INNERVATED AND KEY MUSCLES	AVAILABLE MOVEMENTS	FUNCTIONAL CAPABILITIES (ASSISTIVE EQUIPMENT MAY BE REQUIRED)	EQUIPMENT AND ASSISTANCE REQUIRED

MOST DISTAL NERVE ROOT SEGMENTS INNERVATED AND KEY MUSCLES	AVAILABLE MOVEMENTS	FUNCTIONAL CAPABILITIES (ASSISTIVE EQUIPMENT MAY BE REQUIRED)	EQUIPMENT AND ASSISTANCE REQUIRED
		4. Curb climbing in wheelchair	Able to negotiate curbs using a "wheelie" technique
		5. Wheelchair sports	Full participation
T9 to T12 Lower abdominals All intercostals	Improved trunk control Increased endurance	1. Household ambulation	Bilateral knee-ankle orthoses and crutches or walker (high energy consumption for ambulation) Wheelchair used for energy conservation
		2. Locomotion	
L2,L3,L4 Gracilis Iliopsoas Quadratus lumborum	Hip flexion Hip adduction Knee extension	1. Functional ambulation	Bilateral knee-ankle orthoses and crutches
		2. Locomotion	Wheelchair used for convenience and energy

438

		conservation
Rectus femoris		Bilateral ankle-foot orthoses and crutches or canes
Sartorius		Wheelchair used for convenience and energy conservation
L4,L5	Strong hip flexion	1. Functional ambulation
Extensor digitorum	Strong knee extension	2. Locomotion
Low back muscles	Weak knee flexion	
Medial hamstrings (weak)	Improved trunk control	
Posterior tibialis		
Quadriceps		
Tibialis anterior		
Posterior tibialis		
Quadriceps		
Tibialis anterior		

*This table presents general functional expectations at various lesion levels. Each progressively lower segment includes the muscles from the previous levels. Although the key muscles listed frequently receive innervation from several nerve root segments, they are listed here at the neurologic levels where they add to functional outcomes.

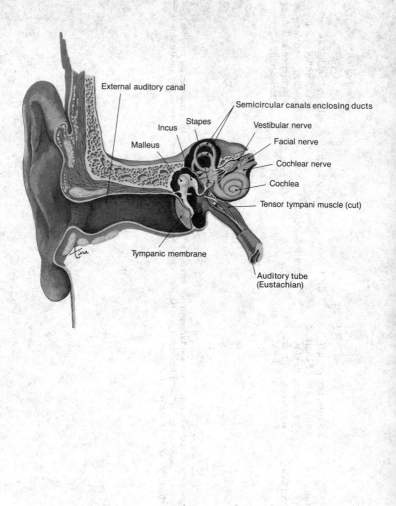

External auditory canal

Semicircular canals enclosing ducts

Stapes

Incus

Vestibular nerve

Malleus

Facial nerve

Cochlear nerve

Cochlea

Tensor tympani muscle (cut)

Tympanic membrane

Auditory tube
(Eustachian)

INNER EAR

The direction of flow of endolymph in the cochlear duct and the direction of flow of the perilymph in the scala tympani and scala vestibuli are shown.

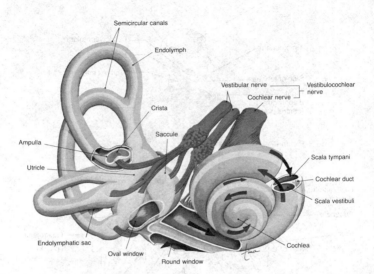

PAIN REFERRED FROM VISCERA

(anterior view)

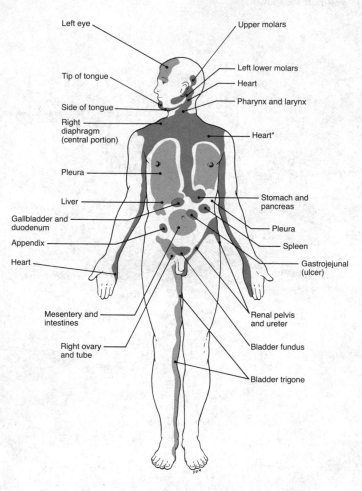

Left eye

Upper molars

Tip of tongue

Left lower molars

Heart

Pharynx and larynx

Side of tongue

Right diaphragm (central portion)

Heart*

Pleura

Liver

Stomach and pancreas

Gallbladder and duodenum

Pleura

Appendix

Spleen

Heart

Gastrojejunal (ulcer)

Mesentery and intestines

Renal pelvis and ureter

Right ovary and tube

Bladder fundus

Bladder trigone

*The pain of coronary insufficiency can involve any aspect of the anterior chest but is more common in the substernal region.

(posterior view)

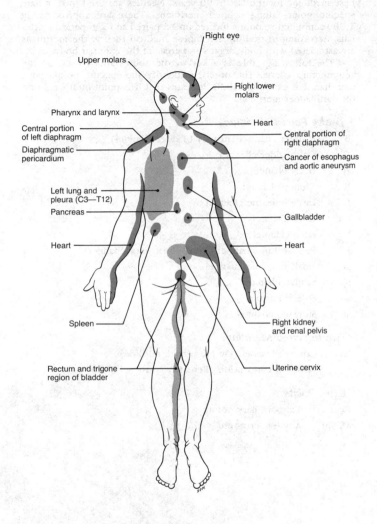

Right eye

Upper molars

Right lower molars

Pharynx and larynx

Heart

Central portion of left diaphragm

Central portion of right diaphragm

Diaphragmatic pericardium

Cancer of esophagus and aortic aneurysm

Left lung and pleura (C3—T12)

Pancreas

Gallbladder

Heart

Heart

Spleen

Right kidney and renal pelvis

Rectum and trigone region of bladder

Uterine cervix

ACUPUNCTURE POINTS

Acupuncture is a technique that has been part of traditional Chinese medicine for the last 5000 years. Needles are used to stimulate specific points along defined meridians. There are approximately 1,000 acupuncture points located on 12 paired and 2 unpaired meridians. According to traditional Chinese medical theory, the meridians are associated with body organs and areas of the external body.

The following table is a key to the abbreviations used on the acupuncture charts. The numbers identify the specific points on a meridian. For example, Gb20 indicates that it is point number 20 on the gallbladder meridian.

Twelve Paired Meridians

B	Bladder channel (urinary bladder channel)
Gb	Gallbladder channel
H	Heart channel
K	Kidney channel
Li	Large intestine channel
Liv	Liver channel
Lu	Lung channel
P	Pericardium channel (heart constrictor channel)
Si	Small intestine channel
Sj	Sanjiao channel
Sp	Spleen channel
St	Stomach channel

Two Unpaired Meridians

Gv	Governor vessel (Du Mo) (back midline)
Vc	Vessel of conception (Ren Mo) (front midline)

Extra Points

Ex	Extraordinary points
Ah Shi	Any tender points

ACUPUNCTURE POINTS

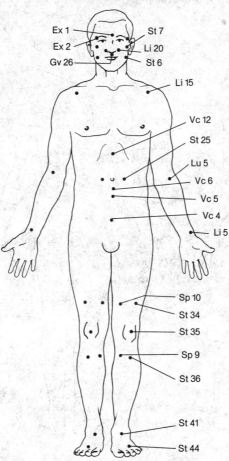

ACUPUNCTURE POINTS

Ex 1
St 7
Ex 2
Li 20
Gv 26
St 6
Li 15
Vc 12
St 25
Lu 5
Vc 6
Vc 5
Vc 4
Li 5
Sp 10
St 34
St 35
Sp 9
St 36
St 41
St 44

ACUPUNCTURE POINTS

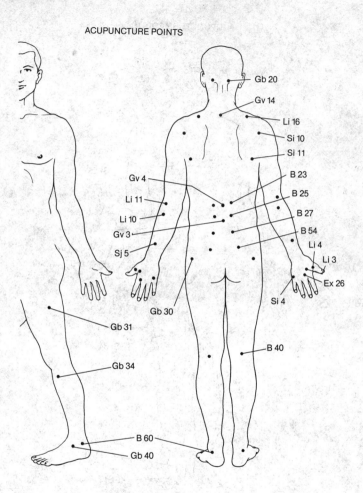

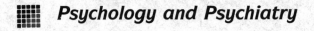

Psychology and Psychiatry

NEUROPSYCHOLOGIC TESTS

Standard Neuropsychologic Tests Listed According to Test Use

A brief description of commonly used tests for neuropsychological evaluations is provided below. Tests are grouped according to function and then listed in alphabetical order. Letters in parentheses following the test names refer to the list of publishers and distributors at the end of the list.

Listing of Tests by Category

Screening Tests
Halstead-Reitan Battery (I)
Luria's Neuropsychological Investigation (K)
Luria-Nebraska Neuropsychological Battery (K)

Tests of Intelligence
Leiter International Performance Scale (LIPS) (K)
Stanford-Binet (S-B) (Houghton Mifflin)
Wechsler Adult Intelligence Scale – Revised (WAIS-R) (G)

Tests of Memory
Auditory Verbal Learning Test (AVLT)
Bender-Gestalt Recall
Benton Visual Retention Test (BVRT) (G)
Memory For Designs (H)
Randt Memory Test
Recurring Figure Test
Russell Revision of the Wechsler Memory Scale
Tactual Performance Test (TPT) (I)
Wechsler Memory Scale (WMS) (G)

Tests of Abstraction and Higher Cognitive Procedures
Category Test (I)
Proverbs Test (H)
Raven's Progressive Matrices (G)
Shipley-Hartford Scale (K)
Trail Making Test (I)
Wisconsin Card Sorting Test (F)

Tests of Perceptual Function

Seashore Rhythm Test (G,I)
Speech Sounds Perception Test (I)

Tests of Constructional Ability

Bender-Gestalt Test (G)
Benton Visual Retention Test (G)
Minnesota Perception Diagnostic Test (K)
Raven's Progressive Matrices (G)

Tests of Visual Sequencing

Symbol Digit Modalities Test
Trail Making Test (I)

Personality Tests

Minnesota Multiphasic Personality Inventory (MMPI) (G)

Test Publishers and Distributors

A. American Guidance Service
   Publisher's Building
   4201 Woodland Road
   Circle Pines, Minnesota 55014
B. Consulting Psychologists Press
   577 College Avenue
   Palo Alto, California 94306
C. Jantak Associates, Inc.
   1526 Gilpin Avenue
   Wilmington, Delaware 19806
D. Lea & Febiger
   200 Chesterfield Parkway
   Malvern, Pennsylvania 19355-9725
E. Department of Psychology
   PO Box 1700
   University of Victoria
   Victoria, British Columbia VAW 2Y2 Canada
F. Psychological Assessment Resources, Inc.
   P.O. Box 998
   Odessa, Florida 33556
G. The Psychological Corporation
   555 Academic Court
   San Antonio, Texas 78204

H. Psychological Test Specialists
   Box 1441
   Missoula, Montana 59801
I. Reitan Neuropsychology Laboratory
   2920 S. 4th Avenue
   Tucson, Arizona 85713
J. Stoelting Co.
   620 Wheat Lane
   Wood Dale, Illinois 60191
K. Western Psychological Services
   12031 Wilshire Boulevard
   Los Angeles, California 90025

References

1. Strub RL and Black, FW: The Mental Status Examination in Neurology, ed 2. FA Davis, Philadelphia, 1986.
2. Strub, RL and Black, FW: Neurobehavioral Disorders: A Clinical Approach. FA Davis, Philadelphia, 1988.
3. Lezak, MD: Neuropsychological Assessment. Oxford University Press, New York, 1983.

STANDARD NEUROPSYCHOLOGICAL TESTS LISTED ALPHABETICALLY

Auditory Verbal Learning Test (AVLT)

An easily administered test of immediate verbal memory span. A 15-word list is administered five times, thus providing a learning curve and documenting learning strategies, retroactive and proactive interferences, and confusion or confabulation tendencies. The test can also measure retention over time when additional delayed trials are administered.

Bender-Gestalt Recall

A test of memory in which patients are asked to recall and reproduce the nine designs that comprise the Bender-Gestalt Test. Unlike other memory tests, patients are not told beforehand that they will be required to recall the designs. The test can be useful in identifying memory deficits in patients who have had a borderline performance on other memory tests where they had the opportunity to make a concerted effort to remember.

Bender-Gestalt Test

A popular, rapid screening test of paper-and-pencil constructional ability. The person being examined reproduces each of nine geometric line and dot drawings. Drawings are scored for errors of integration, distortion, perseveration, and rotation. The test is considered sensitive to neurologic lesions in virtually all quadrants of the brain, especially the nondominant hemisphere.

Benton Visual Retention Test (BVRT)

A test designed to assess visual perception and analysis, short-term visual memory and constructional ability for a wide age range. A series of both simple and complex line drawings are presented to the patient for varying periods. The patient is instructed to reproduce the designs either immediately or after a variable delay. It has explicit scoring instructions and a normative data base.

Category Test

A component of the Halstead-Reiter battery that tests abstract reasoning and problem solving. The patient is required to learn sorting behavior based upon variables such as size, shape, number, color, position, and brightness. Critics say the test is time-consuming and can be frustrating to the patient. The test has been criticized for being highly influenced by the age, education, and intelligence of the person being examined, which can complicate the interpretation of the test.

Halstead-Reiter Battery

Among the most popular and widely reported standardized neuropsychologic research battery in use. The battery is complex and time-consuming and requires special apparatus. It includes tests of general intelligence, concept formation, expressive and receptive language, auditory perception, time perception, verbal and nonverbal memory, perceptual-motor speed, tactile performance, spatial relations, finger agnosis, double simultaneous stimulation, and personality. An impairment index is derived to differentiate most organic from nonorganic conditions. It also may provide information relative to the nature and locus of a lesion, the effect of the neuropsychologic deficit, or the patient's social and adaptive functioning. It is a lengthy test with minimal emphasis on memory or language. This battery also has been criticized for lacking descriptive data functionally relevant to the nonpsychologist.

Leiter International Performance Scale (LIPS)

A test of intelligence that utilizes a pictured stimulus–block-matching paradigm for use with nonverbal children and adults. It is a useful adjunct in those situations when a purely nonverbal test is needed. This test has been criticized for not being well standardized for validity and reliability for ages 14 years to adult.

Luria-Nebraska Neuropsychological Battery

A clinically popular, but controversial battery is primarily used to test patients having suspected brain damage. This battery is an attempt to synthesize the neurologic and psychometric approaches for neuropsychologic assessment. Its advantages are its brevity (1.5 to 2 hours), simplicity of administration and interpretation, and a reporting format that resembles the popular Minnesota Multiphasic Personality Inventory (MMPI). This battery has been criticized for its statistical validity and reliability and the content of certain test items.

Luria's Neuropsychological Investigation

A comprehensive neuropsychologic battery that includes techniques to assess auditory-motor organization, kinesthetic functions, higher visual functions, receptive and expressive language, reading and writing, mathematical skill, memory, and intellectual processes. The test is readily adaptable to individual cases. It is limited in the testing of attention and vigilance, visual memory, and nonverbal abstract reasoning. The test has been criticized for lacking a normative base.

Memory for Designs

A memory test comprised of 15 line drawings of variable complexity that are displayed to the patient one at a time for 5 seconds. The patient must then reproduce the design immediately after exposure. An objective scoring system is provided.

Minnesota Multiphasic Personality Inventory (MMPI)

The most commonly used standardized test of emotional status. The test consists of 566 statements to which the patient responds *true* or *false*, as applicable. Scoring profiles graphically represent performance in the clinical areas of hypochondriasis, depression, hysteria, psychopathic deviancy, masculinity-femininity interests, paranoia, obsessive-compulsive disorder, schizophrenia, hypomania, and social introversion. Experimental scales also are available.

Minnesota Perception–Diagnostic Test

A copying test for constructional ability similar to the Bender-Gestalt and Benton Visual Retention Test. The patient must copy designs and is scored for the degree of rotation. Normative data are provided for both adults and children.

Proverbs Test

A standardized test of proverbs designed to assess the patient's level of abstract versus concrete thinking. The person being examined is presented with four alternative interpretations for each proverb, one of which is the correct abstract response and another a literal interpretation. The other two interpretations are either of variable levels of inaccuracy or are common misinterpretations. The Proverbs Test is presented in a structured multiple-choice format that can be easily scored and compared to standard norms.

Randt Memory Test

A brief (30-minute) test battery designed to test memory acquisition, storage, and both short-term (minutes) and long-term (24 hours) retrieval. The test includes subtests of general information, recall of five items, digit repetition, paired-associate learning, verbal memory for paragraph-length material, visual recognition of pictured items, and incidental memory. The test is based on current theories of memory function. Full standardization of this test is still in progress.

Raven's Progressive Matrices

A test of visual-spatial analysis, spatial conceptualization, and numerical reasoning. The tasks consist of designs with missing parts. The person being examined chooses from the given options the design that fits best. Advantages are its brevity and ease of administration. The test is particularly useful for patients with perceptual motor deficits and cortically damaged patients. Reported drawbacks are its questionable reliability and validity, its extreme difficulty for young children, and its limited normative data base.

Recurring Figures Test

A test to assess visual recognition memory and rate of forgetting. The patient is initially presented with a set of 20 geometric and irregularly drawn nonsense figures that include 8 stimulus designs. The patient is then shown a total of 140 designs comprised of 7 sets of the original 8 designs interspersed with 84 unique designs. The patient must indicate when a previously seen design is presented. Scoring reflects the total number of correct responses, the total geometric versus nonsense designs as well as a measure of "forgetting" over the seven trials. The test is applicable to differentiate brain-damaged patients from normal patients, to lateralize lesions, and in experimental studies of memory processing.

Russell Revision of the Wechsler Memory Scale

A memory test containing a new administration and scoring procedure of the logical memory paragraphs and visual reproduction subtests of the Wechsler Memory Scale (WMS). Each subtest is first administered according to standard procedures and followed 30 minutes later by a delayed recall trial. A short-term memory score, a 30-minute delayed recall score, and a retained memory score are determined. The test is effective in discriminating the unimpaired from patients with dementia. It is useful for comparing verbal with visual memory and delayed with immediate recall.

Seashore Rhythm Test

A test of perceptual function that is an integral part of the Halstead-Reitan Battery and many of its derivatives. This test requires the patient to discriminate between pairs of musical tones that are either the same or different. It is primarily used to assess right temporal lobe functioning.

Shipley-Hartford Scale

A test to measure verbal logical reasoning. A baseline multiple-choice vocabulary test is contrasted with performance on a subtest of verbal abstract reasoning. The test is based on the premise that abstraction is more readily impaired than vocabulary following organic deficits. Advantages are its time and cost-effectiveness.

Speech Sounds Perception Test

A test of perceptual function that is a subtest of the Halstead-Reitan Battery. The patient is required to identify which of four nonsense speechlike syllables they have heard via tape-recorder headphones. The test is an effective measure of sustained attention and is considered to be sensitive to the effects of brain damage, particularly left temporal lesions.

Stanford-Binet

A test of intelligence that is age-graded and highly verbal, with a wide variety of subtests that are arranged in order of difficulty. It is designed primarily for use with children (ages 2 to adult). The test has been criticized for being of questionable validity, for deficiency in pattern analysis, and for providing only an overall IQ. It is not a part of most neuropsychological test batteries.

Symbol Digit Modalities Test

This test assesses visual searching, visual sequencing, sustained attention, and new-learning abilities. The patient is presented with a series of nine symbols, each of which is associated with a number 1 to 9. The patient must then place as many numbers with the correct randomly ordered symbols within a 90-second time period. Responses can be tested verbally or written for further comparison. Normative data are available for ages 18 to 74 and for groups with different educational backgrounds and clinical diagnoses.

Tactual Performance Test

A test of memory that is a part of the Halstead-Reitan battery. The patient is blindfolded and must complete a form board first with the dominant hand and then with both hands. The blindfold and form are removed, and the patient must draw a picture of the form board with shapes aligned correctly. Scoring reflects the time required to complete each trial, the number of correct shapes remembered during the drawing trial, and the correct position of each shape. Despite its popularity, it has been criticized for its complexity, the time required, and the level of frustration that some patients may experience.

Trail Making Test

A popular test included in the Halstead-Reitan battery for visual sequencing, perceptual-motor speed, and the ability to make alternating conceptual shifts. It contains two parts: one to draw a line connecting 25 pseudo-randomly numbered circles and another part where the patient must alternate between letters and numbers to connect the circles. Standardized norms are available for various age groups. The test is considered sensitive to the effects of many brain dysfunctions.

Wechsler Adult Intelligence Scale – Revised (WAIS-R)

This test is one of the many commonly used psychometric tests and one of the most familiar, particularly for evaluating cognitive functioning. The WAIS-R is regarded as the standard test for intelligence in adults between 16 and 74 years of age. This test provides a measure of global intellectual functioning (full-scale IQ) as well as verbal and performance scale IQs from specific subtests. Those IQs within the range of 90 to 110 are classified as average, between 80 and 89 as low average, between 70 and 79 as borderline, and below 70 as mentally retarded. Discrepancies between Verbal and Performance Scale IQs and the variations among subtest scores are used to determine the patient's specific areas of intellectual strength and weaknesses. A Spanish-language version is available, as is a version for children under 16 years of age.

Wechsler Memory Scale (WMS)

A relatively brief (approximately 30 minutes) series of tests to assess memory-related functions. These functions include personal information, current information, orientation, mental control, logical memory, digit span, visual reproduction, and paired-associate learning. A Memory Quotient (MQ) is determined from the performance on the subtests. Scores are age-corrected for increasing chronological age. For many years this was the only widely available and standardized objective test of memory for clinical use. The WMS has been criticized for its highly verbal nature, emphasis on very basic processes (e.g., personal information), and the procedure of combining widely variable tests to provide a MQ.

Wisconsin Card Sorting Test

A test to assess abstract ability, conceptual shifting, and ability to learn. The patient is required to sort a series of printed cards according to color, form, or number. Each time 10 consecutive correct responses are reached, the corrected category is shifted without notice. The test is considered sensitive to frontal lobe lesions.

References

1. Strub, RL and Black, FW: The Mental Status Examinations in Neurology, ed 2. FA Davis, Philadelphia, 1986.
2. Strub, RL and Black, FW: Neurobehavioral Disorders: A Clinical Approach. FA Davis, Philadelphia, 1988.
3. Lezak, MD: Neuropsychological Assessment. Oxford University Press, New York, 1983.

PSYCHOPHARMACOLOGICAL AGENTS

Commonly Prescribed Psychopharmacological Agents: Drugs Used as Antipsychotic Agents

DRUG	TYPE OF SIDE EFFECT		
GENERIC NAME	"EXTRAPYRAMIDAL"	SEDATIVE	ANTICHOLINERGIC
Phenothiazines			
Chlorpromazine (Thorazine)	Mild	Strong	Strong
Fluphenazine (Permitil)	Strong	Weak	Weak
Mesoridazine (Serentil)	Weak to moderate	Moderate to strong	Moderate
Perphenazine (Triavil, Trilafon)	Strong	Weak to moderate	Moderate
Prochlorperazine (Compazine)	Strong	Moderate	Weak
Thioridazine (Mellaril)	Weak	Strong	Strong
Trifluoperazine (Stelazine)	Strong	Weak	Weak
Triflupromazine (Vesprin)	Mild to strong	Mild to strong	Strong

Cont. on the following page(s)

459

Commonly Prescribed Psychopharmacological Agents: Drugs Used as Antipsychotic Agents *Continued*

DRUG	TYPE OF SIDE EFFECT		
GENERIC NAME	"EXTRAPYRAMIDAL"	SEDATIVE	ANTICHOLINERGIC
Thioxanthenes Chlorprothixene (Taractan)	Strong	Weak	Weak
Thiothixene (Navane)	Strong	Weak	Weak
Butyrophenones Haloperidol (Haldol)	Strong	Weak	Weak
Dihydroindolones Molindone (Moban)	Strong	Weak	Weak
Dibenzoxapines Loxapine (Loxitane)	Strong	Weak	Weak

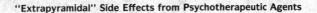

"Extrapyramidal" Side Effects from Psychotherapeutic Agents

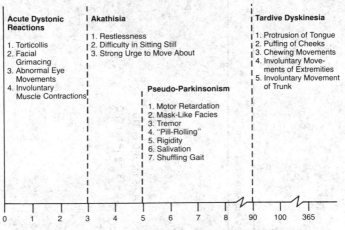

Acute Dystonic Reactions

1. Torticollis
2. Facial Grimacing
3. Abnormal Eye Movements
4. Involuntary Muscle Contractions

Akathisia

1. Restlessness
2. Difficulty in Sitting Still
3. Strong Urge to Move About

Pseudo-Parkinsonism

1. Motor Retardation
2. Mask-Like Facies
3. Tremor
4. "Pill-Rolling"
5. Rigidity
6. Salivation
7. Shuffling Gait

Tardive Dyskinesia

1. Protrusion of Tongue
2. Puffing of Cheeks
3. Chewing Movements
4. Involuntary Movements of Extremities
5. Involuntary Movement of Trunk

0   1   2   3   4   5   6   7   8   90   100   365

TIME FROM ONSET OF NEUROLEPTIC THERAPY (DAYS)

Extrapyramidal side effects and their relative onset after beginning antipsychotic drug therapy (from Carpenter, W and Rudo, A: Tardive dyskinesis. Behavioral Medicine 6:35, 1979. As appearing in Mathewson, MK: Pharmacotherapeutics: A Nursing Process Approach. FA Davis, Philadelphia, 1986).

Commonly Prescribed Psychopharmacologic Agents: Drugs Used as Anti-anxiety Drugs

Benzodiazepine Antianxiety Drugs

GENERIC NAME	TRADE NAME	DOSAGE*	PEAK EFFECT
Chlordiazepoxide	Librium	5–10 mg TID or QID	1–4 hr
Diazepam	Valium (and others)	2–10 mg BID–QID	1–2 hr
Lorazepam	Ativan	1–3 mg BID or TID	2–3 hr
Oxazepam	Serax	10–15 mg TID or QID	3–21 hr

*Indicates usual adult anxiolytic dosage; oral administration.

Commonly Prescribed Psychopharmacologic Agents: Drugs Used as Sedative-Hypnotics			
GENERIC NAME	TRADE NAME	ONSET OF EFFECTS*	DURATION OF ACTION*
Benzodiazepines			
Flurazepam	Dalmane	20–45 min	7–8 hr
Temazepam	Restoril	20–40 min	7–8 hr
Triazolam	Halcion		
Barbiturates			
Pentobarbital	Nembutal	30 min	3–6 hr
Secobarbital	Seconal	30 min	3–5 hr

*Indicates usual single oral hypnotic dose. Doses are usually administered at or just before bedtime.

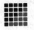

Vascular Anatomy, Cardiology, and Cardiac Rehabilitation

ARTERIES OF THE BODY

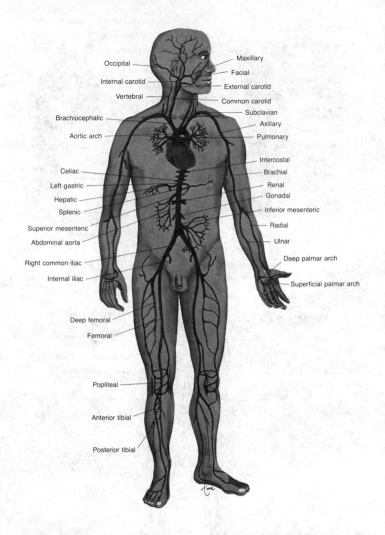

Occipital
Maxillary
Facial
Internal carotid
External carotid
Vertebral
Common carotid
Brachiocephalic
Subclavian
Aortic arch
Axillary
Pulmonary
Intercostal
Celiac
Brachial
Left gastric
Renal
Hepatic
Gonadal
Splenic
Inferior mesenteric
Superior mesenteric
Radial
Abdominal aorta
Ulnar
Right common iliac
Deep palmar arch
Internal iliac
Superficial palmar arch
Deep femoral
Femoral
Popliteal
Anterior tibial
Posterior tibial

BRANCHES OF THE AORTA

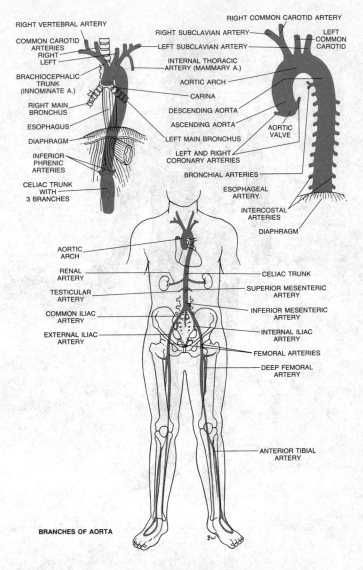

RIGHT VERTEBRAL ARTERY

COMMON CAROTID ARTERIES
RIGHT
LEFT

BRACHIOCEPHALIC TRUNK (INNOMINATE A.)

RIGHT MAIN BRONCHUS

ESOPHAGUS

DIAPHRAGM

INFERIOR PHRENIC ARTERIES

CELIAC TRUNK WITH 3 BRANCHES

RIGHT COMMON CAROTID ARTERY

RIGHT SUBCLAVIAN ARTERY

LEFT SUBCLAVIAN ARTERY

INTERNAL THORACIC ARTERY (MAMMARY A.)

AORTIC ARCH

CARINA

DESCENDING AORTA

ASCENDING AORTA

LEFT MAIN BRONCHUS

LEFT AND RIGHT CORONARY ARTERIES

BRONCHIAL ARTERIES

ESOPHAGEAL ARTERY

LEFT COMMON CAROTID

AORTIC VALVE

INTERCOSTAL ARTERIES

DIAPHRAGM

AORTIC ARCH

RENAL ARTERY

TESTICULAR ARTERY

COMMON ILIAC ARTERY

EXTERNAL ILIAC ARTERY

CELIAC TRUNK

SUPERIOR MESENTERIC ARTERY

INFERIOR MESENTERIC ARTERY

INTERNAL ILIAC ARTERY

FEMORAL ARTERIES

DEEP FEMORAL ARTERY

ANTERIOR TIBIAL ARTERY

BRANCHES OF AORTA

468 VASCULAR ANATOMY, AND CARDIAC REHAB

BRANCHES OF THE AORTA

LOCATION	NAME	STATUS
Thorax		
Ascending aorta	Right and left coronary arteries	One pair
Aortic arch	Brachiocephalic trunk	Unpaired
	Right subclavian	
	Right common carotid	
	Left common carotid	Unpaired
	Left subclavian	Unpaired
Descending aorta	Visceral branches	Unpaired
	Esophageal	
	Left upper and lower bronchial	
	Right bronchial	
	Pericardial	
	Mediastinal	
	Parietal branches	Paired
	Posterior intercostal (T3–T11)	
	Subcostal (T12)	
	Superior phrenic	
Abdominal	Visceral branches	Unpaired
	Celiac	
	Superior mesenteric	
	Inferior mesenteric	
	Glandular/visceral branches	Paired
	Suprarenal	
	Renal	
	Testicular (ovarian)	
	Parietal branches	
	Inferior phrenic	Paired
	Lumbar (L1–L4)	Paired
	Median sacral	Unpaired

Reference

1. Clemente, CD (ed): Gray's Anatomy, ed 30. Lea & Febiger, Philadelphia, 1985.

ARTERIES OF THE PELVIS AND PERINEUM

PARENT VESSEL	PRIMARY BRANCH	SECONDARY BRANCHES	ANASTOMOSES	AREA SUPPLIED
Internal iliac (visceral)	Umbilical	Superior vesical	Artery of ductus Deferens to testicular	Bladder
		Ductus deferens	Testicular	Ductus deferens
		Middle vesical	Branches from the opposite side	Fundus of bladder, seminal vesicles
	Inferior vesicular		Branches from opposite side	
	Middle rectal		Inferior vesical, superior and inferior rectal	
	Uterine		Ovarian	
		Vaginal	Inferior vesical	
Internal iliac (anterior parietal)	Obturator	Iliac	Iliolumbar	Iliacus muscle
		Vesical		Bladder
		Pubic	Inferior epigastric, and its opposite side	
		Anterior	Posterior branch, femoral circumflex	Obturator externus, pectineus, gracilis, and adductor muscles

Artery			Distribution
	Posterior	Anterior branch, inferior gluteal	Hip joint, buttocks
Internal pudendal (listings here are for the male; in the female the artery is smaller and supplies homologous structures)	Muscular	Inferior gluteal	Levator ani, obturator internus, piriformis, coccygeus, and gluteus maximus muscles and other lateral rotators
	Inferior rectal	Perineal, superior and middle rectal, and vessels on the opposite side	Muscles and integument of the anal region
	Perineal	Inferior rectal and vessels on the opposite side	Bulbospongiosus, ischiocavernosus, scrotum
	Artery of the bulb of the penis		Bulb of the penis
	Urethral		Urethra
	Deep artery of the penis	Terminal branch of internal pudendal	Erectile tissue
	Dorsal artery of the penis	Deep artery of the penis	Glans, prepuce

Cont. on the following page(s)

ARTERIES OF THE PELVIS AND PERINEUM *Continued*

PARENT VESSEL	PRIMARY BRANCH	SECONDARY BRANCHES	ANASTOMOSES	AREA SUPPLIED
Internal iliac (posterior parietal)	Iliolumbar	Lumbar	Last lumbar	Psoas major and quadratus lumborum muscles
		Iliac	Iliac of obturator, superior gluteal, iliac circumflex, lateral femoral circumflex	Iliacus and gluteal and abdominal muscles
	Lateral sacral	Superior	Middle sacral, superior gluteal	Skin and muscles on the dorsum of the sacrum
		Inferior	Middle sacral and opposite branch of the lateral sacral	Skin and muscles on the dorsum of the sacrum
	Superior gluteal	Superficial	Inferior gluteal, posterior branches of lateral sacral	Gluteus maximus, skin over the dorsal sacrum
		Deep	Deep iliac circumflex, ascending branch	Gluteal muscles, hip joint

		of lateral femoral circumflex	
Inferior gluteal	Muscular	Superior gluteal, internal pudendal, posterior branch of obturator, medial femoral circumflex	Gluteus maximus, lateral rotator muscles, upper part of hamstring muscles
	Coccygeal	Medial and lateral circumflex	Gluteus maximus and skin over the coccyx
	Artery of sciatic nerve		Runs in the sciatic nerve and supplies that nerve
	Articular	Obturator	Capsule of the hip joint
	Cutaneous		Skin of buttock and posterior thigh
External iliac	Inferior epigastric	Superior epigastric of internal thoracic, lower intercostals	
	Cremasteric (in males)	Testicular, external pudendal, perineal	Cremaster muscle
	Artery of the round ligament (in females)	(Corresponds to cremasteric in women)	Round ligament

Cont. on the following page(s)

ARTERIES OF THE PELVIS AND PERINEUM *Continued*

PARENT VESSEL	PRIMARY BRANCH	SECONDARY BRANCHES	ANASTOMOSES	AREA SUPPLIED
		Pubic	Obturator	
		Muscular	Iliac circumflex, lumbar, superficial epigastric of femoral	Abdominal muscles
	Deep iliac circumflex		Ascending branch of lateral femoral circumflex, iliolumbar, superior gluteal, lumbar, inferior epigastric	

Reference

1. Clemente, CD (ed): Gray's Anatomy, ed 30. Lea & Febiger, Philadelphia, 1985.

ARTERIES OF THE TRUNK

PARENT VESSEL	PRIMARY BRANCH	SECONDARY BRANCHES	ANASTOMOSES	AREA SUPPLIED
Thoracic aorta (visceral)	Pericardial		Pericardiophrenic of internal thoracic	Pericardium, pleura, diaphragm
	Bronchial			Bronchial tubes, areolar tissue of lung, bronchial lymph nodes
	Esophageal		Esophageal branches of inferior thyroid, ascending branches of left inferior phrenic and left gastric	
	Mediastinal			Lymph nodes, vessels, nerve and loose areolar tissue in the posterior mediastinum
Thoracic aorta (parietal)	Posterior intercostal	Dorsal branch		Muscles of the back, dorsal ramus of the spinal nerve
		Collateral intercostal	Internal thoracic	
		Muscular	Highest and lateral thoracic of axillary	Intercostal, pectoral, and serratus anterior muscles

Cont. on the following page(s)

ARTERIES OF THE TRUNK *Continued*

PARENT VESSEL	PRIMARY BRANCH	SECONDARY BRANCHES	ANASTOMOSES	AREA SUPPLIED
		Lateral cutaneous		Skin and superficial fascia overlying the intercostal space
				Breasts
	Subcostal	Mammary	Superior epigastric, caudal intercostal, and lumbar	
	Superior phrenic		Musculophrenic and pericardiophrenic	Dorsal part of the upper surface of the diaphragm
Abdominal aorta (visceral)	Celiac			
		Left gastric	Dorsal branch with right gastric; cardioesophageal branch with esophageals	Cardiac portion of the stomach, lower esophagus, stomach
		Common hepatic (branches listed below)		
		Gastroduodenal	Vessels to stomach and pancreas from superior mesenteric	Pylorus, pancreas, duodenum
		Right gastric	Dorsal branch of left gastric	Pylorus, stomach

	Branch	Anastomoses	Distribution
	Right hepatic		Liver and via the cystic artery to the gallbladder
	Left hepatic		Capsule of the liver, caudate lobe of the liver
	Middle hepatic		Quadrate lobe of liver
Splenic (lienal)	Pancreatic	Gastroduodenal, inferior pancreaticoduodenal of superior mesenteric	Pancreas
	Left gastroepiploic	Gastric and epiploic branches of the right gastroepiploic	Stomach
	Short gastrics	Left gastric, left gastroepiploic, inferior phrenic	Fundus and cardia of stomach
	Splenic	Other splenic branches	Spleen
	Inferior pancreatico-duodenal	Superior and posterior branches of the pancreaticoduodenal of celiac	Pancreas, duodenum
Superior mesenteric	Intestinal (jejunal and ileal)		Small intestine
	Ileocolic	End of superior mesenteric and right colic	Ascending colon, cecum, appendix, termination of ileum
	Right colic	Ileocolic, middle colic	Ascending colon
	Middle colic	Right colic, left colic of inferior mesenteric	Transverse colon

Cont. on the following page(s)

ARTERIES OF THE TRUNK *Continued*

PARENT VESSEL	PRIMARY BRANCH	SECONDARY BRANCHES	ANASTOMOSES	AREA SUPPLIED
	Inferior mesenteric			Left half of transverse colon and descending colon
		Left colic	Middle colic, highest sigmoid	Descending colon, left part of transverse colon
		Sigmoid	Left colic and superior rectal	Caudal part of descending colon, sigmoid colon
		Superior rectal	Middle rectal branches of internal iliac; inferior rectal branches of internal pudendal	Rectum
	Middle suprarenal		Suprarenal branches of inferior phrenic and renals	Suprarenal glands
	Renal			Kidneys
	Testicular (ovarian)		Artery of ductus deferens (ovarian: uterine of internal iliac)	Epididymis (ovaries, round ligament, skin of inguinal region, labia majora)
Abdominal aorta (parietal)	Inferior phrenic	Medial branch	Medial branch of	

		opposite side, musculo-phrenic, pericardio-phrenic	Inferior vena cava, esophagus
	Lateral branch	Lower inter-costals, musculo-phrenic	
Lumbar		Lower intercostals, subcostal, iliolumbar, deep iliac circumflex, inferior epigastric	Muscles and skin of the back
		Lumbar branch of iliolumbar, lateral sacral	
Middle sacral			
Common iliacs (see arteries of the pelvis)			
Abdominal aorta (terminal branch)			

Reference

1. Clemente, CD (ed): Gray's Anatomy, ed 30. Lea & Febiger, Philadelphia 1985.

ARTERIES OF THE HEAD AND UPPER EXTREMITY

PARENT VESSEL	PRIMARY BRANCH	SECONDARY BRANCHES	ANASTOMOSES	AREA SUPPLIED BY SECONDARY BRANCHES
Subclavian	Vertebral	Spinal	Other spinal arteries	Periosteum and bodies of vertebrae
		Muscular	Occipital, ascending and deep cervical arteries	Deep muscles of neck
		Meningeal	Small branches	Falx cerebelli
		Posterior spinal	Vessels on opposite side	
		Anterior spinal	Inferior thyroid, intercostals, lumbar, iliolumbar, and lateral sacral	Pia mater and spinal cord
		Posterior inferior cerebellar	Anterior inferior cerebellar, superior cerebellar of basilar	Medulla and choroid plexus of IV ventricle, inferior surface of the cerebellum to the lateral border
		Basilar	Pontine	Pons and midbrain
			Labyrinthine (internal auditory)	Internal ear
			Anterior inferior cerebellar	Lateral aspect of the pons, anterolateral and anteromedial parts of the inferior surface of the cerebellum

	Superior cerebellar	Superior surface of the cerebellum, midbrain, pineal body, anterior medullary velum, tela choroidea of the III ventricle
	Posterior cerebral	Temporal and occipital lobes
Thyrocervical trunk	Inferior thyroid	Inferior thyroid on the opposite side	Inferior part of thyroid gland
Inferior thyroid	Inferior thyroid on the opposite side	Inferior part of thyroid gland
Suprascapular	Scapular circumflex, descending scapular, thoracoacromial, and subscapular	Supraspinatus and infraspinatus muscles and sternocleidomastoid and surrounding muscles, skin of anterior superior chest, and structures of the shoulder joint, clavicle, and scapular
Transverse Cervical	Descending branch of occipital, subscapular, suprascapular, circumflex scapular, and, through its descending scapular branch, with posterior intercostals	Trapezius, levator scapulae and deep cervical muscles, rhomboid and serratus posterior superior, subscapularis, supraspinatus, and infraspinatus muscles
Internal thoracic		
Pericardiophrenic	Musculophrenic and inferior phrenic	Pleura and Pericardium

Cont. on the following page(s)

ARTERIES OF THE HEAD AND UPPER EXTREMITY *Continued*

PARENT VESSEL	PRIMARY BRANCH	SECONDARY BRANCHES	ANASTOMOSES	AREA SUPPLIED BY SECONDARY BRANCHES
		Mediastinal		Lymph nodes and areolar tissue in the anterior mediastinum
		Thymic		Thymus
		Sternal	Intercostal and bronchial	Transversus thoracis muscle and posterior surface of the sternum
		Anterior intercostals	Posterior intercostals	Intercostal muscles
		Musculophrenic	Pericardiophrenic, mediastinal, intercostals	Diaphragm, abdominal muscles
		Superior epigastric	Superior epigastric on opposite side, inferior epigastric; the right superior epigastric connects with the hepatic	Abdominal muscles and overlying skin
	Costocervical trunk	Highest (supreme) intercostal	Second intercostal	

Artery	Branch	Subbranch	Distribution to	Structures supplied
		Deep cervical	Vertebral, descending occipital	Semispinalis capitis, cervicis and adjacent muscles
		Descending scapular	(Variable artery; when found, its distribution is similar to the deep branch of the transverse cervical)	
Axillary	Highest thoracic		Internal thoracic, intercostals	Pectoral muscles
	Thoracoacromial	Pectoral	Internal and lateral thoracic, intercostals	Pectoral muscles and breast
		Acromial	Suprascapular, thoracoacromial, posterior humeral circumflex	Deltoid muscle
		Clavicular		Pectoralis major and deltoid muscle
		Deltoid		
		Suprascapular		Sternoclavicular joint and subclavius muscles

Cont. on the following page(s)

ARTERIES OF THE HEAD AND UPPER EXTREMITY *Continued*

PARENT VESSEL	PRIMARY BRANCH	SECONDARY BRANCHES	ANASTOMOSES	AREA SUPPLIED BY SECONDARY BRANCHES
	Lateral thoracic		Internal thoracic, subscapular, intercostal, pectoral branch of thoracoacromial	Serratus anterior, pectoral, and subscapularis, and axillary lymph nodes
	Subscapular	Scapular circumflex	Suprascapular, descending scapular	Infraspinatus, teres major and minor muscles long head of the triceps and deltoid muscles
		Thoracodorsal	Circumflex scapular, descending scapular, intercostal, lateral thoracic, thoracoacromial	Subscapularis, latissimus dorsi, Serratus anterior, and intercostal muscles
	Posterior humeral circumflex		Anterior humeral circumflex, deep brachial	Deltoid muscle and shoulder joint
	Anterior humeral circumflex		Posterior humeral circumflex	Head of humerus and shoulder joint
Brachial	Deep Brachial			

		Radial collateral	Posterior humeral circumflex, radial recurrent of radial	
		Middle collateral	Interosseous recurrent	
		Deltoid (ascending)	Posterior humeral circumflex	Brachialis and deltoid muscles
		Nutrient		Humerus
	Principal nutrient of the humerus			Humerus
	Superior ulnar collateral		Posterior ulnar recurrent, inferior ulnar collateral	
	Inferior ulnar collateral		Anterior ulnar recurrent, superior ulnar collateral, posterior ulnar recurrent	
	Muscular			Coracobrachialis, biceps brachii, and brachialis muscles
Radial	Radial recurrent		Radial collateral of deep brachial	Supinator, brachioradialis and brachialis muscles, elbow joint

Cont. on the following page(s)

ARTERIES OF THE HEAD AND UPPER EXTREMITY *Continued*

PARENT VESSEL	PRIMARY BRANCH	SECONDARY BRANCHES	ANASTOMOSES	AREA SUPPLIED
	Muscular			Brachioradialis and pronator teres muscles
	Palmar carpal		Palmar carpal of ulnar, palmar interosseous, deep palmar arch	Carpal bones
	Superficial palmar		Terminal ulnar branches	Muscles of the thenar eminence
	Dorsal carpal		Dorsal carpal branch of ulnar, palmar interosseous, and dorsal interosseous	Fingers
	First dorsal metacarpal			Thumb and index finger
	Princeps pollicis			Skin and subcutaneous tissue of the thumb
	Radial indicis		Proper digital, princeps pollicis	Ulnar aspect of the index finger
	Deep palmar arch		Deep palmar arch of ulnar	

Ulnar	Palmar metacarpal		Common digital branches of the superficial palmar arch	
	Perforating		Dorsal metacarpal	
	Recurrent		Palmar carpal network	Intercarpal articulations
	Anterior ulnar recurrent		Superior and inferior ulnar collaterals	Brachialis and pronator teres muscles
	Posterior ulnar recurrent		Superior and inferior ulnar collaterals, interosseous recurrents	Elbow joint and muscles near the elbow joint
	Common interosseous	Palmar (anterior) interosseous	Dorsal interosseous	Flexor digitorum profundus and flexor pollicis longus muscles, radius and ulna
		Dorsal (posterior) interosseous	Palmar interosseous, dorsal carpal network	Superficial and deep muscles of the posterior compartment of the forearm
	Muscular			Superficial and deep flexors of the finger and muscles on the ulnar aspect of the forearm

Cont. on the following page(s)

ARTERIES OF THE HEAD AND UPPER EXTREMITY *Continued*

PARENT VESSEL	PRIMARY BRANCH	SECONDARY BRANCHES	ANASTOMOSES	AREA SUPPLIED BY SECONDARY BRANCHES
	Palmar carpal		Corresponding palmar carpal branch of the radial	
	Dorsal carpal		Corresponding dorsal carpal branch of the radial	Ulnar aspect of dorsal surface of the little finger
	Deep palmar		Radial to complete the deep palmar arch	
	Superficial palmar arch		Superficial palmar branch of the radial	
	Common palmar digital		Dorsal digital	Soft parts on the dorsum of the middle and distal phalanges
		Proper palmar digital	Dorsal branches to dorsal digital	

Reference

1. Clemente, CD (ed): Gray's Anatomy, ed 30. Lea & Febiger, Philadelphia, 1985.

ARTERIES OF THE LOWER EXTREMITY

PARENT VESSEL	PRIMARY BRANCH	SECONDARY BRANCHES	ANASTOMOSES	AREA SUPPLIED
Femoral	Superficial epigastric		Inferior epigastric and superficial epigastric on the opposite side	Superficial subinguinal lymph nodes
	Superficial iliac circumflex		Deep circumflex iliac, superior gluteal, lateral femoral circumflex	Skin of the groin and superficial subinguinal lymph nodes
	Superficial external pudendal		Internal pudendal	Skin of the lower part of the abdomen, scrotum, and penis (labia majora in female)
	Deep external pudendal		Posterior scrotal (labial), branches of the perineal	Skin of the scrotum (labial majora in Female)
	Muscular			Sartorius, vastus medialis, adductor muscles
	Deep femoral	Medial femoral circumflex	Ascending branch with obturator; superficial branch with inferior	Ascending to adductor muscles, gracilis and obturator externus

Cont. on the following page(s)

ARTERIES OF THE LOWER EXTREMITY *Continued*

PARENT VESSEL	PRIMARY BRANCH	SECONDARY BRANCHES	ANASTOMOSES	AREA SUPPLIED
			gluteal, lateral femoral circumflex, first perforating; deep branch with gluteals; acetabular branch with obturator	muscles; transverse branch to the adductor magnus and brevis muscles; acetabular branch to the fat in the acetabular fossa
		Lateral femoral circumflex	Ascending branch with superior gluteal and deep iliac circumflex; descending branch with superior lateral genicular branch of popliteal; transverse branch with medial femoral circumflex, inferior gluteal, first perforating	
		Perforating	First perforating with inferior gluteal, medial and lateral femoral circumflex, and second	First perforating to adductor brevis and magnus muscles, biceps femoris and gluteus maximus

			perforating; second with first and third perforating; third with second perforating, deep femoral terminal branches and popliteal	muscles; second perforating to posterior femoral muscles
	Muscular		Medial femoral circumflex, superior branches of popliteal	Adductor muscles, hamstring muscles
	Descending genicular	Saphenous	Medial inferior genicular	Skin on the upper and medial leg
		Articular branch	Medial superior genicular and anterior recurrent tibial	Knee joint
Popliteal	Superior muscular		Terminals of deep femoral	Lower parts of the adductor magnus and hamstring muscles
	Sural			Gastrocnemius, soleus, and plantaris muscles
	Cutaneous			Skin on the back of the leg
	Superior genicular	Medial superior genicular	Descending and medial inferior geniculars, lateral superior genicular	Vastus medialis muscle, femur, knee joint

Cont. on the following page(s)

ARTERIES OF THE LOWER EXTREMITY *Continued*

PARENT VESSEL	PRIMARY BRANCH	SECONDARY BRANCHES	ANASTOMOSES	AREA SUPPLIED
		Lateral superior genicular (superficial and deep branches)	Descending branch of lateral femoral circumflex and lateral inferior genicular	Vastus lateralis muscle, femur, knee joint
	Middle genicular			Ligaments and synovial membrane of the knee joint
	Inferior genicular			Popliteus muscle, upper end of tibia, knee joint
		Medial inferior genicular	Lateral inferior and medial superior geniculars	
		Lateral inferior genicular	Medial inferior and lateral superior geniculars, anterior and posterior recurrents of tibial, circumflex fibular	
Anterior tibial	Posterior tibial recurrent		Inferior genicular of popliteal	Popliteus muscle
	Anterior tibial recurrent		Genicular branches of popliteal, circumflex fibular, and	

		descending genicular	
Muscular			Muscles along the vessel
Anterior medial malleolar		Posterior tibial and peroneal	
Anterior lateral malleolar		Posterior tibial, medial plantar	Lateral aspect of the ankle
Dorsal pedis	Arcuate, anterior lateral malleolar, lateral plantar, peroneal	Perforating branch of the peroneal and lateral tarsal	Extensor digitorum brevis muscle
Lateral tarsal			
Medial tarsal		Medial malleolar network	
Arcuate		Lateral tarsal and plantars to yield the second through fourth dorsal metatarsals and two dorsal digital arteries	
First dorsal metatarsal			
Deep plantar		Unites with terminals of lateral plantar to complete plantar arch; produces first plantar metatarsal artery	Medial border of the great toe

Cont. on the following page(s)

493

ARTERIES OF THE LOWER EXTREMITY Continued

PARENT VESSEL	PRIMARY BRANCH	SECONDARY BRANCHES	ANASTOMOSES	AREA SUPPLIED
Posterior tibial	Circumflex fibular		Vessels around knee joint	Soleus and peroneal muscles
	Peroneal	Muscular		Soleus, tibialis posterior, flexor hallucis longus, and peroneal muscles
		Nutrient (fibular)		Fibular
		Perforating	Anterior lateral malleolar, lateral metatarsal	Tarsal bone
		Communicating	Communicating of posterior tibial	
		Lateral malleolar	Lateral malleolar network	
		Lateral calcaneal	Anterior lateral malleolar, medial calcaneal	
	Nutrient (tibial)			Tibialis posterior muscle, tibia

Branch	Subdivision	Distribution
Muscular		Soleus and deep muscles along the back of the leg
Medial malleolar		Medial malleolar network
Communicating		Joins communicating branch of the peroneal
Medial calcaneal		Peroneal, medial malleolar, lateral calcaneal
Medial plantar		First dorsal or plantar metatarsal
Lateral plantar		Muscles on the tibial side of the sole of the foot
	Perforating	Dorsal metatarsals to yield plantar digital arteries; anterior perforating branch to join dorsal metatarsal
		Digits

Reference

1. Clemente, CD (ed): Gray's Anatomy, ed 30. Lea & Febiger, Philadelphia, 1985.

VEINS OF THE BODY

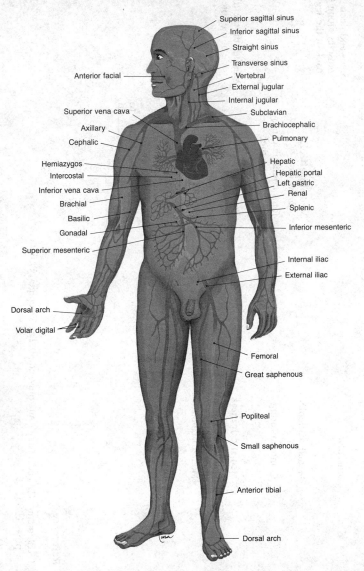

Superior sagittal sinus
Inferior sagittal sinus
Straight sinus
Transverse sinus
Vertebral
External jugular
Internal jugular
Subclavian
Brachiocephalic
Pulmonary
Hepatic
Hepatic portal
Left gastric
Renal
Splenic
Inferior mesenteric
Internal iliac
External iliac
Femoral
Great saphenous
Popliteal
Small saphenous
Anterior tibial
Dorsal arch

Anterior facial
Superior vena cava
Axillary
Cephalic
Hemiazygos
Intercostal
Inferior vena cava
Brachial
Basilic
Gonadal
Superior mesenteric
Dorsal arch
Volar digital

Venous Drainage from the Lungs

VEIN	PRIMARY TRIBUTARY	AREA DRAINED
Right pulmonary veins (2)	Right superior pulmonary	Right superior and middle lobes
	Apical segmental	Apex and anterior segments
	Posterior segmental	Posterior middle and superior lobes
	Anterior segmental	Right superior lobe
	Right middle lobe	Middle lobe
	Right inferior pulmonary	Right inferior hilum
	Superior segmental	Medial middle lobe
	Common basal	Anterior basal, lateral basal, and posterior basal segments
Left pulmonary veins (2)	Left superior pulmonary	Apicoposterior, anterior segments
	Apicoposterior segmental	Apicoposterior segments
	Posterior segmental	Intrasegmental and intersegmental areas
	Lingular division	Superior and inferior lingular segments
	Left inferior pulmonary	Intrasegmental and intersegmental areas
	Superior basal	Anterior basal segments
	Inferior basal	Posterior and lateral basal segments

Venous Drainage of the Heart

VEIN	PRIMARY TRIBUTARY	AREA DRAINED
Coronary sinus	Great cardiac	Left atrium, both ventricles
	Small cardiac	Posterior right atrium and ventricle
	Middle cardiac	Both ventricles
	Posterior vein of left ventricle	Left ventricle
	Oblique vein of left atrium	Left atrium
Anterior cardiac		Anterior right ventricle
Small cardiac (thebesian)		Both atria

Venous Drainage of the Face — Deep

VEIN	PRIMARY TRIBUTARY	AREA DRAINED
Maxillary	Confluence of veins of pterygoid plexus	Cavernous sinus
Pterygoid plexus	Veins accompanying maxillary artery	Muscles of mastication

Venous Drainage of the Face — Superficial

VEIN	PRIMARY TRIBUTARY	AREA DRAINED
Facial	Angular, which is formed by the following:	
	Frontal	Anterior scalp
	Supraorbital	Forehead

VEIN	PRIMARY TRIBUTARY	AREA DRAINED
	Deep facial	Muscles of facial expression
	Superficial temporal	Vertex and side of head
	Posterior auricular	Back of ear
	Occipital	Superior sagittal and transverse sinuses
	Retromandibular	Parotid gland and masseter

Venous Drainage of the Cranium — The Brain

VEIN	PRIMARY TRIBUTARY	AREA DRAINED
External cerebral	Superior cerebral (8 to 12 veins)	Superior, lateral, and medial surfaces of hemisphere and opens into the superior sagittal sinus
	Middle cerebral	Lateral hemispheric surfaces into cavernous and sphenoparietal sinuses
	Inferior cerebral	Inferior hemispheric surfaces into superior sagittal sinus
Internal cerebral	Great cerebral (Galen's)	Interior of hemispheres into inferior sagittal sinus
	Internal cerebral, which is formed by:	
	Thalamostriate	Corpus striatum, thalamus

Cont. on the following page(s)

VEIN	PRIMARY TRIBUTARY	AREA DRAINED
	Choroid	Choroid plexus, hippocampus, fornix, corpus callosum
	Basal	Insula, corpus striatum
Cerebellar	Superior cerebellar	Superior vermis into the straight sinus
	Inferior cerebellar	Lower cerebellum into transverse, occipital, and superior petrosal sinuses

Venous Drainage of the Cranium—Sinuses of the Dura Mater

VEIN	PRIMARY TRIBUTARY	AREA DRAINED
Posterior superior sinuses	Superior sagittal sinus	Superior cerebral veins, dura mater
	Inferior sagittal sinus	Falx cerebri and medial surfaces of the hemispheres
	Straight sinus	Inferior sagittal sinus, great cerebral vein
	Transverse sinuses	Right drains superior sagittal and the left straight sinuses; also receives blood from the superior petrosal sinuses

VEIN	PRIMARY TRIBUTARY	AREA DRAINED
	Sigmoid sinuses	Transverse sinuses
	Occipital sinus	Posterior internal vertebral venous plexus into the confluence of sinuses
	Confluence of sinuses	Superior sagittal, straight, occipital, and both transverse sinuses
Anterior inferior sinuses	Cavernous sinus	Superior and inferior ophthalmic veins, some cerebral veins, sphenoparietal sinus
	Superior ophthalmic vein	Corresponding branches of ophthalmic artery
	Inferior ophthalmic vein	Muscles of eye movements
	Intercavernous sinuses	Connects the two cavernous sinuses across the midline
	Superior petrosal sinus	Cerebellar and inferior cerebral veins, veins from tympanic cavity; connects cavernous and transverse sinuses
	Inferior petrosal sinus	Internal auditory veins, veins from medulla, pons, and inferior

Cont. on the following page(s)

VEIN	PRIMARY TRIBUTARY	AREA DRAINED
		surface of cerebellum; drains into the internal jugular bulb
	Basilar plexus	Connects inferior petrosal sinuses

Reference

1. Clemente, CD (ed): Gray's Anatomy, ed 30. Lea & Febiger, Philadelphia, 1985.

VEIN	PRIMARY TRIBUTARY	AREA DRAINED
Diploic	Frontal	Communicates with supraorbital vein and superior sagittal sinus
	Anterior temporal	Temporal communicates with the sphenoparietal sinus and the deep temporal veins
	Posterior temporal	Transverse sinus
	Occipital	Occipital vein, transverse sinus, or confluence of sinuses
Emissary	Mastoid	Connects transverse sinus with the posterior auricular or occipital veins
	Parietal	Connects superior sagittal sinus with veins of the scalp
	Rete hypoglossal canal	Joins transverse sinus with vertebral vein and deep veins of the neck
	Rete foramen ovalis	Connects cavernous sinus with pterygoid plexus through foramen ovale
	Internal carotid plexus	Connects cavernous sinus and internal jugular vein via carotid canal
	Vein of foramen cecum	Connects superior sagittal sinus with veins of nasal cavity

Venous Drainage of the Neck

VEIN	PRIMARY TRIBUTARY	AREA DRAINED
External jugular	Posterior external jugular	Skin and superficial muscles in cranium and posterior neck
	Anterior jugular	Inferior thyroid veins by way of jugular venous arch, internal jugular
	Transverse cervical	Trapezius and surrounding muscles
	Suprascapular	Supraspinatus and feeds into the external jugular near the subclavian
Internal jugular	Inferior petrosal sinus	Internal auditory veins and veins of brainstem
	Lingual	Tongue
	Pharyngeal	Pharynx and vein of pterygoid canal
	Superior thyroid	Thyroid gland and receives superior laryngeal and cricothyroid veins
	Middle thyroid	Inferior thyroid gland
Vertebral	Anterior vertebral	Upper cervical vertebrae
	Accessory vertebral	Cervical vertebrae
	Deep cervical	Suboccipital muscles and cervical vertebrae

VEIN	PRIMARY TRIBUTARY	AREA DRAINED
Azygos	Posterior intercostals	Dorsal spinal musculature and thoracic vertebrae
	Subcostal	Musculature about the twelfth rib and thoracic vertebrae
	Hemiazygos	Four or five intercostal veins, left subcostal vein, some esophageal and mediastinal veins
	Accessory hemiazygos	Intercostal veins on the left side
	Bronchial	Bronchi of lungs
Brachiocephalic	Right brachiocephalic	Right vertebral, internal thoracic, inferior thyroid, and first intercostal veins
	Left brachiocephalic	Same as right brachiocephalic, except it drains left side
Internal thoracic		Drainage corresponds to arterial blood supply of internal thoracic
Inferior thyroid		Lower portion of thyroid gland and receives esophageal, tracheal, and inferior laryngeal veins
Highest intercostal		Upper two or three intercostal spaces; right drains into azygos and left into brachiocephalic

Cont. on the following page(s)

VEIN	PRIMARY TRIBUTARY	AREA DRAINED
Veins of vertebral column	External vertebral venous plexus	Mostly cervical vertebrae and connects with vertebral, occipital, and deep cervical veins
	Internal vertebral venous plexus	Posterior aspects of vertebrae, including ligaments and arches and connects with vertebral veins, occipital sinus, and basilar plexus
	Basivertebral	Foramina of dorsal vertebral bodies and communicates with anterior external vertebral plexuses
	Intervertebral	Internal and external vertebral plexuses and ends in vertebral, intercostal, lumbar, and lateral sacral veins
	Veins of spinal cord	Spinal cord into vertebral veins

Venous Drainage of the Abdomen

VEIN	PRIMARY TRIBUTARY	AREA DRAINED
Inferior vena cava	Lumbar	Posterior wall muscles, vertebral plexuses, and into azygos system via ascending lumbar veins

VEIN	PRIMARY TRIBUTARY	AREA DRAINED
	Testicular (in males)	Epididymis, testis, spermatic cord; right testicular enters the inferior vena cava and left into the renal vein
	Ovarian (in females)	Ovaries, broad ligament; right enters the inferior vena cava and left into the renal vein
	Renal	Kidneys and receives left testicular (or ovarian), inferior phrenic, and suprarenal veins
	Suprarenal	Suprarenal glands
	Inferior phrenic	Undersurface of diaphragm and ending in renal or suprarenal vein on left and inferior vena cava on right
	Hepatic	Liver

Venous Drainage of the Liver — Portal Venous Drainage

VEIN	PRIMARY TRIBUTARY	AREA DRAINED
Portal	Lienal (splenic)	Spleen and entering superior mesenteric vein to form the portal vein
	Branches: Short gastric	Greater curvature of the stomach
	Left gastro-epiploic	Stomach and greater omentum
	Pancreatic	Body and tail of pancreas
	Inferior mesenteric	Rectum, sigmoid and descending colon and receives sigmoid, and inferior rectal veins

Cont. on the following page(s)

VEIN	PRIMARY TRIBUTARY	AREA DRAINED
	Superior mesen- teric	Small intestine, cecum, ascending and transverse colon
	Branches: Right gastro- epiploic	Stomach and greater omentum
	Pancreatico- duodenal	Pancreas and duodenum
	Coronary	Stomach and its lesser curvature, lesser omentum ending in portal vein
	Pyloric	Pyloric portion of lesser curvature of stomach and ending in portal vein
	Cystic	Gallbladder ending in right branch of portal vein
	Paraumbilical	Ligamentum teres of liver and connecting veins of anterior abdominal wall to portal, internal, and common iliac veins

Venous Drainage of the Pelvis and Perineum

VEIN	PRIMARY TRIBUTARY	AREA DRAINED
Common iliac	Iliolumbar	Posterior pelvis and lumbar vertebrae
	Lateral sacral	Anterior sacrum
	Middle sacral	Additional sacral drainage to left common iliac vein
Internal iliac	Superior gluteal	Buttocks
	Inferior gluteal	Posterior thigh and buttocks
	Internal pudendal	Penis, urethral bulb

VEIN	PRIMARY TRIBUTARY	AREA DRAINED
	Obturator	Adductor region of the thigh
	Lateral sacral	Anterior surface of sacrum
	Middle rectal	Rectal plexus, bladder, prostate, seminal vesicle, and levator ani
	Inferior rectal	Lower rectum draining into the internal pudendal vein
	Dorsal vein of penis	Superficial drains prepuce and skin while deep vein drains glans penis, corpora cavernosa
	Vesical	Bladder and base of prostate
	Uterine	Uterus
	Vaginal	Vagina

Venous Drainage of the Lower Extremity — Boundary of Abdomen and Lower Extremity

VEIN	PRIMARY TRIBUTARY	AREA DRAINED
External iliac	Inferior epigastric	Internal surface of lower abdominal wall
	Deep iliac circumflex	Deep tissue around anterior superior iliac spine and inner pelvic brim
	Superficial external pudendal	Superficial lower abdomen, scrotum, and labia and upper thigh

VEIN	PRIMARY TRIBUTARY	AREA DRAINED
Great saphenous		Medial aspect of leg from ankle upward across medial knee and thigh to enter femoral vein at femoral ring
	Accessory saphenous	Medial and posterior thigh
Small saphenous		Lateral to Achilles tendon up posterior leg to popliteal vein
Dorsal digital		Clefts between toes
Intercapitular		Form short common digital veins to produce dorsal venous arch
Plantar cutaneous venous arch		Sole of the foot

VEIN	PRIMARY TRIBUTARY	AREA DRAINED
Plantar digital		Plantar surface of toes of foot to drain into plantar metatarsal veins
Plantar metatarsal		Along metatarsal bones to ankle and contributing to deep plantar venous arch
Medial plantar		Medial aspect of sole of foot and upward to form posterior tibial vein
Lateral plantar		Lateral aspect of sole of foot and upward to form posterior tibial vein
Posterior tibial		Medial portion of deep muscles of leg and draining into popliteal vein
Peroneal		Venous plexus of heel along lateral leg to drain into posterior tibial vein
Anterior tibial		Anterior compartment of leg to drain into popliteal vein
Popliteal		Posteromedial muscles of thigh to become femoral vein
Femoral		Anterior compartment of thigh to drain into external iliac
Femoral profunda		Deep muscles of anterior, anteromedial, and anterolateral thigh to drain into femoral vein

VEIN	PRIMARY TRIBUTARY	AREA DRAINED
Palmar digital		Palmar surface of digits and connected to dorsal digital veins by oblique intercapitular veins
Dorsal digital venous network		Tissues of fingers and along fingers dorsally to back of hand
Median ante-brachial		Superficial veins of hand up forearm to basilic vein below elbow
Basilic		Back of hand to anterior surface of arm above elbow to upper third of arm, draining into brachial vein
Accessory cephalic		Ulnar side of dorsal venous network to cephalic at elbow
Cephalic		Drains hand, forearm, and arm by extending up lateral aspect of arm to axillary vein near clavicle

VEIN	PRIMARY TRIBUTARY	AREA DRAINED
Superficial and deep palmar venous arches		Fingers
Palmar and dorsal metacarpal		Metacarpals
Brachial		From the elbow on each side of forearm, draining deep tissues to form the axillary in the arm
Axillary		Axillary and clavicular join to drain into subclavian vein
Subclavian		Drains external jugular and anterior jugular and enters the internal jugular vein, along with thoracic duct on left and right lymphatic duct on right

Reference

1. Clemente, CD (ed): Gray's Anatomy, ed 30. Lea & Febiger, Philadelphia, 1985.

BLOOD PRESSURE

Systole

The period of cardiac contraction.

Diastole

The period of cardiac relaxation, or cardiac filling.

Procedure for Measuring Blood Pressure: The cuff is placed 1 to 2 inches above the antecubital fossa, inflated until no radial pulse is palpable, and then the brachial artery is auscultated over the fossa during deflation of the cuff. The sounds heard vary in intensity and quality during deflation and are called Korotkoff's sounds. Five phases of Korotkoff's sounds are described.

phase 1: First sounds that are heard, clear tapping sounds that increase in intensity. Systolic blood pressure is when rhythmic tapping is first heard.

phase 2: The clear tapping sound of phase 1 is replaced with a softer muffled sound or murmur.

phase 3: A less clear but louder and crisper tapping sound replaces the muffled sound of phase 2.

phase 4: Tapping of phase 3 changes to muffled, soft blowing sound. This is sometimes called the *first diastolic pressure*.

phase 5: Disappearance of all sounds. Diastolic blood pressure generally measured as this phase if only two values are recorded. If three pressures are recorded, phase 5 is the *second diastolic pressure*.

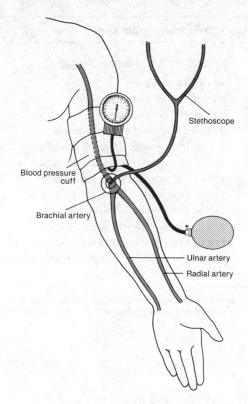

Stethoscope

Blood pressure
cuff

Brachial artery

Ulnar artery

Radial artery

Placement of the blood pressure cuff and stethoscope for monitoring brachial artery pressure.

Variations in Blood Pressure with Age*

AGE	NORMAL BLOOD PRESSURE (mmHg)
Newborn	40 to 70 systolic
1 month	80 systolic, 45 diastolic
6 months	90 systolic, 60 diastolic
2 years	80 to 90 systolic, 55 to 65 diastolic
4 years	100 to 115 systolic, 55 to 75 diastolic
6 years	105 to 125 systolic, 60 to 80 diastolic
8 years	105 to 125 systolic, 65 to 80 diastolic
10 years	110 to 135 systolic, 65 to 80 diastolic
12 years	115 to 135 systolic, 65 to 80 diastolic
14 years	120 to 140 systolic, 70 to 85 diastolic
Adult	110 to 140 systolic, 60 to 80 diastolic
Elderly	Same as for an adult, or slightly higher systolic and slightly lower diastolic

*(From Kozier and Erb: Techniques of Clinical Nursing. Addison-Wesley, Redwood City, CA, 1989, p 487, with permission.)

LYMPHATIC SYSTEM

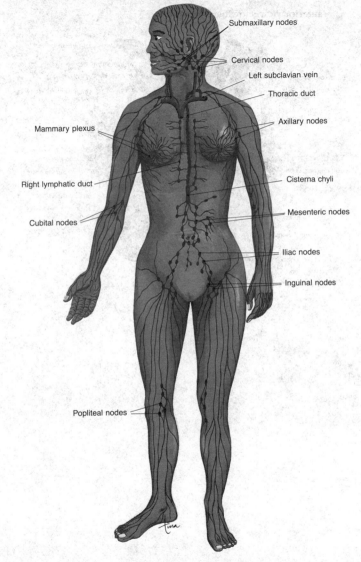

The lymphatic system, with major nodes illustrated.

THE HEART—EXTERNAL ANATOMY

(anterior view showing circulation)

- Left subclavian artery
- Left subclavian vein
- Left internal jugular vein
- Left common carotid artery
- Aortic arch
- Left pulmonary artery (to lungs)
- Left atrium
- Left pulmonary veins (from lungs)
- Circumflex artery
- Left coronary artery
- Left coronary vein
- Left anterior descending artery
- Left ventricle

- Brachiocephalic (trunk) artery
- Superior vena cava
- Right pulmonary artery
- Right pulmonary veins
- Right atrium
- Right coronary artery
- Inferior vena cava
- Right ventricle
- Aorta

THE HEART—EXTERNAL ANATOMY

(posterior view showing circulation)

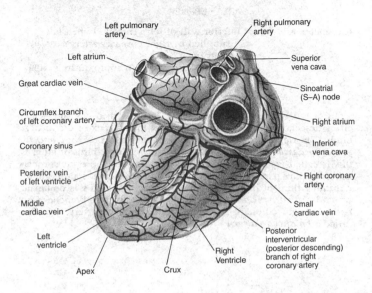

Left pulmonary artery

Left atrium

Great cardiac vein

Circumflex branch of left coronary artery

Coronary sinus

Posterior vein of left ventricle

Middle cardiac vein

Left ventricle

Apex

Crux

Right Ventricle

Right pulmonary artery

Superior vena cava

Sinoatrial (S–A) node

Right atrium

Inferior vena cava

Right coronary artery

Small cardiac vein

Posterior interventricular (posterior descending) branch of right coronary artery

ARTERY | AREA SUPPLIED

Circumflex Artery — Inferior wall of left ventricle (when not supplied by right coronary artery)

Left atrium

Sinoatrial (SA) node (in approximately 40% of humans)

Coronary artery dominance is a term used to describe which artery descends posteriorly from the crux to the apex of the myocardium. The right coronary artery is dominant and branches into the *posterior descending branch* in approximately two thirds of humans; this is called *right dominance*. In these persons the right coronary artery supplies part of the left ventricle and ventricular septum. In the remaining third of humans, a branch of the circumflex is dominant, which is called *left dominance*, or dominance is from branches from both the right coronary artery and the circumflex artery, which is called a *balanced pattern*.

VASCULAR SUPPLY TO THE CONDUCTION SYSTEM

There is considerable variation in the arterial venous branches to the myocardium. The table below lists the most common distributions.

ARTERY	AREA SUPPLIED
Right coronary artery (RCA)	Right atrium Right ventricle Inferior wall of left ventricle (in most humans) Atrioventricular (AV) node Bundle of His Sinoatrial (SA) node (in approximately 60% of humans)
Left anterior descending artery (LAD)	Left ventricle Interventricular septum Right ventricle Inferior areas of the apex Inferior areas of both ventricles

References

1. Brannon, FJ, Geyer, MJ, and Foley, MW: Cardiac Rehabilitation. FA Davis, Philadelphia, 1988.
2. Netter, FJ: The CIBA Collection of Medical Illustrations, Vol 5, Heart. CIBA, Summit, NJ 1978.

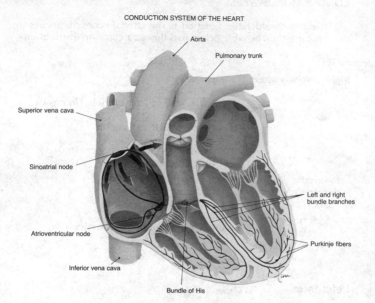

CONDUCTION SYSTEM OF THE HEART

Aorta

Pulmonary trunk

Superior vena cava

Sinoatrial node

Atrioventricular node

Inferior vena cava

Left and right bundle branches

Purkinje fibers

Bundle of His

ELECTROCARDIOGRAPHIC (EKG) WAVES, SEGMENTS, AND INTERVALS

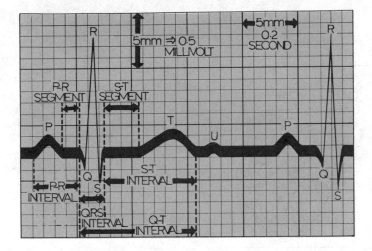

Normal Ranges of EKG Components

	DURATION	AMPLITUDE
P wave	<.10 s	1 – 3 mm
PR interval	0.12 – 0.20 s	Isoelectric after the P-wave deflection
QRS	0.06 – 0.10 s	25 – 30 mm (maximum)
ST segment	0.12 s	−½ to +1 mm
T wave	0.16 s	5 – 10 mm

ELECTROCARDIOGRAPHIC (EKG)
RECORDING OF MYOCARDIAL ACTIVITY

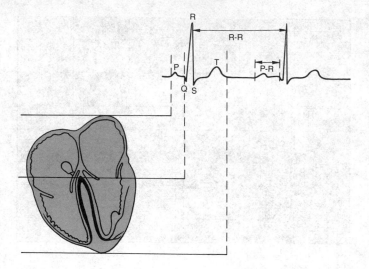

EKG COMPONENT	MYOCARDIAL EVENT
P wave	Atrial depolarization
QRS complex	Ventricular depolarization
T wave	Ventricular repolarization

INTERPRETING THE ELECTROCARDIOGRAPH

Steps to Follow When Interpreting an EKG Rhythm Strip

1. Calculate the rate.
2. Examine the rhythm and determine if regular or irregular.
3. Identify P waves.
4. Evaluate P-R interval for duration and relationship of P wave to QRS complex.
5. Evaluate QRS complex for shape and duration.
6. Identify extra waves or complexes.
7. Determine clinical significance of a dysrhythmia.

Abbreviations Used in EKG Interpretation

APC (APB)	Atrial premature contraction (beat)
CHB	Complete heart block
JPC (JPB)	Junctional premature contraction (beat)
LBBB	Left bundle branch block
NPC (NPB)	Nodal premature contraction (beat)
NSR	Normal sinus rhythm
PAC (PAB)	Premature atrial contraction (beat)
PAT	Paroxysmal atrial tachycardia
PJC (PJB)	Premature junctional contraction (beat)
PNC (PNC)	Premature nodal contraction (beat)
PVC (PVB)	Premature ventricular contraction (beat)
RBBB	Right bundle branch block
RSR	Regular sinus rhythm
SVT	Supraventricular tachycardia
VPC (VPB)	Ventricular premature contraction (beat)

Reference

1. Brown, JR and Jacobson, S: Mastering Dysrhythmias: A Problem-Solving Guide. FA Davis, Philadelphia, 1988.

METHODS USED TO CALCULATE HEART RATES

Calculating the Rate

Four methods can be used to calculate rates with regular cardiac rhythms. When conduction is normal, both atrial and ventricular rates are identical.

Heart Rate Normal Values

Normal	60 to 100 beats per minute
Bradycardia	less than 60 beats per minute
Tachycardia	greater than 100 beats per minute

When the rhythm is irregular, each beat in a 30 or 60 second rhythm strip should be counted to estimate the rate.

First Method for Calculating Rate: Multiply the number of QRS complexes in a 6 second strip (most EKG paper has markers every 1, 3, or 6 seconds) by 10 (chart speed = 25 mm/s). Estimate the portion of an R-R interval when only a portion of one is contained at the end of 6 seconds.

Second Method for Calculating Rate: Divide 300 by the number of whole or partial large boxes between two consecutive R waves.

Third Method for Calculating Rate: Find an R wave that falls on a large box line and count how many large boxes are in the interval before the next R wave. Memorize the values for each large box interval.

Heart Rate	Number of Large Boxes
300	1
150	2
100	3
75	4
60	5
50	6
43	7

Fourth Method for Calculating Rate: Divide 1500 by the number of small boxes between consecutive R waves.

CARDIAC RATES: EXAMPLES

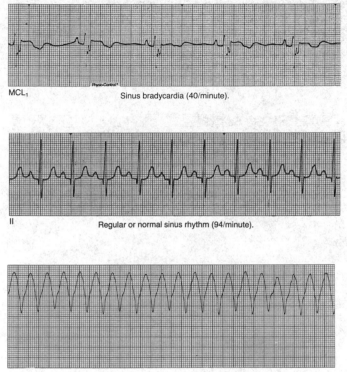

MCL₁   Physio-Control®

Sinus bradycardia (40/minute).

II

Regular or normal sinus rhythm (94/minute).

Ventricular tachycardia (180/minute).

ASSESSING THE REGULARITY OF AN EKG RHYTHM STRIP

Examine the Rhythm and Determine if Regular or Irregular: Assess the regularity of the R-R intervals. A regular rhythm has equally sized spaces between all intervals. An intermittently irregular rhythm is generally regular with occasional disruptions (extra beats, for example). A regularly irregular rhythm has a cyclical pattern of varying R-R intervals. An irregularly irregular rhythm has no recurring pattern; R-R intervals vary in an inconsistent manner.

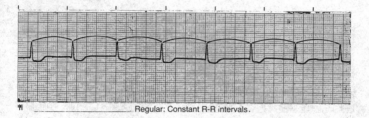

Regular: Constant R-R intervals.

Examples of Irregular Rhythms

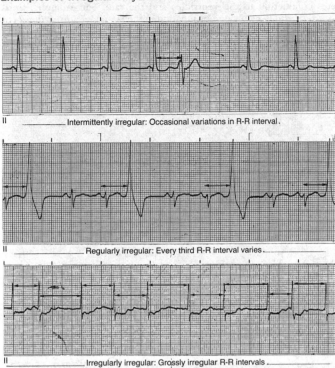

II — Intermittently irregular: Occasional variations in R-R interval.

II — Regularly irregular: Every third R-R interval varies.

II — Irregularly irregular: Grossly irregular R-R intervals.

Naming Rhythms: Rhythms are generally named by the beat that initiates conduction to the ventricles and the rate. For example, *sinus bradycardia* is a slow rate originating in the S-A node, a *junctional* (or *nodal*) *rhythm* is a normal rate originating in the A-V junction, and *ventricular tachycardia* is a rapid rhythm originating in the ventricles.

Examples of Named Rhythms

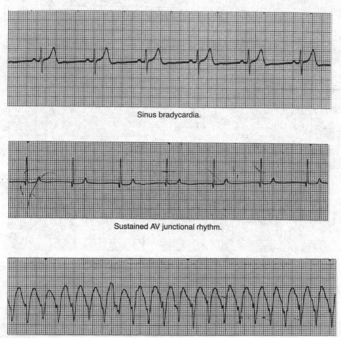

Sinus bradycardia.

Sustained AV junctional rhythm.

Ventricular tachycardia.

IDENTIFYING P WAVES

The presence of P waves indicates that myocardial conduction is initiated in the atria. A normal impulse initiated in the S-A node has a P wave that is upright, rounded, and 1 to 3 mm tall. The P waves that are abnormally shaped include *flutter* (F) waves, which are also called *saw-toothed* and have a regular pattern; *fibrillation* (f), which are small, grossly irregular deflections on the baseline; and *premature* P waves, which look different and usually have a different P-R interval than the regular P waves in a rhythm strip. (Premature beats are discussed under extra beats.)

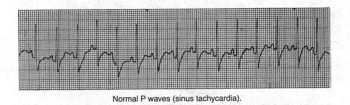

Normal P waves (sinus tachycardia).

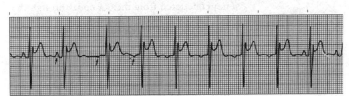

Alterations in P wave shapes.

Evaluating the P-R Interval for Duration and Relationship of P Wave to QRS Complex

The normal P-R interval is between 0.12 and 0.20 seconds (3 to 5 small boxes). A shorter-than-normal P-R interval indicates increased A-V conduction or an atrial impulse that does not originate in the S-A node. A longer-than-normal P-R interval indicates a slowing of conduction from the S-A node into the A-V junction. A prolonged P-R interval defines *atrioventricular heart block*. With normal conduction, a QRS complex should follow each P wave.

TYPE OF BLOCK	CHARACTERISTICS
First degree	Prolonged P-R interval; all P waves are followed by a QRS complex
Second degree Mobitz Type I (Wenckebach)	Progressive lengthening of the P-R interval until one P wave is not conducted (no QRS follows a P wave). Occurs as a regular irregularity.
Mobitz Type II	Atrial rate is regular, but some impulses are not conducted from the S-A node through the A-V junction. Ratio of conduction (e.g., 2 : 1 or 3 : 1) is regular. Occurs as a regular irregularity.
Third degree (complete)	No conduction of impulse through the A-V junction; no relationship between atrial and ventricular activity. Atrial and ventricular rhythms may be regular, but the ventricular rate is initiated below the A-V node and is slow and independent of atrial activity.

TYPES OF ATRIOVENTRICULAR
HEART BLOCKS

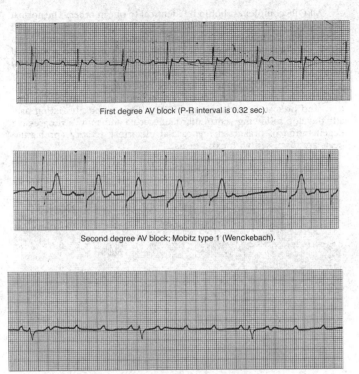

First degree AV block (P-R interval is 0.32 sec).

Second degree AV block; Mobitz type 1 (Wenckebach).

Second degree AV block; Mobitz type 2; 4:1 AV conduction ratio.

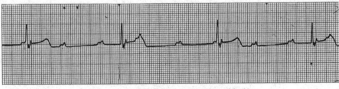

Third degree AV block (complete heart block).

EVALUATION OF QRS COMPLEX FOR SHAPE AND DURATION

All QRS complexes should be identical to one another. The normal duration of a QRS complex is 0.10 to 0.60 seconds (1.5–2.5 small boxes). Bundle branch blocks signify conduction interference down either the right or left bundle. Although both demonstrate a widened QRS complex, a right bundle branch block (RBBB) has a notched and widened R component, and a left bundle branch block (LBBB) has only a widened R. Bundle branch blocks are best diagnosed with a 12-lead EKG. Irregularities in ventricular conduction include flutter, fibrillation, and premature contractions (PVCs). Flutter and fibrillation usually develop following ventricular tachycardia and show a progressive degeneration of organized myocardial electrical activity (premature beats are discussed with extra beats).

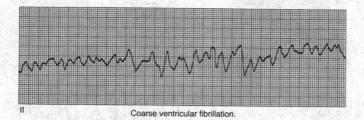

II

Coarse ventricular fibrillation.

IDENTIFYING EXTRA WAVES OR COMPLEXES

Extra waves or complexes signify myocardial irritability. The problem may be atrial, junctional (nodal), and/or ventricular. The severity of an arrhythmia is related to the location, frequency, and number of sites where extra beats are initiated.

Supraventricular Dysrhythmias

Premature atrial contractions (PACs) arise from an ectopic atrial focus. Their P waves look different from normal and also usually have a different P-R interval. *Premature junctional (nodal) contractions (PJCs)* originate in the A-V junction; the P wave may be inverted due to retrograde conduction and may occur before, following, and buried within the QRS complex. Both PACs and PJCs have normally shaped QRS complexes and are generally not dangerous unless frequent or associated with signs and symptoms of altered hemodynamics.

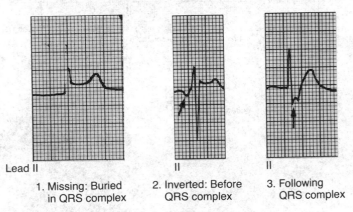

Lead II   II   II

1. Missing: Buried in QRS complex   2. Inverted: Before QRS complex   3. Following QRS complex

Position of P wave in AV junctional complexes.

Premature Contractions

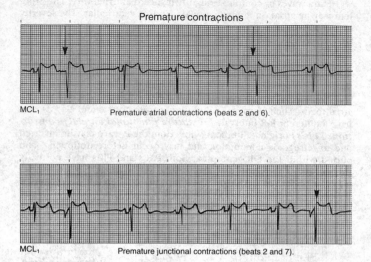

Premature contractions

MCL₁

Premature atrial contractions (beats 2 and 6).

MCL₁

Premature junctional contractions (beats 2 and 7).

Ventricular Dysrhythmias

Premature ventricular contractions (PVCs) are the most dangerous and are classified by frequency and irritable foci. The PVCs are not preceded by a P wave, are conducted abnormally through the ventricles, and are characterized by wide, bizarre QRS complexes. *Unifocal PVCs* arise from a single irritable focus and are identically shaped; *multifocal PVCs* come from different sites and do not look alike. Frequency of PVCs is described by the terms *single, quadrigeminy* (one PVC every fourth beat), *trigeminy* (one every third beat), and *bigeminy* (every other beat is a PVC). Paired PVCs are called *couplets* and a run of PVCs is called a *salvo*. As PVCs signify ventricular irritability, multiple sites and increasing frequency are potentially lethal because the cardiac rhythm may disintegrate into ventricular tachycardia, fibrillation, or asystole. More than six PVCs per minute is considered dangerous. Particularly lethal is a PVC that falls on a T wave (R on T phenomenon). It does not allow the ventricle to repolarize, and ventricular fibrillation is likely to ensue.

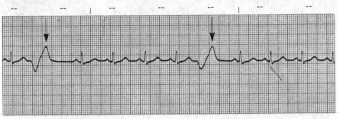

Two unifocal premature ventricular contractions (PVCs) (beats 2 and 7).

Ventricular Dysrhythmias

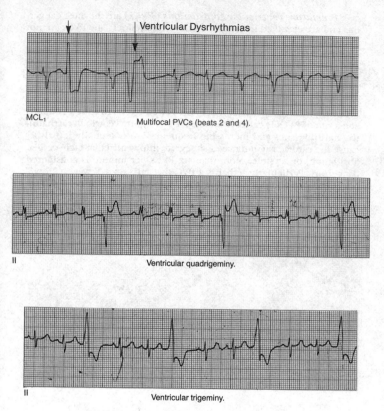

MCL₁   Multifocal PVCs (beats 2 and 4).

II   Ventricular quadrigeminy.

II   Ventricular trigeminy.

Ventricular Dysrhythmias

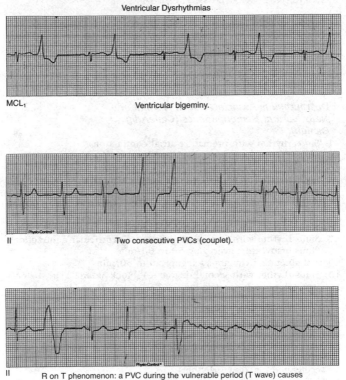

Ventricular Dysrhythmias

MCL₁   Ventricular bigeminy.

II   Two consecutive PVCs (couplet).

II   R on T phenomenon: a PVC during the vulnerable period (T wave) causes
                              ventricular fibrillation.

DETERMINING THE CLINICAL
SIGNIFICANCE OF A DYSRHYTHMIA

Dysrhythmias result in varying degrees of abnormal hemodynamics. Cardiac output is decreased with very slow or very rapid rates.

Dysrhythmias Classified by Their Effect on Cardiac Output*

Dysrhythmias Associated with Normal or Near Normal Hemodynamics (Generally Benign)

1. Sinus rhythm with premature atrial contractions
2. Sinus rhythm with premature junctional contractions
3. Artificial pacemaker rhythm with 1 : 1 capture
4. Atrial fibrillation with an average ventricular response between 60 and 100/min
5. Atrial flutter with an average ventricular response between 60 and 100/min
6. Sinus rhythm with first degree A-V block
7. Sinus rhythm with occasional premature ventricular contractions
8. Sinus bradycardia averaging 50 to 60/min
9. A-V junctional rhythm averaging 50 to 60/min
10. Sinus rhythm with second degree A-V block Mobitz Type 1
11. Isorhythmic A-V dissociation

Dysrhythmias with Normal or Near Normal Hemodynamics but Potentially Dangerous

1. Sinus rhythm with short episodes of ventricular tachycardia
2. Sinus rhythm with short episodes of paroxysmal supraventricular tachycardia
3. Accelerated junctional rhythms
4. Artificial pacemaker rhythm with premature ventricular contractions that are new, multifocal, or couplets
5. Sinus rhythm with second degree A-V block Mobitz Type 2
6. Atrial flutter or fibrillation with tachycardia ventricular rates
7. Sinus rhythm with sinus arrest
8. Sinus bradycardia with rates below 50/min

Dysrhythmias with Significantly Altered Hemodynamics

1. Ventricular tachycardia (with pulses)
2. Sinus rhythm or atrial fibrillation with complete heart block
3. Very slow (40/min or below) sinus, junctional, or idioventricular rhythms
4. Malfunctioning artificial pacemakers with idioventricular rhythms

Dysrhythmias Associated with Absent Hemodynamics — Lethal Conditions

1. Ventricular fibrillation
2. Asystole
3. Pulseless ventricular tachycardia or flutter
4. Agonal idioventricular complexes
5. Electromechanical dissociation
6. Third-degree A-V heart block with ventricular standstill

---

*Classification devised by Fritz Streuli, M.D.

CARDIAC EXAMINATION

auscultation: Listening to the intensity and quality of heart sounds as they vary over the surface of the chest. Four primary areas are identified over which to auscultate the cardiac valves.

Area to Auscultate for the Cardiac Valves	
VALVE	AREA TO AUSCULTATE
Aortic	Second right intercostal space at right sternal border (base of heart)
Pulmonic	Second left intercostal space at left sternal border
Tricuspid	Fourth left intercostal space along lower left sternal border
Mitral	Fifth left intercostal space at midclavicular line (apical area)

References

1. Seidel, HM, et al: Mosby's Guide to Physical Examination. CV Mosby, St. Louis, 1987.
2. Sokolow, M and McIlroy, MB: Clinical Cardiology. Lange Medical Publications, Los Altos, CA, 1981.

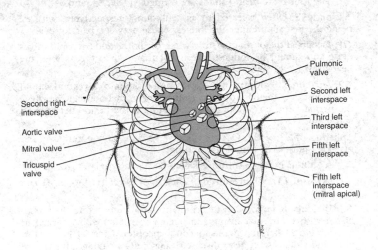

Second right interspace

Aortic valve

Mitral valve

Tricuspid valve

Pulmonic valve

Second left interspace

Third left interspace

Fifth left interspace

Fifth left interspace (mitral apical)

BASIC HEART SOUNDS

The four basic heart sounds are termed S1, S2, S3, and S4.

S1 and S2: Often referred to as "lub-dub," respectively, with S1 being the first sound after the longest pause between pairs of beats.

S1: Occurs at the onset of systole when the mitral and tricuspid valves close and should be loudest when auscultated over the apex of the heart (left lower sternal border).

S2: Attributed to closure of the aortic and pulmonic valves and should be loudest over the base of heart (left upper sternal border). Systole is the period between S1 and S2, and diastole is the period between S2 and the next S1.

splitting of S1 or S2: Occurs when valves close asynchronously and may be a normal or pathologic finding.

A2 and P2: When splitting is heard, S2 is referred to as A2 and P2.

M1 and T1: When splitting is heard, S1 is referred to as M1 and T1.

S3: Difficult or impossible to hear without a stethoscope. It is associated with ventricular filling and occurs soon after S2. A normal or physiologic S3 is often found in young people. When S3 is heard in older individuals with heart disease, it may indicate congestive failure and is called a *ventricular gallop*.

S4: Difficult or impossible to hear without a stethoscope. It is associated with ventricular filling as well as atrial contraction and occurs just before S1. An audible S4 is generally pathologic and may indicate hypertensive cardiovascular disease, coronary artery disease, postmyocardial infarction, aortic stenosis, or cardiomyopathy.

summation gallop: May be present with severe myocardial disease. It is a long heart sound that occurs when S3 and S4 blend together.

ventricular gallop: See S3.

EXTRA HEART SOUNDS (murmurs)

Described as *snaps, clicks, rubs,* and *murmurs*. Extra sounds are generally pathologic. Murmurs are caused by disturbances in the normal blood flow through the cardiac chambers and are usually classified based on their duration (timing), intensity, quality, pitch, location, and radiation. The following criteria are used for classification.

timing: During systole, diastole, or both. A murmur may be described as lasting an entire time period (holosystolic or pansystolic) or during a portion of a time period (early diastolic).

intensity: The system for evaluating the intensity of extra sounds is:

grade 1: Softest audible murmur.

grade 2: Murmur of medium intensity.

grade 3: Loud murmur without thrill.

grade 4: Murmur with thrill.

grade 5: Loudest murmur that cannot be heard with stethoscope off the chest.

grade 6: Audible with stethoscope off the chest.

quality: This describes the tone of the murmur, such as harsh, musical, blowing, rumbling. A crescendo murmur increases in intensity, a decrescendo murmur falls, and a crescendo-decrescendo murmur rises and then falls.

pitch: High, medium, or low pitched.

location: Area of the precordium in which the murmur is heard: aortic, pulmonic, tricuspid, mitral.

radiation: Described when the sound of the murmur is transmitted to other regions of the body, such as across the chest, into the axilla or neck, or down the left sternal border.

THE CARDIAC CYCLE

The events of the cardiac cycle are depicted below, showing changes in left atrial pressure, left ventricular pressure, aortic pressure, ventricular volume, the electrocardiogram, and the phonocardiogram.

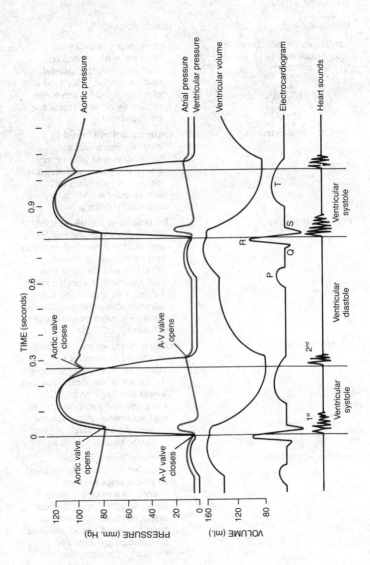

DIAGNOSTIC TESTS FOR CARDIAC DYSFUNCTION

PROCEDURE	DESCRIPTION
Cardiac catheterization (for angiography)	The coronary arteries are injected with a contrast material, and the arterial system can be visualized with cinefluoroscopy: narrowing or occlusion of arteries can be evaluated
Cardiac catheterization	Catheterization is used to measure intracardiac, transvalve, and pulmonary artery pressures and measure blood gas pressures to determine cardiac output and evaluate shunting
Echocardiography	The reflections of ultrasound waves from cardiac surfaces are analyzed; used to evaluate left ventricular systolic function and the structure and function of cardiac walls, valves, and chambers; can identify abnormal conditions such as tumors or pericardial effusion
Electrocardiogram	Surface electrodes record the electrical activity of the heart; 12-lead EKG provides 12 views of the heart; used to assess cardiac rhythm, diagnose the location, extent, and acuteness of myocardial ischemia and infarction, and evaluate changes with activity
Exercise stress tests	Numerous protocols for exercise tests have been used to assess responses to increased workloads with steps, treadmills, or bicycle ergometers; in conjunction with EKG and blood pressure recordings, patients are evaluated for exercise

PROCEDURE	DESCRIPTION
	capacity, cardiac dysrhythmias, and diagnosis, prognosis, and management of coronary artery disease.
Holter monitoring	Continuous ambulatory EKG monitoring done by tape recording the cardiac rhythm for up to 24 hours; used to evaluate cardiac rhythm, efficacy of medications, transient symptoms that may indicate cardiac disease, and pacemaker function, and to correlate symptoms with activity
Phonocardiography	Records cardiac sounds; used to time the events of the cardiac cycle and to confirm auscultatory findings
Radionuclide angiography	Red blood cells tagged (marked) with a radionuclide are injected into blood; ventricular wall motion can be evaluated and the ejection fraction determined; abnormal blood flow with valve and congenital defects can also be detected; techniques include gated-pool equilibrium studies and first-pass techniques
Technetium 99m scanning (hot spot imaging)	Technetium 99m injected into blood is taken up by damaged myocardial tissue; this identifies and localizes acute myocardial infarctions
Thallium-201 myocardial perfusion imaging (cold spot imaging)	Thallium-201 injected into blood at peak exercise; scanning identifies ischemic and infarcted myocardium,

Cont. on the following page(s)

PROCEDURE   DESCRIPTION

which does not take up
thallium-201; used to
diagnose coronary artery
disease and perfusion,
particularly when EKG is
equivocal

Reference

1. Warren, JV and Lewis, RP: Diagnostic Procedures in Cardiology: A
   Clinician's Guide. Year Book Medical Publishers, Chicago, 1985.

DIAGNOSIS OF ACUTE MYOCARDIAL INFARCTION

Signs and Symptoms. Signs and symptoms of acute myocardial infarction (AMI) include pain similar to that for angina pectoris. There is a heaviness, squeezing, or tight feeling in the chest, nausea and vomiting, light-headedness, dyspnea and hypotension, sweating, weakness, and apprehension. There may be fever, shock, and cardiac failure.

Myocardial Enzymes: Tissue necrosis causes enzymes to be released into the blood. Enzymes released by myocardial damage demonstrate a characteristic pattern and duration of presence in the blood.

ABBREVIATION FOR ENZYME	ENZYME (NORMAL VALUE)	DESCRIPTION
AST (formerly called SGOT)	Aspartate aminotransferase (serum glutamic-oxaloacetic transaminase) (<45 U/ml)	Appears in serum within hours, peaks at 12 to 24 hours, falls to normal within 2 to 7 days; AST is also released due to damage to muscle, brain tissue, and other internal organs
CPK (CK)	Creatine phosphokinase (<30) U/ml	Appears in serum within hours, peaks within 24 hours, falls to normal within 3 to 5 days; CPK is also released due to damage to brain tissue and skeletal muscle
CK-MB	Creatine kinase myocardial band isoenzyme ($<5\%$ CPK)	Isoenzyme of CPK more specific for myocardial damage; appears in serum at 4 to 6 hours, peaks at 12 to 24 hours, falls to normal within 48 hours

Continued on the following page(s)

LDH (LD)	Lactate dehydrogenase (<600 U/ml)	Begins to rise 12 to 24 hours, peaks by day 3, and returns to normal within 8 to 12 days; also released due to damage to brain, red blood cell tisue, kidney, lung, and spleen

---

Functional and Therapeutic Classifications of Patients with Diseases of the Heart

---

FUNCTIONAL	PERMISSIBLE WORK LOADS CONTINUOUS – INTERMITTENT	MAXIMAL
Class I	4.0 – 6.0 cal/min	6.5 METs

Patients with cardiac disease but without resulting limitations of physical activity. Ordinary physical activity does not cause undue fatigue, palpitation, dyspnea, or anginal pain.

| Class II | 3.0 – 4.0 cal/min | 4.5 METs |

Patients with cardiac disease resulting in slight limitation of physical activity. Patients are comfortable at rest. Ordinary physical activity results in fatigue, palpitation, dyspnea, or anginal pain.

| Class III | 2.0 – 3.0 cal/min | 3.0 METs |

Patients with cardiac disease resulting in marked limitation of physical activity. Patients are comfortable at rest. Less than ordinary physical activity causes fatigue, palpitation, dyspnea, or anginal pain.

| Class IV | 1.0 – 2.0 cal/min | 1.5 METs |

Patients with cardiac disease resulting in inability to carry on any physical activity without discomfort. Symptoms of cardiac insufficiency or of the anginal syndrome may be present even at rest. If any physical activity is undertaken, discomfort is increased.

FUNCTIONAL	PERMISSIBLE WORK LOADS CONTINUOUS – INTERMITTENT	MAXIMAL
THERAPEUTIC		
Class A	Patients with cardiac disease whose physical activity need not be restricted in any way.	
Class B	Patients with cardiac disease whose ordinary physical activity need not be restricted but who should be advised against severe or competitive efforts.	
Class C	Patients with cardiac disease whose ordinary physical activity should be moderately restricted and whose more strenuous efforts should be discontinued.	
Class D	Patients with cardiac disease whose ordinary physical activity should be markedly restricted.	
Class E	Patients with cardiac disease who should be at complete rest or confined to bed or chair.	

Reprinted by permission of the American Heart Association, New York.

ELEVATION OF ENZYMES FOLLOWING
ACUTE MYOCARDIAL INFARCTION

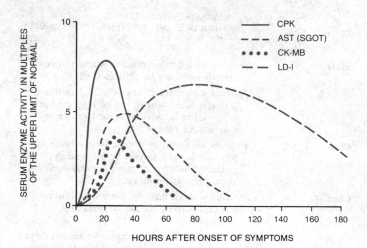

Stylized depiction (assembled from multiple sources) of the time-activity curves of CPK, CK-MB, LD-1, and AST (SGOT), following onset of acute myocardial infarction (defined on the basis of sentinel-persistent chest pain). (From Warren and Lewis: Diagnostic Procedures in Cardiology. Year Book Medical Publishers, Chicago, 1985, p. 214 with permission.)

ELECTROCARDIOGRAPHIC CHANGES
FOLLOWING MYOCARDIAL INFARCTION

Serial 12-lead EKG recordings are used to diagnose the presence and evolution of acute myocardial infarction (AMI). Injury is localized by the presence of abnormal waves on specific EKG leads.

A. Sequential phases in infarction

1. Acute	ST elevation (earliest change) Tall, hyperacute T waves New Q or QS wave
2. Evolving	Deep T wave inversions may persist; usually returns to normal (months) ST elevation returns to baseline (days) Q or QS waves may decrease in size, rarely disappear

B. Infarction type

1. Subendocardial intramural	ST-T changes: ST depression or T wave inversion Without QRS changes
2. Transmural	Abnormal Q or QS waves in leads overlying the infarct ST-T changes

C. Infarction Site

1. Anterior infarction:	Q or QS in V1 to V4
2. Lateral infarction:	Q or QS in lead I, aV1
3. Inferior infarction:	Q or QS in leads II, III, aVf
4. Posterior infarction:	Large R waves in V1-V3 ST depression V1, V2, or V3

Standard 12-lead electrocardiogram: leads I to III, aVr, aV1, and aVf are limb leads; V1 to V6 are chest leads.

Adapted from Goldberger, A and Goldberger, E: Clinical Electrocardiography —A Simplified Approach, ed 2. CV Mosby, St. Louis, 1985; also adapted from Conover, MB: Understanding Electrocardiography—Physiological and Interpretive Concepts, ed 3. CV Mosby, St. Louis, 1980.

ANGINA PECTORIS

Angina pectoris is a manifestation of myocardial ischemia due to coronary artery disease.

Types of Angina

stable: Predictable in appearance; after exercise, eating, or emotional stress and relieved by rest, nitrates, or other coronary artery vasodilators. The discomfort is most often substernal, precordium, epigastrium with radiation to the left arm, jaw, or neck (C8 to T4 dermatomes); ST segment depression (horizontal or downsloping) occurs during ischemic episodes.

unstable: Also called *preinfarction* or *crescendo angina.* Unstable angina can occur at rest or with activity. The pain is similar to that with typical stable angina but may be more intense and may last several hours; ST segment depression or elevation occurs.

Prinzmetal (variant): Occurs principally at rest and may occur in a circadian manner, at a similar time of day, often in the early morning hours. An ST segment elevation is seen on EKG, and sometimes painless episodes of ST segment elevation occur. A less frequent finding is ST segment depression. It is more common in women (under 50). Coronary artery spasm in normal or obstructed arteries has been found with this type of angina.

syndrome X: Chest pain that is seemingly ischemic in origin but with a normal arteriogram and normal EKG. It may be referred pain.

Levels of Angina

1+	Light or barely noticeable.
2+	Moderate, bothersome.
3+	Severe and very uncomfortable.
4+	Most severe pain ever experienced.

Reference

Irwin, S and Tecklin, JS: Cardiopulmonary Physical Therapy, ed 2. CV Mosby, St. Louis, 1990.

CARDIAC DISORDERS: TYPES OF VALVULAR DYSFUNCTION

TERM	DESCRIPTION
Atresia	Congenital absence or closure
Prolapse	Typically of the mitral valve; valve cusp falls back into atrium during systole
Regurgitation	Incompetent valve closure allows blood to flow backwards; this is also called *insufficiency*
Stenosis	Valve becomes stiff and fibrotic, obstructing the passage of blood through the valve

CONGENITAL CARDIAC LESIONS

The incidence of congenital cardiac anomalies is 8 per 1000 live births. Rubella is the most common infection related to congenital cardiovascular defects. Other possible causes include exposure to x-rays, alcohol, infections or drugs, maternal diabetes, family history, and some hereditary dysplasias such as Down's syndrome. Cardiac defects can be classified as cyanotic or acyanotic and then further categorized by whether pulmonary circulation is normal or increased.

Cyanotic lesions are present when the abnormality causes deoxygenated blood to enter the systemic circulation without passing through the lungs. This can result from admixture, as occurs with right-to-left shunts, pulmonary hypoperfusion, or transposition of the great vessels which results in poor communication between the systemic and pulmonary circulations.

COMMON CONGENITAL DEFECTS

Acyanotic Defects with Increased Pulmonary Blood Flow

patent ductus arteriosus (PDA): Persistence of a communication between the main pulmonary artery and the aorta. Usually blood flow through the ductus arteriosus stops within 1 day following birth, and it closes within a few weeks.

atrial septal defect (ASD): A communication between the atria. Septal defects are classified according to their location. Defects in the ostium secundum (foramen ovale region) account for 85 to 95 percent of ASDs. Ostium primum defects affect the lower midseptum and are also called *endocardial cushion defects*; they account for 25 percent of ASDs in neonates and have a higher mortality. Sinus venosus defects are 5 to 10 percent of ASDs.

ventricular septal defect (VSD): This is a communication between the ventricles that permits left-to-right shunts.

Acyanotic Defects with Normal Pulmonary Blood Flow

pulmonic stenosis: Obstruction of right ventricular outflow due to narrowing of the pulmonic valve.

coarctation of aorta: Congenital constriction of the aorta that reduces blood flow to the extremities. It can be preductal or postductal (proximal or distal to the ductus arteriosus); blood pressure in the arms is greater than in the legs (and left arm if the coarctation is proximal to the left subclavian orifice).

Cyanotic Defects with Decreased Pulmonary Blood Flow

tetralogy of Fallot: Consists of four components — ventricular septal defect (VSD), right ventricular outflow obstruction, dextropositioned aorta, and right ventricular hypertrophy. A right-to-left shunt results in cyanosis. Sympathetic activity that raises systemic vascular resistance will increase the shunt, so excitement is contraindicated. A child may squat during exertion or excitement, which probably raises arterial oxygenation by raising systemic arterial resistance.

transposition of the great vessels: The pulmonary artery arises from the left ventricle and the aorta (and coronary arteries) from the right ventricle. This condition would be incompatible with life except that there are usually septal defects present: patient ductus arteriosus (PDA), and/or atrial septal defect (ASD) and/or ventricular septal defect (VSD) and/or dilated bronchial arteries.

SIGNS AND SYMPTOMS OF CONGESTIVE HEART FAILURE (CHF) IN THE INFANT

Respirations greater than 60 per minute (tachypnea is the most common manifestation of left ventricular failure), dyspnea, wheezing, expiratory grunting, nonproductive irritative cough, resting tachycardia (160 – 200 bpm), failure to thrive, irritability, hepatomegaly (from right ventricular failure), and slow neuromotor development are typical of congestive heart failure in infants.

Reference

Merck Manual, ed. 15. Merck Sharp & Dohme, Rahway, New Jersey, 1987.

HEART FAILURE

Heart failure results when the myocardium is unable to maintain adequate circulation of the blood for respiration and metabolism. There may be failure of the right or left ventricle or both.

Types of Heart Failure

TYPE	DESCRIPTION
Backward	Venous return to the heart is reduced, with resulting venous stasis and congestion
Congestive	Systemic congestion (edema, enlarged liver, elevated venous pressure) due to right heart failure and/or pulmonary congestion due to left heart failure
Forward	Cardiac output is greatly reduced due to left ventricular failure, as after myocardial infarction when the ventricle has lost contractility
High output	Cardiac failure that results from conditions that increase the amount of circulation, as with a large arteriovenous fistula or anemia
Low output	Failure of the heart to maintain adequate cardiac output due to insufficient venous return, as with hemorrhage

Comparisons of Right and Left-Sided Heart Failure

RIGHT

Elevated end-diastolic right
  ventricular pressure

Systemic congestion:
  Enlarged liver
  Ascites
  Jugular venous distention
  Dependent (pitting) edema

Fatigue
Anorexia and bloating

Oliguria, nocturia

Cyanosis (capillary stasis)

Pleural effusion (R>L)

Unexplained weight gain

Etiology:
  Mitral stenosis
  Pulmonary parenchymal or
    vascular disease
  Pulmonic or tricuspid
    valvular disease
  Infective endocarditis

LEFT

Elevated end-diastolic left
  ventricular pressure

Pulmonary congestion:
  Pulmonary edema
  Dyspnea, orthopnea
  Paroxysmal nocturnal dyspnea
  Cough
  Bronchospasm
  (Cardiac asthma)

Fatigue

Oliguria

Cyanosis (central)

Tachycardia

Etiology:
  Hypertension
  Coronary artery disease
  Aortic valve disease
  Cardiomyopathies
  Congenital heart defects
  Infective endocarditis
  High-output conditions
  Various connective tissue
    disorders

Reference

Merck Manual, ed. 15. Merck, Sharp & Dohme, Rahway, New Jersey, 1987.

Sample In-Patient Rehabilitation: Seven-Step Myocardial Infarction Program*			
STEP	SUPERVISED EXERCISE	ACTIVITY	EDUCATIONAL-RECREATIONAL ACTIVITY
	In Cardiac Care Unit		
1	Active and passive ROM all extremities, in bed Teach patient ankle plantar and dorsiflexion—repeat hourly when awake	Partial self-care Feed self Dangle legs on side of bed Use bedside commode Sit in chair 15 min 1–2 times/day	Orientation to CCU Personal emergencies, social service aid as needed
2	Active ROM all extremities, sitting on side of bed.	Sit in chair 15–30 min 2–3 times/day Complete self-care in bed	Orientation to rehabilitation team, program Smoking cessation Educational literature if requested Planning transfer from CCU
	On Hospital Ward		
3	Warm-up exercises. 2 METs: Stretching Calisthenics Walk 50 ft and back at slow pace	Sit in chair ad lib To ward class in wheelchair Walk in room	Normal cardiac anatomy and function Development of atherosclerosis What happens with myocardial infarction 1–2 METs craft activity
4	ROM and calisthenics, 2.5 METs Walk length of hall (75 ft) and	Out of bed as tolerated Walk to bathroom	Coronary risk factors and their control

Step	Exercise	Ward activity	Educational and craft activity
	back, average pace Teach pulse counting	Walk to ward class, with supervision	Diet Energy conservation Work simplification techniques (as needed) 2–3 METs craft activity
5	ROM and calisthenics, 3 METs Check pulse counting Practice walking few stairsteps Walk 300 ft bid	Walk to waiting room or telephone Walk in ward corridor prn	
6	Continue above activities Walk down flight of steps (return by elevator) Walk 500 ft bid Instruct in home exercise	Tepid shower or tub bath, with supervision To occupational therapy, cardiac clinic teaching room, with supervision	Heart attack management: Medications Exercise Surgery Response to symptoms Family, community adjustments on return home Craft activity prn
7	Continue above activities Walk up flight of steps Walk 500 ft bid Continue home exercise instruction; present information regarding outpatient exercise program	Continue all previous ward activities	Discharge planning: Medications, diet, activity Return appointments Scheduled tests Return to work Community resources Educational literature Medication cards Craft activity prn

*From Wenger, N: Rehabilitation of the Patient with Symptomatic Atherosclerotic Coronary Disease. In Hurst, JW (ed): The Heart, ed 5. McGraw-Hill, New York, 1982, p 1151, with permission.

Cardiac and Noncardiac Drug Interventions and Their Possible Effect on Exercise Regimens
Major Arrows Next to Drug Names Indicate the Effect on the Variable

	EXERCISE PERFORMANCE	EFFECT ON HEART RATE	EFFECT ON BLOOD PRESSURE	EFFECT ON EKG	EFFECT ON GRADED EXERCISE TESTING
Antianginal nitrate agents	↑Nitro-Bid ↑Isordil ↑Isordil Tembids ↑Cardilate ↑Peritrate	↑Nitro-Bid ↑Sorbitrate ↑Ointment	↓Nitro-Bid ↓Sorbitrate ↓Ointment	Reduces evidence of myocardial ischemia	May delay onset of ischemic response (lower double product)
Beta blockers	↓↑Inderal ↓↑Lopressor	↓Inderal ↓Lopressor	↓Inderal ↓Lopressor	U waves may become prominent due to bradycardia	May delay onset of ischemic response (lower double product)
Antihypertensive diuretics		→Diuril, Esidrix →Enduron, Lasix →Edecrin, Aldactone →Dyrenium	↓Diuril, Esidrix ↓Enduron, Lasix ↓Edecrin, Aldactone ↓Dyrenium	Prolongs QT interval, accentuates U waves if hypokalemic	May cause false-positive if hypokalemic
Vasodilator		↑Apresoline	↓Apresoline		

Central nervous system		↓Serpasil ↓Ismelin ↓Inderal	↓Serpasil ↓Ismelin ↓Inderal, Minipress →Aldomet, Catapres		May delay onset of ischemic response
Digitalis glycosides	↑Strophanthin-G ↑Crystodigin ↑Lanoxin	↑With toxicity or may ↓ if blocks A-V node		May produce ST depression or sagging change accentuated with exercise	False-positive
Antiarrhythmics	↑Lanoxin ↑Dilantin ↑↓Xylocaine ↑Pronestyl ↓Inderal ↓Lopressor ↑↓Quinaglute	↑Pronestyl ↑Quinaglute ↑Norpace		ST-T wave changes, U-wave changes, widening of QRS, QT changes	Lanoxin—false-positive Quinaglute, Inderal—may delay onset of ischemic response
Tranquilizers (phenothiazines)	Minor antiarrhythmic effect	↑	→	T and U wave changes	May cause false-positive
Antidepressants		↑	→	ST-T wave changes	May cause false-positive

Continued on the following page(s)

Cardiac and Noncardiac Drug Interventions and Their Possible Effect on Exercise Regimens
Major Arrows Next to Drug Names Indicate the Effect on the Variable *Continued*

	EXERCISE PERFORMANCE	EFFECT ON HEART RATE	EFFECT ON BLOOD PRESSURE	EFFECT ON EKG	EFFECT ON GRADED EXERCISE TESTING
Antianxiety (lithium)		No change	No change	ST-T wave changes	May cause false-positive
Others					
Nicotine		↑	↑		
Broncho-dilators		↑	↑		May cause false-positive
Antihistamines with decon-gestants		↑	↑	No change	?
Thyroid Drugs		↑	↔	No change	No change
Cold Remedies				?	?
Alcohol				?	?

From American College of Sport Medicine: Guidelines for Graded Exercise Testing and Exercise Prescription, ed. 2. Lea & Febiger, Philadelphia, 1980.

ENERGY CONSUMPTION

METs. Metabolic equivalents (METs) are used to compare the energy cost of various activities to the resting state. Oxygen consumption in a resting state is estimated to be approximately 3.5 ml O_2/kg/min, which is 1 MET. The oxygen consumption of an individual for a given activity is usually expressed in liters per minute or milliliters per kilogram per minute. Energy expenditure in calories depends on the weight of the individual. When the individual's weight and oxygen consumption are known, the energy expenditure in calories can be estimated.

Conversions

$$1 \text{ MET} = 3.5 \text{ ml } O_2/\text{ml/min}$$
$$1 \text{ MET} = 1 \text{ kcal/kg/min}$$
$$1 \text{ l } O_2/\text{min} = 5 \text{ kcal}$$

Example: A 110-pound person performs a 5-MET activity for 20 minutes.

$$110 \text{ lbs} = 50 \text{ kg } (2.2 \text{ lbs} = 1 \text{ kg})$$

Oxygen consumption =

$$5 \times 3.5 \text{ ml } O_2/\text{kg/min} = 17.5 \text{ ml } O_2/\text{kg/min}$$

Expressed in l/min = 5×3.5 ml O_2/kg/min $\times 50$ kg
$$= 875 \text{ ml } O_2/\text{min}$$

divided by 1000 (to convert milliliters to liters) = 0.875 l O_2/min)

Calories consumed = 0.875×5 kcal/min = 4.375 kcal/min

Total caloric consumption = 4.375 kcal/min $\times$ 20 min = 87.5 calories

Approximate Energy Requirements in METs for Horizontal and Grade Walking

% GRADE	mi·h⁻¹ 1.7	2.0	2.5	3.0	3.4	3.75
	m·min⁻¹ 45.6	53.7	67.0	80.5	91.2	100.5
0	2.3	2.5	2.9	3.3	3.6	3.9
2.5	2.9	3.2	3.8	4.3	4.8	5.2
5.0	3.5	3.9	4.6	5.4	5.9	6.5
7.5	4.1	4.6	5.5	6.4	7.1	7.8
10.0	4.6	5.3	6.3	7.4	8.3	9.1
12.5	5.2	6.0	7.2	8.5	9.5	10.4
15.0	5.8	6.6	8.1	9.5	10.6	11.7
17.5	6.4	7.3	8.9	10.5	11.8	12.9
20.0	7.0	8.0	9.8	11.6	13.0	14.2
22.5	7.6	8.7	10.6	12.6	14.2	15.5
25.0	8.2	9.4	11.5	13.6	15.3	16.8

Approximate Energy Requirements in METs for Horizontal and Uphill Jogging/Running

Outdoors on Solid Surface

% GRADE	mi·h⁻¹	5	6	7	7.5	8	9	10
	m·min⁻¹	134	161	188	201	215	241	268
0		8.6	10.2	11.7	12.5	13.3	14.8	16.3
2.5		10.3	12.3	14.1	15.1	16.1	17.9	19.7
5.0		12.0	14.3	16.5	17.7	18.8		
7.5		13.8	16.4	18.9				
10.0		15.5	18.5					

On a Treadmill

% GRADE	5	6	7	7.5	8	9	10
0	8.6	10.2	11.7	12.5	13.3	14.8	16.3
2.5	9.5	11.2	12.9	13.8	14.7	16.3	18.0
5.0	10.3	12.3	14.1	15.1	16.1	17.9	19.7
7.5	11.2	13.3	15.3	16.4	17.4	19.4	
10.0	12.0	14.3	16.5	17.7	18.8		
12.5	12.9	15.4	17.7	19.0			
15.0	13.8	16.4	18.9				

Approximate Energy Expenditure in METs during Bicycle Ergometry*

BODY	WEIGHT	EXERCISE RATE (kg·m·min⁻¹ AND WATTS)							
kg	lbs	300 50	450 75	600 100	750 125	900 150	1050 175	1200 200	(kg·m·min⁻¹) (WATTS)
50	110	5.1	6.9	8.6	10.3	12.0	13.7	15.4	
60	132	4.3	5.7	7.1	8.6	10.0	11.4	12.9	
70	154	3.7	4.9	6.1	7.3	8.6	9.8	11.0	
80	176	3.2	4.3	5.4	6.4	7.5	8.6	9.6	
90	198	2.9	3.8	4.8	5.7	6.7	7.6	8.6	
100	220	2.6	3.4	4.3	5.1	6.0	6.9	7.7	

*VO$_2$ for zero load pedaling is approximately 550 ml·min⁻¹ for 70- to 80-kg subjects.
(From ACSM: Guidelines For Graded Exercise Testing and Exercise Prescription, ed 2.)

APPROXIMATE MET VALUES FOR VARIOUS ACTIVITIES

These values should be used as guidelines only. There is much individual variation in energy expenditure depending on how an activity is performed (e.g., speed, technique). One MET equals 3.5 ml O_2 per kg per min.

ACTIVITY	METs
Ambulation, braces and crutches	6.5
Archery	3 – 4
Auto, radio, TV repair	2 – 3
Backpacking	5 – 11
Badminton	4 – 9+
Basketball (game)	7 – 12+
Basketball (nongame)	3 – 9
Beating carpets	4
Bedside commode	3
Billiards	2.5
Bowling	2 – 4
Boxing (sparring)	8.3
Boxing (in ring)	13.3
Bricklaying	3.5
Canoeing, rowing, kayaking	3 – 8
Carpentry	2 – 7
Carrying 80-lb load	7 – 8
Cleaning windows	3
Climbing hills	5 – 10+
Cricket	4.6 – 7.4
Cycling (pleasure)	3 – 8+
Cycling, 5.5 mph	3.5
Cycling, 10 mph	7
Cycling, 11 mph	6 – 7
Cycling, 12 mph	7 – 8
Cycling, 13 mph	9
Dancing (aerobic)	6 – 9
Dancing (social, square, tap)	3.7 – 7.4

Continued on the following page(s)

ACTIVITY	METs
Desk work	1.5 – 2
Digging ditches	7 – 8
Dressing, undressing	2 – 2.3
Driving car	2
Fencing	6 – 10+
Field Hockey	8
Fishing (stream wading)	5 – 6
Fishing (from bank)	2 – 4
Gardening (wheelbarrow)	4 – 10
Gardening (weeding)	3 – 5
Gardening (raking)	3 – 6
Gardening (hoeing, digging)	4 – 8
Golf (power cart)	2 – 3
Golf (walk, carry bag)	4 – 7
Hand sewing	1
Handball	8 – 12+
Hiking (cross-country)	3 – 7
Horse ploughing	5
Horseback riding (galloping)	8.2
Horseback riding (trotting)	6.6
Horseback riding (walking)	2.4
Horseshoe pitching	2 – 3
Housework (heavy: scrubbing, making beds)	3 – 6
Housework (light: sweeping, ironing, polishing)	2 – 4
Hunting (big game, dragging)	3 – 14
Hunting (bow or gun, small game)	3 – 7
Ironing, standing	3.5
Jogging, 5 mph	7 – 8
Judo	13.5
Kneading dough	2.5
Machine sewing	1.5
Mopping	3.5
Mountain climbing	5 – 10+
Mowing lawn, on cart	2

ACTIVITY	METs
Mowing lawn, power mower	4 – 5
Mowing lawn, hand mower	4 – 6
Music playing	2 – 3
Paddleball, racquetball	8 – 12
Painting, plumbing (home)	3 – 8
Painting (recreational)	1.5
Paperhanging	4 – 5
Peeling potatoes	2.5
Plastering	3.5
Playing piano	2
Radio assembly	2.5
Rope jumping (120 to 140 skips/min)	11 – 12
Rope jumping (60 to 80 skips/min)	9
Running, 6 min/mile	16.3
Running, 7 min/mile	14.1
Running, 8 min/mile	12.5
Running, 9 min/mile	11.2
Running, 10 min/mile	10.2
Running, 11 min/mile	9.4
Running, 12 min/mile	8.7
Sailing	2 – 5
Sawing hardwood	7 – 8
Scrubbing, standing	2.5
Scuba diving	5 – 10
Sexual intercourse	5 – 5.5+
Shoveling	6 – 10+
Showering	3.5 – 4.2
Shuffleboard	2 – 3
Skating, ice and roller	5 – 8
Skiing, cross-country	6 – 12+
Skiing, downhill	5 – 8
Sledding, tobogganing	4 – 8
Snow shoveling (wet snow)	8 – 15
Snow shoveling (powder snow)	6 – 9

Continued on the following page(s)

Approximate MET Values for Various Activities 573

ACTIVITY	METs
Snowshoeing	7 – 14
Soccer	5 – 12+
Splitting/sawing wood, cutting trees (hand saw)	5 – 10
trees (power saw)	2 – 4
Squash	8 – 12+
Stair climbing	4 – 8
Stairs, carrying 24 lb, up 8 steps	10
Stairs, up 8 steps	5 – 5.5
Stairs, down flight	4.5 – 5.2
Swimming	4 – 8+
Table tennis	3 – 5
Tending furnace	8.5
Tennis	4 – 9+
Touch football	6 – 10
Tractor ploughing	3.5
Using bedpan	4
Volleyball	3 – 6
Walking, 1.7 mph	2.3
Walking, 2 mph	2.5
Walking, 2.5 mph	2.9
Walking, 3 mph	3.3
Walking, 3.4 mph	3.6
Walking, 3.75 mph	3.9
Walking, 4 mph	4.6
Walking, 4.5 mph	5.4
Walking, 5 mph	6.9
Walking, 5.5 mph	8.6
Walking upstairs	4 – 8
Walking downstairs	4 – 5
Washing face, hands	2
Washing/hanging clothes	2.5 – 3.5
Watch repairing	1.5
Water skiing	5 – 7
Wheelchair propulsion	2
Woodworking (light)	2 – 3

EXERCISE PRESCRIPTION

Intensity. For healthy individuals, 65 to 90 percent of age-adjusted maximum heart rate or 50 to 85 percent of maximum oxygen consumption. Cardiac patients should have a stress test or exercise at lower intensities initially.

Duration: Fifteen to 60 minutes per exercise session should be scheduled.

Frequency: Three to 5 days per week should be scheduled. No more than 2 days off should occur between exercise sessions.

Exercise Prescription by Heart Rate

The age-adjusted maximum heart rate (AAMHR) for an individual can be estimated by subtracting age from 220. The training heart rate (THR) can then be calculated.

$$\text{THR range} = 0.65 \ (220 - \text{age}) \text{ to } 0.90 \ (220 - \text{age})$$

The Karvonen equation uses the individual's resting heart rate to establish a THR range:

$$\text{THR range} = 0.65 \text{ to } 0.9 \ (\text{AAMHR} - \text{resting HR}) + \text{resting HR}$$

Reference

1. American College of Sports Medicine: Guidelines for Exercise Testing and Prescription. Lea & Febiger, Philadelphia, 1986.

Exercise Prescription by Relative Perceived Exertion: Borg Scale

Individual variability and medications influence the maximum heart rate and heart rate response to exercise. Borg devised a scale that correlates subjective relative perceived exertion (RPE) with intensity measured by heart rate or other variables. Ratings of 12 to 16 on the original Borg scale correspond to approximately 60 to 90 percent of the AAMHR, although it is more accurate to correlate an individual's ratings with heart rate at appropriate intensities during a stress test. The new Borg scale is designed to have ratio properties for use in research. The original scale is more commonly used for exercise prescription.

ORIGINAL BORG SCALE		NEW BORG SCALE	
6		0	Nothing at all
7	Very, very light	0.5	Very, very weak
8		1	Very weak
9	Very light	2	Weak
10		3	Moderate
12		4	Somewhat strong
13	Somewhat hard	5	Strong
14		6	
15	Hard	7	Very strong
16		8	
17	Very hard	9	
18		10	Very, very strong
19	Very, very hard	·	Maximal

Reference

1. Borg, GAV: Psychophysical bases of perceived exertion. *Med Sci Sports Exercise 14:*377, 1982.

Exercise Prescription by METs

Activities of appropriate intensity can be selected if an individual's functional capacity in METs is known. An intensity of 60 to 70 percent of the functional capacity is considered an appropriate training range. If 60 percent of maximum MET is used, add the maximum MET level to 60, divide this by 100, and multiply this value by maximum METs.

Example for an individual with a 5 MET maximum:

$$\frac{(60 + 5)}{100} = 0.65$$

0.65×5 METs $= 3.25$ METs (average training intensity)

TREADMILL PROTOCOLS USED IN CARDIAC REHABILITATION

Bruce Protocol

STAGE	TIME (min)	ELEVATION (%)	SPEED (mph)
1	3.0	10	1.7
2	3.0	12	2.5
3	3.0	14	3.4
4	3.0	16	4.2
5	3.0	18	5.0
6	3.0	20	5.5
7	3.0	22	6.0

Balke Protocol

STAGE	TIME (min)	ELEVATION (%)	SPEED (mph)
1	2.0	2	3.3
2	2.0	4	3.3
3	2.0	6	3.3
4	2.0	8	3.3
5	2.0	10	3.3
6	2.0	12	3.3
7	2.0	14	3.3
8	2.0	16	3.3
9	2.0	18	3.3
10	2.0	20	3.3

Ellestad 1 Protocol

STAGE	TIME (min)	ELEVATION (%)	SPEED (mph)
1	3.0	10	1.7
2	2.0	10	3.0
3	2.0	10	4.0
4	3.0	10	5.0
5	2.0	15	6.0
6	2.0	15	7.0
7	2.0	15	8.0

Naughton Protocol

STAGE	TIME (min)	ELEVATION (%)	SPEED (mph)
1	3.0	0	2.0
2	3.0	3.5	2.0
3	3.0	7.0	2.0
4	3.0	10.5	2.0
5	3.0	14.0	2.0
6	3.0	17.5	2.0
7	3.0	21.0	2.0

Oxygen Requirements for Step, Treadmill, and Bicycle Ergometer

FUNCTIONAL CLASS	METS	O₂ REQUIREMENTS ml O₂/kg/min	STEP TEST *Nagle Balke Naughton* 2 min stages 30 steps min, Step height increased 1.4 cm q 2 min — Height (cm)	Bruce 3 min stages mph%gr		Kattus 3 min stages mph%gr		Balke %grade at mph	Balke %grade at 3 mph	BICYCLE ERGOMETER For 70 kg body weight 1 kg·m/min
	16	56.0						26		
	15	52.5				4	22	24		
	14	49.0						22		
Normal and I	13	45.5		4.2	16			20		1500
	12	42.0	40			4	18	16	22.5	1350
	11	38.5	36					16	20.0	1200

580

	10	35.0	32					14	17.5	1050
II	9	31.5	28	3.4	14			12	15.0	900
	8	28.0	24					10	12.5	
	7	24.5	20	2.5	12	4	14	8	10.0	750
	6	21.0	16			4	10	6	7.5	600
	5	17.5	12	1.7	10	3	10	4	5.0	450
III	4	14.0	8			2	10	2	2.5	300
	3	10.5	4						0.0	
	2	7.0								150
IV	1	3.5								

From American Heart Association: The Exercise Standards Book. American Heart Association, Dallas, 1979.

Indications for Stopping an Exercise Test

1. Subject requests to stop.
2. Failure of the monitoring system.
3. Progressive angina (stop at 3 level or earlier on a scale of 1 to 4).
4. Two millimeters horizontal or downsloping ST depression or elevation.
5. Sustained supraventricular tachycardia.
6. Ventricular tachycardia.
7. Exercise induced left or right bundle branch block.
8. Any significant drop (≥ 10 mm Hg) of systolic blood pressure, or failure of the systolic blood pressure to rise with an increase in exercise load after the initial adjustment period.
9. Lightheadedness, confusion, ataxia, pallor, cyanosis, nausea, or signs of severe peripheral circulatory insufficiency.
10. Excessive rise in blood pressure: systolic greater than 250 mm Hg: diastolic greater than 120 mm Hg.
11. R on T premature ventricular complexes.
12. Unexplained inappropriate bradycardia — pulse rise slower than two standard deviations below age-adjusted normals.
13. Onset of second- or third-degree heart block.
14. Multifocal premature ventrical contractions [PVCs].
15. Increasing ventricular ectopy.

Criteria for an Abnormal Exercise Test*

1. One millimeter or more of exercise induced ST-segment depression or elevation relative to the Q-Q line, lasting 0.08 seconds or more from the J-point.
2. Chest discomfort typical of angina induced or increased by exercise.
3. Ventricular tachycardia or frequent ($>30\%$) premature ventricular contractions, or multifocal premature ventricular contractions.
4. Exercise-induced left or right bundle branch block.
5. Significant drop (greater than 10 mm Hg) in systolic blood pressure during exercise, or failure of the systolic blood pressure to rise with an increase in exercise intensity after the initial adjustment period.
6. Sustained supraventricular tachycardia.
7. R on T premature ventricular contractions (PVCs).
8. Exercise-induced second- or third-degree heart block.
9. Postexercise U-wave inversion.
10. Inappropriate bradycardia.

---

*From ACSM: Guidelines for Graded Exercise Testing and Exercise Prescription, ed 2.

Contraindications for Entry into Inpatient and Outpatient Exercise Programs*

The following criteria may be used as contraindications for program entry:

1. Unstable angina.
2. Resting systolic blood pressure over 200 mm Hg or resting diastolic blood pressure over 100 mm Hg.
3. Significant drop (20 mm Hg or more) in resting systolic blood pressure from the patient's average level that cannot be explained by medications.
4. Moderate to severe aortic stenosis.
5. Acute systemic illness or fever.
6. Uncontrolled atrial or ventricular arrhythmias.
7. Uncontrolled tachycardia (greater than 100 bpm).
8. Symptomatic congestive heart failure.
9. Third-degree heart block.
10. Active pericarditis or myocarditis.
11. Recent embolism.
12. Thrombophlebitis.
13. Resting ST displacement (greater than 3 mm).
14. Uncontrolled diabetes.
15. Orthopedic problems that would prohibit exercise.

---

*From ACSM: Guidelines for Graded Exercise Testing and Exercise Prescription, ed 2.

Criteria for Termination of an Inpatient Exercise Session*

The following guidelines may be used to terminate the exercise session for cardiac inpatients:

1. Fatigue.
2. Failure of monitoring equipment.
3. Light-headedness, confusion, ataxia, palor, cyanosis, dyspnea, nausea, or any peripheral circulatory insufficiency.
4. Onset of angina with exercise.
5. Symptomatic supraventricular tachycardia.
6. ST displacement (greater than 3 mm horizontal or down sloping from rest).
7. Ventricular tachycardia (3 or more consecutive premature ventricular contractions [PVCs]).
8. Exercise induced left or right bundle branch block.
9. Onset of second and or third degree heart block.

Criteria for Termination of an Inpatient Exercise Session* *(Con't.)*

10. R on T premature ventricular contractions (PVCs) toned.
11. Frequent unifocal premature ventricular contractions (PVCs) (greater than 30% of the complexes).
12. Frequent multifocal premature ventricular contractions (PVCs) (greater than 30% of the complexes).
13. Couplets (greater than 2 per minute).
14. Increase in heart rate over 20 bpm above standing resting heart rate for myocardial infarct patients.
15. Drop of 10 mm Hg or more in systolic blood pressure.
16. Excessive blood pressure rise systolic greater than or equal to 220 or diastolic greater than or equal to 110 mm Hg.
17. Inappropriate bradycardia drop in heart rate greater than 10 bpm with increase or no change in work load.

---

*From ACSM: Guidelines for Graded Exercise Testing and Exercise Prescription, ed 2.

Pulmonary Anatomy and Pulmonary Therapy

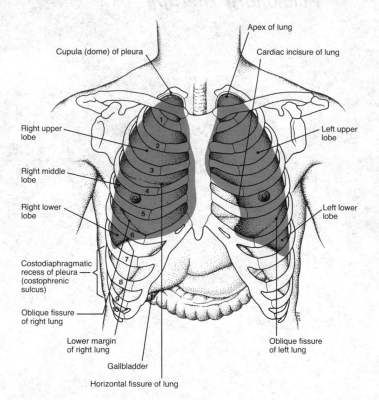

Cupula (dome) of pleura

Apex of lung

Cardiac incisure of lung

Right upper lobe

Left upper lobe

Right middle lobe

Right lower lobe

Left lower lobe

Costodiaphragmatic recess of pleura — (costophrenic sulcus)

Oblique fissure of right lung

Left lower lobe

Lower margin of right lung

Oblique fissure of left lung

Gallbladder

Horizontal fissure of lung

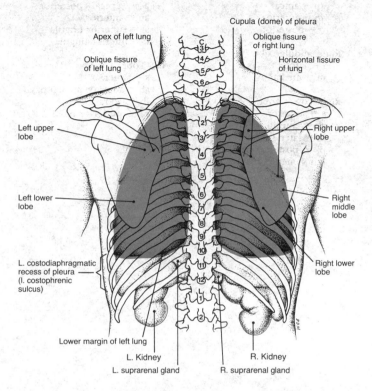

Cupula (dome) of pleura

Oblique fissure of right lung

Horizontal fissure of lung

Apex of left lung

Oblique fissure of left lung

Left upper lobe

Right upper lobe

Left lower lobe

Right middle lobe

L. costodiaphragmatic recess of pleura (l. costophrenic sulcus)

Right lower lobe

Lower margin of left lung

L. Kidney

L. suprarenal gland

R. Kidney

R. suprarenal gland

RIGHT LUNG

Right Upper Lobe
   ap = apical
   an = anterior
   p = posterior

Right Middle Lobe
   l = lateral
   m = medial

Right Lower Lobe
   s = superior
   ab = anterior basal
   lb = lateral basal
   pb = posterior basal
   mb = medial basal

LEFT LUNG

Left Upper Lobe
   a-p = apical – posterior
   an = anterior
   sl = superior lingula
   il = inferior lingula

Left Lober Lobe
   s = superior
   ab = anterior medial basal
   lb = lateral basal
   pb = posterior basal

ANATOMY OF THE BRONCHOPULMONARY TREE

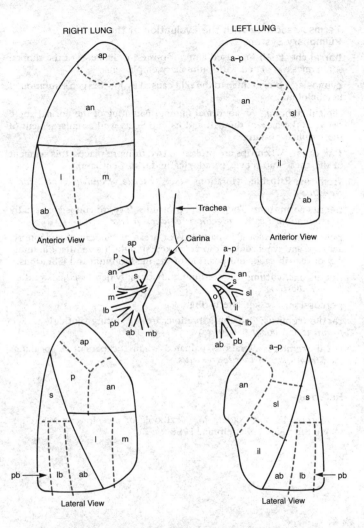

RIGHT LUNG

LEFT LUNG

RIGHT LUNG — Anterior View: ap, an, l, m, ab

LEFT LUNG — Anterior View: a-p, an, sl, il, ab

Trachea

Carina

ap, p, an, l, m, lb, pb, ab, mb, s

a-p, an, s, sl, il, lb, ab, pb, o

RIGHT LUNG — Lateral View: ap, p, an, s, l, m, pb, lb, ab

LEFT LUNG — Lateral View: a-p, an, sl, s, il, ab, lb, pb

PHYSICAL EXAMINATION OF THE PULMONARY SYSTEM

Terms Associated with the Evaluation of the Pulmonary System

barrel chest: An increased anterior-posterior diameter of the thorax; sometimes associated with pulmonary emphysema.

cyanosis: A bluish tinge to the skin caused by low oxygen saturation of hemoglobin.

digital clubbing: An abnormal finding; flattening of the normal angle between the base of the nail and its cuticle as well as enlargement of the terminal phalanx.

flail chest: When ribs are broken in two or more places, this segment of the chest wall moves paradoxically during ventilation.

fremitus: Palpable vibrations (see *tactile fremitus* and *vocal fremitus*).

pectus carinatum: The sternum protrudes forward and is abnormally prominent; also called *pigeon* or *chicken breast*.

palpation: The chest is palpated for areas of tenderness, symmetry, amount, and synchrony of thoracic excursion during ventilation, integrity of the rib cage, and position of the mediastinum and vibrations.

pectus excavatum: The sternum is abnormally depressed; also called *funnel chest*.

percussion: See separate listing.

tactile fremitus: Palpable vibrations are felt during ventilation. (See *fremitus* and *vocal fremitus*.)

vocal fremitus: Vibrations palpated when the patient is speaking. (See *fremitus* and *tactile fremitus*.)

Reference

1. Murray, JF and Nadel, JA: Textbook of Respiratory Medicine. WB Saunders, Philadelphia, 1988.

TERMS USED TO DESCRIBE BREATHING

Terms Used to Describe Breathing	

TERM	EXPLANATION
Apnea	Absence of breathing
Apneusis	Cessation of respiration in the inspiratory position
Biot's	Several short breaths or gasps followed by irregular periods of apnea
Bradypnea	Abnormally slow rate
Cheyne-Stokes	Cycles of gradual increase in rate and depth of respiration with apneic pauses between cycles
Dyspnea	Subjective complaint of shortness of breath
Eupnea	Normal rate and rhythm
Hyperpnea	Increased breathing; increased depth with or without increased rate
Hyperventilation	Increased ventilation; technically a decrease in $paCO_2$
Hypoventilation	Decreased ventilation; technically an increase in $paCO_2$
Kussmaul's	Deep gasping respirations associated with diabetic acidosis and coma ("air hunger")
Orthopnea	Dyspnea that occurs when patient assumes recumbent position
Paroxysmal nocturnal dyspnea (PND)	Dyspnea that comes on at night and suddenly awakens the patient
Tachypnea	Abnormally rapid rate

PERCUSSION OF THE PULMONARY SYSTEM

Percussion: An evaluation technique where the examiner strikes the distal end of the middle finger of one hand over the middle finger of the other hand, which is placed firmly over the chest wall. The resonance created by this maneuver has a variable pitch and feel, depending on the density of the underlying tissue. Four different percussion notes are described.

Percussion Sounds		

NOTE (SOUND)	NORMAL LOCATION	CHARACTERISTIC OF UNDERLYING TISSUE
Fat	Muscle on extremity	No underlying air
Dull	Liver, heart, viscera	Primarily soft tissue, some air
Normal resonance	Lung	Air and soft tissue
Hyper-resonant (tympanic)	Stomach	Primarily air

AUSCULTATION

Breath sounds are classified as normal or abnormal and with or without accompaniments (adventitious breath sounds). Normal breath sounds vary, depending on what area is being auscultated.

Location of Normal Breath Sounds

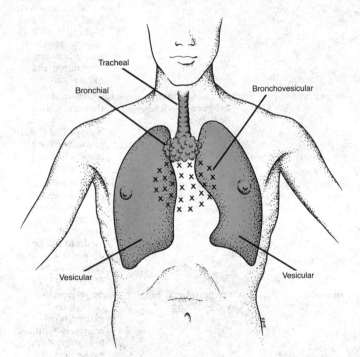

Definitions of breath sounds are on the following pages.

	Normal Breath Sounds	
TYPE	LOCATION AUSCULTATED	DESCRIPTION OF SOUND
Tracheal	Trachea	Inspiration and expiration are equal in duration; loud, high-pitched, and hollow; short pause between inspiration and expiration
Bronchial	Over manubrium, between clavicles, or between scapulae	Inspiration shorter than expiration; loud, high-pitched, short pause between inspiration and expiration
Bronchovesicular	Over large airways near sternum and between scapulae	Inspiration should equal expiration in duration, lower intensity than bronchial; medium-pitched, no pause between inspiration and expiration
Vesicular	Over peripheral lung tissue	Long inspiration with short expiration; relatively faint and low-pitched; no pause between inspiration and expiration

ABNORMAL BREATH SOUNDS

When tracheal, bronchial, or bronchovesicular breath sounds are auscultated over a lung that should sound vesicular, the breath sound is abnormal. Sound is transmitted better through solid or consolidated lung tissue, and increased transmission is indicative of pathology. Sometimes these abnormal breath sounds are termed *tubular*. An abnormal intensity of a breath sound is also noted when present.

egophony: The nasal, bleating sound of spoken or whispered words auscultated over consolidated lung tissue.

bronchophony: Abnormal transmission of spoken words; typically, the patient is asked to say the letter *E* or *99*; with bronchophony, the *E* will sound like an *A* and is sometimes noted as "E to A change."

pectoriloquy: Abnormal transmission of whispered syllables that normally cannot be heard distinctly; examining for pectoriloquy usually involves asking the patient to whisper, "One, two, three."

ADVENTITIOUS BREATH SOUNDS

Adventitious breath sounds are accompaniments to normal or abnormal breath sounds. Adventitious breath sounds are always abnormal and should be described by name and by when they are heard during respiration (inspiration, expiration, early, late, etc.). They are further classified into three major categories: continuous and noncontinuous breath sounds and rubs.

continuous breath sounds: Most prominent during expiration, they are thought to be caused by the vibrations of air passing through airways narrowed by inflammation, bronchospasm, or secretions. Frequently they are present in asthma and chronic bronchitis. The noises of wheezes are described as squeaky, snoring, or groaning.

wheezes: high-pitched, sibilant, and musical.

rhonchi: Low-pitched and sonorous.

noncontinuous breath sounds: Most common during inspiration, they are thought to be caused by the sound of gas bubbling through secretions or by the opening of alveoli and small airways that have collapsed because of fluid, poor aeration, or inflammation. These sounds are frequently associated with congestive heart failure, atelectasis, and pulmonary fibrosis. Noncontinuous breath sounds are described as sounding like soda pop fizzing or hair rubbed through the fingers next to the ear. They should be called *crackles;* other terms used are *rales* and *crepitations.* Descriptive terms used with crackles are *fine* or *coarse.*

friction rub: Caused by the rubbing of pleural surfaces against one another, usually as a result of inflammation or neoplastic processes. A friction rub sounds similar to footsteps on packed snow or creaking old leather and is more commonly heard during inspiration, but this can be highly variable. A friction rub may be accompanied by pain during inspiration.

TERMS USED IN PULMONARY FUNCTION TESTING

Pulmonary Function Terminology

ABBREVIATION	TERM AND DEFINITION
ABG	Arterial blood gas: Study of the pH and concentrations of O_2 and CO_2 in arterial blood. Hemoglobin, O_2 saturation, and HCO_3^- concentration are also usually calculated.
ERV	Expiratory reserve volume: Volume of air that can be voluntarily expired from the resting end-expiratory level
$FEF_{25-75\%}$	Forced expiratory flow: Air flow during the middle two quarters of a forced expiration (synonymous with MEF)
FEV_1	Forced expiratory volume: Volume of air expired during the first second of a FVC. Different subscripts are used to denote the duration of the expiratory volume from the onset of expiration.
FEV_1/FVC	Ratio of volume of air expired in the first second to the vital capacity
FRC	Functional residual capacity: Volume of air in the lungs at the resting end-expiratory level
FVC	Forced vital capacity: Volume of air in a VC when subject expires with maximal voluntary effort
IC	Inspiratory capacity: Volume of air that can be inspired from the resting end-expiratory level
IRV	Inspiratory reserve volume: Volume of air that can be inspired from the end-inspiratory level (peak of a tidal breath)
MBC	Maximal breathing capacity: Synonymous with MVV
MEF	Maximal mid-expiratory flow: Synonymous with $FEF_{25-75\%}$
MV	Minute volume: Total volume of air expired during one minute (respiratory rate $\times$ TV)

Continued on the following page(s)

ABBREVIATION	TERM AND DEFINITION
	Pulmonary Function Terminology *Continued*
MVV	Maximum voluntary ventilation: Estimate of the maximal volume of air a subject can breath in a minute based on the volume breathed with maximal voluntary ventilatory effort for a given time (synonymous with MBC)
PEF	Peak expiratory flow: Most rapid flow rate of air during expiration
$\dot{Q}$	Perfusion: Volume of blood that circulates through the heart and lungs in 1 minute
RV	Residual volume: Volume of air remaining in lungs following full expiration
TLC	Total lung capacity: Total volume of air in the lungs following a full inspiration
TV	Tidal volume: Volume of air contained in one breath during normal quiet breathing
$\dot{V}$	Ventilation: Amount of air exchanged in 1 minute
$\dot{V}/\dot{Q}$	Ratio of ventilation to perfusion. Normal value for the lungs as a whole is about 0.8.
VC	Vital capacity: Maximal volume of air measured on complete expiration after full inspiration
V_T	Synonymous with tidal volume (TV)

Reference

1. Murray, JF and Nadel, JA: Textbook of Respiratory Medicine. WB Saunders, Philadelphia, 1988.

COMMON PULMONARY FUNCTION TESTS

spirometry: Measures lung volumes and capacities (with the exception of RV and TLC), flow rates, and the MVV; used as a general screening test for detection of abnormal breathing patterns, lung obstruction and/or restriction, efficacy of medication (bronchodilation), estimate ventilatory reserve, and patient compliance.

Spirograms and Lung Volumes

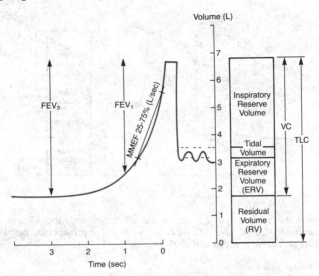

Normal. RV ≃ 25% of TLC; FRC ≃ 40% of TLC. FEV_1 = >75% of FVC; FEV_3 = >95% of FVC.

COMMON PULMONARY FUNCTION TESTS:

Spirograms and Lung Volumes:
Restrictive Disease

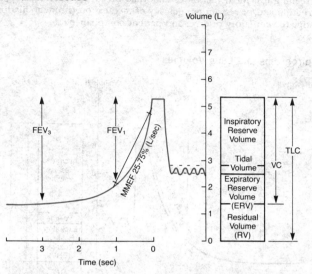

Restrictive disease. Lung volumes are all diminished, the RV less so than the FRC, FVC, and TLC. $FEV_{1\%FVC}$ is normal or greater than normal. Tidal breathing is rapid and shallow.

COMMON PULMONARY FUNCTION TESTS:

Spirograms and Lung Volumes:
Obstructive Disease

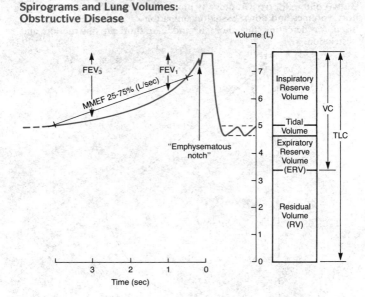

Obstructive disease. RV and FRC are increased. TLC is also increased, but to a lesser degree, so that VC is decreased. There is prolongation of expiration. $FEV_1 = <75\%$ of VC. Note the "emphysematous notch."

COMMON PULMONARY FUNCTION TESTS

flow-volume loops: Graphically plot maximal inspiratory and expiratory volumes and flows; visual examination of the shape of the loop used for detecting intrathoracic and extrathoracic obstruction and restriction.

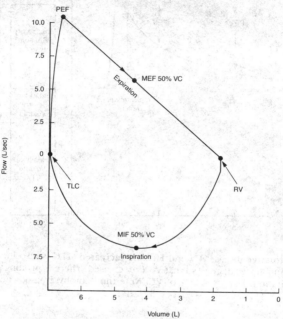

Normal. (Left) Inspiratory limb of loop is symmetric and convex. Expiratory limb is linear. Flow rates at midpoint of VC are often measured. $MIF_{50\%VC} > MEF_{50\%VC}$ because of dynamic compression of the airways. Peak expiratory flow is sometimes used to estimate degree of airways obstruction but is very dependent on patient effort. Expiratory flow rates over lower 50% of VC (i.e., approaching RV) are sensitive indicators of small airway status.

Restrictive disease (e.g., sarcoidosis, kyphoscoliosis). (Right) Configuration of loop is narrowed because of diminished lung volumes. Flow rates are normal (actually greater than normal at comparable lung volumes because increased elastic recoil of lungs and/or chest wall holds airways open).

diffusing capacity (DL_{CO}): The patient inspires a small amount of CO; the CO in the end-expired gas is analyzed and the amount of CO that diffused into the blood is calculated. Low DL_{CO} may indicate thickening of alveolar-capillary membranes and/or abnormal ventilation/perfusion relationships.

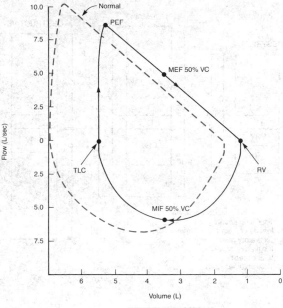

FLOW-VOLUME LOOPS

body plethysmography: Measures total lung capacity and airway resistance. It allows the RV to be accurately determined and is most useful for diagnosing obstructive disorders.

nitrogen washout test: Measures the distribution of ventilation and closing volume (the volume during expiration when small airways collapse). Concentration of N_2 is measured over complete expiration after breathing 100 percent O_2. An abnormal curve of N_2 concentration reflects asynchronous alveolar emptying and small airway closure, characteristic of obstructive disorders.

ventilation/perfusion scan: A radioactive tracer is injected into the circulation and/or the patient inhales a radioactive gas or aerosol. Distribution and matching of ventilation to perfusion can then be examined. Disorders that might be detected by a V/Q scan include vascular occlusion (pulmonary embolism), lung consolidation, and obstructive and restrictive diseases.

From The Merck Manual of Diagnosis and Therapy, ed 15. pp. 586–587, edited by Robert Berkow. Copyright 1987 by Merck & Co., Inc. with permission.

LUNG VOLUMES AND CAPACITIES

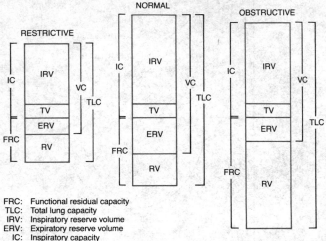

FRC: Functional residual capacity
TLC: Total lung capacity
IRV: Inspiratory reserve volume
ERV: Expiratory reserve volume
 IC: Inspiratory capacity
 VC: Vital capacity
 TV: Tidal volume
 RV: Residual volume

CLASSIFICATION OF PULMONARY IMPAIRMENTS

restrictive: Characterized by a decreased vital capacity (VC) with normal expiratory air flows.

obstructive: Characterized by reductions in air flows with or without reductions in the vital capacity (VC).

Severity of Impairment (percent of predicted normal)						
SEVERITY	VC	FEV_1	FEV_1/FVC	MEF	TLC	DL_{CO}
Normal	>80	>80	>70	>65	>80	>80
Mild	66–80	66–80	60–70	50–65	66–80	61–80
Moderate	50–65	50–65	45–59	35–49	50–65	40–60
Severe	<50	<50	<45	<35	<50	<40

Reference

1. Murray, JF and Nadel, JA: Textbook of Respiratory Medicines. WB Saunders, Philadelphia, 1988.

Typical Signs and Symptoms of Pulmonary Diseases				
PATHOLOGICAL PROCESS	CHEST WALL MOVEMENT	MEDIASTINAL POSITION	PERCUSSION NOTE	BREATH SOUNDS
Atelectasis	Reduced on affected side	Shifted toward affected side	Dull or flat	Decreased or absent
Asthma	Normal or symmetrically decreased	Midline	Normal or hyper-resonant	Vesicular with prolonged expiration
Chronic or acute bronchitis	Normal or symmetrically decreased	Midline	Normal	Vesicular with prolonged expiration
Bronchiectasis	May be reduced over affected area	Midline or toward affected area	Abnormal, may be dull or hyperresonant	Bronchial or broncho-vesicular
Pulmonary effusion or empyema	Reduced or absent on affected side	Away from affected side	Dull or flat	Decreased or absent; high-pitched bronchial may be present

VOCAL SOUNDS	ADVENTITIOUS SOUNDS	COUGH—SPUTUM	MISCELLANEOUS
Reduced or absent with large area collapsed; egophony and whispering pectoriloquy with smaller collapse	None or coarse rales	None, hacking or productive, particularly if atelectasis is due to mucous plugging	May have fever; may have pain
Normal or diminished	Wheezing cough	Dry or productive of tenacious mucoid sputum with plugs	Anxiety, severe broncho- spasm may restrict air flow to the extent that no wheezing is heard
Normal	Wheezing and rhonchi	Productive of mucoid or purulent sputum with infection	May have fever
Increased	Coarse rales, rhonchi	Usually copious amounts of purulent sputum; possibly foul-smelling; hemoptysis may occur	Physical exam depends on amount of fluid in bronchi- ectatic areas
Reduced or absent	May have pleural rub	Absent or nonpro- ductive	

Continued on the following page(s)

PATHOLOGICAL PROCESS	CHEST WALL MOVEMENT	MEDIASTINAL POSITION	PERCUSSION NOTE	BREATH SOUNDS
Pneumonia (lung consolidation)	Reduced on affected side	Midline	Dull	Broncho-vesicular, bronchial
Lung abcess, cavitation	Normal or reduced on affected side	Normal or toward affected side	Abnormal (dull or hyperresonant)	Bronchial, amphoric
Emphysema	Normal or symmetrically decreased	Midline	Normal or hyperresonant	Harsh vesicular with prolonged expiration; may be decreased or distant
Pulmonary edema	Normal or symmetrically reduced	Midline	Normal, may be dull at lung bases	Vesicular
Pulmonary embolism	Reduced on affected side	Midline	Normal or dull	May be reduced

VOCAL SOUNDS	ADVENTITIOUS SOUNDS	COUGH— SPUTUM	MISCELLANEOUS
Egophony, whispering pectoriloquy	Fine rales early; coarse later	Dry, hacking, or productive; sputum may be purulent, bloody	Fever; may have pleuritic pain
Increased, egophony, whispering pectoriloquy	Coarse rales	Productive of purulent, foul-smelling sputum	Physical exam depends on amount of fluid in affected area; abscess may develop distal to bronchial obstruction; lung cancer should be ruled out; may have fever
Normal or reduced	None, rhonchi, rales	Variable	
Normal	Rales, generally symmetrical	Irritating, frothy white or pink sputum	
Normal	Rales, wheezing, pleural friction rub	Dry, hacking, or productive; may have hemoptysis	May have pleuritic pain, apprehension

Continued on the following page(s)

PATHOLOGICAL PROCESS	CHEST WALL MOVEMENT	MEDIASTINAL POSITION	PERCUSSION NOTE	BREATH SOUNDS
Cystic fibrosis	Normal or reduced	Midline	Normal, dull or hyperresonant	Vesicular, bronchovesicular, bronchial
Pneumothorax	Reduced on affected side (but hemithorax may be enlarged)	Away from affected side	Hyperresonant, tympanic	Decreased, distant, or absent
Laryngotracheobronchitis (Croup)	Retractions	Midline	Normal	Vesicular, prolonged inspiration
Bronchiolitis	Retractions	Midline	Hyperresonant	Vesicular, prolonged expiration

Reference

1. Seidel, HM, Ball, JW, Dains, JE, Benedict, GW: Mosby's Guide to Physical Examination. CV Mosby, St. Louis, 1987.

VOCAL SOUNDS	ADVENTITIOUS SOUNDS	COUGH— SPUTUM	MISCELLANEOUS
May have egophony	Rales, wheezing	Productive of large amounts of tenacious mucoid, muco-purulent, or purulent sputum; may have hemoptysis	Physical exam depends on extent of disease and amount of retained secretions
Decreased	None	Dry	May have local or referred pain
Normal	Stridor, wheezing, rales	Barking, productive of viscous sputum	Low-grade fever
Normal	Wheezing, rales	Hacking, productive of mucoid to purulent sputum	Typically follows a URI

Differential Features of COPD

FEATURE	EMPHYSEMA	CHRONIC BRONCHITIS	ASTHMA
Family history	Occasional (α_1 antitrypsin deficiency)	Occasional (cystic fibrosis)	Frequent
Atopy	Absent	Absent	Frequent
Smoking history	Usual	Usual	Infrequent
Sputum character	Absent or mucoid	Predominantly neutrophilic	Predominantly eosinophilic
Chest x-ray	Useful if bullae, hyperinflation, or loss of peripheral vascular markings are present	Often normal; occasional hyperinflation	Often normal; hyperinflation during acute attack
Spirometry	Obstructive pattern unimproved with bronchodilator	Obstructive pattern improved with bronchodilator	Obstructive pattern usually shows good response to bronchodilator

Physical Signs in COPD

STAGE	SIGNS
Early	Examination may be negative or show only slight prolongation of forced expiration (which can be timed while auscultating over the trachea—normally 3 seconds or less); slight diminution of breath sounds at the apices or bases; scattered rhonchi or wheezes, especially on expiration, often best heard over the hila anteriorly. The rhonchi often clear after cough.

Moderate	Above signs are usually present and more pronounced, often with decreased rib expansion in addition there is:
	    use of the accessory muscles of respiration
	    retraction of the supraclavicular fossae in inspiration
	    generalized hyperresonance
	    decreased area of cardiac dullness
	    diminished heart sounds at base
	    increased anteroposterior distance of the chest*

Advanced	Examination usually shows the above findings to a greater degree and often shows:
	    evidence of weight loss
	    depression of the liver
	    hyperpnea and tachycardia with mild exertion
	    low and relatively immobile diaphragm
	    contraction of abdominal muscles on inspiration
	    inaudible heart sounds, except in the xiphoid area cyanosis

Continued on the following page(s)

613

Physical Signs in COPD *Continued*

STAGE	SIGNS
Cor pulmonale	Increased pulmonic second sound and close splitting
	Right-sided diastolic gallop
	Left parasternal heave (right ventricular overactivity)
	Early systolic pulmonary ejection click, with or without systolic ejection murmur
	With failure:
	distended neck veins, functional tricuspid insufficiency
	V-waves, and hepatojugular reflux
	hepatomegaly
	peripheral edema

*Misplaced confidence may be placed in relating the shape of the thorax to the presence or absence of obstructive lung disease. It has been shown that the classic "barrel chest" with poor rib separation may be due solely or largely to dorsal kyphosis. In such patients ventilatory function may nonetheless be normal because of good diaphragmatic motion.

Classes of Respiratory Impairment*

	CLASS 1 0% IMPAIRMENT	CLASS 2 20–30% IMPAIRMENT	CLASS 3 40–50% IMPAIRMENT	CLASS 4 60–90% IMPAIRMENT
Roentgenographic appearance	Usually normal but there may be evidence of healed or inactive chest disease including, for example, minimal nodular silicosis or pleural scars	May be normal or abnormal	May be normal but usually is not	Usually is abnormal
Dyspnea	When it occurs, it is consistent with the circumstances of activity	Does not occur at rest and seldom occurs during the performance of the usual activities of daily living. The patient can keep pace with persons of same age and	Does not occur at rest but does occur during the usual activities of daily living. However, the patient can walk a mile at his own pace without dyspnea although	Occurs during such activities as climbing one flight of stairs or walking 100 yards on the level, on less exertion, or even at rest

Continued on the following page(s)

615

Classes of Respiratory Impairment* Continued

	CLASS 1 0% IMPAIRMENT	CLASS 2 20–30% IMPAIRMENT	CLASS 3 40–50% IMPAIRMENT	CLASS 4 60–90% IMPAIRMENT
		body build on the level without breathlessness but not on hills or stairs	he cannot keep pace on the level with others of the same age and body build	
Tests of ventilatory function (at least two should be performed)				
FEV FVC MMV	Not less than 85% of predicted	70–85% of predicted	55–70% predicted	Less than 55% of predicted
Arterial oxygen saturation	Not applicable	Not applicable	Usually 88%+ or greater at rest and after exercise	Usually less than 88% at rest and after exercise

*From Guides to the Evaluator of Permanent Impairment–The Respiratory System, J.A.M.A., 1965, pp. 194, 919.
+88% saturation corresponds to an arterial Po_2 of 58mm, assuming the arterial pH is in the normal range.

ARTERIAL BLOOD GASES AND OXYGENATION

arterial blood gas (ABG) studies: Provide information about how well the lungs are functioning to provide oxygen, eliminate carbon dioxide, and, with the kidneys, regulate the blood's acid-base balance. Serious consequences can result from abnormal ABGs.

Normal Arterial Blood Gas Values

ARTERIAL	PREMATURE	TERM INFANT	CHILD	ADULT
pH	7.35 to 7.39	7.26 to 7.41	7.35 to 7.45	7.35 to 7.45
paCO$_2$	38 to 44 mm Hg	34 to 54 mm Hg	35 to 45 mm Hg	35 to 45 mm Hg
paO$_2$	65 to 80 mm Hg	60 mm Hg	75 to 100 mm Hg	75 to 100 mm Hg
O$_2$ sat	40 to 90%	40 to 95%	95 to 98%	95 to 98%
CO$_2$ content	19 to 27 mEq/L	20 to 28 mEq/L	18 to 27 mEq/L	23 to 29 mEq/L
Base excess	−1 to −2 mEq/L	−7 to −1 mEq/L	−4 to +2 mEq/L	−2 to +2 mEq/L

Reference

1. West, JB: Respiratory Physiology—the essentials, ed. 3. Williams & Wilkins, Baltimore, 1985.

Gas Pressure (mm Hg)

GAS	DRY AIR	MOIST TRACHEAL AIR	ALVEOLAR GAS	ARTERIAL BLOOD	MIXED VENOUS BLOOD
pO_2	159.1	149.2	104	100	40
pCO_2	0.3	0.3	40	40	46
pH_2O	0.0	47.0	47	47	47
pN_2	600.6	563.5	569	573	573
P_{TOTAL}	760	760	760	760	706

Interpretation of Abnormal Acid-Base Balance

TYPE	pH	$paCO_2$	CO_2	CAUSES	SIGNS AND SYMPTOMS
Respiratory alkalosis	↑	→	WNL	Alveolar hyperventilation	Dizziness, syncopy, tingling, numbness, early tetany
Respiratory acidosis	→	↑	WNL	Alveolar hypoventilation	Early: anxiety, restlessness, dyspnea, headache; late: confusion, somnolence, coma
Metabolic alkalosis	↑	WNL	↑	Bicarbonate ingestion, vomiting, diuretics, steroids, adrenal disease	Vague symptoms: weakness, mental dullness, possibly early tetany
Metabolic acidosis	→	WNL	→	Diabetic, lactic, or uremic acidosis, prolonged diarrhea	Secondary hyperventilation (Kussmaul breathing), nausea and vomiting, cardiac arrhythmias, lethargy, and coma

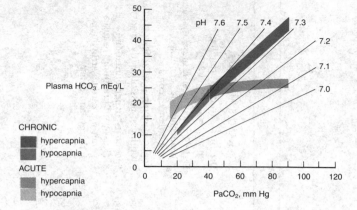

This nomogram, adapted from McLean, relates the values of the pH, P_{CO_2}, and bicarbonate concentration in the plasma of arterial blood. If two of these are known, a line drawn through the corresponding points will intersect the third column at the point of the desired value. The values shown are only approximate because there are normal differences between men and women, and because variations in the levels of hematocrit, blood buffer base, oxygen saturation of the blood, and temperature at which the determinations are made also affect these relationships.

OXYGENATION

The paO_2 and the hemoglobin oxygen saturation (O_2 sat) provide information about how well the lungs are functioning as an oxygenator.

hypoxemia: An abnormally low amount of oxygen in the blood.

hypoxia: Refers to a low amount of oxygen, usually at the tissue level.

Causes of Hypoxemia

TYPE	DESCRIPTION	CAUSES
Hypoventilation	Low level of ventilation causes increase in $paCO_2$ with concomitant decrease in paO_2	Drug overdose, anesthesia, pathology of medulla, abnormalities of spinal pathways, poliomyelitis, diseases and pathology of respiratory muscles, chest wall trauma, kyphoscoliosis, upper airway obstruction
Diffusion impairment	Blood-gas barrier is thickened	Asbestosis, sarcoidosis, interstitial fibrosis, collagen diseases, alveolar cell carcinoma
Shunt	Blood reaches arterial system without passing through ventilated regions of the lungs; can be anatomic or physiologic	Congenital cardiac defects, infectious and inflammatory processes
V/Q inequality	Mismatching of ventilation to blood flow	Chronic obstructive lung disease, interstitial lung disease, vascular disorders

Continued on the following page(s)

TYPE	DESCRIPTION	CAUSES
Decreased inspired oxygen	Partial pressure of oxygen lowers as barometric pressure decreases	High altitudes

noninvasive oxygen monitoring: Ear oximetry is useful for monitoring oxygen saturation during exercise. Capillary oxygen saturation is measured by spectrophotometry using a device that attaches to the ear. Transcutaneous skin electrodes are also used to assess oxygen saturation in pediatric patients; transcutaneous oxygen pressure (TcO_2) correlates well with the paO_2, although the TcO_2 value tends to be lower.

high-flow: All of the gas the patient breathes is delivered by a mask or tube, which allows for precise control of the fraction of inspired oxygen (FIO_2). Venturi or "Venti" masks are high-flow systems that mix room air with oxygen to provide a precise FIO_2.

low-flow: Provides only part of the patient's minute volume and uses masks, nasal cannula, or prongs. The tidal volume should be between 300 and 700 ml and the ventilatory rate below 25 per minute to use a low-flow system. Due to variability in ventilation, the FIO_2 can only be estimated.

Estimated Fraction of Inspired Oxygen (FIO_2) with Low-Flow Devices

LOW-FLOW DEVICE	ESTIMATED FIO_2
Room air	21%
Nasal prongs	
1 L/min	24%
3 L/min	28%
3 L/min	32%
4 L/min	36%
5 L/min	40%
6 L/min	44%
Osygen mask	
5 – 6 L/min	40%
6 – 7 L/min	50%
7 – 8 L/min	60%
Mask with reservoir bag	
6 L/min	60%
7 L/min	70%
8 L/min	80%
9 L/min	90%
10 L/min	99+%

BRONCHIAL DRAINAGE

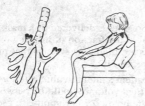

UPPER LOBES Apical Segments

Bed or drainage table flat.

Patient leans back on pillow at 30° angle against therapist.

Therapist claps with markedly cupped hand over area between clavicle and top of scapula on each side.

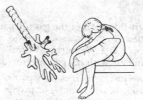

UPPER LOBES Posterior Segments

Bed or drainage table flat.

Patient leans over folder pillow at 30° angle.

Therapist stands behind and claps over upper back on both sides.

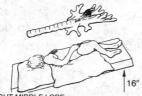

16"

RIGHT MIDDLE LOBE

Foot of table or bed elevated 16 inches.

Patient lies head down on left side and rotates ¼ turn backward. Pillow may be placed behind from shoulder to hip. Knees should be flexed.

Therapist claps over right nipple area. In females with breast development or tenderness, use cupped hand with heel of hand under armpit and fingers extending forward beneath the breast.

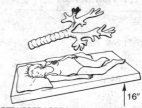

16"

LEFT UPPER LOBE Lingular Segments

Foot of table or bed elevated 16 inches.

Patient lies head down on right side and rotates ¼ turn backward. Pillow may be placed behind from shoulder to hip. Knees should be flexed.

Therapist claps with moderately cupped hand over left nipple area. In females with breast development or tenderness, use cupped hand with heel of hand under armpit and fingers extending forward beneath the breast.

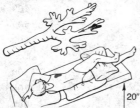

20"

LOWER LOBES Lateral Basal Segments

Foot of table or bed elevated 20 inches.

Patient lies on abdomen, head down, then rotates ¼ turn upward. Upper leg is flexed over a pillow for support.

Therapist claps over uppermost portion of lower ribs. (Position shown is for drainage of right lateral basal segment. To drain the left lateral basal segment, patient should lie on his right side in the same posture).

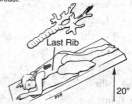

Last Rib

20"

LOWER LOBES Posterior Basal Segments

Foot of table or bed elevated 20 inches.

Patient lies on abdomen, head down, with pillow under hips. Therapist claps over lower ribs close to spine on each side.

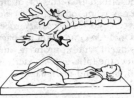

UPPER LOBES Anterior Segments

Bed or drainage table flat.

Patient lies on back with pillow under knees.

Therapist claps between clavicle and
nipple on each side.

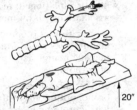

20″

LOWER LOBES Anterior Basal Segments

Foot of table or bed elevated 20 inches.

Patient lies on side, head down, pillow under knees.

Therapist claps with slightly cupped hand over lower
ribs. (Position shown is for drainage of <u>left</u> anterior
basal segment. To drain the right anterior basal
segment, patient should lie on his left side in same
posture).

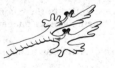

LOWER LOBES Superior Segments

Bed or table flat.

Patient lies on abdomen with two pillows under hips.

Therapist claps over middle of back at tip of scapula
on either side of spine.

SPUTUM ANALYSIS

Sputum is described in terms of quantity, viscosity, color, and odor. The frequency, time of day, and ease of expectoration is also noted. Laboratory analysis is necessary to establish a definitive diagnosis. These tests include Gram-stain for bacteria, culture and sensitivity for infectious agent, and appropriate antibiotic, acid-fast bacillus stain (AFB) to detect the tuberculosis bacillus, and cytology to examine for cellular constituents and malignancy.

TERM	DESCRIPTION
Fetid	Foul-smelling, typical of anaerobic infection; typically occurs with bronchiectasis, lung abscess, or cystic fibrosis
Frothy	White or pink-tinged, foamy, thin sputum associated with pulmonary edema
Hemoptysis	Expectoration of blood or bloody sputum; amount may range from blood-streaked to massive hemorrhage and is present in a variety of pathologies
Mucoid	White or clear, not generally associated with bronchopulmonary infection but is present with chronic cough (acute or chronic bronchitis, cystic fibrosis)
Mucopurulent	Mixture of mucoid sputum and pus, yellow to pale green, associated with infection
Purulent	Pus, yellow or greenish sputum, often copious and thick, common with acute and chronic infection
Rusty	Descriptive of the color of sputum; classic for pneumococcal pneumonia (also called *prune juice*)
Tenacious	Thick, sticky sputum

Reference

1. Irwin, S and Techlin, JS: Cardiopulmonary Physical Therapy, ed. 2. CV Mosby, St. Louis, 1990.

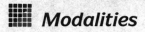
Modalities

ELECTROMAGNETIC MODALITIES

The Electromagnetic Spectrum

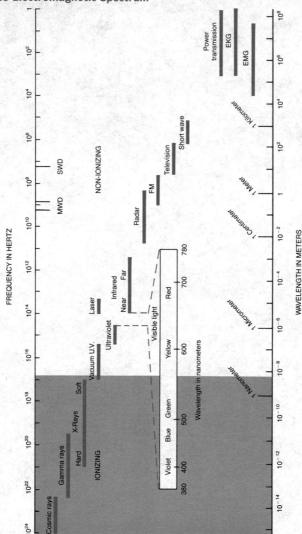

A graphic representation of the electromagnetic spectrum. (Adapted from *H:S Lighting Handbook,* ed 5, 1972.)

RADIATION	WAVELENGTH
Long wave diathermy	300 meters
Short wave diathermy	30 – 3 meters
Infrared rays	15,000 – 770 nm
Visible rays*	770 – 390 nm
red	650 nm
orange	600 nm
yellow	580 nm
green	530 nm
blue	475 nm
violet	400 nm
Ultraviolet	390 – 13.6 nm
Roentgen rays	13.6 – 0.14 nm

*Values are for the purest forms of the colors.

Physical Laws Relating to the Application of Electromagnetic Modalities

inverse square law: The intensity of the electromagnetic radiation received (RR) varies inversely with the square of the distance (D) from the source of the radiation. The following formula predicts the radiation received from a single source; it is not applicable to reflected radiation.

$$RR = \frac{\text{Radiation Source}}{D^2}$$

cosine law: Maximal radiation is applied when the source of radiation is at a right angle to the patient. The applied radiation is directly proportional to the cosine of the angle formed by the patient's body with the source of radiation.

INFRARED RADIATION

Sources of Infrared Radiation

All bodies above absolute zero ($-273\,°C$) emit infrared radiation. The higher the temperature above absolute zero, the greater the emitted infrared radiation.

Nonluminous Sources of Infrared Radiation

These emit infrared via the heat generated in a high-resistance electrical coil. The coil heats and in turn heats a covering element that causes the generation of infrared radiation. This is primarily long wave radiation. Although these sources emit a dull glow, their primary source is nonluminous. These generators must be warmed before use.

Luminous Sources of Infrared Radiation

These are primarily incandescent lights that emit mostly short wave radiation. Emission is instantaneous.

Effects of Infrared Radiation

Exposure leads to capillary dilation, which causes an erythema. Infrared radiation also serves as a possible counterirritant.

Types of Infrared Radiation and Penetration Depths		
TYPES	PENETRATION	SOURCE
Visible spectrum, 390–760 nm	1–10 mm	Luminous
Near infrared (short wave), 760–1500 nm	1–10 mm	Luminous
Far infrared (long wave), 1500–12,000 nm	0.05–1 mm	Nonluminous

References

1. Michlovitz, SL: Thermal Agents in Rehabilitation. FA Davis, Philadelphia, 1986.
2. Lehmann, JF: Therapeutic Heat and Cold, ed 3. Williams & Wilkins, Baltimore, 1982.

TERMS RELATED TO THE
USE OF DIATHERMY

applicator: In short wave diathermy, the applicator is an electrode through which a current flows.

capacitance: The ability to store electric charge. A property of a structure that consists of two or more conductors separated by a dielectric. This arrangement permits the storage and release of electric charge. In the case of diathermy, the conductors are usually flat metal plates.

capacitive applicator (short wave diathermy): Applicators that employ two air-spaced metal plates 7.5 to 17.5 cm in diameter (see *capacitance*).

capacitor: A device capable of storing and releasing electric charge (see *capacitance*).

diathermy: A therapeutic deep-heating modality that uses high-frequency electromagnetic radiation.

dielectric: A nonconducting substance; an insulator. In the case of therapeutic diathermy, the patient's tissues serve as the dielectric.

direct-contact applicator (microwave diathermy): Applicators that are spaced 1 cm or less from the body.

eddy currents: In diathermy these are the heat-producing currents in the body that are formed by a magnetic field applied externally.

electrode: A material through which a current flows (see *applicator*).

inductive applicator (short wave diathermy): Drum or cable magnetic field applicators.

magnetic field: A region in which a force is exerted along a magnetic pole. Units are amperes per meter (A/m). In diathermy, magnetic fields are formed around eddy currents.

magnetron: The vacuum tube that is used to produce microwave radiation.

microwave diathermy: A modality that produces electromagnetic radiation with a frequency above 300 MHz and a wavelength shorter than 1 m.

patient circuit: The part of a diathermy device that transfers electrical energy to the patient.

short wave diathermy: A modality which produces electromagnetic radiation by means of an oscillating electromagnetic field with a frequency between 10 and 100 MHz and a wavelength between 3 and 30 m.

spaced applicators (microwave diathermy): Applicators that are placed 3 to 6 cm from the body. These applicators usually produce nonuniform heating patterns.

specific absorption rate: The rate of energy absorbed per unit mass of tissue (expressed in watts per kilogram).

References

1. Therapeutic Microwave and Shortwave Diathermy: A Review of Thermal Effectiveness, Safe Use, and State of the Art: 1984. U.S. Department of Health and Human Services, Washington, DC, 1984.
2. Michlovitz, SL: Thermal Agents in Rehabilitation. ed. 2 FA Davis, Philadelphia, 1990.

Frequencies Used in Diathermy (FCC Approved)		
FREQUENCY	WAVELENGTH	TYPE OF DIATHERMY
13.56 Hz	22.0 m	Short wave
27.12 Hz*	11.0 m	Short wave
40.68 Hz	7.5 m	Short wave
915 Hz	33.0 cm	Microwave
2450 Hz*	12.0 cm	Microwave

*Most widely used frequencies.

References

1. Therapeutic Microwave and Shortwave Diathermy: A Review of Thermal Effectiveness, Safe Use, and State of the Art: 1984. U.S. Department of Health and Human Services, Washington, DC, 1984.
2. Michlovitz, SL: Thermal Agents in Rehabilitation. ed. 2 FA Davis, Philadelphia, 1990.

TERMS RELATED TO THE
USE OF ULTRASOUND

duty cycle: The term used in ultrasound to describe the time that sound waves are being emitted during one pulse period. Duty cycle is the duration of the pulse of sound waves in seconds divided by the pulse period. Duty cycle can also be expressed as a percentage.

$$\text{Duty cycle} = \frac{\text{Pulse duration (time on)}}{\text{Pulse period (time on + time off)}}$$

effective intensity (spatial average intensity: The ratio of the ultrasonic power to the effective radiating area of the applicator. Effective intensity is expressed in watts per square centimeter (W/cm^2).

effective radiating area: The area of the applicator that emits ultrasound (expressed in cm^2).

piezoelectric effect (direct): The generation of an electrical voltage across a crystal when the crystal is compressed.

piezoelectric effect (indirect or reverse): The contraction or expansion of a crystal when voltage is applied to the crystal. In ultrasound the reverse piezoelectric effect is used to generate sound waves.

pulse average intensity (temporal peak intensity): The maximum output of energy that is produced during the on phase of a pulsed ultrasound cycle.

pulse duration: In pulsed ultrasound it is the time interval during which ultrasound is being emitted.

pulse period: In pulsed ultrasound the duration of one cycle (the sum of the time on and the time off).

pulse repetition rate: The repetition frequency of the ultrasonic waveform expressed in pulses per second (pps).

pulsed ultrasound: Ultrasound that is intermittently interrupted by brief periods of time in which no ultrasound energy is produced.

reverse piezoelectric effect: See *piezoelectric effect.*

spatial average intensity: See *effective intensity.*

temporal peak intensity (pulsed average intensity): See *pulsed average intensity.*

ultrasonic frequency: The frequency of the ultrasound wave, expressed in hertz (Hz), kilohertz (KHz), or megahertz (MHz).

ultrasonic power: The average power emitted from the sound head during each cycle of the sound wave (expressed in watts).

ultrasonic transducer: A device designed to convert electrical energy into ultrasonic waves.

ultrasound: Sound waves with a frequency of greater than 20,000 Hz. Therapeutic ultrasound is in the frequency range of 0.9 MHz to 3 MHz.

References

1. Michlovitz, SL: Thermal Agents in Rehabilitation. FA Davis, Philadelphia, 1986.
2. U.S. Department of Health and Human Services: A Practitioner's Guide to The Ultrasonic Therapy Equipment Standard. HHS Publication FDA 85-8240, Washington DC, 1985.

		MOST EFFECTIVE
EFFECT	WAVELENGTH	WAVELENGTH
Erythema	250 – 297 nm	297 nm
Pigmentation	300 – 400 nm	340 nm
Antirachitic	240 – 300 nm	283 nm
Bactericidal	230 – 280 nm	245.3 nm
Carcinogenic	230 – 320 nm	300 nm
Antipsoriatic	280 – 400 nm	360 nm

Effects of Different Ultraviolet Wavelengths (Approximate Values)

Definitions of Erythemal Doses

Two systems of classifying erythemal doses have been used. In one classification, the level where erythema first appears is called the *minimal erythemal dose* (MED). In the other system, the first level is called *first-degree erythema*. When the term MED is used, there will be three degrees of erythemal doses. When the minimum level of erythema is called *first-degree erythema*, there will be four degrees of erythemal doses.

suberythemal dose (SED): Ultraviolet exposure insufficient to cause reddening.

minimal erythemal dose (MED): (Also called *first-degree*) slight reddening of skin, without desquamation; possible slight itching sensation.

first-degree erythemal (1D): (Also called *second-degree*) more reddening than occurs with an MED and slight desquamation (peeling); itching and burning as with sunburn.

second-degree erythemal (2D): (Also called *third-degree*) marked reddening with considerable itching, burning, and desquamation (peeling) of epidermis, some edema; similar to severe sunburn.

third-degree erythemal (3D): (Also called *fourth-degree*) intense reaction with edema, swelling, blister formation.

Characteristics of Erythemal Doses			
DOSE	CHARACTERISTIC EFFECT	APPEARS	DISAPPEARS
SED	No visible reaction		
MED	Slight reddening	4–6 hrs	24 hrs
1D	Mild sunburn	4–6 hrs	3–4 days
2D	Severe sunburn	2 hrs	Several days
3D	Edema and blistering	2 hrs	Several days

Reference

1. Forster, A and Palastanga, N: Clayton's Electrotherapy Theory and Practice, ed 9. Bailliere Tindall, New York, 1985.

PARAFFIN CHARACTERISTICS

Temperatures

In most clinical applications paraffin is applied at temperatures between 118°F to 126°F (47.8°C to 52.2°C). This temperature range is set on most commercial units; if higher temperatures are desired, there is frequently an adjustment screw that can be used.

Paraffin melts rapidly at 130°F (54.4°C) and sterilizes at 200°F (93.3°C).

Mixture Ratio

For clinical use, paraffin is usually mixed using the following ratio: 7 parts paraffin to 1 part mineral oil. A small amount of oil of wintergreen is often added if the paraffin is used frequently.

References

1. Michlovitz, SL: Thermal Agents in Rehabilitation. FA Davis, Philadelphia, 1986.
2. Lehmann, JF: Therapeutic Heat and Cold, ed 3. Williams & Wilkins, Baltimore, 1982.

MASSAGE

A review of the literature on massage reflects the very inexact nature of the field. The definitions and categories given below are by no means universal. Massage strokes are listed in the order of increasing vigor.

stroking (effleurage): Passing of the hands over a large body area with constant pressure.

> **superficial effleurage:** Extremely light form, using palms of hands, described as little more than a caress.

> **deep effleurage:** Strong enough stroking to evoke a mechanical as well as reflex effect on muscles.

compression: Use of intermittent pressure to lift, roll, press, squeeze, and stretch tissue and to hasten venous and lymphatic flow.

kneading (petrissage): Hands take a large fold of skin and underlying tissue and forcefully roll, raise, and squeeze it.

> *Pinching* (pincement)

> *Rolling* (roulement): rolling of muscle belly

> *Wringing*: like wringing a towel

> *Fulling*: rippling of deeper muscle caused by asynchronous movement of hands

> *Fist kneading*: compression via knuckles of a partially closed fist

> *Digital kneading*: use of a single finger or three positioned triangularly.

friction: Firm contact over a limited area to loosen adherent tissue.

> *Crushing* (ecrasement): localized and vigorous

> *Tearing* (dilaceration): intense deep pressure, like connective tissue massage (CTM)

> *Pleating* (pleissate): ends of finger perpendicular to veins

> *Sawing* (sciage): rapid and deep transverse movement of the ulnar border

> *Come-and-go*: reciprocal movement of the two index fingers or the thumbs

vibration and shaking: Hands are kept in contact with the patient, and movement originates with the therapist's body and is transmitted to the patient via the therapist's outstretched arms. Shaking (secousses) is characterized by the alternate flexion and extension of the therapist's elbows, whereas in vibration the elbows remain fully extended.

point vibration: Use of a single digit.

percussion: Brief, brisk, rapid contacts reciprocally applied with relaxed wrists.

tapping (tapotement): Rapid series of blows, hands parallel and partially flexed, with the ulnar borders of the hand striking the patient. Sometimes *tapping* is used to describe percussion with the fingertips.

hammering (martelage): Soft percussion with the ulnar edges of the hand of the slightly flexed last four fingers, so that the little finger strikes first.

clapping (claquement): Using fingers, palm, and thumb to form a concave surface.

hacking (hachure): Chopping strokes made by the ulnar surface hitting the patient; more vigorous than tapping.

beating (frappement): Striking with half-closed fists so that the ulnar side of the hand makes contact.

References

1. Tappan, F: Healing Massage Techniques: Holistic, Classic and Emergency Methods. Appleton & Lange, East Norwalk, CT, 1988.
2. Wood, EC: Beards Massage Principles and Treatment, ed 2. WB Saunders, Philadelphia, 1974.

ELECTROTHERAPEUTIC STIMULATION MODES

TYPE OF STIMULATION	INTENSITY	WAVEFORM	DURATION	FREQUENCY
Low voltage	<150 volts	DC or sine wave	Variable	2–2000 Hz
High voltage	Peak 2000–2500 mA; total 1.2–1.5 mA	Twin peak pulses	5–65 uSec	1–150 Hz (depending on purpose)
Russian mode	90–100 mA	Continuous sine wave	400 uSec	2500 Hz carrier modulated to 50 Hz pulses with 10 mSec intervals
Interferential	70–90 mA	Sine wave	250 uSec	4000 Hz (medium)

References

1. Wolf, SL (ed): Electrotherapy. Churchill Livingstone, New York, 1981.
2. Nelson, R and Currier, DP, eds: Clinical Electrotherapy. Appleton-Croft, New York, 1986.

CHARACTERISTICS OF TRANSCUTANEOUS ELECTRICAL NERVE STIMULATION (TENS)

TYPE OF STIMULATION	INTENSITY (AMPLITUDE)	PULSE DURATION (WIDTH)	FREQUENCY (RATE)
Conventional	Perceptible paresthesia (low)	20–60 uSec (narrow)	50–500 Hz (high)
Acupuncturelike	To tolerance (high)	150–250 uSec (wide)	1–4 Hz (low)
Pulse train	To tolerance (high)	100–200 uSec (wide)	2–3 Hz carrier with 70–100 Hz internal frequency (high and low carrier)
Brief intense	To tolerance (high)	150–250 uSec (wide)	100 Hz (high)

Reference

1. Mannheimer, JS and Lampe, GN: Clinical Electrical Nerve Stimulation. FA Davis, Philadelphia, 1984.

RHEOBASE AND CHRONAXIE

rheobase: The minimal strength of current that stimulates a muscle when the current is permitted to flow for an infinite period of time. *Infinite time* is considered by convention to be 300 ms of current flow. Rheobase is described in units of current (e.g., milliamps).

chronaxie: The minimum duration of current flow that is needed to stimulate a muscle at twice the current intensity of the rheobase current. Chronaxie is described in units of time (e.g., milliseconds).

Reference

1. Kimura, J: Electrodiagnosis in Diseases of Nerve and Muscle. ed. 2 FA Davis, Philadelphia, 1989.

REACTION TO DEGENERATION

Reaction to degeneration occurs when a muscle contracts in response to stimulation with galvanic (direct current, or DC) but not in response to faradic (alternating, or AC) current. Response to DC in the absence of a response to AC stimulation indicates that the muscle is denervated. This is because muscle tissue is less excitable than nervous tissue. Therefore, for a response to occur in muscle, the duration of current flow must be prolonged. There is prolonged current flow with DC stimulation but not with AC stimulation. The contraction produced in denervated muscle by DC stimulation is typically slow and wormlike.

Reference

1. D'Ambrosia, RD: Musculoskeletal Disorders: Regional Examination and Differential Diagnosis. JB Lippincott, Philadelphia, 1972.

MOTOR POINTS

Motor points are sites on the skin surface where the underlying muscle can be electrically stimulated to contract by lower levels of electricity than are needed in surrounding areas. The motor point overlies the innervation zone(s) of a muscle. This is where motor nerve endings are concentrated or where the nerve trunk enters the muscle. The motor point is often used as a placement site for surface electrodes used to stimulate muscle. The accompanying figures should be considered only as approximate locations of motor points for major muscle groups. The exact location, extent, and number of motor points can vary.

References

1. Walthard, KM and Tchicaloff, M: Motor points. In Licht, S (ed): Electrodiagnosis and Electromyography, ed 2. Waverly Press, Baltimore, 1970.
2. Coers, C and Woolf, AL: The Innervation of Muscle: A Biopsy Study. Charles C. Thomas, Springfield, IL, 1959.

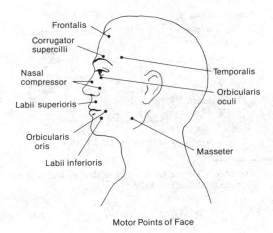

Motor Points of Face

The motor point table is adapted from: Watkins, AL: A Manual of Electrotherapy, ed 3. Lea & Febiger, Philadelphia, 1972.

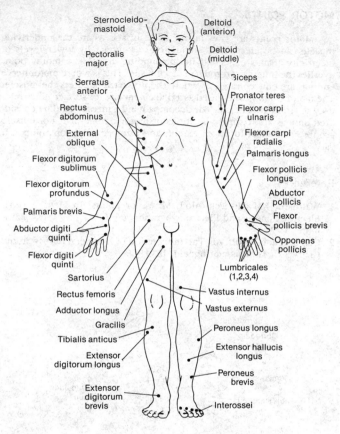

MOTOR POINTS OF ANTERIOR BODY

The motor point table is adapted from: Watkins, AL: A Manual of Electrotherapy, ed. 3. Lea & Febiger, Philadelphia, 1972.

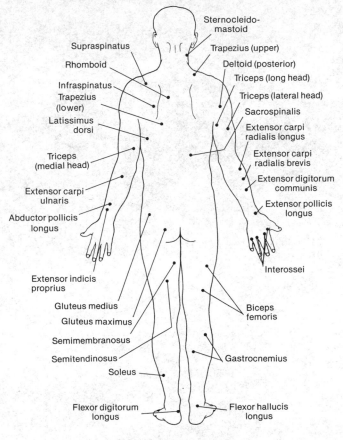

MOTOR POINTS OF POSTERIOR BODY

The motor point table is adapted from: Watkins, AL: A Manual of Electrotherapy, ed. 3. Lea & Febiger, Philadelphia, 1972.

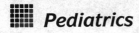
Pediatrics

CLASSIFICATION OF BIRTH INJURIES

Cerebral Birth Injury: Damage to the nervous system by complications during pregnancy, labor, delivery, or the immediate neonatal period. Associated with a number of predisposing factors related to maternal health, maternal age, social status, labor and delivery, birth weight, gestation, and parity. Most common mechanisms are asphyxia (which may be chronic or acute) and trauma.

Intracranial Hemorrhage

intraventricular hemorrhage — not related to trauma: More common in premature infants and with respiratory distress syndrome (RDS).

compression head injury — compression of the head: Most likely in full-term or postmature infants, many of whom are large for their gestational age. May present as subarachnoid, subdural, or (infrequently) cerebellar hemorrhage.

Fractures

Most of these lesions heal without treatment; however, the infant may be more comfortable when the fracture is immobilized.

skull fractures: Fissure fractures are not uncommon but are usually of little significance. Depressed fractures (a "pond" fracture) may result from pressure on the sacral promontory. The majority resolve spontaneously.

clavicle fractures: May occur during breech delivery if the baby's arms become displaced or may be the result of a difficult vertex delivery. Recovery is likely without treatment; however, it is usual to immobilize the upper arm against the chest. The baby should always be examined for a concurrent brachial plexus injury.

humeral fractures: May occur when a displaced arm is pulled down during a breech delivery. The baby should always be examined for nerve damage.

femoral fractures: May occur when a leg is pulled down during delivery of a breech presentation with extended legs. The fracture may be immobilized by bandaging the affected limb to the abdomen.

Nerve Lesions

abducens palsy: Transient abducens palsy occurs in a significant proportion of children born after prolonged labor and those who are delivered by forceps. Usually there is full recovery after a few days or weeks.

facial palsy: Pressure from a forceps blade may injure the extracranial part of the facial nerve. Facial palsy occasionally occurs following a spontaneous vaginal delivery. Recovery may be expected within 2 to 3 weeks.

Erb's palsy: Trauma to the C5 and C6 spinal roots due to excessive traction on the neck during a delivery, such as a difficult breech extraction or vertex delivery, where there has been difficulty with delivery of the shoulders. The affected arm lies limply at the infant's side, with the hand pronated and wrist slightly flexed. Recovery is usually complete within 2 weeks.

other brachial plexus injuries: The C4 root may be implicated in addition to Erb's palsy, thereby affecting function of the diaphragm with possible resultant acute respiratory distress. Much less common are damage to the lower roots (C7–T1).

radial palsy: Involvement of the radial nerve usually by subcutaneous fat necrosis or spontaneously due to pressure as a result of malposition in utero. Complete recovery is expected.

spinal cord injuries: These lesions are rare; however, they may occur following a breech delivery or with spinal fractures or subluxations. They occur most commonly in the cervical and thoracic region and are produced by traction on the vertebral column during delivery. There may also be an additional lesion to the brachial plexus due to tearing of the cervical roots from the spinal cord.

Reference

1. Forfar, JO and Arniel, GC (eds): Textbook of Pediatrics, ed 2, Vol. 1. 1982.

DEVELOPMENTAL ASSESSMENT: REFLEX TESTING

REFLEXES	STIMULUS	RESPONSE
Primitive/Spinal		
Flexor withdrawal	Noxious stimulus (pinprick) to sole of foot; Tested in supine or sitting position	Toes extend, foot dorsiflexes, entire leg flexes uncontrollably. Onset: 28 weeks gestation Integrated: 1 – 2 months
Crossed extension	Noxious stimulus to ball of foot of extremity fixed in extension; tested in supine position	Opposite lower extremity flexes, then adducts and extends Onset: 28 weeks gestation Integrated: 1 – 2 months
Traction	Grasp forearm and pull up from supine into sitting position	Grasp and total flexion of the upper extremity Onset: 28 weeks gestation Integrated: 2 – 5 months
Moro	Sudden change in position of head in relation to trunk: drop patient backward from sitting position	Extension, abduction of upper extremities, hand opening, and crying followed by flexion, adduction of arms across chest Onset: 28 weeks gestation Integrated: 5 – 6 months
Startle	Sudden loud or harsh noise	Sudden extension or abduction of arms, crying Onset: birth Integrated: persists

Continued on the following page(s)

651

DEVELOPMENTAL ASSESSMENT: REFLEX TESTING *Continued*

REFLEXES	STIMULUS	RESPONSE
Grasp	Maintained pressure to palm of hand (palmer grasp) or to ball of foot under toes (plantar grasp)	Maintained flexion of fingers or toes Onset: palmar: birth; plantar: 28 weeks gestation Integrated: palmar: 4–6 months; plantar: 9 months
Tonic/Brainstem		
Asymmetrical tonic neck (ATNR)	Rotation of the head to one side	Flexion of skull limbs, extension of the jaw limbs, "bow and arrow" or "fencing" posture Onset: birth Integrated: 4–6 months
Symmetrical tonic neck (STNR)	Flexion or extension of the head	With head flexion: flexion of arms, extension of legs; with head extension: extension of arms, flexion of legs Onset: 4–6 months Integrated: 8–12 months
Symmetrical tonic labyrinthine (TLR or STLR)	Prone or supine position	With prone position: increased flexor tone/flexion of all limbs; with supine: increased extensor tone/extension of all limbs

Reaction	Test	Onset / Integrated
Positive supporting	Contact to the ball of the foot in upright standing position	Onset: birth Integrated: 6 months Rigid extension (cocontraction) of the lower extremities Onset: birth Integrated: 6 months
Associated reactions	Resisted voluntary movement in any part of the body	Involuntary movement in a resting extremity Onset: birth–3 months Integrated: 8–9 years
Neck righting action on the body (NOB)	Passively turn head to one side; tested in supine	Body rotates as a whole (log rolls) to align the body with the head Onset: 4–6 months Integrated: 5 years
Body righting acting on the body (BOB)	Passively rotate upper or lower trunk segment; tested in supine	Body segment not rotated follows to align the body segments Onset: 4–6 months Integrated: 5 years
Labyrinthine head righting (LR)	Occlude vision; alter body position by tipping body in all directions	Head orients to vertical position with mouth horizontal Onset: birth–2 months Integrated: persists
Optical righting (OR)	Alter body position by tipping body in all directions	Head orients to vertical position with mouth horizontal Onset: birth–2 months Integrated: persists
Body righting acting	Place in prone or supine position	Head orients to vertical position with mouth

Continued on the following page(s)

DEVELOPMENTAL ASSESSMENT:
REFLEX TESTING *Continued*

REFLEXES	STIMULUS	RESPONSE
on head (BOH)		horizontal Onset: birth–2 months Integrated: 5 years
Protective extension (PE)	Displace center of gravity outside the base of support	Arms or legs extend and abduct to support and to protect the body against falling Onset: arms: 4–6 months; legs: 6–9 months Integrated: persists
Equilibrium reactions —tilting (ER)	Displace the center of gravity by tilting or moving the support surface (e.g., with a movable object such as an equilibrium board or ball)	Curvature of the trunk toward the upward side along with extension and abduction of the extremities on that side; protective extension on the opposite (downward) side Onset: prone 6 months; supine 7–8 months; sitting 7–8 months; quadruped 9–12 months; standing 12–21 months Integrated: persists
Equilibrium reactions —postural fixation	Apply a displacing force to the body, altering the center of gravity in its relation to the base of support; can also be observed during voluntary activity	Curvature of the trunk toward the external force with extension and abduction of the extremities on the side to which the force was applied Onset: prone 6 months; supine 7–8 months; sitting 7–8 months; quadruped 9–12 months; standing 12–21 months Integrated: persists

NORMAL DEVELOPMENT: POSTURAL CONTROL

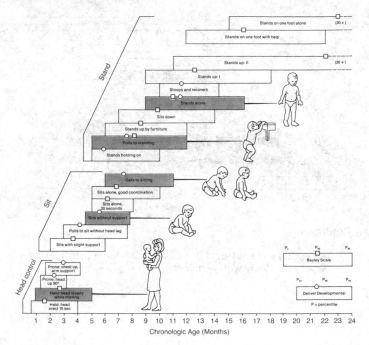

Reference

(From Keogh, J and Sugden, D: Movement Skill Development. Macmillan, New York, 1985, with permission.)

NORMAL DEVELOPMENT: LOCOMOTOR SKILLS

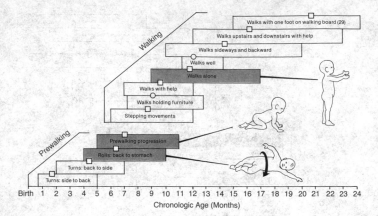

Reference

(From Keogh, J and Sugden, D: Movement Skill Development. Macmillan, New York, 1985, with permission.)

NORMAL DEVELOPMENT: MANUAL SKILLS
(control of prehension)

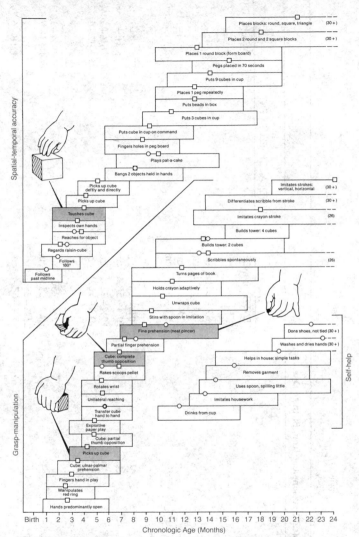

Places blocks: round, square, triangle (30 +)

Places 2 round and 2 square blocks (30 +)

Places 1 round block (form board)

Pegs placed in 70 seconds

Puts 9 cubes in cup

Places 1 peg repeatedly

Puts beads in box

Puts 3 cubes in cup

Puts cube in cup on command

Fingers holes in peg board

Plays pat-a-cake

Bangs 2 objects held in hands

Picks up cube deftly and directly

Picks up cube

Touches cube

Inspects own hands

Reaches for object

Regards raisin-cube

Follows 180°

Follows past midline

Spatial-temporal accuracy

Imitates strokes: vertical, horizontal (30 +)

Differentiates scribble from stroke (30 +)

Imitates crayon stroke (26)

Builds tower: 4 cubes

Builds tower: 2 cubes

Scribbles spontaneously (26)

Turns pages of book

Holds crayon adaptively

Unwraps cube

Stirs with spoon in imitation

Fine prehension (neat pincer)

Partial finger prehension

Cube: complete thumb opposition

Rakes-scoops pellet

Rotates wrist

Unilateral reaching

Transfer cube hand to hand

Explositive paper play

Cube: partial thumb opposition

Picks up cube

Cube: ulnar-palmar prehension

Fingers hand in play

Manipulates red ring

Hands predominantly open

Grasp-manipulation

Dons shoes, not tied (30 +)

Washes and dries hands (30 +)

Helps in house: simple tasks

Removes garment

Uses spoon, spilling little

Imitates housework

Drinks from cup

Self-help

Birth 1 2 3 4 5 6 7 8 9 10 11 12 13 14 15 16 17 18 19 20 21 22 23 24
Chronologic Age (Months)

Normal Development: Manual Skills 657

Physical Development from Birth to One Year

AGE	PHYSICAL DEVELOPMENT		
	LENGTH RANGE		WEIGHT RANGE
Birth			
boys	18¼–21½	in.	5½–9¼	lb
	46.4–54.4	cm	2.54–4.15	kg
girls	17¾–20¾	in.	5¼–8½	lb
	45.4–52.9	cm	2.36–3.8	kg
1 month			
boys	19¾–23	in.	7–11¾	lb
	50.4–58.6	cm	3.16–5.38	kg
girls	19¼–22½	in.	6½–10¾	lb
	49.2–56.9	cm	2.97–4.92	kg
3 months			
boys	22¼–25¾	in.	9¾–16¼	lb
	56.7–65.4	cm	4.43–7.37	kg
girls	21¾–25	in.	9¼–14¾	lb
	55.4–63.4	cm	4.18–6.74	kg

6 months

boys 25–28½ in. 63.4–72.3 cm   13¾–20¾ lb 6.20–9.46 kg

girls 24¼–27¾ in. 61.8–70.2 cm   12¾–19¼ lb 5.79–8.73 kg

9 months

boys 26¾–30¼ in. 68.0–77.1 cm   16½–24 lb 7.52–10.93 kg

girls 26–29½ in. 66.1–75.0 cm   15½–22½ lb 7.0–10.17 kg

12 months

boys 28¼–32 in. 71.7–81.2 cm   18½–26½ lb 8.43–11.99 kg

girls 27½–31¼ in. 69.8–79.1 cm   17¼–24¾ lb 7.84–11.24 kg

APGAR SCORE

SIGN	SCORE (for each item)		
	0	1	2
Heart rate	Absent	Slow (less than 100)	Greater than 100
Respiratory effort	Absent	Slow, irregular	Good; crying
Muscle tone	Limp	Some flexion of extremities	Active motion
Reflex irritability	No response	Grimace	Cough or sneeze
Color	Blue, pale	Body pink; extremities blue	Completely pink

FONTANELS

The fontanels of the infant are shown in the figure. The posterior fontanel closes between 2 and 3 months of age; the anterior fontanel closes between 16 and 18 months of age.

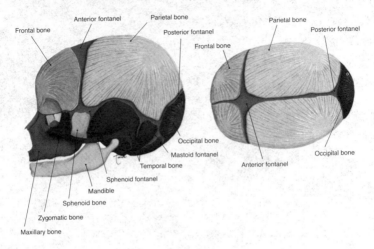

Reference

1. Rang, M: The Growth Plate and Its Disorders. Williams & Wilkins, Baltimore, 1969.

▦ Amputees, Prosthetics, and Orthotics

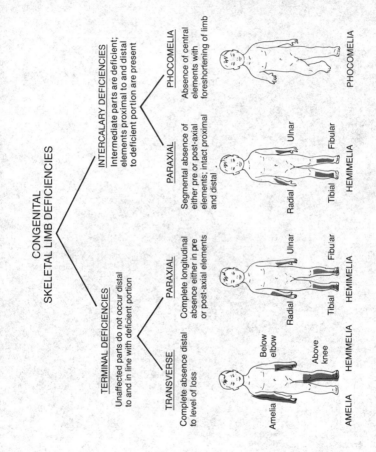

CONGENITAL
SKELETAL LIMB DEFICIENCIES

TERMINAL DEFICIENCIES
Unaffected parts do not occur distal to and in line with deficient portion

INTERCALARY DEFICIENCIES
Intermediate parts are deficient; elements proximal to and distal to deficient portion are present

TRANSVERSE
Complete absence distal to level of loss

PARAXIAL
Complete longitudinal absence either in pre or post-axial elements

PARAXIAL
Segmental absence of either pre or post-axial elements; intact proximal and distal

PHOCOMELIA
Absence of central elements with foreshortening of limb

Amelia

Below elbow

Above knee

AMELIA   HEMIMELIA

Radial

Tibial

Ulnar

Fibular

HEMIMELIA

Radial

Tibial

Ulnar

Fibular

HEMIMELIA

PHOCOMELIA

Classification of longitudinal and transverse defects in limb bud development. Adapted from Hall, CB, Brooks, MD, and Dennis, JF: Congenital skeletal deficiencies of the extremities: Classification and fundamentals of treatment. JAMA 181:591, 1962.

Guide for Preprosthetic Evaluation

ITEM TO BE EVALUATED	OBSERVE FOR:
Skin	1. Scar (location; healed, unhealed; adherent, mobile; invaginated, flat, thickened, keloid; from other surgery or a burn)
	2. Open lesions (size, shape, exudate)
	3. Moisture (moist, dry, crusting)
	4. Sensation (absent, diminished, hypersensitive to touch or pressure)
	5. Grafts (location, type, degree of healing)
	6. Dermatologic lesions (psoriasis, eczema, acne vulgaris, dermatitis, boils, epidermoid cysts)
Length	Bone length; soft tissue, redundant tissue length; the length of the below-knee limb is usually measured from the medial tibial plateau, and the above-knee limb from the ischial tuberosity or the greater trochanter
Shape	Cylindrical, conical, hourglass, "dog-ears," bulbous, above-knee adductor roll
Vascularity (Both limbs if cause of amputation is vascular disease)	1. Pulses (femoral, popliteal, dorsalis pedis, posterior tibial)
	2. Color (cyanotic, redness)
	3. Temperature (cool, warm)
	4. Edema (circumference measurements, water displacement measurement, diameter measurement using calipers)
	5. Pain (in dependent position, throbbing, claudication)
	6. Tropic changes (shininess, dryness, loss of hair)
Range of motion (ROM)	1. Hips (flexion, abduction, or external rotation contracture)
	2. Knee (flexion, extension contracture)
	3. Ankle (plantar flexion contracture)

ITEM TO BE EVALUATED	OBSERVE FOR:
Strength	Major muscle groups; adaptation must be made for shortened lever arm
Neurologic	1. Neuroma (location, tenderness) 2. Phantom (sensation; pain; description: throbbing, burning, electrical; duration) 3. Diabetic neuropathy (touch, joint proprioception, nerve conduction velocity, electromyogram) 4. Mental status (alert, senile; intelligent, limited ability to understand)
Activities of daily living	1. Transfers (bed to wheelchair, to toilet, to tub, to automobile; independent, dependent) 2. Ambulatory status (with crutches, walker; type of gait; independent, dependent) 3. Home (architectural barriers, safety rails; stairs; other hazards, such as small rugs, unsturdy rails) 4. Self-care (independent, dependent; includes residual limb care)
Psychological	1. Emotional status (depression, denial, cooperativeness, enthusiasm, motivation) 2. Family situation (interest, support, level of understanding, ability to help) 3. Work situation (job opportunity) 4. Prosthetic goals (desire for a prosthesis, anticipated activity level and life-style)
Medical status	1. Cause of amputation (disease, tumor, trauma, congenital) 2. Associated diseases/symptoms (neuropathy, visual disturbances, cardiopulmonary disease, renal disease, congenital anomalies) 3. Medications

Continued on the following page(s)

ITEM TO BE EVALUATED	OBSERVE FOR:
Prior prosthesis	Type, components, problems, gait deviations

Reference

1. Sanders, GT: Lower Limb Amputations: A Guide to Rehabilitation. FA Davis, Philadelphia, 1986.

BELOW-KNEE PROSTHETIC EVALUATION

The following table lists the various elements that should be checked as part of the evaluation of a below-knee prosthesis. Elements to be checked (standards) are in the left column and possible causes of a failure to meet the standards are in the right column.

STANDARD	POSSIBLE DEFICIENCIES
Dons prosthesis easily	1. Socket too small; residual limb edematous 2. Technique improper 3. Medial wedge contour unsatisfactory (supracondylar suspension)
Stands comfortably 1. Anterior heel and sole flat on floor	1. Socket too far anterior, causing knee to flex and weight to be borne primarily on sole 2. Socket too far posterior, causing knee to feel forced backward and weight to be borne primarily on heel
2. Medial and lateral borders of sole flat on floor	1. Socket too abducted, causing excessive loading laterally 2. Socket too adducted, causing excessive loading medially
Stands with pelvis level, both knees extended	Pelvis may tilt toward prosthetic side and/or contralateral hip and knee may flex if: 1. Heel cushion or prosthetic foot bumper too soft 2. Prosthetic foot dorsiflexed 3. Socket too flexed 4. Socket too loose, causing residual limb to lodge too deeply 5. shank too short
Minimal (less than 0.5 cm, ¼ inch) slippage when prosthesis is lifted during standing	1. Suspension inadequate 2. Socket too large
Stands with thigh corset, if present, well fitted 1. Uprights conform to thigh contour	1. Uprights improperly contoured 2. Joints set too far or too close to the thigh 3. Joints set too far proximal or distal to the epicondyles, interfering with sitting comfort

Continued on the following page(s)

STANDARD	POSSIBLE DEFICIENCIES
2. Mechanical knee joints close to the thigh, in line with the epicondyles	4. Corset improperly set on uprights
	5. Corset shape unsuitable for wearer's thigh
	6. Corset too large
3. Corset flat on thigh, without gapping or pinching	
4. Corset edges not touching each other	
Appearance satisfactory	Shank does not match contour or color of contralateral limb

Sits comfortably with knees flexed 90°	1. Posterior socket brim inadequate:
	  a. Too sharp
	  b. Too high
	  c. Insufficient provision for hamstring tendons

	2. Cuff suspension attached to the socket too far anterior or distal (cuff suspension)
	3. Mechanical knee joints attached to the socket too far anterior or distal (thigh corset suspension)
	4. Medial wedge contour unsatisfactory (supracondylar suspension)
Kneels comfortably	Because kneeling requires acute knee flexion, the same deficiencies that interfere with sitting hamper kneeling
Walks comfortably with minimal deviation	See "Below Knee Prostheses: Gait Deviations and Their Causes"
Walks with adequate suspension	1. Cuff attached to the socket too far anteriorly (cuff suspension)
	2. Socket loose (supracondylar suspension)
Walks quietly	1. Prosthetic foot improperly fitted to shoe
	2. Prosthetic foot joints loose (articulated assembly)
	3. Mechanical knee joints loose (thigh corset suspension)
With prosthesis removed, construction satisfactory	1. Plastic lamination not uniform
	2. Edges rough
	3. Foot not joined to shank with smooth transition

STANDARD	POSSIBLE DEFICIENCIES
	4. Stitching inadequate
	5. Rivets not flush with surface
	6. Cosmetic cover inadequate
Skin unblemished by prosthesis 10 minutes after removal	1. Socket too tight
	2. Socket too loose, sliding during walking and/or causing residual limb to bear too much load distally
	3. Corset too tight (thigh corset suspension)
	4. Medial wedge contour unsatisfactory (supracondylar suspension)
Wearer satisfied	1. Any deficiency noted above
	2. Discomfort within residual limb or proximal joints
	3. Psychosocial dysfunction
	4. At final evaluation, insufficient training

References

1. Prosthetics and Orthotics Staff: Lower Limb Prosthetics, rev ed. New York University, New York, 1981.
2. American Academy of Orthopedic Surgeons: Atlas of Limb Prosthetics. CV Mosby, St. Louis, 1981.

BELOW KNEE PROSTHESES: GAIT DEVIATIONS AND THEIR CAUSES

DEVIATION	PROSTHETIC CAUSES	BIOLOGICAL CAUSES
Excessive knee flexion in early stance	Insufficient plantar flexion Stiff heel cushion or plantar bumper Excessive socket flexion Socket malaligned too far anteriorly Excessive posterior placement of cuff tabs	Knee flexion contracture Weak quadriceps
Insufficient knee flexion in early stance	Excessive plantar flexion Soft heel cushion or plantar bumper Insufficient socket flexion Socket malaligned too far posteriorly	Pain at anterodistal aspect of residual limb Weak quadriceps Extensor hyper-reflexia Arthritis of the knee
Excessive lateral thrust	Excessive inset of foot Excessive socket adduction	
Medial thrust	Outset of foot Insufficient socket adduction	

Early knee flexion in late stance "drop off"	Insufficient plantar flexion Distal end of keel or toe break misplaced posteriorly Soft dorsiflexion stop Excessive socket flexion Socket malaligned too far anteriorly Excessive posterior placement of cuff tabs	Knee flexion contracture
Delayed knee flexion in late stance "walking uphill"	Excessive plantar flexion Distal end of keel or toe break misplaced anteriorly Stiff dorsiflexion stop Insufficient socket flexion Socket malaligned too far posteriorly	Extensor hyper-reflexia Knee arthritis

References

1. Prosthetics and Orthotics Staff: Lower Limb Prosthetics, rev ed. New York University, New York, 1981.
2. American Academy of Orthopedic Surgeons: Atlas of Limb Prosthetics. CV Mosby, St. Louis, 1981.

ABOVE-KNEE PROSTHETIC EVALUATION

The following table lists the various elements that should be checked as part of the evaluation of an above-knee prosthesis. Elements to be checked (standards) are in the left column and possible causes of a failure to meet the standards are in the right column.

STANDARD	POSSIBLE DEFICIENCIES
Dons prosthesis easily	1. Socket too small; residual limb edematous 2. Suction valve not located below residual limb or at bottom of anterior surface of socket 3. Technique improper

Stands comfortably	1. Proximal flesh roll caused by improper donning or too small a socket
	2. Greater trochanter and/or distal femoral socket concavities inadequate
	3. Quadrilateral socket
	  a. Adductor longus tendon not in channel
	    Socket too large; anteromedial discomfort
	    Socket too small
	  b. Medial brim sharp
	  c. Ischial tuberosity not on posterior brim
	    Socket too large, causing residual limb to lodge too deeply and impinge anteromedially
	    Socket too small, causing posterior discomfort
	  d. Posterior brim not parallel to floor
	4. Ischial containment socket
	  a. Socket too small; posteromedial corner does not cover ischial tuberosity
	  b. Socket too large: posterior wall gaps

STANDARD	POSSIBLE DEFICIENCIES
	c. Socket impinges on coccyx and/or pubis
Stands with pelvis level, both knees extended (Note: if prosthesis has a manually locked knee unit, shank should be 1 cm (½ inch) short to provide for clearance during swing phase)	Pelvis may tilt toward prosthetic side and/or contralateral hip and knee may flex if: 1. Heel cushion or prosthetic foot bumper too soft 2. Prosthetic foot dorsiflexed 3. Socket too loose, causing residual limb to lodge too deeply 4. Shank too short
Stands relaxed with prosthetic knee extended	1. Unlocked prosthetic knee unit: knee bolt too far anterior to line from hip to anterior border of heel, or ankle bolt of articulated foot-ankle assembly 2. Locked prosthetic knee unit: defective lock
Appearance satisfactory	Shank and/or thigh section do not match contour or color of contralateral limb
Sits comfortably with knees flexed 90°; should be able to lean forward to touch shoe	1. Anterior wall too high, impinging on abdomen 2. Posterior wall too thick or not parallel with chair seat 3. Insufficient posteromedial socket concavity (quadrilateral socket) 4. Mechanical hip joint not superior and anterior to greater trochanter (pelvic band suspension) 5. Pelvic band not contoured to torso (pelvic band suspension)
Walks comfortably with minimal deviation	See next table Above-Knee Prosthetic Gait Analysis
Walks with adequate suspension	1. Suction suspension a. Socket too large b. Lateral socket wall not contacting thigh

Continued on the following page(s)

	c. Lateral socket wall too short
	d. Greater trochanter concavity inadequate
	e. Suction valve clogged with glue, powder, or perspiration
	2. Silesian bandage auxiliary suspension
	a. Lateral attachment not superior and posterior to greater trochanter
	b. Anterior attachment (single attachment or midpoint between double anterior attachment) too high
	3. Pelvic band suspension
	a. Band not between iliac crest and greater trochanter
	b. Mechanical hip joint not superior and anterior to greater trochanter
Walks quietly	1. Prosthetic foot improperly fitted to shoe
	2. Prosthetic foot joints loose (articulated assembly)
	3. Extension stop in the knee unit insufficiently padded
	4. Loose mechanism in knee unit
	5. Fluid-controlled knee unit leaking
With prosthesis removed, construction satisfactory	1. Socket interior rough
	2. Knee and ankle clearance excessive or insufficient
	3. Posterior thigh and shank not contoured to permit acute knee flexion
	4. Posterior thigh and shank not congruent when prosthetic knee is flexed fully

STANDARD	POSSIBLE DEFICIENCIES
	5. Rigid socket lacks resilient backpad to absorb noise when sitting and reduce clothing abrasion
	6. Knee lock, if present, malfunctions
	7. Plastic lamination or molding not uniform
	8. Foot not joined to shank with smooth transition
	9. Stitching inadequate
	10. Rivets not flush with surface
	11. Cosmetic cover inadequate
Skin unblemished by prosthesis 10 minutes after removal	1. Socket too tight
	2. Socket too loose, sliding during walking and/or causing residual limb to bear too much load distally
	3. Socket does not cover proximal medial thigh, permitting fleshy bulge
	4. Socket edges too sharp
Wearer satisfied	1. Any deficiency noted above
	2. Discomfort within amputation limb or proximal joints
	3. Psychosocial dysfunction
	4. At final evaluation, insufficient training

ABOVE-KNEE PROSTHESES: GAIT DEVIATIONS AND THEIR CAUSES

DEVIATION	PROSTHETIC CAUSES	BIOLOGICAL CAUSES
Lateral trunk bending	Short prosthesis	Weak abductors
	Inadequate lateral wall adduction	Abduction contracture
	Sharp or excessively high medial wall	Hip pain
	Malalignment in abduction	Very short residual limb
		Instability
Wide walking base (abducted gait)	Long prosthesis	Abduction contracture
	Excessive abduction of hip joint	Adductor tissue roll
	Inadequate lateral wall adduction	Instability
	Sharp or excessively high medial wall	
	Malalignment in abduction	
Circumduction	Long prosthesis	Abduction contracture
	Excessive stiffness of knee unit	Poor knee control
	Inadequate suspension	
	Small socket	
	Excessive plantarflexion	
Medial (lateral) whip	Faulty socket contour	
	Malrotation of knee unit	
Rotation of foot on heel strike	Stiff heel cushion or plantar bumper	
	Malrotation of foot	

Uneven heel rise	Inadequate knee friction
	Lax or taut extension aid
	Excessively forceful hip flexion
Terminal swing impact	Insufficient knee friction
	Taut extension aid
Foot slap	Soft heel cushion or plantar bumper
Uneven step length	Faulty socket contour
	Inadequate knee friction
	Lax or taut extension aid
	Weak hip musculature
	Hip flexion contracture
	Instability
Lordosis	Inadequate support from posterior brim
	Inadequate socket flexion
	Hip flexion contracture
	Weak hip extensors
Vaulting	Long prosthesis
	Inadequate suspension
	Inadequate knee friction
	Excessive plantarflexion
	Small socket
	Walking speed exceeding that for which friction in a sliding friction knee unit was adjusted

References

1. Prosthetics and Orthotics Staff: Lower Limb Prosthetics, rev ed. New York University, New York, 1981.
2. American Academy of Orthopedic Surgeons: Atlas of Limb Prosthetics. CV Mosby, St. Louis, 1981.

The following table lists the various elements that should be checked as part of the evaluation of a hip-disarticulation prosthesis. Elements to be checked (standards) are in the left column and possible causes of a failure to meet the standards are in the right column.

STANDARD	POSSIBLE DEFICIENCIES
Dons prosthesis easily	1. Socket too small; residual limb edematous 2. Technique improper
Stands comfortably	1. Socket improperly contoured over the iliac crests 2. Residual limb not sufficiently lateral in socket 3. Ischial tuberosity not covered by socket 4. Perineal flesh roll below socket
Stands with pelvis almost level. Pelvis should tilt slightly toward prosthetic side; a 1 cm (½ inch) lift under the prosthesis should restore level pelvic alignment. Slight shortness aids clearance during swing phase	1. Heel cushion or prosthetic foot bumper too soft 2. Prosthetic foot dorsiflexed 3. Shank or thigh section too short
Stands relaxed, with prosthetic hip and knee extended	1. A straight line joining the mechanical hip and knee joint fails to pass at least 3.5 cm (1½ inches) posterior to the heel 2. Hip extension stop too thick
Minimal (less than 0.5 cm or ¼ inch) slippage when prosthesis is lifted during standing	1. Socket too large 2. Residual limb not sufficiently lateral in socket 3. Socket depressions over the iliac crests too shallow or too high
Appearance satisfactory	Shank and/or thigh section do not match contour or color of contralateral limb

STANDARD	POSSIBLE DEFICIENCIES
Sits comfortably with knees flexed 90°	1. Hip extension stop too thick 2. Mechanical hip joint is displaced too far posteriorly or too far distally 3. Posterior wall of thigh section not parallel with chair seat 4. Socket too large 5. Socket improperly contoured over the ischium 6. Residual limb not sufficiently lateral in socket 7. Waistband inadequately flared or too low 8. Proximal socket brim inadequately flared or too low 9. Knee extension aid fails to swively to permit full knee flexion
Walks comfortably with minimal deviation	1. See previous table; because prosthesis is intentionally short, the wearer may bend laterally 2. Hip instability, caused by failure of hip extension stop to contact socket in early stance, because either the stop is too thin or the mechanical hip joint is too posterior 3. Knee instability, caused by failure of knee extension in early stance, because either the hip extension stop is too thick or the mechanical hip joint is displaced anteriorly
Walks with adequate suspension	1. Socket too large 2. Socket depressions over the iliac crests too shallow or too high 3. Contralateral side of socket provides insufficient support 4. Lateral waistband too loose

Continued on the following page(s)

STANDARD	POSSIBLE DEFICIENCIES
Walks quietly	1. Prosthetic foot improperly fitted to shoe 2. Prosthetic foot joints loose (articulated assembly) 3. Extension stop in knee unit insufficiently padded 4. Loose mechanism in knee or hip unit 5. Fluid-controlled knee unit leaking
With prosthesis removed, construction satisfactory	1. Socket interior rough 2. Knee and ankle clearance excessive or insufficient 3. Posterior thigh and shank not contoured to permit acute knee flexion 4. Posterior thigh and shank not congruent when prosthetic knee is flexed fully 5. Plastic lamination not uniform 6. Foot not joined to shank with smooth transition 7. Stitching inadequate 8. Rivets not flush with surface 9. Cosmetic cover inadequate
Skin unblemished by prosthesis 10 minutes after removal	1. Socket too tight 2. Socket too loose, sliding during walking 3. Socket edges too sharp
Wearer satisfied	1. Any deficiency noted above 2. Discomfort within amputated limb or proximal joints 3. Psychosocial dysfunction 4. At final evaluation, insufficient training

References

1. Prosthetics and Orthotics Staff: Lower Limb Prosthetics, rev ed. New York University, New York, 1981.
2. American Academy of Orthopedic Surgeons: Atlas of Limb Prosthetics. CV Mosby, St. Louis, 1981.

UPPER LIMB PROSTHETIC EVALUATION

The following table lists the various elements that should be checked as part of the evaluation of an upper limb prosthesis. Elements to be checked (standards) are in the left column and possible causes of a failure to meet the standards are in the right column.

STANDARD	POSSIBLE DEFICIENCIES
Dons prosthesis easily	1. Socket too tight 2. Harness too complex 3. Technique improper
Wearing prosthesis, move upper limb through satisfactory excursion comfortably	Below-elbow, above-elbow, and shoulder prostheses: chest strap too tight (chest strap suspension); Below-elbow and above-elbow prostheses: 1. Axilla loop too small and/or unpadded 2. Front support strap not in deltopectoral groove (figure-of-eight suspension) Below-elbow prosthesis: 1. Socket anterior brim restricts elbow flexion 2. Socket posterior brim restricts elbow extension 3. Socket too loose, reducing transmission of forearm pronation and supination to the socket 4. Elbow hinge pinches flesh 5. Triceps pad or cuff improperly aligned Above-elbow prosthesis: 1. Socket anterior brim restricts shoulder flexion to less than 90° 2. Socket lateral brim restricts shoulder abduction to less than 90° 3. Socket posterior brim restricts shoulder hyperextension to less than 30°

Continued on the following page(s)

STANDARD	POSSIBLE DEFICIENCIES

Terminal device opens and closes satisfactorily. Active opening and closing should equal passive excursion when forearm is perpendicular to torso. Below-elbow prosthesis: full excursion should be obtained also with terminal device at waist and at mouth. Above-elbow and shoulder prostheses: active excursion at waist and at mouth should be at least half of the mechanical range.

1. Cable-controlled terminal device
   a. Cable malaligned
   b. Cable too long or too short
   c. Cable path has sharp bends
   d. Cable housing too long
   e. Cross of figure-of-eight harness too far toward residual side
   f. Control attachment strap on or above scapular spine
   g. Chest strap too loose (chest strap suspension)
   h. Leather lift loop too large or too distal
   i. Terminal device adjustments, e.g., two-position thumb, malfunctioning
2. Myoelectrically controlled terminal device
   a. Electrodes improperly located
   b. Socket too loose, preventing electrode contact with skin
   c. Battery inadequately charged

Prosthesis operates efficiently. Below-elbow prosthesis: force at terminal device should equal at least 80 percent of force measured at control attachment strap of harness. Above-elbow and shoulder prostheses: terminal device force should be at least 70 percent of force measured at control attachment strap.

1. Cable malaligned
2. Cable too long
3. Cable path has sharp bends

Minimal slippage when 23 kg (50 pounds) axial stress is applied to prosthesis. Below-elbow supracondylar socket should not slip more than 1 cm (½ inch). All

1. Socket too loose
2. Harness attachments insecure
3. Shoulder saddle too small (chest strap suspension)

STANDARD	POSSIBLE DEFICIENCIES

other sockets should not slip more than 2.5 cm (1 inch).

Limbs equal in length when elbows are extended
1. Prosthetic hand: should be at same level as sound hand
2. Hook: should be at same level as thumb of sound hand

1. Below-elbow, above-elbow, and shoulder prostheses:
   a. Forearm too short or too long
   b. Terminal device too small or too large
2. Above-elbow and shoulder prostheses: Humeral section too short or too long

Wrist unit rotates and, if lock is present, locks satisfactorily

1. Friction adjustment too tight or too loose
2. Locking mechanism malfunctions

Above-elbow and shoulder prostheses: Elbow unit moves and locks satisfactorily. Maximum of 45° shoulder flexion needed to flex elbow fully

1. Cable malaligned
2. Cable too long
3. Cable housing too long
4. Cable housing ends abut before full elbow flexion is achieved
5. Cross of figure-of-eight harness too far toward residual side
6. Control attachment strap on or above scapular spine
7. Chest strap too loose (chest strap suspension)
8. Leather lift loop too large, too short, or improperly located
9. Leather lift loop folds or does not pivot
10. Elastic suspensor strap too loose or too taut
11. Locking mechanism malfunctioning
12. Turntable too loose or too tight

Appearance satisfactory

1. Terminal device too large or too small
2. Prosthetic hand
   a. Glove improperly installed
   b. Glove stained or torn

Continued on the following page(s)

	c. Glove color does not match contralateral limb
	3. Forearm and humeral section, if present, does not match contour or color of contralateral limb
With prosthesis removed, construction satisfactory	1. Plastic lamination not uniform
	2. Edges of socket or housing rough
	3. Stitching inadequate
	4. Rivets not flush with surface
	5. Cosmetic cover inadequate
Skin unblemished by prosthesis 10 minutes after removal	1. Socket or harness too tight
	2. Socket edges rough
	3. Axilla loop too small or unpadded
Wearer satisfied	1. Any deficiency noted above
	2. Discomfort within residual limb or proximal joints
	3. Psychosocial dysfunction
	4. At final evaluation, insufficient training

References

1. Prosthetics and Orthotics Staff: Upper-Limb Prosthetics. New York University, New York, 1986.
2. Atkins, DJ and Meier, RH (eds): Comprehensive Management of the Upper-Limb Amputee. Springer-Verlag, New York, 1989.

LOWER LIMB ORTHOTIC EVALUATION

The following table lists the various elements that should be checked as part of the evaluation of a lower limb orthosis. Elements to be checked (standards) are in the left column and possible causes of a failure to meet the standards are in the right column.

STANDARD	POSSIBLE DEFICIENCIES
Don orthosis easily	1. Shoe or proximal components too small
	2. Fastenings unsuitable
	3. Shoe does not open sufficiently. Blucher design, in which anterior borders of lace stays are not attached, provides maximum opening.
	4. Shoe does not detach from proximal components. Shoe insert, split stirrup, and caliper are easier to don than solid stirrup.
Stand comfortably	1. Shoe too tight, especially at metatarsophalangeal joints
	2. Shoe too short, contacting toetips
	3. Shoe insert or foot valgus/varus correction strap contour unsatisfactory
	4. Knee valgus/varus correction strap contour unsatisfactory
	5. Shells, bands, and uprights too tight
	6. Calf band presses on fibular head
	7. Medial and lateral uprights not at midline of leg: if too posterior, reduces area of calf shell or band; if too anterior, may permit unstable knee to hyperextend
	8. Posterior upright not at posterior midline of leg
	9. Mechanical ankle and knee joint stops set improperly

Continued on the following page(s)

STANDARD	POSSIBLE DEFICIENCIES
	10. Medial upright impinges into perineum
	11. Lateral upright contacts greater trochanter
Stand with pelvis level, both knees extended (Note: if orthosis has a locked knee joint, 1 cm (1/2 inch) shortening provides for clearance during swing phase)	Shoe elevation inadequate to compensate for limb shortness
Stands relaxed	Knee and hip locks not engaged securely
Patellar-tendon bearing or proximal thigh brim, if included, reduces weight bearing at the heel	Brim contour inadequate to support weight proximally
Appearance satisfactory	Orthosis design or construction excessively bulky
Sits comfortably with knees flexed 105° (Note: orthosis limiting dorsiflexion will restrict acute knee flexion)	1. Proximal border of calf shell or band too sharp or too high
	2. Mechanical ankle joints not level with distal tip of medial malleolus
	3. Mechanical knee joints not level with medial femoral epicondyle
	4. Mechanical hip joints not superior and anterior to greater trochanter
	5. Pelvic band not contoured to torso
Walks comfortably with minimal deviation	See Lower Limb Orthoses: Gait Deviations and their Causes
With orthosis removed, construction satisfactory	1. Edges rough
	2. Metal nicked
	3. Stitching inadequate
	4. Rivets not flush with surface
	5. Shoe heel and sole not level, including shoes with wedges
	6. Insert does not fit snugly in shoe
	7. Mechanical ankle, knee, or hip joints bind when moved

STANDARD	POSSIBLE DEFICIENCIES
	8. Mechanical ankle or knee joints do not contact simultaneously at full flexion and at full extension
	9. Lengthening provision inadequate (child's orthosis)
Skin unblemished by orthosis 10 minutes after removal	1. Orthosis too tight
	2. Mechanical ankle joints not level with distal tip of medial malleolus, causing calf band to abrade leg (if orthosis permits dorsiflexion)
Wearer satisfied	1. Any deficiency noted above
	2. Discomfort within the lower limb or back
	3. Psychosocial dysfunction
	4. At final evaluation, insufficient training

References

1. Prosthetics and Orthotics Staff: Lower-Limb Prosthetics, rev ed. New York University, New York, 1981.
2. American Academy of Orthopedic Surgeons: Atlas of Orthotics, ed 2. CV Mosby, St. Louis, 1981.
3. Redford, JB (ed): Orthotics Etcetera. Williams & Wilkins, Baltimore, 1986.

LOWER LIMB ORTHOSES: GAIT DEVIATIONS AND THEIR CAUSES

DEVIATION	ORTHOTIC CAUSES	BIOLOGICAL CAUSES
Lateral trunk bending	Excessive height of medial upright of KAFO	Weak abductors
	Excessive abduction of hip joint	Abduction contracture
	Insufficient shoe lift to compensate for leg shortening	Dislocated hip
		Hip pain
		Instability
Hip hiking	Hip or knee lock uncompensated by contralateral shoe lift	Weak hip flexors
	Pes equinus uncompensated by contralateral shoe lift	Hip extensor hyper-reflexia
	Inadequate plantar flexion stop or dorsiflexion spring	
Internal (external) hip rotation	Transverse plane malalignment	Weak lateral (medial) hip musculature
Circumduction	Hip or knee lock uncompensated by contralateral shoe lift	Weak hip flexors
	Pes equinus uncompensated by contralateral shoe lift	Abduction contracture
	Inadequate plantarflexion stop or dorsiflexion spring	
Wide walking base	Excessive height of medial upright of KAFO	Weak abductors
	Excessive abduction of hip joint	Abduction contracture
	Knee lock uncompensated by contralateral shoe lift	Instability
		Genu valgum

Gait deviation	Orthotic cause	Anatomic cause
Excessive medial (lateral) foot contact	Transverse plane malalignment	Weak invertors (evertors) Pes valgus (varus) Genu valgum (varum)
Anterior trunk bending	Inadequate knee lock	Weak quadriceps
Posterior trunk bending		Weak hip extensors
Lordosis	Inadequate support from the brim of a weight-relieving KAFO	Hip flexion contracture Weak hip extensors
Hyperextended knee	Genu recurvatum inadequately controlled by plantar stop and excessively concave calf band Pes equinus uncompensated by contralateral shoe lift	Weak quadriceps Lax knee ligaments Extensor hyper-reflexia
Knee instability	Inadequate knee lock Inadequate dorsiflexion stop	Knee flexion contracture Weak quadriceps
Inadequate dorsiflexion control	Inadequate plantar flexion stop or dorsiflexion spring	Weak dorsiflexors Extensor hyper-reflexia
Vaulting	Hip or knee lock uncompensated by contralateral shoe lift Pes equinus uncompensated by contralateral shoe lift Inadequate plantar flexion stop or dorsiflexion spring	Weak hip flexors Abduction contracture

References

1. Prosthetics and Orthotics Staff: Lower-Limb Prosthetics, rev ed. New York University, New York, 1981.
2. American Academy of Orthopedic Surgeons: Atlas of Orthotics, ed 2. CV Mosby, St. Louis, 1981.
3. Redford, JB (ed): Orthotics Etcetera. Williams & Wilkins, Baltimore, 1986.

UPPER LIMB ORTHOTIC EVALUATION

The following table lists the various elements that should be checked as part of the evaluation of an upper limb orthosis. Elements to be checked (standards) are in the left column and possible causes of a failure to meet the standards are in the right column.

STANDARD	POSSIBLE DEFICIENCIES
Dons orthosis easily	1. Orthosis too tight 2. Orthosis too complex 3. Technique improper 4. Fastenings unsuitable
Wearing orthosis, move fingers comfortably	1. Mechanical joints not congruent with anatomic joints 2. Components press on bony prominences 3. Wrist strap does not lie between metacarpal bases and wrist crease
Orthosis promotes maximum function (except for orthosis intended to promote rest)	1. Palmar surface of finger tips obstructed 2. Opponens bar does not provide adequate ulnar directed force on thumb metacarpal 3. Opponens bar does not extend to palmar edge of thumb metacarpal 4 Thumb abduction bar does not maintain adequate abduction 5. Thumb abduction bar restricts thumb interphalangeal or index metacarpophalangeal joint motion 6. Palmar or dorsal bars do not conform to contour of distal transverse arch 7. Metacarpophalangeal extension stop ineffective 8. Thumb and index and middle fingers not aligned to provide desired grasp, either three-jaw chuck or lateral grasp

STANDARD	POSSIBLE DEFICIENCIES
	9. Forearm bar too long or too short
	10. Forearm bar does not maintain wrist in desired position
	11. Electric microswitch actuator unsatisfactory
	12. Battery inadequately charged
	13. Utensil holder too large or too small
Appearance satisfactory	Orthosis excessively bulky or complex
With orthosis removed, construction satisfactory	1. Edges rough
	2. Plastic molding not uniform
	3. Rivets not flush with surface
	4. Mechanical joints bind when moved
Skin unblemished by orthosis 10 minutes after removal	1. Orthosis too tight
	2. Orthosis too loose, permitting slippage during function
	3. Edges rough
Wearer satisfied	1. Any deficiency noted above
	2. Discomfort within the upper limb
	3. Psychosocial dysfunction
	4. At final evaluation, insufficient training

References

1. American Academy of Orthopedic Surgeons: Atlas of Orthotics, ed 2. CV Mosby, St. Louis, 1981.
2. Redford, JB (ed): Orthotics Etcetera. Williams & Wilkins, Baltimore, 1986.

SPINAL ORTHOTIC EVALUATION

The following table lists the various elements that should be checked as part of the evaluation of a spinal orthosis. Elements to be checked (standards) are in the left column and possible causes of a failure to meet the standards are in the right column.

STANDARD	POSSIBLE DEFICIENCIES
Dons orthosis easily	1. Orthosis too tight 2. Thoracic band too long 3. Technique improper
Stands comfortably	1. Pelvic or thoracic band too narrow or not conforming to torso 2. Pelvic band at or above posterior superior iliac spines 3. Pelvic band terminates posterior to lateral midline of torso 4. Thoracic band above inferior angles of scapulae 5. Thoracic band not horizonal 6. Posterior uprights press on vertebrae 7. Interscapular band too short, too long, or too high 8. Subclavicular extensions of the thoracic band, if present, too high or too low 9. Abdominal support too small 10. Suprapubic pad, if present, impinges on pelvis 11. Sternal plate, if present, too high 12. Occipital plate, if present, too low
Appearance satisfactory	Orthosis design or construction excessively bulky
Sits comfortably	1. Pelvic band below greater trochanters or contacting chair 2. Thoracic band too high 3. Interscapular band too low

STANDARD	POSSIBLE DEFICIENCIES
	4. Abdominal support too large or inferior border too low or too high
	5. Posterior uprights press on vertebrae
	6. Pads impinge on clavicles
With orthosis removed, construction satisfactory	1. Edges rough
	2. Metal nicked
	3. Stitching inadequate
	4. Rivets not flush with surface
	5. Plastic molding not uniform
Skin unblemished by orthosis 10 minutes after removal	1. Orthosis too tight
	2. Pelvic or thoracic band improperly contoured
Wearer satisfied	1. Any deficiency noted above
	2. Discomfort within the trunk or neck
	3. Psychosocial dysfunction

References

1. American Academy of Orthopedic Surgeons: Atlas of Orthotics, ed 2. CV Mosby, St. Louis, 1981.
2. Redford, JB (ed): Orthotics Etcetera. Williams & Wilkins, Baltimore, 1986.
3. Prosthetics and Orthotics Staff: Spinal Orthotics. New York University, New York, 1987.

EVALUATION OF ORTHOTICS FOR SCOLIOSIS

The following table lists the various elements that should be checked as part of the evaluation of orthoses used to treat scoliosis. Elements to be checked (standards) are in the left column and possible causes of a failure to meet the standards are in the right column.

STANDARD	POSSIBLE DEFICIENCIES
Dons orthosis easily	1. Orthosis too tight 2. Technique improper 3. Pelvic girdle straps too short 4. Pelvic girdle opening insufficient
Stands comfortably	1. Pads too snug or too small 2. Pelvic girdle too tight 3. Pelvic girdle anteroinferior border contacts pubis 4. Pelvic girdle anterosuperior border too low or too high 5. Pelvic girdle superolateral border contacts ribs 6. Pelvic girdle does not accommodate iliac spines 7. Thoracic pad strap not centered on pad 8. Thoracic pad spans fewer than three ribs 9. Lumbar pad impinges on pelvis or vertebrae 10. Shoulder ring or sling improperly contoured 11. Sternal pad too high 12. Pads or frame interfere with deep breathing or arm motion
Appearance satisfactory	1. Pelvic girdle superolateral border gaps 2. Uprights not contoured to the torso 3. Shoulder ring or sling improperly contoured
Sit comfortably	1. Pelvic girdle anteroinferior border too low, contacting chair

STANDARD	POSSIBLE DEFICIENCIES
	2. Pelvic girdle anteroinferior border too low, impinging on thighs
	3. Pelvic girdle lateral border impinges on greater trochanters
With orthosis removed, construction satisfactory	1. Uprights not covered with plastic or leather
	2. Edges rough
	3. Metal nicked
	4. Stitching inadequate
	5. Rivets not flush with surface
	6. Plastic molding not uniform
Skin umblemished by orthosis 10 minutes after removal. Painless reddening is satisfactory just above the ilium and beneath pads.	1. Pads impinge on bony prominences
	2. Pelvic girdle too tight or too loose
Wearer satisfied	1. Any deficiency noted above
	2. Discomfort within the trunk or neck
	3. Psychosocial dysfunction

References

1. American Academy of Orthopedic Surgeons: Atlas of Orthotics, ed 2. CV Mosby, St. Louis, 1981.
2. Redford, JB (ed): Orthotics Etcetera. Williams & Wilkins, Baltimore, 1986.
3. Prosthetics and Orthotics Staff: Spinal Orthotics. New York University, New York, 1987.

Gait

NORMAL GAIT

Phases of the Gait Cycle (Percentages are approximate and velocity dependent)

Right DS 10%	Right SS 40%	Left DS 10%	Left SS 40%
Left Step 50%		Right Step 50%
Right Stance 60%		Right Swing 40%

NORMAL

The figure shows a typical subject during the phases of the *gait cycle*. The subject's right heel touches the ground to begin a phase of *right double support (DS)*. When the left leg comes off the ground *right single support (SS)* begins. Right single support occurs at the same time as *left swing*. The periods of right double support and right single support make up the *left step period*. When the left heel comes in contact with the ground, the period of *left double support (DS)* begins. The periods of right double support, right single support, and left double support make up the *right stance phase*. When the right leg comes off the ground, the period of *left single support (SS)* begins. Left single support occurs at the same time as *right swing*. The periods of left double support and left single support make up the *right step period*. The percentages are averages and vary greatly between subjects and as a function of walking speed.

traditional nomenclature: The events taking place during the phase are named, for the most part, according to the events that take place at the foot, for example, heel strike.

Ranchos Los Amigos nomenclature: The events taking place during the phases are named, for the most part, according to the purpose of the phase, for example, initial contact.

Terms Used to Describe Gait for Observational Analysis

TRADITIONAL	RANCHO LOS AMIGOS
Stance Phase	
Heel strike: The beginning of the stance phase when the heel contacts the ground.	Initial contact: The beginning of the stance phase when the heel or another part of the foot contacts the ground.
Foot flat: Occurs immediately following heel strike, when the sole of the foot contacts the floor.	Loading response: The portion of the stance phase from immediately following initial contact until the contralateral extremity leaves the ground.
Midstance: The point at which the body passes directly over the reference extremity.	Midstance: The portion of the stance phase that begins when the contralateral extremity leaves the ground and ends when the body is directly over the supporting limb.

Continued on the following page(s)

TRADITIONAL	RANCHO LOS AMIGOS
Heel-off: The point following midstance at which time the heel of the reference extremity leaves the ground.	Terminal stance: The portion of the stance phase from midstance to a point just prior to initial contact of the contralateral extremity.
Toe off: The point following heel off when only the toe of the reference extremity is in contact with the ground.	Preswing: The portion of stance from the initial contact of the contralateral extremity to just prior to the lift off of the reference extremity. This portion includes toe off.

Swing Phase

Acceleration: The portion of beginning swing from the moment the toe of the reference extremity leaves the ground to the point when the reference extremity is directly under the body.	Initial swing: The portion of swing from the point when the reference extremity leaves the ground to maximum knee flexion of the same extremity.
Midswing: Portion of the swing phase when the reference extremity passes directly below the body. Midswing extends from the end of acceleration to the beginning of deceleration.	Midswing: Portion of the swing phase from maximum knee flexion of the reference extremity to a vertical tibial position.
Deceleration: The swing portion of the swing phase when the reference extremity is decelerating in preparation for heel strike.	Terminal swing: The portion of the swing phase from a vertical position of the tibia of the reference extremity to just prior to initial contact.

Adapted from O'Sullivan, SB and Schmitz, TJ: Physical Rehabilitation: Assessment and Treatment, ed 2. FA Davis, Philadelphia, 1988, p 197.

Foot and Ankle: Stance Phase (as seen from a lateral view)

PORTION OF PHASE	NORMAL MOTION	NORMAL MOMENT	NORMAL MUSCLE ACTIVITY
Heel strike to foot flat	$0°-15°$ plantar flexion	Plantar flexion	Pretibial group acts eccentrically to oppose plantar flexion moment and thereby to prevent foot slap by controlling plantar flexion
Foot flat through midstance	$15°$ plantar flexion to $10°$ dorsiflexion	Plantar flexion to dorsiflexion	Gastroenemius and soleus act eccentrically to oppose the dorsiflexion moment and to control tibial advance
Midstance to heel off	$10°-15°$ dorsiflexion	Dorsiflexion	Gastroenemius and soleus contract eccentrically to oppose the dorsiflexion moment and control tibial advance
Heel off to toe off	$15°$ dorsiflexion to $20°$ plantar flexion	Dorsiflexion	Gastroenemius, soleus, peroneus brevis, peroneus longus, flexor hallicus longus contract to plantar flex the foot

Continued on the following page(s)

PORTION OF PHASE	RESULT OF WEAKNESS	POSSIBLE COMPENSATION
Heel strike to foot flat	Lack of ability to oppose the plantar flexion moment causes the foot to slap the floor	To avoid foot slap and to eliminate the plantar flexion moment, heel strike may be avoided and either the foot placed flat on the floor or placed with the toes first at initial contact
Foot flat through midstance	Excessive dorsiflexion and uncontrolled tibial advance	To avoid excessive dorsiflexion, the ankle may be maintained in plantar flexion
Midstance to heel off	Excessive dorsiflexion and uncontrolled forward motion of tibia	The ankle may be maintained in plantar flexion; if the foot is flat on the floor, the dorsiflexion moment is eliminated and a step-to gait is produced
Heel off to toe off	No roll off	Whole foot is lifted off the ground

Adapted from O'Sullivan, SB and Schmitz, TJ: Physical Rehabilitation Assessment and Treatment, ed 2. FA Davis, Philadelphia, 1988, p 198.

COMMON GAIT DEVIATIONS

Foot and Ankle: Stance Phase (as seen from a lateral view)

PORTION OF PHASE	DEVIATION	DESCRIPTION	POSSIBLE CAUSES	ANALYSIS
Initial contact	Foot slap	At heel strike, forefoot slaps the ground	Weak dorsiflexors or atrophy of dorsiflexors	Look for low muscle tone at ankle. Look for steppage gait (excessive hip and knee flexion) in swing phase.
	Toes first	Toes contact ground instead of heel. A tiptoe posture may be maintained throughout the phase, or the heel may contact the ground.	Leg length discrepancy; contracted heel cord; plantar flexion contraction; hyper-reflexive plantar flexors; flaccidity of dorsiflexors; painful heel	Compare leg lengths and look for hip and/or knee flexion contractures. Analyze reflex activity and timing of activity in plantar flexors. Check for pain in heel.
	Foot flat	Entire foot contacts the ground at heel strike	Excessive fixed dorsiflexion; flaccid or weak dorsiflexors	Check range of motion at ankle. Check for hyperextension at the knee and persistence of immature gait pattern.

Continued on the following page(s)

705

Foot and Ankle: Stance Phase (as seen from a lateral view) *Continued*

PORTION OF PHASE	DEVIATION	DESCRIPTION	POSSIBLE CAUSES	ANALYSIS
Midstance	Excessive positional plantar flexion	Tibia does not advance to neutral from 10° plantar flexion	No eccentric contraction of plantar flexors; could be due to flaccidity/weakness in plantar flexors; surgical overrelease, rupture, or contracture of Achilles tendon	Check for hyper-reflexive or weak quadriceps; hyperextension at the knee; hip hyperextension; backward- or forward-leaning trunk. Check for weakness in plantar flexors or rupture of Achilles tendon.
	Heel lift in midstance	Heel does not contact ground in midstance	Hyper-reflexive plantar flexors	Check reflexes of plantar flexors, quadriceps, hip flexors, and adductors.
	Excessive positional dorsiflexion	Tibia advances too rapidly over the foot, creating a greater than normal amount of dorsiflexion	Inability of plantar flexors to control tibial advance; knee flexion or hip flexion contractures	Look at ankle muscles, knee and hip flexors, range of motion, and position of trunk.

Toe clawing	Toes flex and "grab" floor	Could be due to a plantar grasp reflex that is only partially integrated; could be due to positive supporting reflex; hyper-reflexive toe flexors	Check plantar grasp reflex, positive supporting reflexes, and range of motion of toes.
Push-off (heel off to toe off)	No roll off	Insufficient transfer of weight from lateral heel to medial forefoot	Mechanical fixation of ankle and foot; flaccidity or inhibition of plantar flexors, inverters, and toe flexors; rigidity/cocontraction of plantar flexors and dorsiflexors; pain in forefoot	Check range of motion at ankle and foot. Check muscle function and reflexes at ankle. Look at dissociation between posterior foot and forefoot.

Adapted from O'Sullivan, SB and Schmitz, TJ: Physical Rehabilitation Assessment and Treatment, ed 2. FA Davis, Philadelphia, 1989, p 203.

NORMAL GAIT

Foot and Ankle: Swing Phase (as seen from a lateral view)

PORTION OF PHASE	NORMAL MOTION	NORMAL MOMENT	NORMAL MUSCLE ACTION	RESULT OF WEAKNESS	POSSIBLE COMPENSATION
Acceleration to midswing	Dorsiflexion to neutral	None	Dorsiflexors contract to bring the ankle into neutral and to prevent the toes from dragging on the floor	Foot drop and/or toe dragging	Hip and knee flexion may be increased to prevent toe drag, or the hip may be hiked or circumducted. Sometimes vaulting on the contralateral limb may occur.
Midswing to deceleration	Neutral	None	Dorsiflexion	Foot drop and/or toe dragging	Hip and knee flexion may be increased to prevent toe drag. The swing leg may be circumducted, or vaulting may occur on the contralateral side.

Adapted from O'Sullivan, SB and Schmitz, TJ: Physical Rehabilitation Assessment and Treatment, ed 2. FA Davis, Philadelphia, 1989, p 198.

COMMON GAIT DEVIATIONS

Foot and Ankle: Swing Phase (as seen from a lateral view)

PORTION OF PHASE	DEVIATION	DESCRIPTION	POSSIBLE CAUSES	ANALYSIS
Swing	Toe drag	Insufficient dorsiflexion (and toe extension) so that forefoot and toes do not clear floor	Flaccidity or weakness of dorsiflexors and toe extensors; hyper-reflexive of plantar flexors; inadequate knee or hip flexion	Check for ankle, hip, and knee range of motion. Check for strength and reflexes at hip, knee, and ankle.
	Varus	The foot is excessively inverted	Hyper-reflexive invertors; flaccidity or weakness of dorsiflexors and evertors; extensor pattern.	Check for muscle reflexes of invertors and plantar flexors. Check strength of dorsiflexors and evertors. Check for extensor pattern of the lower extremity.

Adapted from O'Sullivan, SB and Schmitz, TJ: Physical Rehabilitation Assessment and Treatment, ed 2. FA Davis, Philadelphia, 1988, p 203.

NORMAL GAIT

Knee: Stance Phase (as seen from a lateral view)

PORTION OF PHASE	NORMAL MOTION	NORMAL MOMENT	NORMAL MUSCLE ACTION	RESULT OF WEAKNESS	POSSIBLE COMPENSATION
Heel strike to foot flat	Flexion 0° – 15°	Flexion	Quadriceps contracts initially to hold the knee in extension and then eccentrically to oppose the flexion moment and control amount of flexion	Excessive knee flexion because the quadriceps cannot oppose the flexion moment	Plantar flexion at ankle so that foot flat instead of heel strike occurs. Plantar flexion eliminates the flexion moment. Trunk leans forward to eliminate the flexion moment at the knee and therefore may be used to compensate for quadriceps weakness.

Foot flat through midstance	Extension 15°–5°	Flexion to extension	Quadriceps contracts in early part, and then no activity is required	Excessive knee flexion initially	Same as above in early part of midstance. No compensation required in later part of phase.
Midstance to heel off	5° of flexion to 0° (neutral)	Flexion to extension	No activity required		None required
Heel off to toe off	0°–10° flexion	Extension to flexion	Quadriceps required to control amount of knee flexion		

Adapted from O'Sullivan, SB and Schmitz, TJ: Physical Rehabilitation Assessment and Treatment, ed 2. FA Davis, Philadelphia, 1988, p 199.

COMMON GAIT DEVIATIONS

Knee: Stance Phase (as seen from a lateral view)

PORTION OF PHASE	DEVIATION	DESCRIPTION	POSSIBLE CAUSES	ANALYSIS
Initial contact (heel strike)	Excessive knee flexion	Knee flexes or buckles rather than extends as foot contacts ground	Painful knee; hyper-reflexive knee flexors or weak or flaccid quadriceps; short leg on contralateral side	Check for pain at knee; reflexes of knee flexors; strength of knee extensors; and leg lengths; anterior pelvic tilt
Foot flat	Knee hyperextension (genu recurvatum)	A greater than normal extension at the knee	Flaccid/weak quadriceps and soleus compensated for by pull of gluteus maximus; spasticity of quadriceps; accommodation to a fixed ankle plantar flexion deformity	Check for strength and reflexes of knee and ankle flexors, and range of motion at ankle

Midstance	Knee hyperextension (genu recurvatum)	During single limb support, tibia remains in back of ankle mortice as body weight moves over foot; ankle is plantar flexed	Same as above	Same as above
Push off (heel off to toe off)	Excessive knee flexion	Knee flexes to more than 40° during push off	Center of gravity is unusually forward of pelvis; could be due to rigid trunk, knee/hip flexion contractures; flexion-withdrawal reflex; dominance of flexion synergy in middle of recovery from CVA.	Look at trunk posture, knee and hip range of motion, and flexor synergy
	Limited knee flexion	The normal amount of knee flexion (40°) does not occur.	Overactive quadriceps and/or plantar flexors.	Look at reflexes of hip, knee, and ankle muscles

Adapted from O'Sullivan, SB and Schmitz, TJ: Physical Rehabilitation Assessment and Treatment, ed 2. FA Davis, Philadelphia, 1988, p 204.

NORMAL GAIT

Knee: Swing Phase (as seen from a lateral view)

PORTION OF PHASE	NORMAL MOTION	NORMAL MOMENT	NORMAL MUSCLE ACTION	RESULT OF WEAKNESS	POSSIBLE COMPENSATION
Acceleration to midswing	40°–60° flexion	None	Little or no activity in quadriceps; biceps femoris (short head), gracilis, and sartorius contract concentrically	Inadequate knee flexion	Increased hip flexion, circumduction, or hiking
Midswing	60°–30° extension	None			
Deceleration	30°–0° extension	None	Quadriceps contracts concentrically to stabilize knee in extension in preparation for heel strike	Inadequate knee extension	

Adapted from O'Sullivan, SB and Schmitz, TJ: Physical Rehabilitation Assessment and Treatment, ed 2. FA Davis, Philadelphia, 1988, p 199.

COMMON GAIT DEVIATIONS

Knee: Swing Phase (as seen from a lateral view)

PORTION OF PHASE	DEVIATION	DESCRIPTION	POSSIBLE CAUSES	ANALYSIS
Acceleration to midswing	Excessive knee flexion	Knee flexes more than 65°	Diminished preswing knee flexion, flexor-withdrawal reflex, dysmetria	Look at reflexes of hip, knee, and ankle muscles; test for reflexes and dysmetria
	Limited knee flexion	Knee does not flex to 65°	Pain in knee, diminished range of knee motion, extensor spasticity; circumduction at the hip	Assess for pain in knee and knee range of motion; test reflexes at knee and hip

Adapted from O'Sullivan, SB and Schmitz, TJ: Physical Rehabilitation Assessment and Treatment, ed 2. FA Davis, Philadelphia, 1988, p 204.

NORMAL GAIT

Hip: Stance Phase (as seen from a lateral view)

PORTION OF PHASE	NORMAL MOTION	NORMAL MOMENT	NORMAL MUSCLE ACTION	RESULT OF WEAKNESS	POSSIBLE COMPENSATION
Heel strike to foot flat	30° flexion	Flexion	Erector spinae, gluteus maximus, hamstrings	Excessive hip flexion and anterior pelvic tilt owing to inability to counteract flexion moment	Trunk lean backward to prevent excessive hip flexion and to eliminate the hip flexion moment
Foot flat through midstance	30° flexion to 5° (neutral)	Flexion to extension	Gluteus maximus at beginning of period to oppose flexion moment; then activity ceases as moment changes from flexion to extension	At the beginning of the period, excessive hip flexion and anterior pelvic tilt owing to inability to counteract flexion moment	At beginning of the period, subject may lean trunk backward to prevent excessive hip flexion; however, once the flexion moment changes

Midstance to heel off	Extension	No activity	None	None required
Heel off to toe off	10° of hyperextension to neutral	Extension	Iliopsoas, adductor magnus, and adductor longus	Undetermined	Undetermined

to an extension moment, the subject no longer needs to incline the trunk backward

Adapted from O'Sullivan, SB and Schmitz, TJ: Physical Rehabilitation Assessment and Treatment, ed 2. FA Davis, Philadelphia, 1988, p 199.

COMMON GAIT DEVIATIONS

Hip: Stance Phase (as seen from a lateral view)

PORTION OF PHASE	DEVIATION	DESCRIPTION	POSSIBLE CAUSES	ANALYIS
Heel strike to foot flat	Excessive flexion	Flexion exceeding 30°	Hip and/or knee flexion contractures; knee flexion caused by weak soleus and quadriceps; hyper-reflexive of hip flexors.	Check hip and knee range of motion and strength of soleus and quadriceps. Check reflexes of hip flexors.
Heel strike to foot flat	Limited hip flexion	Hip flexion does not attain 30°	Weakness of hip flexors; limited range of hip flexion; gluteus maximus weakness	Check strength of hip flexors and extensors. Analyze range of hip motion.
Foot flat to midstance	Limited hip extension	The hip does not attain a neutral position	Hip flexion contracture, hyper-reflexive hip flexors	Check hip range of motion and reflexes of hip muscles.
	Internal rotation	An internally rotated position of the extremity	Hyper-reflexive internal rotators; weakness of external rotators; excessive forward rotation of opposite pelvis	Check reflexes of internal rotators and strength of external rotators. Measure range of motion of both hip joints.

External rotation	An externally rotated position of the extremity	Excessive backward rotation of opposite pelvis	Assess range of motion at both hip joints.
Abduction	An abducted position of the extremity	Contracture of the gluteus medius; trunk lateral lean over the ipsilateral hip	Check for abduction pattern.
Adduction	An adducted position of the lower extremity	Hyper-reflexive hip flexors and adductors such as seen in spastic diplegia; pelvic drop to contralateral side	Assess reflexes of hip flexors and adductors. Test muscle strength of hip abductors.

Adapted from O'Sullivan, SB and Schmitz, TJ: Physical Rehabilitation Assessment and Treatment, ed 2. FA Davis, Philadelphia, 1988, p 205.

NORMAL GAIT

Hip: Swing Phase (as seen from a lateral view)

PORTION OF PHASE	NORMAL MOTION	NORMAL MOMENT	NORMAL MUSCLE ACTIVITY	RESULT OF WEAKNESS	POSSIBLE COMPENSATION
Acceleration to midswing	20°–30° flexion	None	Hip flexor activity to initiate swing iliopsoas, rectus femoris, gracilis, sartorius, tensor fascia lata	Diminished hip flexion, causing an inability to initiate the normal forward movement of the extremity and to raise the foot off the floor	Circumduction and/or hip hiking may be used to bring the leg forward and to raise the foot high enough to clear the floor
Midswing to deceleration	30° flexion to neutral	None	Hamstrings	A lack of control of the swinging leg; inability to place limb in position for heel strike	

Adapted from O'Sullivan, SB and Schmitz, TJ: Physical Rehabilitation Assessment and Treatment, ed 2. FA Davis, Philadelphia, 1988, p 202.

COMMON GAIT DEVIATIONS

Hip: Swing Phase (as seen from a lateral view)

PORTION OF PHASE	DEVIATION	DESCRIPTION	POSSIBLE CAUSES	ANALYSIS
Swing	Circumduction	A lateral circular movement of the entire lower extremity consisting of abduction, external rotation, adduction, and internal rotation	A compensation for weak hip flexors or a compensation for the inability to shorten the leg so that it can clear the floor	Check strength of hip flexors, knee flexors, and ankle dorsiflexors. Check range of motion in hip flexion, knee flexion, and ankle dorsiflexion. Check for extensor pattern.
	Hip hiking	Shortening of the swing leg by action of the quadratus lumborum	A compensation for lack of knee flexion and/or ankle dorsiflexion; also may be a compensation for extensor spasticity of swing leg	Check strength and range of motion at knee, hip, and ankle. Also check reflexes at knee and ankle.
	Excessive hip flexion	Flexion greater than 20°–30°	Attempt to shorten extremity in presence of footdrop; flexor pattern	Check strength and range of motion at ankle and foot. Check for flexor pattern.

Adapted from O'Sullivan, SB and Schmitz, TJ: Physical Rehabilitation Assessment and Treatment, ed 2. FA Davis, Philadelphia, 1988, p 205.

COMMON GAIT DEVIATIONS

Trunk: Stance Phase

PORTION OF PHASE	DEVIATION	DESCRIPTION	POSSIBLE CAUSES	ANALYSIS
Stance	Lateral trunk lean	A lean of the trunk over the stance extremity (gluteus medius gait/trendelenberg gait)	A weak or paralyzed gluteus medius on the stance side cannot prevent a drop of pelvis on the swing side, so a trunk lean over the stance leg helps compensate for the weak muscle; a lateral trunk lean also may be used to reduce force on hip if a patient has a painful hip	Check strength of gluteus medius and assess for pain in the hip.
	Backward trunk lean	A backward leaning of the trunk, resulting in hyperextension at the hip (gluteus maximus gait)	Weakness or paralysis of the gluteus maximus on the stance leg; anteriorly rotated pelvis.	Check for strength of hip extensors. Check pelvic position.

| Forward trunk lean | A forward leaning of the trunk, resulting in hip flexion | Compensation for quadriceps weakness; the forward lean eliminates the flexion moment at the knee; hip and knee flexion contractures | Check for strength of quadriceps. |
| | A forward flexion of the upper trunk | Posteriorly rotated pelvis | Check pelvic position. |

Adapted from O'Sullivan, SB and Schmitz, TJ: Physical Rehabilitation Assessment and Treatment, ed 2. FA Davis, Philadelphia, 1988, p 206.

CRUTCH-WALKING GAITS

three-point gait: Both crutches are moved forward with the affected limb. This non-weight-bearing gait can be used if the patient has one normal lower limb that can tolerate full weight bearing. For example, this mode of crutch walking is used after hip or knee operations. A modified three-point gait is the partial-weight-bearing gait during which the affected extremity is allowed to bear some weight when both crutches are on the ground.

four-point gait: One crutch is advanced in this gait pattern, followed by advancement of the opposite lower extremity. Only one leg or crutch is off the floor at a time, leaving three points for support, making this a very stable and safe gait. This gait can be used for the patient who is able to move his legs alternately but who has poor balance or is not able to bear full weight bilaterally without the support of crutches.

partial-weight-bearing gait: See *three-point gait.*

two-point gait: A modification of the four-point gait. The right crutch and left leg move together, and the left crutch and right leg move together. It is close to the natural rhythm of walking.

swing-to gait: Both crutches are moved forward together, and the lower extremities are then swung forward to a position between the crutches. This gait is often used by paraplegic patients who are unable to move their legs alternately.

swing-through gait: Both crutches are moved forward together, and the lower extremities are then swung forward to a position beyond the crutches. This gait is often used by paraplegic patients who are unable to move their legs alternately.

Reference

1. O'Sullivan, SB and Schmitz, TJ: Physical Rehabilitation: Assessment and Treatment, ed 2. FA Davis, Philadelphia, 1988.

TECHNIQUES USED TO CLIMB STAIRS WHILE USING ASSISTIVE DEVICES

I. Cane
  A. Ascending
     1. The unaffected lower extremity leads up.
     2. The cane and affected lower extremity follow.
  B. Descending
     1. The affected lower extremity and cane lead down.
     2. The unaffected lower extremity follows.
II. Crutches: three-point gait (non-weight-bearing gait)
  A. Ascending
     1. The patient is positioned close to the foot of the stairs. The involved lower extremity is held back to prevent "catching" on the lip of the stairs.
     2. The patient pushes down firmly on both handpieces of the crutches and leads up with the unaffected lower extremity.
     3. The crutches are brought up to the stair that the unaffected lower extremity is now on.
  B. Descending
     1. The patient stands close to the edge of the stair such that the toes protrude slightly over the top. The involved lower extremity is held forward over the lower stair.
     2. Both crutches are moved down *together* to the *front* half of the next step.
     3. The patient pushes down firmly on both handpieces and lowers the unaffected lower extremity to the step that the crutches are now on.
III. Crutches: partial-weight-bearing gait
  A. Ascending
     1. The patient is positioned close to the foot of the stairs.
     2. The patient pushes down on both handpieces of the crutches and distributes weight partially on the crutches and partially on the affected lower extremity while the unaffected lower extremity leads up.
     3. The involved lower extremity and crutches are then brought up together.
  B. Descending
     1. The patient stands close to the edge of the stair such that the toes protrude slightly over top of the stair.
     2. Both crutches are moved down *together* to the *front* half of the next step. The affected lower extremity is then lowered (depending on patient skill, these may be combined). *Note:* When crutches are not in floor contact, greater weight must be shifted to the uninvolved lower extremity to maintain a partial-weight-bearing status.
     3. The uninvolved lower extremity is lowered to the step the crutches are now on.

IV. Crutches: two- and four-point gait
  A. Ascending
    1. The patient is positioned close to the foot of the stairs.
    2. The right lower extremity is moved up and then the left lower extremity.
    3. The right crutch is moved up and then the left crutch is moved up (patients with adequate balance may find it easier to move the crutches up together).
  B. Descending
    1. The patient stands close to the edge of the stair.
    2. The right crutch is moved down and then the left (may be combined).
    3. The right lower extremity is moved down and then the left.

---

*The sequences presented here describe stair-climbing techniques without the use of a railing. When a secure railing is available, the patient should be instructed to use it always.

Adapted from O'Sullivan, SB and Schmitz, TJ: Physical Rehabilitation Assessment and Treatment, ed 2. FA Davis, Philadelphia, 1988, p 303.

COMMON GAIT DEVIATIONS
(in alphabetical order)

Gait deviations (limps) take on many forms, and their etiologies may be complex. The list below is not meant to be all-inclusive. Only the most common patterns are listed, and only the most common etiologies for those patterns are noted.

antalgic gait (painful gait): Avoidance of weight bearing on the affected side, shortening of the stance, and an attempt to unload the limb as much as possible. In addition, the painful region is often supported by one hand, while the other arm is outstretched. This pattern is often the result of pain caused by injury to the hip, knee, ankle, or foot.

arthrogenic gait: Elevation of the pelvis and circumduction of the leg on the involved side with exaggerated plantar flexion of the opposite ankle. This pattern is often due to stiffness, laxity, or deformity of the hip or knee and is often seen with fusion of these joints or after the recent removal of a cylinder cast.

ataxic gait: This gait may take two forms, depending on the pathology.

> **spinal ataxia:** Characterized by the patient walking with a broad base and throwing out the feet, which come down first on the heel and then on the toes with a slapping sound or "double tap." It is characteristic for patients to watch their feet while walking. In milder cases, the gait may appear near normal with the eyes open, but when the patient is asked to walk with eyes closed, the patient staggers, becomes unsteady, and may be unable to walk. This gait is thought to result from the disruption of sensory pathways in the CNS, as occurs with tabes dorsalis or multiple sclerosis.

> **cerebellar ataxia:** A gait deviation that is equally severe when the patient walks with eyes open or closed. The gait is wide based, unsteady, and irregular. The patient staggers and is unable to walk tandem or to follow a straight line. This form of ataxia occurs with cerebellar lesions. If the disease is localized to one hemisphere, there is persistent deviation or swaying toward the affected side.

calcaneous gait: See *gastrocnemius-soleus gait.*

dorsiflexor gait: See *footdrop gait.*

dystrophic (penguin) gait: There is a pronounced waddling element to this gait. The patient rolls the hips from side to side during the stance phase of every forward step in order to shift the weight of the body. There is an exaggerated lumbar lordosis while walking or standing. It usually presents as a difficulty in running or climbing stairs. This gait is encountered in various myopathies and is most typical of muscular dystrophy.

flaccid gait: See *hemiplegic gait.*

footdrop (dorsiflexor or steppage) gait: The patient lifts the knee high and slaps the foot to the ground on advancing to the involved side. This gait is typical of patients with weak or paralyzed dorsiflexor muscles.

gastrocnemius-soleus (calcaneus) gait: This deviation is demonstrated best when the patient walks up an incline. At push off, the heel does not come off the ground, and the affected side lags compared to the other side. This gait results from weakness to the gastrocnemius and/or the soleus muscles.

gluteus maximus (hip extensor) gait: A lurching gait characterized by a posterior thrust of the thorax at heel strike to maintain hip extension of the stance leg. The knee is tightly extended in midstance, which slightly elevates the hip on that side. This gait usually results from weakness to the gluteus maximus muscle.

gluteus medius (trendelenburg) gait: In the uncompensated gluteus medius limp, the pelvis dips more when the unaffected limb is in swing phase and there is an apparent lateral protrusion of the stance hip; if necessary, the patient may use a steppage gait to clear the swing leg. The gluteus medius gait commonly occurs due to weakness of the gluteus medius muscle or with congenital dislocations of the hip or with coxa vara. If the gluteus medius is absent or extremely weak, a compensated gait appears where the patient shifts the trunk to the affected side during the stance phase.

hemiplegic or hemiparetic (flaccid) gait: The patient swings the paretic leg outward and ahead in a circle (circumduction) or pushes it ahead. Heel strike is often missing, and the patient strikes with the forefoot. This gait is present when one leg is shorter than the other or with a deformity in one of the bones of the leg.

hip extensor gait: See *gluteus maximus gait*.

painful gait: See *antalgic gait*.

Parkinsonian gait: This is a highly stereotypical gait in which the patient has impoverished movement of the lower limb. There is generalized lack of extension at the ankle, knee, hip, and trunk. Diminished step length and a loss of reciprocal arm swing are noted. Patients have trouble initiating movement, and this results in a slow and shuffling gait characterized by small steps. Because patients with Parkinsonism often exhibit flexed postures, their centers of gravity project forward, causing a festinating gait. The patient, in an attempt to regain his balance, takes many small steps rapidly. The rapid stepping causes the patients to increase his walking speed. In some cases patients will break into a run and can only stop their forward progression when they run into an object. Less common than the forward propulsive gait pattern is a retropulsive pattern that occurs when patients lose their balance in a backward direction (retropulsion is more common in patients with cerebellar lesions).

penguin gait: See *dystrophic gait*.
steppage gait: See *footdrop gait*.
Trendelenburg gait: See *gluteus medius gait*.

TERMS AND MEASUREMENTS USED IN KINETIC AND KINEMATIC ANALYSIS OF GAIT

acceleration: Rate of change in velocity per unit time, for translatory motion expressed in distance per second squared, for angular motion expressed in radians per second squared or degrees per second squared.

angular acceleration: See *acceleration*.

base of support: The distance between left and right foot contacts as measured in a plane transverse to the line of progression during gait.

cadence: Number of steps per unit time.

cycle time: See *stride time*.

degree of toe out or toe in: See *foot angle*.

double support time: The amount of time during the gait cycle when both lower extremities are in contact with the ground; for example, when the right leg is in stance phase and the left heel comes in contact with the ground, the period of left double support begins and continues until the left foot comes off the ground.

foot angle: The angle of foot placement with respect to the line of progression.

ground reaction forces: Forces created as a result of foot contact with supporting surface. These are equal in magnitude and opposite in direction to those applied by the limb to the supporting surface.

joint forces: Forces present at articular surfaces.

moment: See *torque*.

speed: Distance divided by time, the rate of displacement of an object; a scalar quantity.

free speed: Normal walking speed; also called *preferred speed*.

step length: The distance between heel strike of one leg and heel strike of the contralateral leg. Left and right step lengths are usually measured because they may differ.

step time: The time between heel strike of one leg and heel strike of the contralateral leg. Left and right step times are usually measured because they may differ.

step width: See *base of support*.

stride time: The time between successive occurrences of the same phase of gait, usually measured in seconds from heel strike of one leg to heel strike of the same leg. Left and right stride times are usually measured because they may differ.

swing time: The time that a foot is off the ground during one gait cycle. Left and right swing times are usually measured because they may differ.

torque: The product of a force times the perpendicular distance (moment arm) from the axis of rotation to the line of action of the force.

velocity: A vector that describes displacement. The term is often confused with speed (a scalar); however, speed represents only the magnitude of velocity.

   angular velocity: A vector that describes displacement around an axis; units are radians per seconds or degrees per second.

   linear velocity: A vector that describes translation of a body in space; moment in a straight line; in gait, usually expressed in meters per second.

width of walking base: See *base of support.*

work: Force times distance.

COMMON GAIT DEVIATIONS SEEN IN HEMIPLEGIC PATIENTS

Stance Phase

DEVIATION	CAUSE
Ankle and Foot	
Equinus gait	Excessive activity of the gastrocnemius muscle
	Plantar flexion contracture
Varus foot	Excessive activity of the tibialis anterior, tibialis posterior, or toe flexor muscles causes the foot to come down on the lateral surface at heel strike
Painful short steps	Contraction of the toe flexors causes excessive pressure on the toes and results in the patient taking short steps to minimize stance time and rollover
Excessive flexion	Flexion contracture
	Excessive dorsiflexion
	Poor position sense
	Weak knee quadriceps
Hyperextension	Plantar flexion contracture
	Poor position sense
	Excessive activity of the quadriceps muscles
	Compensatory locking of the knee to adjust for weak knee extensors (patient leans forward to mechanically lock the knee)
Lateral (Trendelenberg or gluteus medius) limb	Weak hip abductors
Scissoring	Excessive activity of the adductors
Improper positioning of the hip	Weakness of hip girdle
	Poor position sense

Stance Phase

DEVIATION	CAUSE

Trunk and Pelvis

DEVIATION	CAUSE
Flexed trunk	Compensation for weak knee flexors (the patient brings center of gravity forward)
	Weak hip extensors
Improper positioning	Poor position sense
Lack of pelvic rotation	Weakness and lack of control of pelvic girdle muscle

Swing Phase

DEVIATION	CAUSE

Ankle and Foot

DEVIATION	CAUSE
Equinus gait	Excessive activity of the gastrocnemius
	Plantar flexion contracture
	Weak dorsiflexors
Varus foot	Excessive activity of the tibialis anterior
	Weakness of peroneals and toe extensors
Equinovarus	Excessive activity of the triceps surae
Excessive dorsiflexion	Part of powerful flexor synergy pattern

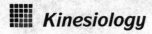 *Kinesiology*

TYPES OF MUSCLE CONTRACTIONS

When excitation-contraction coupling occurs in skeletal muscle, actinomyosin is formed. The formation of the cross-bridges between the two contractile proteins results in a contraction, that is, the actin filaments being pulled toward the middle of the sarcomere. This is what occurs with all muscle contractions. However, depending on the relationship of the external load (resistance) to the tension generated, there may or may not be sliding of the actin filaments with a resultant decrease in the distance between z lines. Therefore, there is only one type of muscle contraction. However, it has become customary to refer to contraction types based on whether or not there is shortening of the whole muscle.

Concentric contractions occur when the external load (resistance) is such that when excitation-contraction coupling occurs there is shortening of the sarcomere leading to a decrease in the length of the whole muscle. In practice this means that a limb segment will be moved in the direction of the muscle tension vector.

Isometric contractions occur when the external load (resistance) is such that when excitation-contraction coupling occurs there is shortening of the sarcomere in order to take up any slack in the muscle or connective tissue, but there will be no observable change in the length of the whole muscle. In practice this means that a limb segment will not move.

Eccentric contractions occur when the external load (resistance) is such that when excitation-contraction coupling occurs there is lengthening of the sarcomere leading to an increase in the length of the whole muscle. In practice this means that a limb segment will be moved in the direction opposite the muscle tension vector.

TYPE OF CONTRACTION	FORCES	FUNCTION	MECHANICAL WORK
Concentric	$M_m > M_r$	Acceleration	Positive ($W = F [+D]$)
Isometric	$M_m = M_r$	Fixation	Zero (no change in length)
Eccentric	$M_m < M_r$	Deceleration	Negative ($W = F [-D]$)

Force Relationships in Different Types of Muscular Contractions

M_r: Resistance moment. This is due to the weight of the limb segment and any load applied to that segment.

M_m: Rotary moment of the muscular force. This is the rotary component that is resolved from the tensile force created when a muscle contracts.

Based on forces and using the above notation, the three types of muscle contractions can be described. This table is based in part on Komi, PV: The stretch-shortening cycle and human power output. In Jones, NL, et al (eds): Human Muscle Power. Human Kinetics, Champaign, IL, 1986, pp 27-39.

References

1. Rodgers, MR and Cavanagh, PR: Glossary of biomechanical terms, concepts and units. J Phys Ther 64:1886, 1984.
2. Soderberg, GL: Kinesiology: Application to Pathological Motion. Williams & Wilkins, Baltimore, 1986.

BIOMECHANICAL, KINESIOLOGICAL, KINETIC, AND KINEMATIC TERMS
(in alphabetical order)

For definitions of terms used in instrumentation, see Glossary of Terms Used to Describe Instruments.

acceleration: Rate of change in velocity; for translatory motion expressed in distance per second squared, for angular motion expressed in degrees per second squared.

action line: See *force*.

active insufficiency: See *muscle insufficiency*.

agonist muscle: A muscle or group of muscles whose contractions may be considered primarily responsible for causing a movement (see *antagonist*).

antagonist muscle: A muscle that can oppose the action of an agonist (see *agonist*); therefore, for a muscle to be an antagonist, it must be referenced to an agonist.

bending: The result of a load applied to a structure such that movement occurs about an axis, with tension and compression occurring on opposite sides of the material bending.

Blix's curve: See *length-tension curve*.

center of gravity: The center of mass, which is also the point where the resultant force of gravity is said to be acting.

center of mass: Same as center of gravity; see *center of gravity*.

composition of forces: Adding two or more forces to show the single resultant force that is formed.

compression: A load in which collinear forces act in opposite directions so as to push a material together.

concentric contraction: See *muscle contractions*.

concurrent force system: See *force systems*.

creep: Progressive deformation over time of a material, even though the load is constant.

density: Mass per unit volume.

derivatives: The process of deriving one quantity from another by analysis of a curve or a function.

differentiation: A calculus technique used in kinematics determine the rate of change of a quantity.

direction of forces: See *force*.

dynamics: The study of bodies in motion and the forces acting on them.

eccentric contraction: See *muscle contractions*.

energy: A fundamental quantity that represents the capacity to do work, expressed in ergs, joules, foot-pounds, or calories.

fatigue: In material science it is the failure of a material due to repetitive loading.

force: The vector quantity that reflects how one body acts on another, that is, attracts, repels, pulls, or pushes. In Newtonian terms, force equals mass times acceleration. Units of force are dynes, newtons, or pounds. Force is a vector and is described like any other vector by the following four characteristics:

> **action line:** The path on which the force is acting.
>
> **direction:** Whether the force is attracting or repelling (pushing or pulling)
>
> **magnitude:** Strength of the force.
>
> **point of application:** Where the force acts on a body.

force couple: Two equal and opposite forces acting from different directions so as to turn an object about a fixed point.

force systems: Ways in which forces may be combined.

> **concurrent:** All the forces meet at one point.
>
> **general:** A collection of forces in a plane that cannot be defined by one of the other systems.
>
> **linear:** All the forces are acting along one line.
>
> **parallel:** All the forces are acting in the same plane but not along the same line.

force-velocity relationship: The relationship between the force a muscle can generate at a given length and the rate at which the muscle shortens. This relationship is present at constant rates of stimulation (i.e., in vitro electrical stimulation) and is inverse for concentric muscle contractions and direct for eccentric contractions up to a point where a plateau is reached.

free body diagram: A graphic representation of all the forces acting upon a body.

friction: A force that is in opposition to movement of two contacting bodies, with the force being parallel to the contacting surfaces.

general force system: See *force systems.*

gravity: The attractive force between two masses as defined by Newton's Law of Universal Gravitation. Force is equal to the gravitational constant (g).

$$g = \frac{mass_1 \times mass_2}{(distance\ between\ masses)^2}$$

ground reaction forces: Forces that act upon the body as a result of the body interacting with the supporting surface.

hysteresis: The property of a material such that the stress-strain relationship is different during loading and unloading; due to internal friction a material exhibiting hysteresis uses energy during loading or unloading.

impulse: The time a force acts on a body, expressed in units of kg × m/s or lb × ft/sec

inertia: The quality that maintains a body at rest or in a constant state of motion (i.e., equilibrium) unless acted upon by an external force (as defined by Newton's First Law).

integration: The technique in calculus that determines the area under a curve (in reference to the x axis).

inversion of muscle action: Used to describe the event where a secondary action of a muscle changes due to joint position; for example, the hip adductors can normally also cause flexion at the hip joint. However, if the femur is fully flexed at the hip, then the adductors can extend the hip because they have undergone inversion of their function.

isokinetic movement: Constant velocity movement.

isometric contraction: See *muscle contractions*.

isotonic contraction: See *muscle contractions*.

joint forces: Forces that act on articular surfaces and are due to muscular action, gravity, and inertia.

kinematics: The branch of dynamics that deals with motion (velocity and acceleration) but excludes consideration of mass and force.

kinetic energy: The mechanical energy in a system that comes from its motion (during translatory motions, K.E. = ½ m × v²).

kinetics: A branch of dynamics that deals with forces.

lengthening contraction: A term originated by physiologists who used it to describe an eccentric contraction; the term is actually an oxymoron (see *muscle contractions*).

length-tension curve: The plotted relationship of a muscle's length and the isometric tension that muscle can generate; because tension is measured directly, length-tension relationships can be measured only in vivo.

levers: A system consisting of two forces and a fulcrum that alters a mechanical advantage.

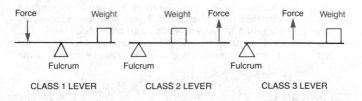

CLASS 1 LEVER   CLASS 2 LEVER   CLASS 3 LEVER

linear force system: See *force systems*.

mass: Defined by Newton's Second Law as equal to the force on an object divided by the acceleration of the object. On earth, weight is a mass divided by the acceleration due to the earth's gravity.

mechanical advantage: A measure of efficiency equal to the ratio formed by dividing the output of a system by the input to the system. Its maximum value is 1 (i.e., 100% efficiency).

mechanics: A branch of physics that deals with energy and forces and their relationship to movement, equilibrium, and deformation.

modulus of elasticity: The ratio of stress to strain.

moment arm: The perpendicular distance from the action of a force to the axis of rotation.

moment of force: The product of a force times the perpendicular distance (moment arm) from the axis of rotation.

momentum: Mass times velocity.

motion types: Motion in space may be divided into two types: rotary movement, where movement occurs in an arc around a fixed point; and translatory movement, where a body moves in space from one point to another.

muscle contractions: Muscles contract in one set manner, that is, muscles create tension due to the formation of actinomyosin cross-bridges. However, depending on the load applied to the muscle, different types of events may occur (see Table of Muscle Contractions).

concentric contraction: A contraction in which the origins and insertions of the contracting muscle are brought closer together due to the action of the muscle.

eccentric contraction: A contraction in which the origins and insertions of a contracting muscle are moved away from each other by an external force, even though the muscle is contracting.

isokinetic contraction: Not really a type of contraction and a term often used incorrectly. There can be an isokinetic movement (i.e., constant velocity movement), but there is no unique contractile event.

isometric contraction: A contraction in which no noticeable shortening of the muscle takes place.

isotonic contraction: Not really a type of contraction, but rather a term that has been used widely to describe many different things. Originally the term was applied to in vivo experiments where a muscle worked against a constant load; therefore, the term cannot be directly applied to moving loads in an intact body. However, the term has been used to describe contractions where the body lifts a given weight, even though the gravitational vector of the weight changes, as does the muscle's moment arm, and as a result the load is not constant.

muscle insufficiency: Occurs when the tension produced by a muscle is reduced because the muscle is contracting from an extremely lengthened or shortened position. Two types of muscle insufficiency were described by Brunnstrom.

> **active insufficiency:** Thought to occur when a two-joint muscle contracts across two joints at the same time. As a result, tension development can be severely compromised because the muscle is at the extreme left (shortened) side of its length-tension curve.

> **passive insufficiency:** Thought to occur when a two-joint muscle is stretched across two joints at the same time. As a result, tension development can be severely compromised because the muscle is at the extreme right (lengthened) side of its length-tension curve.

negative work: A term coined by A. V. Hill to describe the work done by a muscle during an eccentric contraction when the muscle is actually working in opposition to the work being done on a limb segment. Mechanical work is not being performed by the muscle, although physiologic work is taking place.

newton's law:

> **First Law (Law of Inertia):** A body remains at rest or continues to move uniformly unless that body is acted on by a force.

> **Second Law (Law of Momentum):** A change in momentum of a body is proportional to the magnitude and duration of the force acting upon it (proportional to the impulse).

> **Third Law (Law of Reaction):** Action and reaction are equal; therefore, any force acting on one body will be counteracted by an equal and opposite force.

parallel force systems: See *force systems*.

passive insufficiency: See *muscle insufficiency*.

point of application: See *force*.

potential energy: The mechanical energy of a body that is a result of the body's position in space (potential energy = mass × gravitational constant × distance).

power: The rate of doing work (work/time).

pressure: Force divided by the area over which it is applied (force per unit area).

prime mover: A term similar to *agonist* but preferred by some because it does not imply that a muscle is working against an antagonist. See *agonist* and *antagonist*.

resolution of forces: Computing the elements of a force; determining the constituent forces from a single force.

resting length: The length at which the muscle can generate the maximum amount of active tension. Because tension cannot be measured in intact human muscles, we do not know the resting length of any human muscle. Therefore, resting length is not the same as the anatomical position.

rotary motion: See *motion types.*

scalar quantity: A quantity having only magnitude. Scalars can be added arithmetically (e.g., quantified such as speed, time, and temperature).

shear: A force acting tangentially to a surface.

shortening contraction: A term originated by physiologists to describe a concentric contraction as opposed to an eccentric contraction. The term is actually redundant (see *muscle contractions*).

shunt muscles: According to MacConnail and Basmajian, muscles that cause stabilization (or joint compression), or a shunt component is the part of muscle action that causes joint stabilization (see *spurt*).

speed: The magnitude of velocity, expressed as distance per unit time.

spurt muscles: According to MacConnail and Basmajian, muscles that cause rotation, or a spurt component is the part of a muscle action that causes rotation (see *shunt*).

statics: The study of bodies at rest and forces in equilibrium, as contrasted to dynamics, which deals with bodies in motion.

strain: Deformation (lengthening or shortening) of an object due to external loading.

stress: Internal forces developed within a body due to externally applied loads.

stress relaxation: A property of a material such that when that material is suddenly strained and maintained at that strain level it exhibits decreasing stress.

synergist: A muscle that contracts along with an agonist to assist that muscle in performing an action or to stabilize body parts to allow the agonist to cause movement (see *agonist*).

tension: A load in which collinear forces attempt to pull something apart.

torque: Moment of a rotary force; same as *moment*.

translatory motion: See *motion types.*

vector quantity: Has magnitude, direction, and a point and line of application.

velocity: A vector that describes displacement. The term is often confused with *speed* (a scalar); however, speed represents only the magnitude of velocity.

viscoelasticity: The property of a material that exhibits hysteresis, stress relaxation, and creep (see those terms).

volume: Space occupied by an object as measured in cubic units.

weight: The force with which a body is attracted to the earth; mass × g (the gravitational constant), expressed in units of dynes, newtons, and pounds.

work: Force times distance (see *negative work*).

References

1. Rogers, MR and Cavanagh, PR: Glossary of biomechanical terms, concepts and units. J Phys Ther 64:1886, 1984.
2. Soderberg, GL: Kinesiology: Application to Pathological Motion. Williams & Wilkins, Baltimore, 1986.
3. Lehmkuhl, LD and Smith, LK: Brunnstrom's Clinical Kinesiology, ed 4. FA Davis, Philadelphia, 1983.

Temporal Processing of the EMG Signal

Illustration of Several Common Methods of Signal Processing

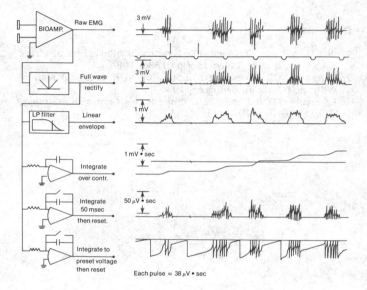

Each pulse = 38 μV • sec

raw EMG: Visual inspection of the raw EMG is the most common way of examining muscle activity as it changes with time. The raw signal allows for visual inspection of the size and shape of individual muscle potentials. The amplitude of the raw EMG when reported should be that seen at the electrodes and should not reflect the gain of any amplifiers in the recording system.

full-wave rectification: The rectifier generates the absolute value of the EMG, usually with a positive polarity.

half-wave rectification: Accomplished by eliminating negative values of the signal. Full-wave rectification is preferred because it retains all of the energy of the signal. Because simple averaging of the signal does not provide useful information, rectification of the signal is commonly used before further signal conditioning (such as moving averages or integration) is conducted. A visual examination of the full-wave rectified signal indicates the changing contraction level of the muscle.

linear envelope: Low-pass filtering of the full-wave rectified signal produces a linear envelope of the signal. It is a type of moving average that follows the trend of the EMG and closely resembles the shape of the muscle tension curve. To represent muscle tension without body movement artifact, the low-pass filter should cut off at about 6 Hz (3 dB) and be at least a second-order type. This form of signal conditioning is often incorrectly confused with integration.

averages: Digital methods for smoothing the random nature of the amplitude of the EMG can be attained through several commonly used techniques.

> **mean (average) of rectified signal:** The mean EMG is the time average of the full-wave rectified EMG over a specified period of time. The shorter this time interval, the less smooth this averaged value will be. By taking the average of randomly varying values of the EMG signal, the larger fluctuations are removed.

> **moving averages:** Several common processing techniques are employed; the most common is low-pass filter, which follows the peaks and valleys of the full-wave rectified signal (see *linear envelope*). Another common procedure is a digital moving-average type defining a "window" that calculates the mean of the detected EMG over the period of the window. The shorter this time interval, the less smooth this average value will be. In order to obtain the time-varying average of a complete EMG record, it is necessary to move the time window T duration along the record; this operation is referred to as a *moving average*. It may be accomplished in a variety of ways that shift the window forward by an amount less than or equal to the time equivalent of the window (T). For typical applications, a value of T ranging from 100 to 200 ms is recommended. Normally the average is calculated for the middle

of the window because it does not introduce a lag in its output; special forms of weighting (exponential, triangular, etc.) can also be applied and should be specified along with the window width, T.

ensemble average: An ensemble average is accomplished digitally for those applications in which the average pattern of the EMG is required for repetitive or evoked responses (e.g., electrically elicited contractions). The time-averaged waveform has an amplitude in mV, and the number of averages is important to report, as well as the standard error at each point in time.

integrated EMG (iEMG or IEMG): A widely used procedure in electromyography that is frequently confused with signal averaging techniques or linear envelope detection. The correct interpretation of integration is purely mathematical and means "area under the curve"; the correct units are $mV \cdot s$ or $\mu V \cdot s$. There are many methods of integrating the EMG; three common procedures are illustrated and described.

integrate over contraction: The simplest form of integration starts at some preset time and continues during the total time of muscle activity. Over any desired period of time, the IEMG can be seen in mV.

resetting of the integrated signal: The integrated signal is reset to 0 at regular intervals of time, usually from 50 to 200 ms (the time should be specified); such a scheme yields a series of peaks that represents the trend of the EMG amplitude with time (similar to a moving average). The sum of all the peaks in any given contraction should equal the IEMG over that contraction.

integration with voltage level reset: The integration begins before the contraction. If the muscle activity is high, the integrator rapidly charges up to the reset level; if low activity occurs, the integrator takes longer to reach reset. Thus the activity level is reflected in the frequency of resets. High frequency of resets (sometimes called *pips*) means high muscle activity; low frequency means low level activity, as seen by the low trace in the illustration above. Each reset represents a value of IEMG and should be specified; the product of the number of resets times this calibration yields the total IEMG over any given time period.

root-mean-square (RMS) value: Not as commonly used as other methods but gaining in popularity with the availability of analog chips that perform the RMS procedure. The RMS is an electronic average representing the square root of the average of the squares of the current or voltage; RMS provides a nearly instantaneous output of the power of the EMG signal.

Terms Used in EMG

TERMINOLOGY	UNITS	COMMENTS/RECOMMENDATIONS
Amplifier gain	Ratio or dB	Sufficient to produce an output of $+/- 1$ V; input bias and offset currents less than 50 pA; input equivalent noise less than $2\ \mu V$ r.m.s.
Input resistance or impedance	ohms	100 to 1000 Mohm; minimum of 100 times skin impedance
Common mode rejection ratio (CMMR)	ratio or dB	90 dB or better
Filter cutoff or bandwidth	Hz	Specify type and order of filter; minimum of $5-500$ Hz (3 dB)
EMG (raw signal)	mV	
EMG (average)	mV	Specify averaging period
EMG (full-wave rectified)	mV	
EMG (nonlinear detector)	mV	Specify nonlinearity (i.e., square law)
EMG (linear envelope)	mV	Cutoff frequency and type of low-pass filter
Integrated EMG (IEMG or iEMG)	mV s	Specify integration period
Integrated EMG with reset every T	mV s or μV s	Specify T (ms)
Integrated EMG to threshold and reset	mV s or μV s	Specify threshold (mV s)

References

1. Winter, DA (Chairman): Units, Terms and Standards in the Reporting of EMG Research. Report of the Ad Hoc Committee of the International Society of Electrophysiological Kinesiology (ISEK), 1980.
2. Winter, DA: Biomechanics of Human Movement. John Wiley & Sons, New York, 1979.
3. Basmajian, JV and De Luca, CJ: Muscles Alive. Williams & Wilkins, Baltimore, 1985.

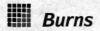 *Burns*

TYPES OF BURNS

The Nature of the Burn Wound: Based on cellular events, a typical burn wound that is more severe than a first-degree burn can be said to have three zones. In the zone of coagulation, there is cell death. In the zone of stasis, cells are injured and will usually die within 24 to 48 hours unless there is adequate treatment. In the zone of hyperemia, there is minimal cell damage. The extent of each zone is dependent on the type of burn.

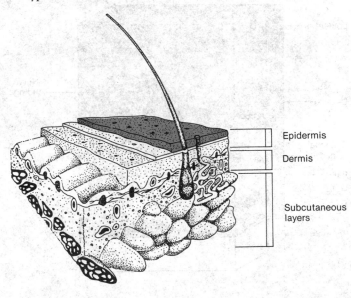

Epidermis

Dermis

Subcutaneous layers

The structure of normal skin and its relationship to underlying tissue is shown in the figure. The colored area indicates the region affected by a first-degree (superficial) burn. Damage is limited to outer epidermis.

Second-Degree (Superficial Partial Thickness)

As can be seen in the figure, the epidermis is damaged, as is the upper part of the dermis. This type of wound is characterized by blister formation and severe pain.

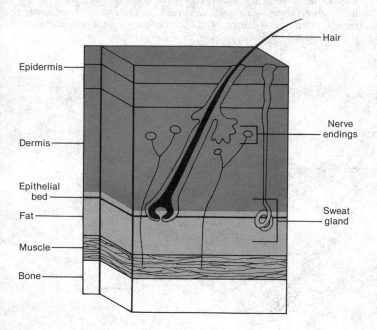

Second-Degree (Deep Partial Thickness)

As can be seen from the figure, this type of burn involves destruction of the epidermis and severe damage to the dermal layer. This type of wound is characterized by eschar formation and pain. The pain may be less severe than with a superficial partial thickness burn because some nerve endings are destroyed by the burn.

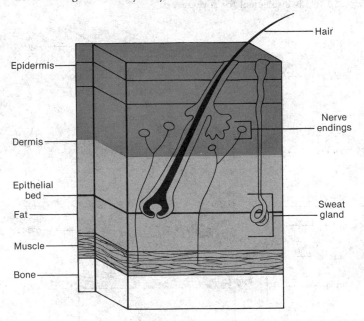

Third-Degree (Full Thickness)

As can be seen from the figure, the epidermal and dermal layers are destroyed. In addition, some of the subcutaneous tissue is damaged. This type of wound is characterized by eschar formation and little pain. Infections are very common with this type of burn. Grafts are necessary because new tissue can only be regenerated from the edges of the burn, and this is insufficient for coverage.

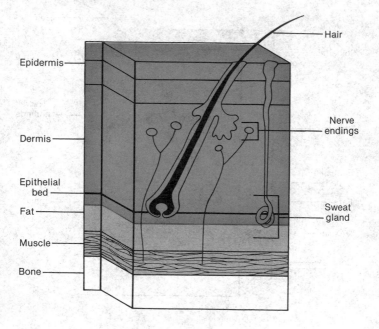

Fourth-Degree (Electrical)

In this type of burn, there is complete destruction of all skin and subcutaneous tissue, and the burn even affects the underlying bone. Extensive surgery is usually necessary to remove necrotic tissue, and for limb burns amputation may be necessary.

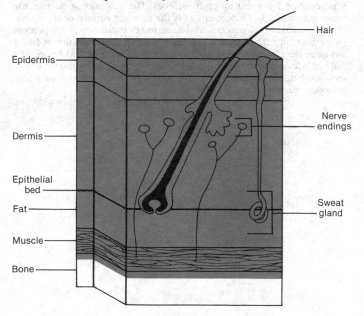

RULE OF NINES FOR ESTIMATING BURN AREA

The Rule of Nines is used to estimate the percentage of body area burned. Body areas are said to constitute either 9 percent of the area or some number divisible by 9. The head and each upper extremity are 9 percent (4.5 percent on each surface). The posterior surface of the trunk (the back) is 18 percent, as is the anterior surface of the trunk. The genital area is 1 percent, and each lower extremity is 18 percent (9 percent on each surface). A modified version of the Rule of Nines has been developed to describe body areas of children. Although the Rule of Nines is very practical, it provides only gross estimates of the areas and has been supplanted for exact estimates by use of Lund-Browder charts (pages 760–761).

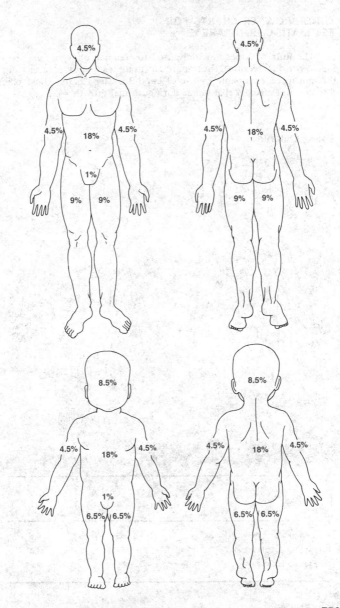

LUND-BROWDER CHARTS FOR ESTIMATING BODY AREAS

The Rule of Nines is widely used to estimate body surface area, (see previous section), but more accurate estimates of areas are thought to be obtainable by use of Lund-Browder Charts. These take into account changes that occur during normal growth.

Young Children

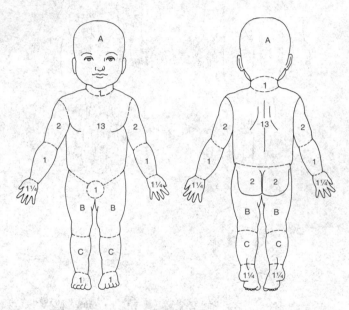

Young Children

	Area	Age in Years		
		0	1	5
A	Each surface of the head	9.5	8.5	6.5
B	Each surface of the thigh	2.75	3.25	4.0
C	Each surface of the leg	2.5	2.5	2.75

Children and Adults

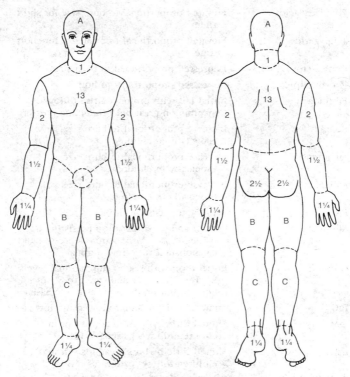

Children and Adults

	Area	Age in Years		
		10	15	Adult
A	Each surface of the head	5.5	4.5	3.5
B	Each surface of the thigh	4.25	4.5	4.75
C	Each surface of the leg	3.0	3.25	3.5

Lund-Browder Charts for Estimating Body Areas 761

BIOLOGICAL EVENTS IN RESPONSE TO BURN INJURIES

Free fatty acids	Elevated proportional to burn size for short time
Triglycerides	Elevated proportional to burn size for short time
Cholesterol	Depressed proportional to burn size
Phospholipids	Depressed proportional to burn size
Fibrinogen	Initial fall with prolonged rise following Consumption great but production greater
Renin	Increase proportional to burn size, especially in children
Angiotensin	Increase proportional to burn size, especially in children
ACTH	Increase proportional to burn size, especially in children
Protein	Rapid and persistent drop
Albumin	Prompt and persistent drop persisting until wound closed; production depressed and catabolism 2 to 3 times normal
Globulin	Initial drop with rise to supranormal levels by 5 to 7 days; catabolism 2 to 3 times normal, but production vastly increased
IgG	Immediate depression followed by slow rise
IgM	Altered little by burn in adults but in children follows pattern of IgG
IgA	Altered little by burn in adults but in children follows pattern of IgG
Red blood cells	Immediate loss proportional to burn size and depth Life span 30% of normal due to plasma factor
White blood cells	Initial and prolonged rise May drop with sepsis
Cardiac output	Precipitous drop to 20 to 40% of normal with slow spontaneous recovery in 24 to 36 hours Myocardial depressant factor demonstrated
Blood viscosity	Sharp rise proportional to hematocrit
Carboxyhemoglobin	Not significant after 72 hours (<2%) Most prominent with inhalation injury (80%) Exists with or without surface burns

BSP	Retention proportional to burn size with rapid rise and persistence for several weeks
Cortisol	Prompt rise to 2 to 4 times normal
Aldosterone	Usually returns to normal by end of first week but may remain elevated for long periods Varied response to ACTH often nil in early period
Peripheral resistance	Rises sharply — slow fall
Pulmonary vascular resistance	Rises sharply — slow fall
Pulmonary artery pressure	Prompt rise and slow return
Left aterial pressure	Normal or low High with failure
pO_2	Low with delay or inadequate therapy
PH	Prompt response to therapy
pCO_2	Initial alkalosis or hyperventilation promptly resolves
Blood lactate	May rise to high levels with hyperventilation or poor perfusion
Excess lactate	Mild elevations characteristic but may rise to high levels with inadequate or delayed resuscitation
SGOT SGPT A–P	Prompt rise with peak at 2 to 3 days and persistence for several weeks owing to liver damage, not release of skin enzymes
Renal function	Renal plasma flow depressed more than glomerular filtration rates Free water clearances down All values promptly return to normal with adequate resuscitation
Evaporative water loss	Donor sites and partial thickness burns have intermediate loss rates Full thickness burns lose at same rate as open pan of water Estimate (25 + % burn) × M² body surface Fifteen to 20 times normal skin rates
Pulmonary function (in absence of pneumonia)	Proportional to magnitude of burn; Independent of inhalation injury Minute ventilation (V_e) increased up to 500%; peak at 5 days

Continued on the following page(s)

Static compliance (C_{stat}) usually normal but may change with onset pneumonia

Lung clearance index (LCI) normal until terminal

Oxygen consumption greatly increased

Forced vital capacity (FVC) normal even with V_e increase; may drop with pneumonia

---

From O'Sullivan, SB and Schmitz, TJ: Physical Rehabilitation: Assessment and Treatment, ed 2. FA Davis, Philadelphia, 1988, p 529.

TOPICAL MEDICATIONS FREQUENTLY USED IN THE TREATMENT OF BURNS

MEDICATION	DESCRIPTION	METHOD OF APPLICATION
Furacin (nitrofurazone)	Antibacterial cream used in less severe burns; indicated to decrease bacteria growth; may be used to prepare wound for graft and/or used prophylactically	Applied directly; may be in rolled form or applied as gauze pad
Garamycin (gentamicin)	Antibiotic used against Gram-negative organism and staphyloccal and streptococcal bacteria	Cream or ointment applied with sterile glove and covered with gauze
Silver sulfadiazine	Topical antibacterial agent effective against *Pseudomonas* infections; it may also cause the adherence of eschar, thus delaying separation	Cream applied with sterile glove in a film 2–4 mm thick; may be left uncovered
Sulfamylon (mafenide acetate)	Topical antibacterial agent effective against Gram-negative and Gram-positive organisms; diffuses easily through eschar; may prevent conversion of burns	Cream applied directly to wound in thin 1/16 inch layer BID; may be left undressed or used with thin layer of gauze; must be completely removed before reapplied or may cause bacterial growth in old Sulfamylon
Silver nitrate	Caustic antiseptic germicide and astringent; penetrates only 1–2 mm of eschar; used only for surface bacteria	Small sticks used to cauterize small areas; dressings or soaks also used every 2 hours; not used with full thickness burns
Travase	Enzyme debrider has no bacterial control action; used with silver sulfadiazine	Applied to eschar with moist occlusive dressing

From O'Sullivan, SB and Schmitz, TJ: Physical Rehabilitation: Assessment and Treatment, ed 2. FA Davis, Philadelphia, 1988, p 532.

GRAFTS USED IN THE TREATMENT OF BURNS

allogenic graft: See *allograft*.

allograft (allogenic): Graft from a genetically nonidentical donor who is a member of the same species.

autodermic graft: See *autogenous graft*.

autogenous graft: Graft taken from part of the recipient's own body.

autograft: See *autogenous graft*.

autologous graft: See *autogenous graft*.

cadaver graft: Graft taken from a body immediately after death.

delayed graft: Skin graft that is partially elevated and then replaced so that it can be moved to another site.

dermal graft: See *split-skin graft*.

full-thickness graft: Graft containing all layers of the skin but no subcutaneous fat.

heterodermic graft: Graft taken from a member of another species.

heterograft: See *heterodermic graft*.

homologous graft: A graft in which the donor is a member of the same species as the recipient.

isologous graft: Graft in which the donor and the recipient are genetically identical.

mesh graft: A graft in which the donor skin has been cut to form a mesh and can be stretched to cover a larger area than would otherwise be possible.

pedicle graft: A skin graft in which one end has been left attached until the free end has begun to receive nourishment from the new site.

split-thickness graft: Graft containing only superficial layers of the dermis.

split thin graft: See *split-thickness graft*.

xenograft: See *heterodermic graft*.

zooplastic graft: See *heterodermic graft*.

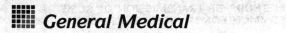
General Medical

METHODS OF TRANSMISSION OF SOME COMMON COMMUNICABLE DISEASES

DISEASE	HOW AGENT LEAVES THE BODY
Acquired immunodeficiency syndrome (AIDS)	Blood, semen, or other body fluids
Cholera	Excreta from intestinal tract
Diphtheria	Sputum and discharges from nose and throat Skin lesions
Gonococcal disease	Lesions Discharges from infected mucous membranes
Hepatitis, infectious viral or serum	Excreta from intestinal tract or from blood or serum
Hookworm	Feces
Influenza	As in pneumonia
Leprosy	Uncertain, may be from lesions Bacilli found in nodules that may break down, forming lesions

HOW ORGANISMS MAY BE TRANSMITTED	METHOD OF ENTRY INTO THE BODY
Inoculation by use of contaminated needles or by direct contact so that infected body fluids can enter the body	Via the bloodstream by blood transfusion or use of contaminated needles for injection of drugs of abuse; or a traumatized mucosal surface, esp. the rectal mucosa
As in typhoid fever	As in typhoid fever
Direct contact Droplet infection from patient coughing Hands of nurse Articles used by and about patient	Through mouth to throat or nose to throat
Direct contact as in sexual intercourse Towels, bathtubs, toilets, etc. Hands of infected persons soiled with their own discharges Hands of attendant	Directly onto mucous membrane Through breaks in membrane
Direct contact with feces of patient Direct contact with equipment contaminated by blood from the patient	Oral route or by inoculation when viral-contaminated equipment such as needles and syringes is used
Direct contact with soil polluted with feces Eggs in feces hatch in sandy soil. Feces may also contaminate food.	Larvae enter through breaks in skin, especially skin of feet, and after devious passage through the body settle in the intestine.
As in pneumonia	As in pneumonia
Uncertain, probably nasal discharges of untreated patients	Uncertain, probably via upper respiratory tract and broken skin

Continued on the following page(s)

DISEASE	HOW AGENT LEAVES THE BODY
Measles (rubella)	As in streptococcal sore throat
Meningitis, meningococcal	Discharges from nose and throat
Mumps	Discharges from infected glands and mouth
Ophthalmia neonatorum (gonococcal infection of eyes of newborn)	Purulent discharges from the eye
Pneumonia	Sputum and discharges from nose and throat
Poliomyelitis	Discharges from nose and throat, and via feces
Rubeola	Secretions from nose and throat
Streptococcal sore throat	Discharges from nose and throat Skin lesions
Syphilis	Infected tissues Lesions Blood Transfer through placenta to fetus

HOW ORGANISMS MAY BE TRANSMITTED	METHOD OF ENTRY INTO THE BODY
As in streptococcal sore throat	As in streptococcal sore throat
Direct contact Hands of nurse or attendant Articles used by and about patient Flies	Mouth and nose
Direct contact with persons affected	Mouth and nose
Direct contact with infected areas such as vagina of infected mother during birth Other infected babies Hands of doctor or nurse Linens	Directly on the conjunctiva
Direct contact Hands of nurse Articles used by and about patient	Through mouth and nose to lungs
Direct contact Hands of nurse or attendant Rarely in milk	Through mouth and nose
Droplet spread from nose or throat by direct contact with nasal or throat secretions Airborne spread is possible.	Through mouth and nose
Direct contact Hands of nurse Articles used by and about patient	Through mouth and nose
Direct contact Kissing or sexual intercourse Contaminated needles and syringes	Directly into blood and tissues through breaks in skin or mucous membranes Contaminated needles and syringes

Continued on the following page(s)

DISEASE	HOW AGENT LEAVES THE BODY
Tetanus	Excreta from infected herbivorous animals and man
Trachoma	Discharges from infected eyes
Tuberculosis, bovine	
Tuberculosis, human	Sputum Lesions Feces
Typhoid fever	Feces and urine
Whooping cough	Discharges from respiratory tract

HOW ORGANISMS MAY BE TRANSMITTED	METHOD OF ENTRY INTO THE BODY
Soil, especially that with manure or feces in it	Directly into bloodstream through wounds (Organism is an anaerobe and prefers deep, incised wound)
Dust, etc.	
Articles used about stables	
Direct contact	Directly on conjunctiva
Hands, towels, handkerchiefs, possibly clothing	
Milk from infected cow	As in tuberculosis, human
Direct contact such as kissing	Through mouth to lungs and intestines
Droplet infection from a person coughing with mouth uncovered	From intestines via lymph channels to lymph vessels and to tissues
Sputum from mouth to fingers, then to food and other things	
Soiled dressings	
Direct contact	Through mouth via infected food or water and thence to intestinal tract
Hands of nurse or attendant	
Linen and all articles used by and about patient	
Hands of carriers soiled by their own feces	
Water polluted by excreta	
Food grown in or washed with such water	
Milk diluted with contaminated water	
Flies	
Direct contact with persons affected	Mouth and nose

Adapted from Taber's Cyclopedic Medical Dictionary, ed 16. FA Davis, Philadelphia, 1989, p 394.

Reference

1. Garner, JS and Simmons, BP: CDC guidelines for isolation precautions in hospitals. Infection Control 4:258, 1983.

SUMMARY OF ISOLATION PRECAUTIONS: PROTECTIVE ASEPSIS*

ISOLATION CATEGORY	PURPOSE	PRIVATE ROOM	GOWNS
Strict isolation, e.g., for diphtheria, pneumonic plague, smallpox, varicella (chicken-pox), zoster	To prevent airborne or contact transmission of highly contagious or virulent micro-organisms	Necessary; door must be kept closed	Must be worn by all persons entering room; for smallpox, coverings for cap and shoes are also recommended
Contact isolation, e.g., for acute respiratory infections and influenza in children, pediculosis, wound infections, herpes simplex, impetigo, rubella, scabies	To prevent highly transmissible infections not requiring strict isolation but spread by close or direct contact	Necessary	Must be worn if soiling is likely
Respiratory isolation, e.g., for epiglottitis, measles, meningitis, mumps, pertussis, pneumonia in children	To prevent infections spread by contaminated articles (e.g., tissues) and respiratory droplets that are coughed, sneezed, or exhaled	Necessary	Not necessary
Tuberculosis isolation (AFB isolation) for pulmonary	To prevent spread of acid-fast bacilli (AFB)	Necessary, with special ventilation	Necessary only if clothing may become contaminated

MASKS	GLOVES	HAND WASHING	DISPOSAL OF CONTAMINATED ARTICLES
Must be worn by all persons entering room	Must be worn by all persons entering room	Necessary after touching client or potentially contaminated articles and before caring for another client	Discard in plastic-lined container or bag and label before sending for decontamination and reprocessing
Must be worn if person comes near client	Worn if touching infected material	Same as for strict isolation	Same as for strict isolation
Must be worn by all persons in close contact	Not necessary	Same as for strict isolation	Same as for strict isolation
Necessary if client is coughing and does not	Not necessary	Same as for strict isolation	Clean and disinfect, although these articles

Continued on the following page(s)

ISOLATION CATEGORY	PURPOSE	PRIVATE ROOM	GOWNS
tuberculosis when clients have positive sputum smear or suggestive chest x-ray film			
Enteric precautions, e.g., for hepatitis A, some gastro-enteritis, typhoid fever, cholera, diarrhea with suspected infectious etiology, encephalitis, meningitis	To prevent infections spread through direct or indirect contact with feces	Necessary if client hygiene is poor, e.g., client is incontinent	Same as for tuberculosis isolation
Drainage/secretion precautions, e.g., for any draining lesion, abscess, infected burn, infected skin, decubitis ulcer, conjunctivitis	To prevent infections, spread through direct or indirect contact with material or drainage from body site	Not necessary unless client hygiene is poor	Same as for tuberculosis isolation

MASKS	GLOVES	HAND WASHING	DISPOSAL OF CONTAMINATED ARTICLES
always cover mouth			rarely transmit disease
Not necessary	Necessary if touching infected material	Same as for strict isolation	Same as for strict isolation
Not necessary	Same as for enteric precautions	Same as for strict isolation	Same as for strict isolation

Continued on the following page(s)

Summary of Isolation Precautions: Protective Asepsis 777

ISOLATION CATEGORY	PURPOSE	PRIVATE ROOM	GOWNS
Blood/body fluid precautions, e.g., for hepatitis B, syphilis, AIDS, malaria	To prevent infections spread through direct or indirect contact with infected blood or body fluids	Necessary if patient hygiene is poor	Same as for tuberculosis isolation

MASKS	GLOVES	HAND WASHING	DISPOSAL OF CONTAMINATED ARTICLES
Not necessary	Necessary if touching infected blood or body fluid	Necessary if hands can become contaminated and before caring for another client	Same as for strict isolation; used needles must be placed in puncture-proof container for disposal

Source: Adapted from J. S. Garner and B. P. Simmons: CDC guidelines for isolation precautions in hospitals, *Infection Control,* July/August 1983, 4(4):258–60. Used by permission.

Reference

1. Garner, JS and Simmons, BP: CDC guidelines for isolation precautions in hospitals. Infection Control 4:258, 1983.

METHODS OF DISINFECTION*

METHOD	CONCENTRATION OR TEMPERATURE	USE	LIMITATIONS
Moist heat			
Autoclaving	250°–270°F (121°–132°C)	Sterilize instruments not harmed by heat and water pressure	Moisture will not permeate some materials Cannot be used for heat-sensitive items
Boiling water	212°F (100°C)	Kill non-spore-forming pathogenic organisms	Does not kill spores Probably not effective against hepatitis virus
Radiation			
Ultraviolet light		Air and surface disinfection	Penetrates poorly Harmful to unprotected skin and eyes
Ionizing		Sterilize medicines, some plastics, sutures, and biologicals	Expensive May alter the medicine or material
Filtration			
Membrane		Water purification	Slow and expensive
Fiberglass filters		Air disinfection	Only cleans incoming air; does not prevent recontamination

Physical cleaning			
Ultrasonic		Disinfect instruments	Aids in cleaning but not effective alone
Washing		Disinfect hands and surfaces	Does not remove all organisms
Chemicals			
Alcohols	70%–90%	Skin degerming	Sometimes irritating Does not kill spores
Chlorines	100–200 parts per million	Water disinfection Food surface sanitization	Inactivated by inorganic matter Does not kill spores Ineffective at certain pH values
Iodines, tincture	2%	Skin degerming	Not sporicidal Sometimes irritating
Iodines, iodophors	74–450 parts per million	General disinfectant	Not sporicidal
Phenols	1%–4%	General disinfectant	Ineffective against some bacteria
Quaternary ammonia compounds, tincture	0.1%	Skin degerming	Neutralized by soap Not sporicidal
Quaternary ammonia compounds, aqueous	Diluted one part to 750 parts	General disinfectant	May be incompatible with some water Ineffective against some bacteria
Mercurials	0.1%	Skin degerming	Slow acting May be irritating

Continued on the following page(s)

METHODS OF DISINFECTION* *Continued*

METHOD	CONCENTRATION OR TEMPERATURE	USE	LIMITATIONS
Formaldehyde (formalin)	5%	Drastic disinfection	Irritating, corrosive
Glutaraldehyde	2%	Instrument sterilization	Irritates mucous membranes Unstable
Germicidal soaps (hexachlorophene)	2%–3%	Skin degerming	Bacteriostatic rather than bactericidal
Gasseous Ethylene oxide	450 mg/liter of air	Sterilization of heat-sensitive materials or those that must be kept dry	Temperature, time, humidity critical Treated materials need to air for varying periods of time (depending on composition) following treatment
Formaldehyde gas		Fumigation Sterilization of heat-sensitive materials	Irritating, corrosive, toxic

*Adapted from Benarde, M. A. (ed.): *Disinfection: A Treatise*. Marcel Dekker, Inc., New York, 1970.

DIABETES

Comparison of Type I Insulin-Dependent Diabetes Mellitus and Type II Non-Insulin-Dependent Diabetes Mellitus

	TYPE I	TYPE II
Age at onset	Usually under 25	Usually over 40
Type of onset	Abrupt	Gradual
HLA association	Positive	Negative
Insulin in blood	Little to none	Some usually present
Islet cell antibodies	Present at onset	Absent
Symptoms	Polyuria, polydipsia, polyphagia, weight loss, ketoacidosis	Polyuria, polydipsia, pruritus, peripheral neuropathy
Control	Insulin and diet	Diet (sometimes only diet control), hypoglycemic agents, sometimes insulin
Vascular and neural changes	Eventually develop	Usually develops
Stability of condition	Fluctuates, difficult to control	Fairly stable, usually easy to control

Adapted from Taber's Cyclopedic Medical Dictionary, ed 16. FA Davis, Philadelphia, 1989, p 492.

Diabetic and Hypoglycemic Comas

	DIABETIC COMA	HYPOGLYCEMIC COMA
Onset	Gradual	Often sudden
History	Often of acute infection in a diabetic or insufficient insulin intake. Previous history of diabetes may be absent.	Recent insulin injection, inadequate meal, or excessive exercise after insulin
Skin	Flushed, dry	Pale, sweating
Tongue	Dry or furred	Moist
Breath	Smell of acetone	Acetone odor rare
Thirst	Intense	Absent
Respiration	Deep (air hunger) (Kussmaul)	Shallow
Vomiting	Common	Rare
Pulse	Rapid, feeble	Full and bounding
Eyeball Tension	Low	Normal
Urine	Sugar and acetone present	No sugar or acetone, unless bladder has not been emptied for some hours
Blood Sugar	Raised (over 200 mg/dl)	Subnormal (20–50 mg/dl)
Blood Pressure	Low	Normal
Abdominal Pain	Common and often acute	Absent

From Taber's Cyclopedic Medical Dictionary, ed 16. FA Davis, Philadelphia, 1989, p 391.

References

1. Sussman, KE, Druznin, B and James, WE: A Clinical Guide to Diabetes Mellitus. Liss, New York, 1987.
2. Jarrett, RJ: Diabetes Mellitus. PGS Publishers, Littleton, Massachusetts, 1980.
3. Diabetes Mellitus, ed. 8. Lilly Research Laboratory, Indianapolis, Indiana, 1980.

AIDS

RISKS OF ACQUIRING HIV INFECTION

Estimates of Risk of Acquiring HIV Infection by Portals of Entry

ENTRY SITE	TYPE OF RISK	RISK VIRUS GETS TO ENTRY SITE	RISK VIRUS ENTERS	RISK INOCULATED
Conjunctiva	Random	Moderate	Moderate	Very low*
Oral mucosa	Random	Moderate	Moderate	Low*
Nasal mucosa	Random	Low	Low	Very low*
Lower respiratory	Low	Very low	Very low	Very low
Anus	High	Very high	Very high	Very high
Skin, intact	Low	Very low	Very low	Very low
Skin, broken	High	Low	High	High
Sexual:				
Vagina	Choice	Low	Low	Medium
Penis	Choice	High	Low	Low
Ulcers (STD)	Choice	High	High	Very high

Blood:				
products	Choice	High	High	High
shared needles	Choice	High	High	Very high
accidental needle	Accident	Low	High	Low
Traumatic wound	Accident	Modest	High	High
Perinatal	Accident	High	High	High

*Based on data summarized in Recommendations for prevention of HIV transmission in health-care settings. MMWR 36:3S, August 21, 1987 and Update: Universal precautions for prevention of transmission of HIV, hepatitis B virus, and other bloodborne pathogens in health-care settings. MMWR 37:377, June 24, 1988. Adapted from Hopp, JW, Rogers, EA: AIDS and the Allied Health Professions. FA Davis, Philadelphia, 1989, p 68.

RISKS OF ACQUIRING HIV INFECTION

Estimates of Risk of Acquiring HIV Infection by Portals of Exit*

PORTAL OF EXIT	VIRUS CONTENT	POTENTIAL FOR SPREAD	CHANCE TO BE INOCULATED
Respiratory nasal:	Very low	Efficient	Very low
		Efficient	Very low
Sputum	Very low	Efficient	Very low
Saliva	Very low	Inefficient	Very low
Tears	Low	Dependent	Very low
GI:			
Vomitus	Very low	Dependent	Very low
Stool	Very low	Dependent	Very low
Urine	Very low	Inefficient	Very low
Sweat	Very low	Inefficient	Very low
Skin fomites	Very low	Inefficient	Very low
Intact skin		Dependent	Low
Broken skin	Low	Dependent	Med–high
Bleeding wound	High	Efficient	Very high

Sexual:			
Ejaculate	Very high	Efficient	Low–mod
Vaginal secretions	Moderate	Efficient	Very high
Purulent	Very high	Efficient	Very high
Blood:			
Transfusion	Very high	Efficient	Very high
Shared needles	High	Efficient	Low
Accidental needle	Low	Inefficient	Very low
Body fluids (usually blood tinged):			
Cerebrospinal fluid	Low	Inefficient	Very low
Synovial fluid	Low	Inefficient	Very low
Pleural fluid	Very low	Inefficient	Very low
Peritoneal fluid	Very low	Inefficient	Very low
Pericardial fluid	Very low	Inefficient	Very low
Amniotic fluid	Low	Efficient	Very high
Perinatal:	High	Dependent	Low
Breast milk	Low	Unknown	Low

*Based on data summarized in Recommendations for prevention of HIV transmission in health-care settings. MMWR 36:3S, August 21, 1987; and Update: Universal precautions for prevention of transmission of HIV, hepatitis B virus, and other bloodborne pathogens in health-care settings. MMWR 37:377, June 24, 1988. Adapted from Hopp, JW, Rogers, EA: AIDS and the Allied Health Professions. FA Davis, Philadelphia, 1989, p 66.

AIDS RESOURCES: ORGANIZATIONS AND HOTLINES

These organizations, which have been active with AIDS-related issues, may be helpful in locating local programs, materials, and general or specific information on AIDS.

AIDS Action Council
(202) 547-3101
729 8th Street SE, Suite 200
Washington, DC 20003

AIDS Crisisline
800-221-7044 (out of NY state)
National Gay and Lesbian Task Force: Referral to nearest AIDS service organization anywhere in U.S.; for reporting of AIDS-related discrimination

AIDS Hotline for Kids
(415) 435-5022
Center for Attitudinal Healing: Psychological support to those with AIDS and cancer, family members, lovers, or friends of AIDS victims. Bereavement support groups for all age groups

AIDS Information
(202) 245-6867
U.S. Public Health Services
Office of Public Affairs, Room 721-H
200 Independence Avenue SW
Washington, DC 20201

AIDS Information Exchange
(202) 293-7330
U.S. Conference of Mayors
1620 Eye Street NW
Washington, DC 20006

The AIDS Institute
800-462-1884
New York State Health Department
Empire State Plaza
Corning Tower, Room 1931
Albany, NY 12237

AIDS Public Education Program
(202) 737-8300
American Red Cross
1730 D Street NW
Washington, DC 20003

AIDS-Related Discrimination Unit
(212) 944-9800
Civil Liberties Union
123 West 43rd Street
New York, NY 10036

AIDS Task Force
(404) 639-2891
Centers for Disease Control
1600 Clifton Road NE
Atlanta, GA 30333

American Association of Marriage and Family Therapy
(202) 429-1825
Families of people with AIDS

American Association of Physicians for Human Rights (AAPHR)
(415) 558-9353
2940 16th Street, Room 309
San Francisco, CA 94103

American Foundation for AIDS Research (AmFAR)
(212) 333-3118
40 West 57th Street, Suite 406
New York, NY 10019

(213) 857-5900
5900 Wilshire Blvd., 2nd Floor – East Satellite
Los Angeles, CA 90036

AZT and Related Drugs
800-843-3988

Computerized AIDS Information Network (CAIN)
(213) 464-7400 ext. 277; (213) 854-3006
Gay and Lesbian Community Service Center
1213 N. Highland Ave.
P.O. Box 38777
Hollywood, CA 90038
Subscription-based computer database on AIDS, updated monthly;
anonymous communication enabling those with AIDS to contact
each other via computer

Federal Centers for Disease Control/American Social Health Association National AIDS Hotline
800-342-AIDS (24 hr)

Gay Men's Health Crisis
(212) 807-6655
Box 274
132 West 24th Street
New York, NY 10011

Lambda Legal Defense and Education Fund
(212) 944-9488
132 West 43rd Street
New York, NY 10036

Mothers of AIDS Patients (MAP)
(619) 426-1317; (619) 282-3987
P.O. Box 3132
San Diego, CA 92103

National AIDS Network (NAN)
(202) 347-0390
1012 14th Street NW, Suite 601
Washington, DC 20005

National Association of People with AIDS
(202) 429-2856
2025 Eye Street NW, Suite 415
Washington, DC 20006

National Child Abuse Hotline
800-422-4553 (24 hr)
Trained psychologist; deals with all sexual assaults, some AIDS-related

National Coalition of Gay Sexually Transmitted Disease Services (NCGSTDS)
(414) 277-7671
P.O. Box 239
Milwaukee, WI 53201

National Council of Churches AIDS Task Force
(212) 870-2385
475 Riverside Dr., Room 572
New York, NY 10115

National Gay/Lesbian Task Force
800-221-7044 (M–F, 3 P.M.–9 P.M.)
Information about AIDS, assistance for victims of antigay violence, and gay/lesbian concerns of any kind

National Hemophilia Foundation
(212) 219-8180
110 Greene Street, Room 406
New York, NY 10012

National Institute on Drug Abuse

800-662-HELP
Drug treatment information

National Leadership Coalition on AIDS
(202) 429-0930

1150 17th Street NW, Suite 202
Washington, DC 20036
Provides information on AIDS in the workplace for corporations and businesses

National Lesbian and Gay Health Foundation
(202) 797-3708
P.O. Box 65472
Washington, DC 20035

Pan American Health Organization (W.H.O. U.S. Chapter)
(202) 861-3200
Information for travel to other countries

Project Inform
800-822-7422 (in CA 800-334-7422)
Latest *experimental* drug information

San Francisco AIDS Foundation
(415) 864-4376
333 Valencia Street, 4th Floor
San Francisco, CA 94103

Sex Information and Education Council of the U.S. (SIECUS)
(212) 673-3850
32 Washington Place
New York, NY 10003

U.S. Hotlines

Please Note: The 800 numbers listed for each state or province can only be used within that state or province. Times given pertain only to that state or province.

National AIDS Hotline (accessible from all states in the U.S.)
800-342-AIDS

Sexually Transmitted Diseases National Hotline
800-227-8922

Alabama
Birmingham
(205) 322-0757
AIDS Outreach

Mobile
(205) 476-9142
AIDS Buddy Program

Montgomery
(205) 284-2273 (6 P.M.–9 P.M., M–F); 800-342-AIDS
AIDS Outreach

Alaska
Anchorage
800-478-AIDS
Alaska AIDS Project

Arizona
Phoenix
(602) 277-1929; (602) 249-1749 (5:30 P.M. – 8 A.M.)
Arizona AIDS Project

Tucson
(602) 326-AIDS
AIDS Project

Arkansas
Little Rock
(501) 666-3340 (6:30 P.M. – 10:30 P.M.)
AIDS Foundation

California
Los Angeles
(212) 876-AIDS
AIDS Project

Sacramento
800-367-AIDS

San Diego
(619) 543-0300 (Northern CA only; (415) 863-AIDS (San Francisco)
AIDS Foundation

Colorado
Denver
(303) 800-AIDS 800-333-AIDS
Colorado AIDS Project

Connecticut
Bantan
(203) 567-4111
N.W. Connecticut AIDS Project

New Briton
(203) 225-6789 (M.W.F 6:30 PM. – 8:30 PM.)
AIDS Project

District of Columbia
Washington
(202) 332-AIDS
Whitman Walker Clinic

Delaware
Wilmington
800-422-0429
Delaware Lesbian and Gay Health Advocates AIDS Co.

Florida
Clearwater
(813) 347-7779
ASAP

Ft. Lauderdale
800-325-5371
AIDS Center One

Miami
(305) 634-4636
Health Crisis Network

Polk County
(813) 665-7071
PASS

St. Petersburg
(813) 786-5139
CARES

St. Petersburg
(813) 323-5857
AM Project

Sarasota
(813) 365-4292
AIDS Support

Tampa
(813) 221-6420
AIDS Network

Georgia
Atlanta
(800) 551-2728
AID Atlanta

Illinois
Chicago
(800) 243-AIDS
AIDS Foundation

Indiana
Indianapolis
(317) 257-HOPE (7 P.M.)
AIDS Task Force

Iowa
Des Moines
(800) 445-AIDS
Central Iowa AIDS Project

Iowa City
(619) 351-0140
Iowa City Crisis Intervention Center: General counseling in all areas including AIDS, information on AIDS testing

Kansas
Topeka
(800) 255-1382, (800) 365-0219 ext. 333
Kansas AIDS Network

Kentucky
Louisville
(502) 637-4342 (6 P.M. – 1 A.M.)
Community Trust Health

Louisiana
New Orleans
(800) 992-4379
NO/AIDS Task Force

Maine
Cumberland County
(807) 775-1267

Portland
(800) 851-AIDS
AIDS Project

Maryland
Baltimore
(800) 638-6252; (301) 945-AIDS
H.E.R.O.

Massachusetts
Boston
(800) 235-2324
AIDS Action

Michigan
Detroit
(800) 522-0399; (313) 567-0399
AIDS Phone Network

Grand Rapids
(616) 459-9177
AIDS Task Force

Minnesota
Minneapolis
(800) 248 AIDS
AIDS Project

Mississippi
(800) 826-2961
Mississippi Board of Health

(800) 537-0851
HIV Information

Jackson
(601) 355-7611
Mississippi Gay Alliance

Missouri
Kansas City
(816) 561-8784
Good Samaritan Project

Kansas City
(800) 234-TEEN (M – Sat. 4 P.M. – 8 P.M.) CST
Teens Teaching AIDS Prevention (TEENS-TAP)

St. Louis
(314) 531-7400
Effort For AIDS

Montana
Billings
(406) 252-1212
AIDS Support Network

Nebraska
Omaha
(402) 342-4236 (800) 782-AIDS
Nebraska AIDS Program

Nevada
Las Vegas
(702) 362-5637
Aid for AIDS of Nevada

Reno
(702) 329-AIDS
Nevada AIDS Foundation, Information and referral

New Hampshire
Concord
(603) 595-0218
New Hampshire Buddy System

New Jersey
New Brunswick/Newark
(201) 837-8125
New Jersey Buddies

New Mexico
Albuquerque
(505) 266-0911
New Mexico AIDS Services: Information and referral

New York
Albany
(518) 445-AIDS
AIDS Council

Buffalo
(716) 847-AIDS
Western New York AIDS Program

Onconta
(607) 432-6654
Southern Tier AIDS Program, Inc.

New York
(212) 867-6655
Gay Men's Health Crisis

New York
(718) 485-8111
New York City Department of Health: HIV hotline and antibody testing
  information

Rochester
(716) 232-4430
AIDS Rochester, Inc.

Syracuse
(315) 475-AIDS; (800) 543-AIDS
AIDS Task Force

North Carolina
Charlotte
(704) 333-AIDS (M–F, 7 P.M.–10 P.M.) EST
Metrolina AIDS Project

Ohio
Cincinnati
(513) 352-3139
AIDS Program, Cincinnati Health Department

Cincinnati
(513) 421-AIDS
AIDS Volunteers of Cincinnati

Cleveland
(216) 621-0776
Health Issues Task Force

Cleveland
(216) 781-6736
Lesbian and Gay Community Service Center

Oklahoma
Oklahoma City
(800) 522-9054; (405) 525-AIDS (M – Thur. 12 P.M. – 5 P.M.; Fri & Sat,
   7 P.M. – 10 P.M.) CST
Oasis Community Center

Oregon
Portland
(800) 777-AIDS; (503) 223-AIDS
Cascade AIDS Project

Pennsylvania
Altoona
(800) 445-6262
AIDS Intervention Project

Lancaster
(717) 394-9900 (M & W, 12 P.M. – 3 P.M.; M – Sat, 6 P.M. – 9 P.M.) EST
AIDS Project

Philadelphia
(215) 732-AIDS (M – F, 11 A.M. – 11 P.M.; most weekends, 3 P.M. – 11
   P.M.) EST
AIDS Task Force

Pittsburgh
(412) 363-AIDS
AIDS Task Force

Rhode Island
Providence
(401) 277-6502
Project AIDS

South Carolina
Statewide
(800) 868-PALS
Palmetto AIDS Life Support Services of South Carolina

South Dakota
Sioux Falls
(605) 332-4599 (Information and referral line)
Sioux Empire Gay and Lesbian Coalition

Tennessee
Knoxville
(615) 523-AIDS
AIDS Response

Nashville
(615) 385-AIDS
Nashville Cares

Texas
Dallas
(214) 559-AIDS
AIDS Resource Center

El Paso
(915) 541-4266
Southwestern AIDS Committee

Houston
(713) 524-AIDS
AIDS Foundation

Vermont
Statewide Hotline
(800) 882-AIDS

Virginia
Statewide Hotline
(800) 533-4148

Richmond
(804) 358-6343; (804) 358-AIDS
AIDS Information Network

Washington
Seattle
(206) 329-6923 (Info)
Northwest AIDS Foundation

Seattle
(206) 323-1229 (Info)
AIDS Action Committee

Wisconsin
Milwaukee
(800) 334-AIDS
AIDS Project

Canada: Hotlines and Other Resources

Alberta
Calgary
(403) 228-0155 (Info); (403) 228-0198 (Office)
AIDS Calgary Awareness

Edmonton
(403) 424-4767 (Office, 9 A.M.–9 P.M.); (403) 429-AIDS (Info)
AIDS Network of Edmonton Society

British Columbia
Vancouver
(604) 687-AIDS (Info); (604) 687-5220 (Office)
AIDS Vancouver

Vancouver
(604) 683-3381
Vancouver PWA Coalition

Victoria
(604) 384-4554; (604) 384-2366
AIDS Vancouver Island

Manitoba
(204) 945-AIDS; Toll Free: (800) 782-AIDS
Manitoba Health: I&R to medical and counseling facilities

Winnipeg
(204) 453-2114 (Info); (204) 453-0045 (Administration)
Village Health Clinic/Winnipeg AIDS Advocacy Council: Medical care
  and counseling

New Brunswick
Fredericton
(800) 561-4009 (Info. M and Thurs, 7:30 P.M.–10:30 P.M.);
  (506) 459-7518 (Office)
SIDAIDS Nouveau Brunswick/New Brunswick

Newfoundland
St. John's
(709) 739-7975
Newfoundland and Labrador AIDS Association

Northwest Territories
(403) 920-8646
Infectious Disease Control, Department of Health, Government of Northwest Territories: Provides services related to testing and treatment

Nova Scotia
Halifax
(902) 425-4882
Metro Area Committtee on AIDS (MAC-AIDS)

Ontario
Guelph
(519) 763-2255
AIDS Committee of Guelph and Wellington County

Hamilton
(416) 528-0584
Hamilton AIDS Network for Dialogue and Support (HANDS)

Kingston
(613) 545-1414; (613) 549-1232
Kingston AIDS Project

Kitchener
(519) 576-2127
AIDS Committee of Cambridge, Kitchener, Waterloo and Area

London
(519) 434-1601
AIDS Committee of London

Ottawa
(613) 237-6726 (Grant); (613) 234-3687 (Office); (613) 238-1717 (Gay Line)
AIDS Committee of Ottawa/la Comite du SIDA d'Ottawa

Ottawa
(613) 957-1772
Federal Center for AIDS, Department of National Health and Welfare: Community and education services, clinical trials, epidemiology, laboratory, and research

Thunder Bay
(807) 345-1516
AIDS Committee of Thunder Bay (ACT-B)

Toronto
(416) 591-8489
AIDS Action Now

Toronto
(416) 926-1626 (Info); (416) 926-0063 (Office)
AIDS Committee of Toronto (ACT)

Toronto
(416) 962-7600
Casey House Hospice, Inc.

Toronto
(416) 392-AIDS
Ontario Ministry of Health: Information, provides phone numbers of
    medical clinics

Toronto
(416) 925-7112
Toronto PWA Foundation

Toronto
(800) 268-6066
Toronto AIDS Hotline

Windsor
(519) 258-AIDS (Info); (519) 973-0222 (Office)
AIDS Committee of Windsor

Quebec
Magog
(819) 843-2853
Intervention regionale Information sur le SIDA (IRIS)

Montreal
(514) 937-7596
Montreal AIDS Resource Centre (MARC/ARMS)

Montreal
(514) 282-9888
Comite SIDA-Aide Montreal (C-SAM)

Montreal
(514) 722-1511; (514) 722-5655
Groupe pour la prevention du SIDA Haitian

Quebec
(418) 687-3032 (Info); (418) 687-4310 (Office)
Mouvement d'information et d'entraide pour la lutte contre le SIDA a
  Quebec (MIELS)

Saskatchewan
Regina
(306) 525-0905 (Info); (306) 525-0902 (Office)
AIDS Regina, Inc.

Saskatoon
(800) 667-6876; (306) 242-5005
AIDS Saskatoon

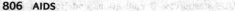

Adapted from Taber's Cyclopedic Medical Dictionary, ed 16. FA Davis, Philadelphia, 1989, p 2305.

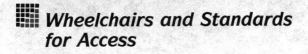

Wheelchairs and Standards for Access

WHEELCHAIR COMPONENTS

General characteristics of chairs are listed, including the optional components for that characteristic. The options are listed in alphabetical order.

Style of Chair

amputee: Rear wheels are set back to compensate for a change in the rider's center of gravity; recommended for bilateral lower extremity amputees.

indoor: Large front wheels provide shorter turning radius to help maneuver in confined areas; difficult to use outdoors.

outdoor: Large wheels in rear.

posture 90: Has 14° backward cant and solid seat with fixed sides; helps to improve posture.

prone cart: Self-propelled stretcher.

sportsman: Lighter weight construction and special design for greater speed and maneuverability; for participation in wheelchair sports.

Construction

active-duty lightweight: Frame made of a strong, lightweight alloy, reducing chair weight by 10 lb while maintaining durability.

heavy duty: Reinforced axles, seat, and back upholstery; greater stability without significant weight increase.

lightweight: Lighter upholstery and frame; one-piece wheel and handrim; chair weight about 35 lb less than standard.

Size

See table with "Standard Wheelchair Dimensions."

Frame

Fowler back: Gatched back for inclines of 10° increments; found on stretchers to elevate the head.

Goldwater (nonfolding): Solid frame with cross-bracing eliminated to allow a full tray (for batteries, charger, etc.); for motorized units only.

Narrowmatic: See *Reduce-A-Width*.

nonfolding: See *Goldwater*.

Reduce-A-Width (Narrowmatic): A detachable device attached to seat and armrest to narrow the wheelchair to allow passage through doorways.

Wheels

one-inch solid rubber: Most common type. The tire is mounted on 22- or 24-inch spoked rim.

cast aluminum: Tubed, pneumatic, 2-inch, treated tire with cast-aluminum spokes; used on motorized wheelchairs and outdoors (Everest and Jennings).

endurance: Magnesium die-cast in web design with 1-inch solid-rubber tire (Invacare), 24-inch wheel.

handrim projections (pegs): Eight (or 12) rubber-tipped projections welded onto handrims (may be either horizontal, vertical, or oblique); for those who have difficulty grasping standard handrims.

one-arm drive: Both handrims are on the same side of the wheelchair, and each controls a different wheel; used for patients who have functional use of only one upper extremity.

pegs: See *handrim projections*.

slick pneumatic: Same as *treaded pneumatic*, without the tread.

treaded pneumatic: Air-filled tube tire absorbs shocks and improves traction on soft ground; more difficult to propel.

casters: Small wheels that assist steering. Normally wheels are 8 or 5 inches, located in the front of the wheelchair.

eight-inch pneumatic: Air filled, providing a cushioned ride but easily punctured and harder to push.

eight-inch semipneumatic: Two-inch-wide, solid-rubber wheel that provides cushioned ride, is puncture-proof and less likely to be caught in elevator or sidewalk cracks, and is harder to push.

82 position: Caster housing is set forward for greater forward stability; has special antiflutter bearings.

solid caster: Five- or eight-inch-diameter, solid-rubber wheel used on children's or sports wheelchairs to decrease turning radius; more difficult to maneuver outdoors.

Wheel locks

Grade-Aid: A device used with toggle lock to assist ascent and roll-back on inclines; allows the wheel to roll forward for propelling but not backward.

lever: Long-handled braking lever used with latched plate; may be used as a braking mechanism for descending ramps.

lock extension: A long extension to the lock handle that makes it easier to reach; often used by hemiplegics on the affected side.

toggle: Standard equipment; normally comes as a pushing lock device but can be ordered as a pull mechanism.

Backs

detachable: Upholstery can be opened by means of swivel locks, Velcro, or zipper; for patients who perform back transfers; can be ordered with opening on right or left side.

full recliner: Back reclines from 90° to within approximately 20° to 0° supine position.

Goldwater: Headrest with 2-inch cushion with Velcro strap fasteners to allow for raising and lowering the cushion.

head extension: Removable headrest.

sectional height: Adjustable height from 125 to 205 inches by 2-inch increments; available only on active-duty lightweight models with detachable or wraparound arms.

self-centering headrest: A headrest with high sides to help stabilize the head and neck.

semirecliner: Reclines 30° (from 90°) and is held in any intermediate position by screw knobs on either side.

spreader bar: Adds stability to frame between back posts; always present on recliners and should be used for backs higher than 22 inches.

Upholstery 3-inch cap: Additional leather reinforcement to the top edge of the upholstery; for the heavy patient who leans excessively against the backrest or hooks an arm over the back for balance.

upright straight back: Seat and back angle is 90°.

Seat

commode: Padded board that rests on seat rails with opening for a commode.

sling: Seat upholstery suspended between seat rails, allowing chair to fold; standard wheelchair seat unless otherwise specified.

solid insert: Padded and upholstered board placed upon seat rails of a sling seat to provide firmer support; raises the sitting height.

Armrests

armpad: Upholstered or plastic attachment to armrest to provide comfort and additional arm support.

desk length: Cut away in front to allow wheelchair to fit under tables.

detachable: See *removable*.

fixed: Nonremovable, directly incorporated into the frame.

full length: Extends from rear upright to front upright.

offset-fix: Rear of armrest is welded to the back post of wheelchair;

allows for increased width between uprights without increasing the overall width of the chair; available for upright backs only.

removable (detachable): Armrest detaches to allow for transfers; increases overall width of chair by 1 to 15 inches.

variable height: Removable armrest that can be adjusted in height by 1-inch increments from 9 to 13 inches; available in wraparound or space-saver.

wraparound/space-saver: Removable armrest designed to maintain the overall width to fixed armrest width; available on upright back only.

Footrests and Leg Rests

cam lock: Spring-loaded latch to lock and release swinging detachable footrest or leg rest.

footplate: A metal support for the foot, available in three sizes:

> no. 1 — smaller size: standard for footrests; must be ordered specially for leg rests.
>
> no. 2 — larger size: standard for leg rests; must be ordered specially for footrests.
>
> no. 3 — large footplate: with additional length of plate toward rear; has cutout for caster clearance.

footrest: Supports only the feet (no calf board): may be swinging, detachable or fixed; includes No. 1 footplate unless otherwise specified.

heel loop: Strap of webbing attached to footplate to prevent feet from slipping backward.

leg rest: Includes a calf board and No. 2 footplate; may be swinging, detachable, elevating, or fixed-elevating.

one-piece parallel foot assembly: One continuous board used instead of two separate foot plates; one side of the board is detachable for folding chair.

pin lock: Pin-type latch to lock and release swinging, detachable footrest and leg rest.

antitips: Right-angled extensions to tipping lever to prevent backward tipping of chair.

cushion-seat: various thicknesses, materials, and cutouts to meet different needs.

forward stabilizers: Attachments to front of frame to prevent forward tipping.

roller bar: Attachment to foot plates on sportsman model to prevent forward tipping; must be ordered with sportsman model footplate.

safety belt: nylon strap attached to the back post; fastened either by Velcro or an automobile seatbelt buckle.

Reference

1. Ruskin, A (ed): Current Therapy in Physiatry, Physical Medicine and Rehabilitation. WB Saunders, Philadelphia, 1984.

STANDARD WHEELCHAIR DIMENSIONS

TYPE OF CHAIR	SEAT WIDTH	SEAT DEPTH	SEAT HEIGHT	ARM HEIGHT	BACK HEIGHT
Adult: designed for full-grown adults of average size and build	18 in 45.72 cm	16 in 40.64 cm	20 in 50.80 cm	10 in 25.40 cm	16.5 in 41.91 cm
Narrow adult: for relatively slender full-grown adults; combines dimensions of both adult and junior models	16 in 40.64 cm	16 in 40.64 cm	20 in 50.80 cm	10 in 25.40 cm	16.5 in 41.91 cm
Tall adult: For tall, full-grown adults	18 in 45.72 cm	17 in 43.18 cm	20 in 50.80 cm	10 in 25.40 cm	18 in 45.72 cm
Tall narrow adult: for tall, slender full-grown adults	16 in 40.64 cm	17 in 43.18 cm	20 in 50.80 cm	10 in 25.40 cm	18 in 45.72 cm
Slim adult: for thin, tall adult youths	14 in 35.56 cm	16 in 40.64 cm	20 in 50.80 cm	10 in 25.40 cm	16.5 in 41.91 cm
Junior: for full-grown adults with smaller than average body sizes	16 in 40.64 cm	16 in 40.64 cm	18.5 in 46.99 cm	10 in 25.40 cm	16.5 in 41.91 cm
Low seat: for persons who desire a lower seat height or who propel the chair with their foot	18 in 45.72 cm	16 in 40.64 cm	17.5 in 44.45 cm	10 in 25.40 cm	16.5 in 41.91 cm

Kid or 13 in junior: For children between ages 9 and 12 years	16 in 40.64 cm	13 in 33.02 cm	18.5 in 46.99 cm	8.5 in 21.59 cm	16 in 40.64 cm
Growing chair*: for children between ages 6 and 8 years; a 13-in junior model with special features; upholstery and footrest can be changed as the child grows	14 in 35.56 cm	11.5 in 29.21 cm	20 in 50.80 cm	6.5 in 16.51 cm	14.5 in 36.83 cm
Child's chair: all features of adult models but specially scaled down for children	14 in 35.56 cm	11.5 in 29.21 cm	18.75 in 47.62 cm	8.5 in 21.59 cm	16.5 in 41.91 cm
Tiny tot-hi: For children between ages 4 and 6 years; scaled to size, the hi and lo determines the seat height most functional for either the attendant or patient	12 in 30.48 cm	11.5 in 29.21 cm	19.5 in 49.53 cm	6 in 15.24 cm	17.5 in 44.45 cm
Tiny tot-lo	12 in 30.48 cm	11.5 in 29.21 cm	17 in 43.18 cm	6 in 15.24 cm	17.5 in 44.45 cm
Pre-school pediatric: for children between the ages 2 and 4 years	10 in 25.40 cm	8 in 20.32 cm	19.5 in 49.53 cm	5 in 12.70 cm	15 in 38.10 cm

*Dimensions are for detachable arm chairs. Refer to catalog for complete dimensions.

815

WHEELCHAIRS FOR THE SEVERELY MULTIPLY IMPAIRED PATIENT

EQUIPMENT	DESCRIPTION	SIZE	INDICATION	CONSIDERATIONS	DISTRIBUTOR
Gunnel relaxation chair	Fiberglass bucket seat on wheeled metal frame with footrests; scoliosis pads, headrests, and reclining-angle seat adjustments	Small: for children up to 5 years Medium: for children 5–10 years Large: for children 10–14 years Adult: (small, medium, and large frames)	Severely impaired with poor head and trunk control with extensor thrusting	1. Comfortable for long-term seating 2. Easy to clean 3. Bulky, hard to push 4. Not designed for transportation	Gunnell Manufacturing Company, Inc.
Wooden relaxation chair	Reclining wooden chair on wheeled frame; safety straps, headrest, and a tray	Small: 10.5 in × 10.5 in Standard: 13.5 in × 13.5 in Adult: 16.5 in × 16 in	Poor head control, poor trunk control, and sitting balance with extensor thrust	1. Adjustable seat angle helps to reduce extensor thrust 2. Tray useful at home or in classroom 3. Somewhat difficult to clean	Hausmann Industries, Inc.

Device	Description	Size	Population	Considerations	Manufacturer
Achiever seat	Padded plastic molded chair on stainless steel base; Headrests, footrest, thigh separator, safety belt, tray and six adjustable back angles; chair converts to seat by removing metal base	For short children weighing up to 45 lbs	Short children with poor trunk balance and head control	4. Bulky, not designed for transportation 1. Seat can be used alone in bathtub or placed on another chair 2. Can be used as a mobile chair 3. Seat alone can be used as a stationary chair 4. Child may quickly outgrow chair 5. Not designed for transportation	Contourpedic Corporation
Mancino learning center	Padded vinyl on steel-wheeled frame; removable arm scaffolding,	Small: toddlers and small children Large: adults up to 5 ft, 9 in tall	Severely impaired with poor sitting balance, strong primitive reflex	1. Many adjustable features to help in positioning	Adaptive Therapeutics Systems, Inc.

Continued on the following page(s)

817

WHEELCHAIRS FOR THE SEVERELY MULTIPLY IMPAIRED PATIENT *Continued*

EQUIPMENT	DESCRIPTION	SIZE	INDICATION	CONSIDERATIONS	DISTRIBUTOR
	safety straps, footrests with divider, adjustable back, movable headrest, and tilting detachable desk		patterns, and poor head and trunk control	2. Special head control, eating and writing systems available to reduce need for supervision 3. Bulky, not designed for transportation 4. Numerous controls can be time-consuming to adjust	
Ortho-Kinetic care chair	Padded vinyl seat and back on wheeled frame; eight position back angles, adjustable seat	Small: for children 18 months – 16 years Large: for children older	Designed for prolonged use by severely handicapped	1. Adaptation and variety make it well suited for long-term class or home use	Ortho-Kinetics, Inc.

	angle and depth, adjustable footrests and wheel brakes; also has headrest, scoliosis system, lap belt, chest belt, tray, abductor and adductor pads, toilet, and wheelchair wheels	than 10 years and adults	2. Bulky, not designed for transportation 3. Sometimes difficult to push or maneuver	Ortho-Kinetics, Inc.
Ortho-Kinetic care chair II	Padded vinyl back and seat on metal frame with wheels; can get wheelchair-type back wheels; seat-to-back angle is 90°; adjustable reclining positions and	Same as Ortho-Kinetic care chair	1. Collapsible for storage or transportation 2. Sturdy for classroom or home use 3. Can fit in station wagon or van but not designed for placement on a car seat	

Continued on the following page(s)

819

WHEELCHAIRS FOR THE SEVERELY MULTIPLY IMPAIRED PATIENT *Continued*

EQUIPMENT	DESCRIPTION	SIZE	INDICATION	CONSIDERATIONS	DISTRIBUTOR
Ortho-Kinetic travel chair	attachable lap tray. Padded vinyl seat and back on a metal frame with elevating back wheels that convert chair to a car seat; adjustable footrests, headrest, scoliosis system, abductor and adductor pads, trunk restraining straps, and adjustable tray	Small: for children 2 to 10 years; 12 in × 12 in seat Medium: for children 8 to 14 years; 14 in × 15 in seat	Good support while able to accommodate travel requirements	1. Excellent multipurpose chair for school, home, and transportation 2. Easily handled in tight spaces 3. Suitable for car or bus travel 4. Can be used as car seat	Ortho-Kinetics, Inc.
Trans-A-Chair	Padded vinyl seat and back	Small: 12.5 in × 14 in	Good sitting support while	1. Excellent multipurpose	Palmco Engineering

					Company
	mounted on metal frame with elevating back wheels that convert chair into a car seat. Adjustable footrests, headrest, scoliosis system, knee abductor system, tray, and trunk-restraining system.	Junior: 15 in × 14 in	adjustable to reduce extensor thrust	chair for home, school, and transportation 2. Easily handled in limited space 3. Suitable for car or bus travel 4. Can be used as car seat	
Patient transport chair	Foam and leatherette seat and nylon woven back on a metal frame with back wheels and stationary front legs; straight back or reclined; footrests and headrest	Nonreclining model—small: 10.5 in × 11 in Large: 13.5 in × 14 in Reclining model—small: 11 in × 10.5 in Large: 12 in × 11.5 in	Outdoor-indoor transportation chair for handicapped child	1. Easily manipulated over uneven terrain and curbs 2. Not designed for prolonged sitting because chair lacks padding or scoliosis support system	J. A. Preston Corporation

Continued on the following page(s)

WHEELCHAIRS FOR THE SEVERELY MULTIPLY IMPAIRED PATIENT *Continued*

EQUIPMENT	DESCRIPTION	SIZE	INDICATION	CONSIDERATIONS	DISTRIBUTOR
Pogon buggy	Folding metal frame with fabric seat and back and plastic footrests	One size for children up to 75 lbs	To provide temporary transportation for nonambulatory children	1. Folding, lightweight chair provides temporary transportation 2. Easy to store in car trunk or at home 3. Good temporary transportation for children without orthopedic problems 4. Not recommended for scoliosis or other postural problems because it	Genac, Inc.

Postura wheelchair	A standard wheelchair with addition of a scoliosis system and headrest	Available in child, junior, narrow adult, and adult sizes	Generalized wheelchair function with addition of postural support system for scoliosis	Scoliosis system adds extra weight to chair, making it more difficult to move than standard wheelchair lacks firm support	Everest & Jennings
Posture 90 wheelchair	90° seat back angle with a built-in 14° tilt; adjustable headrest, side armrest panels, and leg rest panels.	Junior, adult, and narrow adult sizes	Designed to reduce extensor spasm and maintain patient at a 14° backward tilt.	Adjustments to reduce extensor spasm	Everest & Jennings

Reference

1. Fraser, BA, Galka, G, and Hensinger, RN: Gross Motor Management of Severely Multiply Impaired Students, Vol. 1, Evaluation Guide. University Park Press, Baltimore.

SPECIFICATIONS FOR THE ACCOMMODATION OF THE HANDICAPPED

Size of Adult Wheelchair

Seat height	19 in (48.5 cm)
Armrest height	30 in (76 cm)
Push handle height	36 in (91.5 cm)
Toe height	8 in (20.5 cm)
Lap height	27 in (68.5 cm)
Eye level	43–51 in (109–129.5 cm)
Chair width	26 in (66 cm)
Chair width plus hands	30 in (76 cm)
Chair length	42 in (106.5 cm)
Chair length plus feet	48 in (122 cm)
Footrest width	18 in (45.5 cm)

Space Required for Turns

U turn between walls	60 in (152.5 cm) minimum
U turn completion length	78 in (196.5 cm)
Turning space (180° to 360°)	60 in (152.5 cm) diameter minimum
Aisle width (T shape)	36 in (91.5 cm) minimum each

Passageway Widths

Doorways (clear space)	32 in (81.5 cm) minimum
Aisle (1 wheelchair)	36 in (91.5 cm) minimum
Aisle (1 wheelchair plus 1 walking person)	48 in (122 cm) minimum
Aisle (2 wheelchairs)	60 in (152.5 cm) minimum

824 WHEELCHAIRS AND STANDARDS FOR ACCESS

Ramps

Slope 1:12 rise	30 in (76 cm) maximum
Slope 1:12 run	30 ft (9 m) maximum
Slope 1:16 rise	30 in (76 cm) maximum
Slope 1:16 run	40 ft (12 m) maximum
Slope 1:20 rise	30 in (76 cm) maximum
Slope 1:20 run	50 ft (15 m) maximum
Curb spacing	36 in (91.5 cm) minimum
Curb height	2 in (5 cm) minimum (width to suit)
Clearance between 2 handrails	36 in (91.5 cm) minimum
Clearance between handrail and ramp edge	12 in (30.5 cm) minimum (no curb); 1.5 in (3.8 cm) minimum (with curb or wall)
Handrail size (diameter)	1.9 in (4.8 cm) maximum
Curb ramps:	
Slope	1:12
Width	48 in (122 cm) minimum

Elevator Floor Space

Width (center opening)	80 in (203 cm) minimum
Width (side opening	68 in (173 cm) minimum
Back to door	54 in (137 cm) minimum
Back to wall	51 in (129.1 cm) minimum
Door opening	32 in (81.5 cm) minimum

Reach Heights

Controls (side reach)	54 in (137 cm) maximum (ANSI); 48 in (122 cm) maximum (federal regulations)

Reach Heights *Continued*

Gross (side reach)	9 in (23 cm) minimum
Over counter (side reach)	46 in (117 cm) maximum
Controls (front reach)	48 in (122 cm) maximum
Over 20 in (51 cm) counter (front reach)	48 in (122 cm) maximum
Over 24 in (61 cm) counter (front reach)	44 in (112 cm) maximum
Clothes rods	54 in (137 cm) maximum

Drinking Fountains

Spout height	36 in (91.5 cm)
Knee clearance	27 in (68.5 cm) minimum
Projection from wall	17 – 19 in (43 – 48.5 cm)

Kitchens

Aisle width	40 in (101.5 cm) minimum
Aisle where U turn is required	60 in (152.5 cm) minimum
Work shelf width	30 in (76 cm) minimum
Work shelf height	36 in (91.5 cm)
Alternate	32 in (81.5 cm) adjustable
Alternate	28 in (71 cm) adjustable
Work shelf thickness	2 in (5 cm) maximum
Wall cabinets (bottom height)	48 in (122 cm) maximum
Leg space (width)	30 in (76 cm) minimum
Leg space (height)	27 in (68.5 cm) minimum
Leg space (depth)	19 in (48.5 cm) minimum

Bathroom Lavatory

Lavatory projection	17 in (43 cm) minimum
Knee clearance (height)	29 in (73.5 cm) minimum
Knee clearance (depth)	8 in (20.5 cm) minimum
Toe clearance (height)	9 in (23 cm) minimum
Toe clearance (depth)	6 in (15 cm) maximum
Mirror height (bottom)	40 in (101.5 cm) maximum
Floor space (width)	30 in (76 cm) minimum
Floor space (depth)	48 in (122 cm) minimum

Bathroom Toilet

Seat height	17–19 in (43–48.5 cm)
Seat center to sidewall	18 in (45.5 cm) minimum
Seat center to lavatory	18 in (45.5 cm) minimum
Toilet paper dispenser height	19 in (48.5 cm) minimum
Toilet paper dispenser from back wall	36 in (91.5 cm) maximum
Standard stall width	60 in (152.5 cm)
Standard stall (depth wall mounting)	56 in (142 cm) minimum
Standard stall (depth floor mounting)	59 in (150 cm) minimum
Alternate stall width	36–48 in (91.5–122 cm)
Alternate stall depth (when wall mounted)	66 in (167.5 cm) minimum
Alternate stall depth (when floor mounted)	69 in (174.5 cm) minimum
Grab bar height	33–36 in (84–91.5 cm)
Grab bar diameter	1.25–1.5 in (3.2–3.8 cm)
Grab bar wall clearance	1.5 in (3.8 cm) minimum

Bathtubs	
Large tub (top seat)	60 in (152.5 cm) minimum
Large tub with built-in end seat	75 in (190.5 cm) minimum
Seat at head end (width)	15 in (38 cm)
Front access to tub	48 in (122 cm) minimum
Side access to tub	30 in (76 cm) minimum
Grab bar height (to floor)	33–36 in (84–91.5 cm)
Grab bar diameter	1.25–1.5 in (3.2–3.8 cm)
Grab bar wall clearance	1.5 in (3.8 cm) minimum

Showers	
Square	36 in (91.5) cm
Seat height (on side wall)	18 in (45.5 cm)
Grab bar height	33–36 in (84–91.5 cm)
Grab bar clearance to wall	1.5 in (3.8 cm) minimum

Safety for the Blind	
Cane range (height)	27 in (68.5 cm)
Cane range (width)	32 in (81.5 cm)
Cane pace	36–60 in (91.5–152.5 cm)
Wall projection (height to floor)	27 in (68.5 cm) maximum
Wall projection (depth)	12 in (30.5 cm) maximum
Wall projection (height to floor)	Over 27 in (68.5 cm)
Wall projection (depth)	4 in (10 cm) maximum
Secondary projection	4 in (10 cm) maximum
Head clearance	80 in (203 cm) minimum

References

1. 1980 American National Standard Institute #ANSI A117.1.
2. 1980 Federal Register Part III.

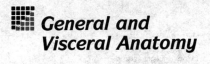

General and
Visceral Anatomy

PLANES OF THE BODY

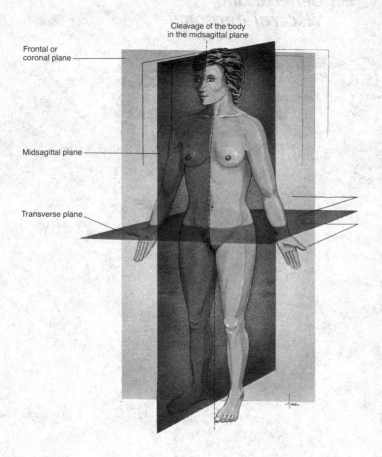

Frontal or coronal plane

Midsagittal plane

Transverse plane

Cleavage of the body in the midsagittal plane

MAJOR ORGANS IN SITU

Major organs of the body as viewed from the front with part of the lungs, small intestine, and colon removed to allow a view of surrounding and underlying structures.

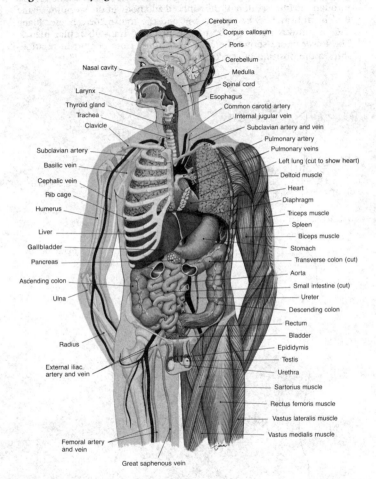

RELATIONSHIP OF SURFACE TOPOGRAPHY
(PLANES) AND VISCERAL STRUCTURES

The upper figure shows the transpyloric and transtubercular planes in relationship to underlying skeletal structure. Plane A-A' is through the intersection of the xiphoid and body of the sternum. Plane B-B' is midway between plane A-A' and the transpyloric plane. Plane C-C' is midway between the transpyloric and transtubercular planes. The lower figure shows the surface anatomy from behind in relationship to the position of the kidneys.

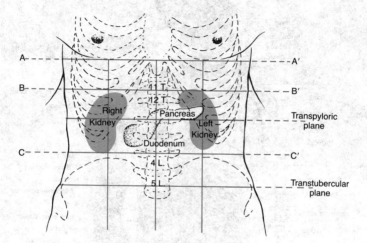

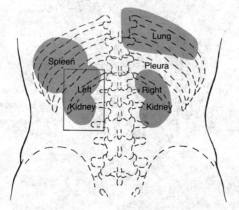

THE BILIARY SYSTEM

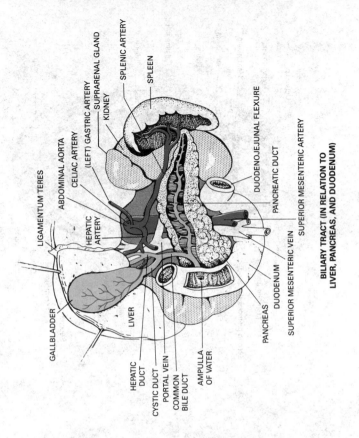

GALLBLADDER

LIGAMENTUM TERES

ABDOMINAL AORTA

CELIAC ARTERY

(LEFT) GASTRIC ARTERY

SUPRARENAL GLAND

KIDNEY

SPLENIC ARTERY

SPLEEN

HEPATIC ARTERY

LIVER

HEPATIC DUCT

CYSTIC DUCT

PORTAL VEIN

COMMON BILE DUCT

AMPULLA OF VATER

PANCREAS

DUODENUM

SUPERIOR MESENTERIC VEIN

DUODENOJEJUNAL FLEXURE

PANCREATIC DUCT

SUPERIOR MESENTERIC ARTERY

BILIARY TRACT (IN RELATION TO
LIVER, PANCREAS, AND DUODENUM)

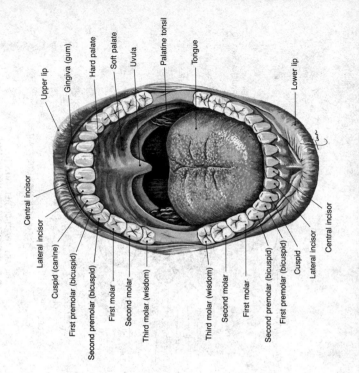

Upper lip
Gingiva (gum)
Hard palate
Soft palate
Uvula
Palatine tonsil
Tongue
Lower lip

Central incisor
Lateral incisor
Cuspid (canine)
First premolar (bicuspid)
Second premolar (bicuspid)
First molar
Second molar
Third molar (wisdom)

Third molar (wisdom)
Second molar
First molar
Second premolar (bicuspid)
First premolar (bicuspid)
Cuspid
Lateral incisor
Central incisor

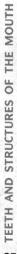

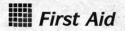

First Aid

HEIMLICH MANEUVER

Techniques

    The Heimlich sign is used to indicate when a person is choking. The choking victim grabs the throat with the thumb on one side of the neck and the index finger on the other side.

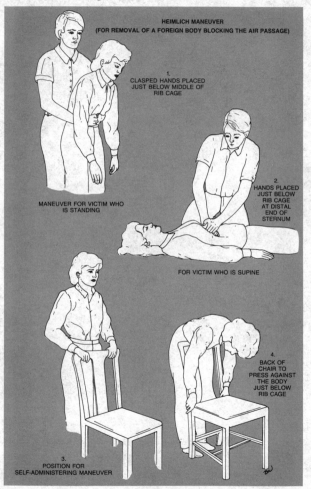

HEIMLICH MANEUVER
(FOR REMOVAL OF A FOREIGN BODY BLOCKING THE AIR PASSAGE)

1. CLASPED HANDS PLACED JUST BELOW MIDDLE OF RIB CAGE

MANEUVER FOR VICTIM WHO IS STANDING

2. HANDS PLACED JUST BELOW RIB CAGE AT DISTAL END OF STERNUM

FOR VICTIM WHO IS SUPINE

3. POSITION FOR SELF-ADMINISTERING MANEUVER

4. BACK OF CHAIR TO PRESS AGAINST THE BODY JUST BELOW RIB CAGE

HEIMLICH MANEUVER

Anatomical Correlates

The illustration below shows the proper hand placement for performing the Heimlich maneuver on a standing victim. The rescuer forms a fist with one hand and places it below the sternum. The rescuer then grasps the wrist of the hand forming the fist. The hands are then rapidly brought inward and upward.

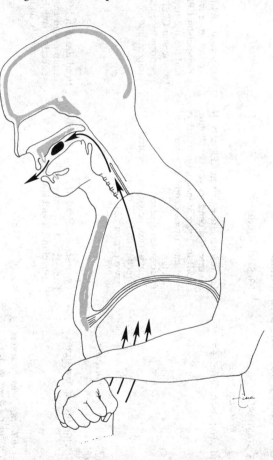

BASIC CARDIAC LIFE SUPPORT STANDARDS

FORMER STANDARD	PRESENT STANDARD	RATIONALE
Training of Rescuers		
One- and two-person CPR	Lay rescuers: one-person CPR only. If present, second lay rescuer should call for professional help. If first rescuer tires, second may provide relief.	One-person CPR improves performance and retention of skills. Two-person CPR may be confusing and has not been used often.
	Professional rescuers (nurses, physicians, emergency medical technicians): Both one- and two-person CPR	Two-person CPR: Less fatiguing; performance may be extended over longer time periods.
Opening Airway (Establishing Breathlessness)		
Head tilt/chin lift and jaw thrust	Lay rescuers: Head tilt/chin lift only. Professional rescuers: Both head tilt/chin lift and jaw thrust	Head tilt/chin lift is safe, effective, simple, and easy to learn. Though effective, jaw thrust is tiring and technically difficult.
After Establishing Breathlessness (Victim Over 1 Year of Age)		
Four quick "staircase" breaths	Two slow breaths of 1 – 1½ seconds each. After delivering first breath,	Slower breaths prevent air entrapment between breaths. Decreased air

pause to inhale before delivering second.

pressure minimizes risk of opening the esophagus and creating gastric distention with possible regurgitation and aspiration. Pause allows rescuer to increase lung volume, enabling more oxygen delivery to lungs.

After Establishing Breathlessness (Infant Victim)

Four quick, full puffs of air

Same as above (two slow breaths of 1 – 1½ seconds each; pause between breaths).

Same as above

After Establishing Complete Airway Obstruction

Four back blows and four abdominal thrusts (Heimlich maneuver)

The abdominal thrust is the only recommended technique for removal of a foreign body causing airway obstruction in victims over 1 year of age. The chest thrust remains the approved technique for obese persons and women in late pregnancy.

Exclusive use of abdominal thrusts is more effective and safer than back blows alone or back blows in combination with abdominal thrusts.

Continued on the following page(s)

BASIC CARDIAC LIFE SUPPORT STANDARDS *Continued*

FORMER STANDARD

PRESENT STANDARD

RATIONALE

Due to risk of abdominal injury, the combination of chest thrusts and back blows remains accepted protocol in infant victims under 1 year of age.

Near-Drowning Victims

No clear guidelines available. Instruction usually in rescue breathing or CPR. Some emphasis on clearing lower airway of water before onset of CPR.

Start rescue breathing as soon as possible. Perform abdominal thrusts only if a foreign object appears to be obstructing the airway or if victim does not respond to mouth-to-mouth ventilation. If necessary, start CPR after abdominal thrusts have been performed.

The necessity of clearing lower airway of aspirated water has not been proved. Attempts to remove water from airway by nonsuctioning techniques are unnecessary and may be dangerous by causing ejection of gastric contents and subsequent aspiration.

After Establishing Lack of Pulse (Infant Victim)

Compress victim's sternum at nipple line with two or three fingers.

Compress victim's sternum one finger-width below nipple line with two or three fingers.

Recent studies demonstrate that an infant's heart lies lower in the chest (in relation to external landmarks) than previously believed.

External Chest Compression,
One-Person CPR

60–80 external chest compressions per minute

80–100 external chest compressions per minute

Rapid chest compressions increase blood flow from the heart. Increase in intrathoracic pressure promotes blood flow from the thoracic cavity to the brain and heart.

Delivering Breaths, Two-Person CPR

One breath on the upstroke of every fifth chest compression, no pause in chest compressions

One breath of 1 – 1½ seconds *during a pause* after every fifth chest compression. Pause may be shorter.

Slower breaths minimize risk of gastric distention, regurgitation, and aspiration.

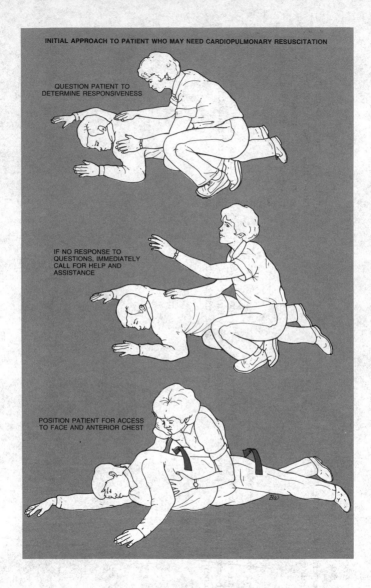

INITIAL APPROACH TO PATIENT WHO MAY NEED CARDIOPULMONARY RESUSCITATION

QUESTION PATIENT TO DETERMINE RESPONSIVENESS

IF NO RESPONSE TO QUESTIONS, IMMEDIATELY CALL FOR HELP AND ASSISTANCE

POSITION PATIENT FOR ACCESS TO FACE AND ANTERIOR CHEST

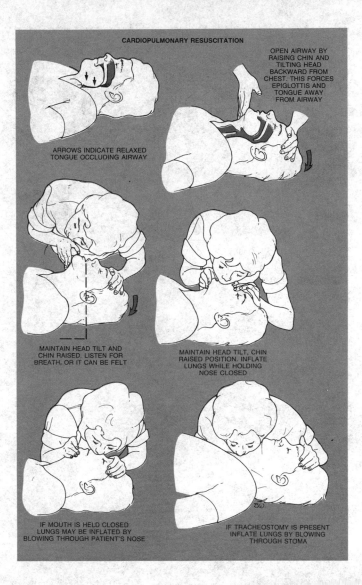

CARDIOPULMONARY RESUSCITATION

ARROWS INDICATE RELAXED TONGUE OCCLUDING AIRWAY

OPEN AIRWAY BY RAISING CHIN AND TILTING HEAD BACKWARD FROM CHEST. THIS FORCES EPIGLOTTIS AND TONGUE AWAY FROM AIRWAY

MAINTAIN HEAD TILT AND CHIN RAISED. LISTEN FOR BREATH, OR IT CAN BE FELT

MAINTAIN HEAD TILT, CHIN RAISED POSITION. INFLATE LUNGS WHILE HOLDING NOSE CLOSED

IF MOUTH IS HELD CLOSED LUNGS MAY BE INFLATED BY BLOWING THROUGH PATIENT'S NOSE

IF TRACHEOSTOMY IS PRESENT INFLATE LUNGS BY BLOWING THROUGH STOMA

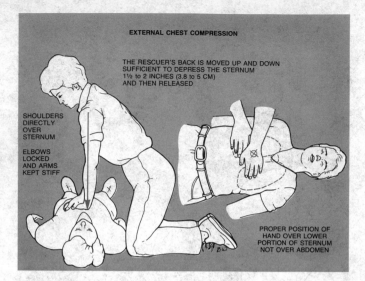

EXTERNAL CHEST COMPRESSION

THE RESCUER'S BACK IS MOVED UP AND DOWN
SUFFICIENT TO DEPRESS THE STERNUM
1½ to 2 INCHES (3.8 to 5 CM)
AND THEN RELEASED

SHOULDERS
DIRECTLY
OVER
STERNUM

ELBOWS
LOCKED
AND ARMS
KEPT STIFF

PROPER POSITION OF
HAND OVER LOWER
PORTION OF STERNUM
NOT OVER ABDOMEN

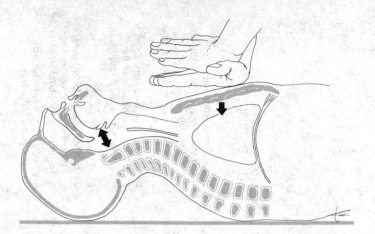

Note the overlapping of the hands and their placement over the lower sternum.

ARREST OF ARTERIAL BLEEDING*

ARTERY	COURSE	BONE AGAINST WHICH PRESSURE IS APPLIED	SPOT TO APPLY PRESSURE
For Wounds of the Face			
Temporal	Upward ½ (13 mm) in front of ear	Temporal bone	Against bony prominence immediately in front of the ear or on temple
Facial	Upward across the jaw diagonally	Lower part of lower maxilla	An inch (2.5 cm) in front of angle of lower jaw
Carotid	From outer upper edge of sternum to angle of jaw	Cervical vertebrae	Deep down and backward an inch (2.5 cm) to the side of the prominence of the windpipe
For Wounds of the Upper Extremity			
Subclavian	Across middle of first rib to armpit	First rib behind clavicle	Deep down and backward over center of clavicle against first rib (depress the shoulder first)
Axillary	Downward across outer side of armpit to inside of humerus	Head of humerus	High up in the armpit against upper part of humerus

Brachial	Along inner side of humerus under edge of biceps muscle	Shaft of humerus	Against shaft of humerus by pulling aside and gripping biceps, pressing tips of fingers deep down against the bone

For Wounds of the Lower Extremity

Femoral	Down the thigh from the pelvis to the knee from a point midway between iliac spine and symphysis pubis to inner side of end of femur at knee joint	Brim of pelvis	Against brim of pelvis, midway between iliac spine and symphysis pubis
Femoral		Shaft of femur	High up on the inner side of the thigh, about 3 in (7.6 cm) below brim of pelvis, over the line given in the direction of the knee
Posterior Tibial	Downward to foot in hollow just behind the prominence of inner ankle	Inner side of tibia, low down above ankle	For wounds in the sole of the foot, against the tibia in center of the hollow behind the inner ankle.

---

*Adapted from Hilda M. Gration, R.N.

Reference, Tables, Conversion Charts and Translations

TEMPERATURE CONVERSIONS

To Convert Centigrade to Fahrenheit

Degrees Fahrenheit = (Degrees Centigrade $\times \frac{9}{5}$) + 32

To Convert Fahrenheit to Centrigrade

Degrees Centigrade = (Degrees Fahrenheit − 32) $\times \frac{5}{9}$

To Convert Centigrade to Absolute (Kelvin)
Degrees Kelvin = Degrees Centigrade − 273

To Convert Absolute (Kelvin) to Centigrade
Degrees Centigrade = Degrees Kelvin + 273

Common Equivalent Temperatures

FAHRENHEIT	CENTIGRADE
−19.4	12.04
32	0
98.6	37
100	37.7
212	100
0	−17.8

METRIC PREFIXES

QUANTITY	MULTIPLES/SUBMULTIPLES	PREFIX	SYMBOL
1,000,000,000,000	10^{12}	tera	T
1,000,000,000	10^9	giga	G
1,000,000	10^6	mega	M
1,000	10^3	kilo	k
100	10^2	hecto	h
10	10^1	deka	da
0.1	10^{-1}	deci	d
0.01	10^{-2}	centi	c
0.001	10^{-3}	milli	m
0.000 001	10^{-6}	micro	μ
0.000 000 001	10^{-9}	nano	n
0.000 000 000 001	10^{-12}	pico	p
0.000 000 000 000 001	10^{-15}	femto	f
0.000 000 000 000 000 001	10^{-18}	atto	a

ENGLISH-TO-METRIC CONVERSIONS

Note: To convert a metric measurement into an English measurement, divide by the factor shown in the tables that follow.

Area

To obtain square meters, multiply:

Sq inches	$\times$ 6.4516^{-4}
Sq feet	$\times$ 0.092903
Sq yards	$\times$ 0.8361274
Sq miles	$\times$ 2,589,988
Acres	$\times$ 4,046.856
Sq millimeters	$\times$ 1.0^{-6}
Sq centimeters	$\times$ 1.0^{-4}
Sq meters	$\times$ 1.0
Sq kilometers	$\times$ 1,000,000
Hectares	$\times$ 10,000

Length

To obtain meters, multiply:

Inches	$\times$ 0.0254
Feet	$\times$ 0.3048
Statute miles	$\times$ 1609.344
Nautical miles	$\times$ 1852
Millimeters	$\times$ 0.001
Centimeters	$\times$ 0.01
Meters	$\times$ 1.0
Kilometers	$\times$ 1000
Newtons	$\times$ 101.9716

Pressure

To obtain pascals (N/m²), multiply:

Inches Hg at 0°C	× 3,386.389
Feet H_2O 4°C	× 2,988.98
Pounds per sq in	× 6,894.757
Pounds per sq ft	× 47.88026
Short tons per sq foot	× 95,760.52
Atmospheres at 760 mm Hg	× 101,325
Centimeters Hg at 0°C	× 1,333.22
Meters H_2O at 4°C	× 9,806.38
Kilograms/sq cm	× 98,066.5
Pascals (N/m²)	× 1.0

Speed and Velocity

To obtain meters per seconds, multiply

Inches/minute	× 4.2333^{-4}
Feet/second	× 0.3048
Feet/minute	× 0.00508
Miles/second	× 1609.344
Miles/hour	× 0.44704
Knots	× 0.5144444
Centimeters/minute	× 1.6667^{-4}
Meters/second	× 1.0
Meters/minute	× 0.0166667
Kilometers/hour	× 0.2777778

Volume and Capacity

To obtain cubic meters, multiply

Cubic inches $\times 1.6387^{-5}$
Cubic feet $\times 0.0283168$
Cubic yards $\times 0.7645549$
Ounces $\times 2.9574^{-5}$
Quarts $\times 9.4635^{-4}$
U.S. gallons $\times 0.0037854$
Imperial gallons $\times 0.0045461$
Cubic cm $\times 1.0^{-6}$
Cubic meters $\times 1.0$
Liters $\times 0.001$

Weight and Mass

To obtain kilograms, multiply:

Grains $\times 6.4799^{-5}$
Ounces (avdp) $\times 0.0283495$
Pounds (avdp) $\times 0.4535924$
Short tons $\times 907.1847$
Long tons $\times 1,016.047$
Milligrams $\times 1.0^{-6}$
Grams $\times 0.001$
Metric tons $\times 1,000,000$
Newtons $\times .1019716$

To obtain newtons, multiply:

Grains $\times 6.3546^{-4}$
Ounces (avdp) $\times 0.2780139$
Pounds (avdp) $\times 4.448222$
Short tons $\times 8896.443$

Tons	× 9964.016
Milligrams	× 9.8067⁻⁶
Grams	× 0.0098067
Kilograms	× 9.80665
Metric tons	× 9806.65
Newtons	× 1.0

Work and Energy

To obtain joules (watt-sec), multiply:

Foot-pounds	× 1.355818
Btu (IT)	× 1055.056
Btu (mean)	× 1055.87
Btu (TC)	× 1054.350
Meter-kilograms	× 9.80665
Kilocalories (IT)	× 4186.8
Kilocalories (mean)	× 4190.02
Kilocalories (TC)	× 4184.0
Joules (watt-sec)	× 1.0
Watt-hours	× 3600

To obtain watts, multiply:

Foot-pounds/second	× 1.355818
Foot-pounds/minute	× 0.0225970
Btu (IT) per hour	× 0.2930711
Btu (TC) per minute	× 17.57250
Horsepower (550 fpps)	× 745.6999
Horsepower (electric)	× 746
Horsepower (metric)	× 735.4988
Kilocalories (TC) per second	× 4184
Watts	× 1.0
Kilowatts	× 1000

SYMBOLS

♏	Minim
℈	Scruple
ʒ	Dram
fʒ	Fluidram
℥	Ounce
f℥	Fluidounce
O	Pint
lb	Pound
℞	Recipe (L. take)
M	Misce (L. mix)
$\overline{aa}$	Of each
A, Å	angstrom unit
C-1,C-2,etc.	Complement
c,c̄	cum (L. with)
Δ	Change; heat
E_o	Electroaffinity
F_1	First filial generation
F_2	Second filial generation
$m\mu$	Millimicron, nanometer
μg	Microgram
mEq	Milliequivalent
mg	Milligram
mg%	Milligrams percent; milligrams per 100 ml
Qo_2	Oxygen consumption
m-	Meta-
o-	Ortho-
p-	Para-
$\overline{p}$	After
Po_2	Partial pressure of oxygen
Pco_2	Partial pressure of carbon dioxide
$\overline{s}$	Without
$\overline{ss}$, ss	[L. *semis*]. One-half
μm	Micrometer
μ	Micron (former term for micrometer)
$\mu\mu$	Micromicron
+	Plus; excess; acid reaction; positive
−	Minus; deficiency; alkaline reaction; negative
±	Plus or minus; either positive or negative; indefinite
#	Number; following a number, pounds
÷	Divided by
×	Multiplied by; magnification
/	Divided by
=	Equals
≈	Approximately equal

>	Greater than; from which is derived
<	Less than; derived from
⊄	Not less than
⊅	Not greater than
≤	Equal to or less than
≥	Equal to or greater than
≠	Not equal to
√	Root; square root; radical
²√	Square root
³√	Cube root
∞	Infinity
:	Ratio; "is to"
::	Equality between ratios; "as"
∴	Therefore
°	Degree
%	Percent
π	3.1416 — ratio of circumference of a circle to its diameter
□, ♂	Male
○, ♀	Female
⇌	Denotes a reversible reaction
n	Subscripted n indicates the number of the molecules can vary from two to greater

ABBREVIATIONS USED IN PRESCRIPTION WRITING AND NOTES (arranged in alphabetical order)

A

a	before
abs feb	while the fever is absent
ac	before meals
ad lib	as desired
ADL	activities of daily living
adv	against
aeg	the patient
alt	alternate
alt die	alternate days
alt hor	every other hour
alt noc	every other night
AMA	against medical advice
ante	before
aq	water
aq ferv	hot water
aq frig	cold water
aq tep	tepid water

B

b	bath
bal	bath
bib	drink
bid	twice a day
bin	twice a night
bis	twice
bol	pill
BR	bedrest
BRP	bathroom privileges

C

c, c̄	with
C/O	complains of
cc	chief complaint
CCW	counterclockwise
cf	compare, refer to
cib	food
CM	tomorrow morning
cms	to be taken tomorrow morning
CN	tomorrow night
cns	to be taken tomorrow night
cont	continue
CV	tomorrow evening
CW	clockwise

D

d	day
D	dose, duration, give, let it be given, right
D/C	discharge
da	give
dc, D/C	discontinue
de d in d	from day to day
decr	decrease
decub	lying down
det	let it be given
dieb alt	on alternate days
dieb tert	every third day
dil	dilute
DISC	discontinue
disch	discharge
div	divide
DP	with proper direction
dur dolor	while the pain lasts

E

ead	the same
EMP	as directed
et	and
eval	evaluation

F

feb dur	while the fever lasts
FLD	fluid
freq	frequent

G

| GRAD | gradually, by degrees |

H

Hd	at bedtime
HOB	head of bed
hor decub	at bedtime
hor interm	at intermediate hours
hor som	at bedtime
hor un spatio	at the end of an hour
hs	at bedtime

I

id	the same
in d	daily
Incr	increase

L

| L | left |
| LIQ | liquid |

| loc dol | to the painful spot |
| lt | left |

M

M&R	measure and record
mit	send
mor dict	as directed
mor sol	in the usual way
mp	as directed

N

NB	note well
NBM	nothing by mouth
noc	night
noct	at night
non rep	do not repeat
NPO/HS	nothing by mouth at bedtime
NOS	not otherwise specified
NPO	nothing by mouth
NR	do not repeat

O

Occ	occasional
OD	once daily
om	every morning
om quar hor	every quarter of an hour
omn bih	every two hours
omn hor	every hour
omn noct	every night
on	every night
OOB	out of bed

P

P	after, position
par aff	the part affected
PC, p.c.	after meals
per	by, for each, through
PO	postoperative
PO, po	by mouth
POD	postoperative day
PP	postpartum, postprandial
prn	as the occasion
pta	prior to admission

Q

q	each, every
q2h	every two hours
q3h	every three hours
q4h	every four hours
qam	every morning
qd	every day
qh	every hour
qhs	every bedtime
qid	four times a day
ql	as much as desired
qm	every morning
qn	every night
qns	quantity not sufficient
qod	every other day
qoh	every other hour
qp	at will
qqh	every four hours
qqhor	every hour
quotid	daily
qv	as much as you like

R	right
REP	let it be repeated
RO/ R/O	rule out
ROM	range of motion
ROS	review of systems
Rot	rotate
RT	right
RX, Rx	prescription, take, treatment

S

S	label, left, sign, without
S/P	status post
si op sit	if it is necessary
simul	at the same time
SOS	if it is necessary, when necessary
s, s̄	without
stat	immediately
std	let it stand

T

Tab	tablet
tds	take three times a day
tid	three times a day
TLC	tender loving care
TO	telephone order

U, V, W

UNK	unknown
ut dict	as directed
VIZ	namely
VO, vo, V/O	verbal order
WNL	within normal limits

NORMAL VALUES FOR BLOOD STUDIES

TEST	NORMAL VALUES
Complete Blood Count (CBC)	
White blood count (WBC) (leukocyte count)	5,000–10,000/cu mm
Differential white blood count (DIFF) (differential leukocyte count)	
Neutrophils	60%–70% (3000–7000/cu mm)
Eosinophils	1%–4% (50–400/cu mm)
Basophils	0.5%–1% (25–100/cu mm)
Lymphocytes	20%–40% (1000–4000/cu mm)
Monocytes	2%–6% (100–600/cu mm)
Red blood count (RBC) (Erythrocyte Count)	Men: 4.2–5.4 million/cu mm (4.8 avg) Women: 3.6–5.0 million/cu mm (4.3 avg)
Hematocrit (HCT) (packed cell volume, PCV)	Men: 40%–54% (varies widely) Women: 37%–47% Newborns: 50%–62%
Hemoglobin (Hgb)	Men: 14–16.5 g/100 mm Women: 12–15 g/100 mm

Red Blood Cell Indices

Mean corpuscular volume (MCV)	87–103 cu mm/red cell
Mean corpuscular hemoglobin concentration (MCHC)	32%–36%
Mean corpuscular hemoglobin (MCH)	27–32 picograms
Stained red cell examination (film) (stained erythrocyte examination)	Size: normocytic (7–8 microns) Color: normochromic Shape: normocyte biconcave disk Structure: normocytes or erythrocytes
Platelet Count	150,000–350,000/cu mm

Erythrocyte Sedimentation Rate (ESR)

Westergren method	Men: 0–15 mm/hr Women: 0–20 mm/hr Children: 0–10 mm/hr
Reticulocyte count	Males: 0.5%–1.5% (of total erythrocytes) Females: 0.5%–2.5% Children: 0.5%–4.0% Infants: 2%–5% Reticulocyte index = one
Periodic acid to Schiff stain (PAS)	Granulocytes stain PAS positive Agranulocytes stain negative
Serum viscosity	1.4–2.0 times that of water

Coagulant Factors

Factor VII	65%–135%
Factor VIII	55%–145%
Factor IX	60%–140%
Factor X	45%–155%
Factor XI	65%–135%
Factor XII	50%–150%
Ristocetin to Willebrand factor	45%–140%
Factor VIII inhibitor	negative
Factor VIII to related antigen	45%–185%
Coagulation time (CT) (whole blood clotting time, Lee- White clotting time)	5–10 minutes
Partial thromboplastin time (PTT)	PTT: 30–45 seconds
Activated partial thromboplastin time (APTT)	10–25 sec
Prothrombin time (ProTime PT)	11–16 sec or 100%
Prothrombin consumption test (PCT) (serum prothrombin time)	15 sec or more, measured 1 hr after coagulation, >80% consumed in 1 hr
Blood pH	Arterial blood: 7.35–7.45 Venous blood: 7.31–7.41

Continued on the following page(s)

NORMAL VALUES FOR BLOOD STUDIES *Continued*

TEST	NORMAL VALUES
Lactic acid	Venous blood: 0.5 – 2.2 mEq/liter Arterial blood: 0.5 – 1.6 mEq/liter
Myoglobin	30 – 90 mg/ml

NORMAL VALUES FOR URINE STUDIES

TEST	NORMAL VALUES
Urine output	1 – 1.5 liters/day
Urine cultures	Negative = less than 10,000 organisms/ml
Color	Yellow: normal color of urine Straw color: normal but indicates low specific gravity Amber: normal but indicates high specific gravity
Specific gravity	Normal: 1.003 – 1.035 (usually between 1.010 and 1.025) Concentrated urine: 1.025 – 1.030 or greater Dilute urine: 1.001 – 1.010
Concentration (Fishberg test)	1.024 or higher (up to 300 ml)
pH	4.6 – 8 (6), can vary widely
Blood or hemoglobin (Heme)	Negative
Protein (albumin)	Negative: 2 – 8 mg/dl, 10 – 100 mg/24 hrs
Sugar (glucose)	Random specimen: negative Quantitative 24 hr: 100 mg
Ketone bodies (acetone)	Negative
Nitrate/bacteria	Negative
Bilirubin	Negative or 0.02 mg/dl
Red cells and red cell casts	1 or 2: LPF Red blood cells: 0 – 1: HPF Red cell casts: 0: LPF
White cells and white cell casts	WBCs: 0 – 4: HPF WBC casts: none – neg: LPF

TEST	NORMAL VALUES
Chlorides (Cl) (quantitative 24 hr)	110–250 mEq/24 hrs 10–20 g NaCl/24 hrs 9 g/liter (0.9 g/ml)
Sodium (Na) (quantitative 24 hr)	130–200 mEq/24 hrs
Potassium (K) (quantitative 24 hr)	40–80 mEq/24 hrs
Uric acid (quantitative 24 hr)	0.4–1.0 g/24 hrs 0.2–0.5 g/24 hrs 2.0 g/24 hr on a high purine diet
Calcium (quantitative 24 hr)	100–250 mg/average diet 150 mg/low calcium diet
Creatinine clearance	100–180 liters/24 hrs
Osmolality	Dilute: <200 milliosmoles Nl: >850 milliosmoles
Myoglobin	0–2 mg MB/ml
Estrogen fractions	Women total: 4–60 mg/24 hrs Estron (E): 2–25 mg/24 hrs Estradiol (E2): 0–10 mg/24 hrs Pregnancy-Estriol (E3): 2–30 mg/24 hrs Men: 4–24 mg/24 hrs

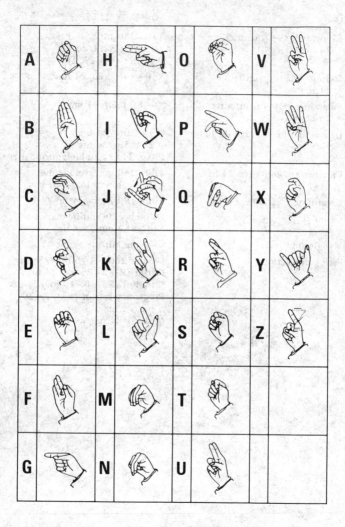

BRAILLE ALPHABET AND NUMERALS

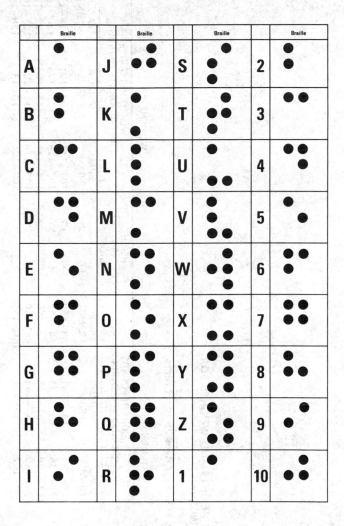

DESIRABLE HEIGHTS AND WEIGHTS FOR MEN AND WOMEN

According to Frame for Ages 25 to 59 years

MEN

HEIGHT (IN SHOES)*		WEIGHT IN POUNDS (IN INDOOR CLOTHING)†		
FT	IN	SMALL FRAME	MEDIUM FRAME	LARGE FRAME
5	2	128–134	131–141	138–150
5	3	130–136	133–143	140–153
5	4	132–138	135–145	142–156
5	5	134–140	137–148	144–160
5	6	136–142	139–151	146–164

WOMEN

HEIGHT (IN SHOES)*		WEIGHT IN POUNDS (IN INDOOR CLOTHING)†		
FT	IN	SMALL FRAME	MEDIUM FRAME	LARGE FRAME
4	10	102–111	109–121	118–131
4	11	103–113	111–123	120–134
5	0	104–115	113–126	122–137
5	1	106–118	115–129	125–140
5	2	108–121	118–132	128–143

Height (ft)	Height (in)			
5	7	138–145	142–154	149–168
5	8	140–148	145–157	152–172
5	9	142–151	148–160	155–176
5	10	144–154	151–163	158–180
5	11	146–157	154–166	161–184
6	0	149–160	157–170	164–188
6	1	152–164	160–174	168–192
6	2	155–168	164–178	172–197
6	3	158–172	167–182	176–202
6	4	162–176	171–187	181–207

Height (ft)	Height (in)			
5	3	111–124	121–135	131–147
5	4	114–127	124–138	134–151
5	5	117–130	127–141	137–155
5	6	120–133	130–144	140–159
5	7	123–136	133–147	143–163
5	8	126–139	136–150	146–167
5	9	129–142	139–153	149–170
5	10	132–145	142–156	152–173
5	11	135–148	145–159	155–176
6	0	138–151	148–162	158–179

*Shoes with 1-inch heels.

†Indoor clothing weighing 5 pounds for men and 3 pounds for women.

Source of basic data: *Build Study, 1979*, Society of Actuaries and Association of Life Insurance Medical Directors of America, 1980.

Copyright 1983 Metropolitan Life Insurance Company. Adapted from Taber's Cyclopedic Medical Dictionary, ed 16. FA Davis, Philadelphia, 1989, p 2017.

MEDICAL WORD ELEMENTS: PREFIXES, ROOT WORDS, AND SUFFIXES

English Meanings of Medical Word Elements

MEDICAL WORD ELEMENT	PRONUNCIATION	MEANING
a-	ăh	without, not, lack of
ab-	ăb	from, away from
-ac	ăk	pertaining to
acr/o-	ăk-rō	extremity
ad-	ăd	to, toward, near
acromi/o	ă-krō-mē-ō	acromion, projection of scapula
aden/o	ăd-ē-nō	gland
adenoid/o	ăd-ē-noid-ō	adenoid
adip/o	ăd-ĭ-pō	fat
adren/o	ăd-rē-nō	adrenal glands
adrenal/o	ă-drĕn-ăl-ō	adrenal glands
agranul/o	ă-grăn-ū-lō	without granules
-al	ăl	pertaining to
albumin/o	ăl-bū-mĭn-ō	white protein, albumin
-algesia	ăl-gē-sē-ah	pain
-algia	ăl-jē-ah	pain
alveol/o	ăl-vē-ōl-ō	alveolus (pl. alveoli)
ambi-	ăm-bĭ	both, both sides
ambly/o	ăm-blē-ō	dull, dim
amphi-	ăm-fĭ	on both sides

an-	ăn	without, not, lack of
an-/o	ā-nō	anus, opening of the rectum
andr/o	ăn-drō	male
angi/o	ăn-jē-ō	vessel
ankyl/o	ăng-kĭ-lō	stiff joint, fusion or growing together of parts
ante-	ăn-tē	before, in front of
anter/o	ăn-tĕr-ō	before, in front of, anterior
anthrac/o	ăn-thrah-kō	coal
anti-	ăn-tĭ	against
aort/o	ā-ōr-tō	aorta
aque/o	ā-kwē-ō	water
ar-	ăr	without, not, lack of
-ar	ĕr	pertaining to
-arche	ăr-kē	beginning
arteriol/o	ăr-tēr-ĭ-ōl-ō	little artery, arteriole
arthr/o	ăr-thrō	joint
-ary	ĕr-ē	pertaining to
-asthenia	ăs-thē-nē-ăh	without strength
atel/o	ăt-ē-lō	incomplete, imperfect
ather/o	ăth-ĕr-ō	fatty deposit, fatty degeneration
atri/o	ā-trē-ō	atrium
audi/o	aw-dē-ō	hearing
bacteri/o	băk-tē-rē-ō	bacteria
balan/o	bah-lăn-ō	glans penis
bas/o	bā-sō	basic or alkaline
bi-	bī	two
bil/i	bĭl-ē	biliary system

873

Continued on the following page(s)

English Meanings of Medical Word Elements *Continued*

MEDICAL WORD ELEMENT	PRONUNCIATION	MEANING
-blast	blăst	germ cell, embryonic, primitive
blast/o	blăs-tō	embryonic, primitive, germ cell
blephar/o	blĕf-ah-rō	eyelid
brachi/o	brăk-ē-ō	arm
brady-	brăd-ē	slow
bronch/o	brŏng-kō	bronchus (pl. bronchi)
bronchi/o	brŏng-kē-ō	bronchus (pl. bronchi)
bucc/o	bŭk-ō	cheek
calc/o	kăl-kō	calcium
calcane/o	kal-kă-nē-ō	calcaneum, heel bone
-capnia	kăp-nē-ah	carbon dioxide, CO_2
carcin/o	kăr-sĭn-ō	cancer
cardi/o	kăr-dē-ō	heart
carp/o	kăr-pō	wrist, carpus
-cele	sēl	hernia, swelling
celi/o	sē-lē-ō	belly, abdomen
-centesis	sĕn-tē-sĭs	surgical puncture
cephal/o	sĕf-ăl-ō	head
cerebell/o	sĕr-ĕ-bĕl-lō	cerebellum
cerebr/o	sĕr-ē-brō	cerebrum
cervic/o	sĕr-vĭ-kō	neck, cervix

cheil/o	kī-lō	lip
chem/o	kē-mō	chemical, drug
chlor/o	klōr-ō	green
-chlorhydria	klōr-hī-drē-ah	hydrochloric acid
chol/e	kō-lē	bile, gall
cholangi/o	kō-lăn-jē-ō	bile vessel
cholecyst/o	kō-lē-sis-tō	gallbladder
choledoch/o	kō-lē-dō-kō	bile duct
chondr/o	kŏn-drō	cartilage
choroid/o	kō-roid-ō	choroid
-chrome	krōm	color
chrom/o	krōm-ō	color
circum-	sĕr-kŭm	around
cirrh/o	sĭr-rō	yellow, tawny
-clasis	klăh-sĭs	a breaking (of), refracture
-clast	klăst	to break
col/o	kō-lō	colon
colp/o	kōl-pō	vagina
condyl/o	kŏn-dĭ-lō	condyle
coni/o	kō-nē-ō	dust
contra-	kŏn-trah	against
cor/e	kō-rē	pupil
core/o	kō-rē-ō	pupil
corne/o	kōr-nē-ō	cornea
coron/o	kōr-ō-nō	heart
cost/o	kōs-tō	ribs
crani/o	krā-nē-ō	skull bones, cranium, skull
-crine	krĭn or krīn	to secrete

Continued on the following page(s)

875

English Meanings of Medical Word Elements *Continued*

MEDICAL WORD ELEMENT	PRONUNCIATION	MEANING
cry/o	krī-o	cold
crypt/o	krĭp-tō	hidden
-cusis	kū-sĭs	hearing
cutane/o	kū-tā-nē-ō	skin
cyan/o	sī-ăn-ō	blue
cycl/o	sī-klō	ciliary body
-cyesis	sī-ē-sĭs	pregnancy
cyst/o	sĭs-tō	bladder, sac of fluid
cyt/o	sī-tō	cell
dacry/o	dăk-rē-ō	tear
dacryoaden/o	dăk-rē-ō-ăd-ĕn-ō	tear gland
dactyl/o	dăk-tĭ-lō	digit (finger or toe)
dent/o	dĕnt-ō	tooth
derm/o	dĕr-mō	skin
dermat/o	dĕr-mah-tō	skin
-desis	dē-sĭs	binding, stabilization, fusion
dextr/o	dĕks-trō	to the right of
di-	dī	two
dia-	dē-ah	through, across
diplo-	dĭp-lō	double
-dipsia	dĭp-sē-ăh	thirst

dist/o	dĭs-tō	distant
dors/o	dŏr-sō	back
duoden/o	dū-ŏd-ĕ-nō	duodenum
-dynia	dĭn-ē-ĭah	pain
dys-	dĭs	bad, painful, difficult
ec-	ĕk	out, out from
-ectasis	ĕk-tĭah-sĭs	dilation, expansion
ecto-	ĕk-tō	outside
-ectomy	ĕk-tĭo-mē	excision, removal
embol/o	ĕm-bŏl-ō	embolus, plug
-emesis	ē-mĭe-sĭs	vomit
-emia	ē-mē-ĭah	blood condition (of)
emmetr/o	ĕm-ē-trō	correct measure
encephal/o	ĕn-sĭef-ah-lō	brain
endo-	ĕn-dō	in, within
enter/o	ĕn-tĭer-ō	intestines
eosin/o	ē-ō-sĭn-ō	red, rosy, dawn-colored
epi-	ĕp-ĭ	upon, over, in addition to
epididym/o	ĕp-ĭ-dĭd-ĭ-mō	epididymis
epiglott/o	ĕp-ĭ-glĭott-ō	epiglottis
episi/o	ē-pĭz-ē-ō	vulva
-er	ĕr	one who
erythem/o	ĕr-ĭ-thē-mō	red
erythr/o	ĕ-rĭth-rō	red
erythrocyt/o	ĕ-rĭth-rō-sĭ-tō	red cell
esophag/o	ē-zĭof-ah-gō	esophagus
-esthesia	ĭes-thē-zĕ-ah	feeling, sensation

Continued on the following page(s)

877

English Meanings of Medical Word Elements *Continued*

MEDICAL WORD ELEMENT	PRONUNCIATION	MEANING
eu-	ū	good, easy
ex-	ĕks	out, out from
exo-	ĕks-ō	outside
extern/o	ĕks-tĕrn-ō	outside
extra-	ĕks-trah	outside
femor/o	fĕm-ō-rō	femur, thigh bone
fibul/o	fĭb-ū-lō	fibula
galact/o	gă-lăk-tō	milk
gangli/o	găng-glē-ō	ganglion (knot)
ganglion/o	găng-glē-ion-ō	ganglion (knot)
gastr/o	găs-trō	stomach
-gen	jĕn	to produce
-genesis	jĕn-ĕ-sĭs	origin, beginning process
gingiv/o	jĭn-jĭ-vō	gum
glauc/o	glaw-kō	gray
gli/o	glī-ō	glue
-globin	glō-bĭn	protein
glomerul/o	glō-mĕr-ū-lō	glomerulus
gloss/o	glŏs-ō	tongue
gluc/o	gloo-kō	sugar, sweetness

gluco/o	gloo-kō-sō	sugar
glyc/o	glī-kō	sugar, sweetness
gonad/o	gō-nǐad-ō	sex glands
-gram	grǐam	a writing, record
granu/o	grǐan-ū-lō	granule
-graph	grǐaf	instrument used for recording
-graphy	grǐa-fē	process of recording
gravica	grǐav-i-dah	pregnancy
gynec/o	jǐn-ē-kō-gǐ-nē-kō	woman, female
hem/o	hēm-o	blood
hemanzj/o	hē-mǐan-jē-ō	blood vessel
hemat/o	hǐem-ah-tō	blood
hemi-	hǐem-ē	half, partial
hepat/o	hǐep-ah-tō	liver
heter/o	hǐet-ǐer-ō	different
hidr/o	hǐ-drō	sweat
hist/o	his-tō	tissue
home/o	hō-mē-ō	likeness, resemblance
homo-	hō-mō	same
humer/o	hū-mǐer-ō	humerus
hydr/o	hǐ-drō	water
hyper-	hǐ-pǐer	over, above, excessive, beyond
hypo-	hǐ-pō	under, below, beneath, less
hyster/o	his-tǐer-ō	uterus, womb
-ia	ē-ah	condition (of), process
-iasis	ǐ-ā-sis	abnormal condition, formation of, presence of

Continued on the following page(s)

879

English Meanings of Medical Word Elements *Continued*

MEDICAL WORD ELEMENT	PRONUNCIATION	MEANING
-ic	ĭk	pertaining to
-ical	ĭk-ĭal	pertaining to
ichthy/o	ĭk-thē-ō	dry, scaly
-icle	ĭk-ĭal	small, little, minute
ile/o	ĭl-ē-ō	ileum
ili/o	ĭl-ē-ō	ilium
im-	ĭm	not
immun/o	ĭm-ū-nō	safe, protected
in-	ĭn	not
infra-	ĭn-frah	under, below, beneath, after
inter-	ĭn-tier	between
intra-	ĭn-trah	in, within
ir/o	ĭr-ō	iris
irid/o	ĭr-ĭ-dō	iris
-is	ĭs	forms noun from root
is/o	ī-sō	equal
ischi/o	ĭs-kē-ō	ischium
-ism	ĭzm	condition, state of being
-ist	ĭst	one who specializes
-itis	ī-tĭs	inflammation
jejun/o	jĕ-joo-nō	jejunum

kary/o	kăr-ē-ō	nucleus
kerat/o	kĕr-ĭah-tō	cornea; hornlike; hard; horny substance
kinesi/o	kĭ-nē-sē-ō	movement
-kinesia	kĭ-nē-zē-iah	movement
labi/o	lā-bē-ō	lip
labyrinth/o	lăb-ĭ-rĭn-thō	labyrinth, inner ear, maze
lacrim/o	lăk-rĭ-mō	tear
lact/o	lăk-tō	milk
lamin/o	lăm-ĭ-nō	lamina
lapar/o	lăp-ĭar-ō	abdominal wall, abdomen
laryng/o	lăh-rĭng-ō	larynx
later/o	lăt-ĕr-ō	side
leiomy/o	lī-ō-mī-ō	smooth (visceral) muscle
-lepsy	lĕp-sē	seizure
leuc/o	loo-kō	white
leuk/o	loo-kō	white
leukocyt/o	loo-kō-sī-tō	white cell
lingu/o	lĭng-gwō	tongue
lip/o	lĭ-pō	fat
-lith	lĭth	stone, calculus
-lithias s	lĭth-ī-ah-sĭs	presence, condition, or formation of calculi
lob/o	lō-bō	lobe
-logy	lō-jē	study of
lumb/o	lŭm-bō	loins
lymph/o	lĭm-fō	lymph, lymph tissue
-lysis	lī-sĭs	separate, destroy, break down
macro-	măk-rō	large

Continued on the following page(s)

881

English Meanings of Medical Word Elements *Continued*

MEDICAL WORD ELEMENT	PRONUNCIATION	MEANING
mal-	măl	ill, bad, poor
-malacia	măh-lā-shē-ĭah	softening
mamm/o	mă-mō	breast
-manometer	măn-ĭom-ĭet-ĭer	instrument to measure pressure
mast/o	măs-tō	breast
mastoid/o	măs-toi-dō	mastoid process
medi-	mē-dē	middle
medull/o	mĕd-ū-lō	medulla
-megaly	mĕg-ĭah-lē	enlargement
melan/o	mĕl-ah-nō	black
mening/o	mĕ-nĭng-gō	meninges, brain covering
meningi/o	mĕ-nĭn-jē-ō	meninges, brain covering
men/o	mĕn-ō	menses, menstruation
mes/o	mĕs-ō	middle
meta	mĕt-ah	after, beyond, over, change
metacarp/o	mĕt-ah-kăr-pō	metacarpus, bones of the hand
-meter	mē-tĕr	measure, instrument for measuring
metr/o	mĕ-trō	uterus, womb
-metry	mĕt-rē	act of measuring, to measure
micro-	mī-krō	small
mid-	mĭd	middle
mono-	mŏn-ō	one

morph/o	mŏr-fō	shape
multi-	mŭl-tē	many, much
my/o	mī-ō	muscle
myc/o	mī-kō	fungus
-mycosis	mī-kō-sĭs	fungal infection
myel/o	mī-e-lō	bone marrow, spinal cord
myring/o	mīe-rĭng-gō	tympanic membrane, eardrum
narc/o	nĭar-kō	sleep
nas/o	nā-zō	nose
nat/a	nā-tia	birth
ne/o	nĕ-ō	new
nephr/o	nĭef-rō	kidney
neur/o	nū-rō	nerve, neuron
neutr/o	nū-trō	neutral dye
noct/o	nĭok-tō	night
nucle/o	nū-klē-ō	nucleus
ocul/o	ĭok-ū-lō	eye
odont/o	ō-dĭon-tō	tooth
-oid	oid	resemble
-ole	iol	small, little, minute
olig/o	ō-lĭ-gō	scanty
-oma	ō-mĭah	tumor
onc/o	ĭong-kō	tumor, mass
onych/o	ĭon-ĭ-kō	nail
oo/o	ō-ō	egg, ovum
oophor/o	ō-ĭof-ō-rō	ovary
ophthalm/o	ĭof-thĭal-mō	eye

883

Continued on the following page(s)

English Meanings of Medical Word Elements Continued

MEDICAL WORD ELEMENT	PRONUNCIATION	MEANING
-opia	ō-pē-ah	vision
-opsia	ŏp-sē-ah	vision
opt/o	ŏp-tō	eye
orch/o	ŏr-kō	testes
orchi/o	ŏr-kē-ō	testes
orchid/o	ŏr-ki-dō	testes
or/o	ŏr-ō	mouth
orth/o	ŏr-thō	straight
-ory	ŏr-ē	pertaining to
-osis	ō-sis	abnormal condition, increase
-osmia	ŏz-mē-ah	smell
oste/o	ŏs-tē-ō	bone
ot/o	ō-tō	ear
-ous	ius	pertaining to
ovari/o	ō-vĭar-ē-ō	ovary
ox/o	ŏks-ō	oxygen, O_2
oxy/o	ŏk-sĭ-ō	oxygen, O_2
pachy/o	păk-ē-ō	thick, heavy
pan-	păn	all
pancreat/o	păn-krē-ĭa-tō	pancreas
papill/o	păp-ĭ-lō	nipple-like protuberance or elevation

para-	păr-ah	near, beside, beyond, abnormal
-para	păar-ah	to bear
parathyroid/o	păar-ah-thī-roi-dō	parathyroid glands
-paresis	pah-rē-sĭs	partial or incomplete paralysis
patell/o	pah-tiel-ō	patella, kneecap
-pathy	pĭah-thē	disease
pector/o	pĭek-tō-rō	chest
ped/i	pĭed-ē	foot
pelv/i	pĭel-vē	pelvis
-penia	pē-nē-iah	decrease, deficiency, lack of
peri-	pĭer-ĭ	around
perine/o	pĭer-ĭ-nē-ō	perineum
peritone/o	pĭer-ĭ-tō-nē-ō	peritoneum
-pexy	pĭek-sē	fixation, suspension
phag/o	fĭag-ō	swallow, eat
-phagia	fā-jē-ah	eating, ingesting, swallowing
phak/o	fā-kō	lens
phalang/o	fĭal-ĭan-jō	phalanges, bones of fingers and toes
pharyng/o	fah-rĭng-gō	pharynx, throat
-phasia	fā-zē-ah	speech
-phil	fĭl	to love, attraction for
-philia	fĭl-ē-ĭah	attraction for, to love
phleb/o	flĭeb-ō	vein
-phobia	fō-bē-ĭah	fear
-phonia	fō-nē-ah	voice
-phoresis	fō-rē-sĭs	borne, carried
phren/o	frĭen-ō	diaphragm, mind
-phylaxis	fĭ-lĭak-sĭs	protection

Continued on the following page(s)

885

English Meanings of Medical Word Elements *Continued*

MEDICAL WORD ELEMENT	PRONUNCIATION	MEANING
-physis	fĭ-sĭs	growth, to grow
pil/o	pī-lō	hair
-plakia	pliak-ē-ĭah	plate
-plasia	plă-zē-ĭah	formation, development, growth
-plasm	plăzm	formation, growth, development
-plasty	plias-tē	formation, plastic repair, surgical repair
-plegia	plē-jē-ĭah	paralysis, stroke
pleur/o	ploo-rō	pleura
-pnea	nē-ah	breathing
pneum/o	nū-mō	lung, air
pneumat/o	nū-mah-tō	air, breath
pneumon/o	nū-mŏn-ō	lung, air
pod/o	pŏ-dō	foot
-poiesis	poi-ē-sĭs	formation, production
poikil/o	poi-kĭ-lō	varied, irregular
polio-	pō-lē-ō	gray
poly-	pŏl-ē	many, much
-porosis	pō-rō-sĭs	pores or cavities
post-	pōst	after, backward, behind
poster/o-	pŏs-tĭer-ō	after, backward, back, behind, posterior
-prandial	prĭan-dē-ĭal	pertaining to a meal
pre-	prē	before, in front of

presby/o	prĕs-bē-ō	old age, elderly
primi-	prĭ-mĭ	first
pro-	prō	before, in front of
proct/o	prŏk-tō	anus, rectum
prostat/o	prŏs-tah-tō	prostate
proxim/o	prŏk-sĭm-ō	near
pseudo-	soo-dō	false
-ptosis	tō-sĭs	prolapse, falling, dropping
-ptysis	tĭ-sĭs	spitting
pub/o	pū-bō	pubis anterior
pulmon/o	pŭl-mŏn-ō	lung
pupill/o	pū-pĭ-lō	pupil
purpur/o	pŭr-pū-rō	purple
py/o	pī-ō	pus
pyel/o	pī-ĕ-lĭo	renal pelvis
pylor/o	pī-lō-rō	pylorus
-pyorrhea	pī-ō-rē-ah	discharge of pus, purulent discharge
quad-	kwŏd	four
quadri-	kwŏd-rĭ	four
rach/o	răk-ō	vertebrae, spinal column
rachi/o	răk-ē-ō	vertebrae, spinal column
rect/o	rĕk-tō	rectum
ren/o	rē-nō	kidney
reticul/o	rē-tĭk-ū-lō	net, mesh (immature RBC)
retin/o	rĕt-ĭ-nō	retina
retro-	rĕt-rō	after, backward, behind
rhabd/o	răb-dō	rod

Continued on the following page(s)

English Meanings of Medical Word Elements *Continued*

MEDICAL WORD ELEMENT	PRONUNCIATION	MEANING
rhabdomy/o	răb-dō-mī-ō	striated (skeletal) muscle
rhin/o	rī-nō	nose
-rrhage	rĭj	burst forth (of)
-rrhagia	ră-jē-ăh	burst forth (of)
-rrhaphy	ră-fē	suture
-rrhea	rē-ăh	discharge, flow
-rrhexis	rek-sĭs	rupture
rube/o	roo-bē-ō	red
salping/o	săl-pĭn-gō/săl-pĭn-jō	fallopian tubes, oviducts, uterine tubes, eustachian tube
-salpinx	săl-pĭnks	fallopian tubes, oviducts, uterine tubes
sarc/o	săr-kō	flesh
scirrh/o	skĭr-rō	hard
scler/o	sklĕ-rō	sclera, hard
-sclerosis	sklĕ-rō-sĭs	abnormal condition (of) hardening
-scope	skōp	instrument to view or examine
-scopy	skō-pē	visual examination
seb/o	sĕb-ō	sebum
semi-	sĕm-ē	half, partial
sial/o	sī-ăh-lō	saliva, salivary gland
sider/o	sĭd-ĕr-ō	iron
sigmoid/o	sĭg-moi-dō	sigmoid colon

sinistr/o	sĭn-ĭs-trō	left
sinus/o	sī-nŭs-ō	sinus, cavity
somat/o	sō-măt-ō	body
-spasm	spăzm	involuntary contraction, twitching
spermat/o	spĕr-mah-tō	sperm
spher/o	sfē-rō	globe, round
sphincter/o	sfĭngk-tĕr-ō	sphincter
sphygm/o	sfĭg-mō	pulse
spir/o	spī-rō	breathe
splen/o	splē-nō	spleen
spondyl/o	spŏn-dĭ-lō	vertebrae, backbone
squam/o	skwā-mō	scale
staped/o	stă-pē-dō	stapes
-stasis	stā-sĭs	standing still, control, stop
steat/o	stē-ă-tō	fat, fatty
-stenosis	stē-nō-sĭs	constriction, narrowing
stern/o	stĕr-nō	sternum, breastbone
steth/o	stĕth-ō	chest
stomat/o	stō-mah-tō	mouth
-stomy	stō-mē	mouth, forming a new opening
sub-	sŭb	under, beneath, below
super-	soo-pĕr	above
supra-	soo-prah	above
sym-	sĭm	union, together
syn-	sĭn	union, together
tachy-	tăk-ē	rapid
-taxia	tăk-sē-ah	muscular coordination

Continued on the following page(s)

English Meanings of Medical Word Elements *Continued*

MEDICAL WORD ELEMENT	PRONUNCIATION	MEANING
ten/o	tĕn-ō	tendon
tend/o	tĕnd-ō	tendon
tendin/o	tĕn-dĭn-ō	tendon
-tension	tĕn-shŭn	pressure
test/o	tĕs-tō	testes
thalam/o	thăl-ăh-mō	thalamus, chamber
thel/o	thē-lō	nipple
-therapy	thĕr-ăh-pē	treatment
therm/o	thĕr-mō	heat
thorac/o	thō-rah-kō	chest
-thorax	thō-răks	chest
thromb/o	thrŏm-bō	clot
thrombocyt/o	thrŏm-bō-sī-tō	platelet, thrombocyte
thym/o	thī-mō	thymus
thyr/o	thī-rō	thyroid
thyroid/o	thī-roi-dō	thyroid
tibi/o	tĭb-ē-ō	tibia
-tic	tĭk	pertaining to
-tocia	tō-sē-ah	childbirth, labor
-tome	tōm	instrument to cut
-tomy	tō-mē	incision, cut into
ton/o	tŏn-ō	tone

Term	Pronunciation	Meaning
tonsill/o	tŏn-sĭl-lō	tonsil
-toxic	tŏks-ĭk	poison
tox/o	tŏks-ō	poison
trache/o	trā-kē-ō	trachea
trans-	trănz	through, across
trich/o	trĭk-ō	hair
tri-	trī	three
-tripsy	trĭp-sē	crush
-trophy	trō-fē	nourishment, development
-tropia	trō-pē-ah	turning
-tropin	trō-pĭn	stimulate
tympan/o	tĭm-pah-nō	tympanic membrane, eardrum
-ula	ūlā	small, little, minute
-ule	yool	small, little, minute
ultra-	ul-trah	beyond, excess
ungu/o	ŭng-gwō	nail
uni-	yoo-nē	one
ur/o	ū-rō	urine
ureter/o	ū-rē-tĕr-ō	ureter
urethr/o	ū-rē-thrō	urethra
-uria	ū-rē-ah	urine
uter/o	ū-tĕr-ō	uterus, womb
vagin/o	vă-jĭn-ō	vagina
vas/o	vah-sō	vas deferens, vessel
ven/o	vē-nō	vein
ventricul/o	vĕn-trĭk-ū-lō	ventricles, little belly

Continued on the following page(s)

English Meanings of Medical Word Elements *Continued*

MEDICAL WORD ELEMENT	PRONUNCIATION	MEANING
ventr/o	vĕn-trō	belly, belly-side
venul/o	vĕn-ū-lō	venule
vertebr/o	vĕr-tĕ-brō	vertebrae, backbone
vesic/o	vĕs-ĭ-kō	bladder
vesicul/o	vĕ-sĭk-ū-lō	seminal vesicle
viscer/o	vĭs-ĕr-ō	organ
vulv/o	vŭl-vō	vulva
xanth/o	zăn-thō	yellow
xer/o	zē-rō	dry
-y	ē	condition, process

Adapted from Gylys, BA and Wedding, ME: Medical Terminology, ed. 2. FA Davis, Philadelphia, 1989, p. 426.

Medical Word Elements for English Terms

ENGLISH TERM	MEDICAL WORD ELEMENT	PRONUNCIATION
abdomen	celi/o	sē-lē-ō
	lapar/o	lăp-ăr-ō
abdominal wall	lapar/o	lăp-ăr-ō
abnormal	para-	păr-ăh
abnormal condition	-iasis	ī-ă-sĭs
(of)	-osis	ō-sĭs
	-sclerosis	sklĕ-rō-sĭs
above	hyper-	hī-per
	super-	soo-per
	supra-	soo-prah
acromion	acromi/o	ă-krō-mē-ō
across	-dia	dē-ăh
	trans-	trănz
adenoid	adenoid/o	ăd-ē-noid-ō
adrenal glands	adren/o	ăd-rē-nō
	adrenal/o	ă-drĕn-ăl-ō
after	infra-	ĭn-frăh
	meta-	mĕt-ăh
	post-	pōst
	postero-	pōs-ter-ō
	retro-	rĕt-rō

Continued on the following page(s)

893

Medical Word Elements for English Terms *Continued*

ENGLISH TERM	MEDICAL WORD ELEMENT	PRONUNCIATION
against	anti-	ăn-tĭ
	contra-	kŏn-trăh
air	pneum/o	nū-mō
	pneumat/o	nū-măh-tō
	pneumon/o	nū-mŏn-ō
albumin	albumin/o	ăl-bū-mĭn-ō
alkaline	bas/o	bā-sō
all	pan-	păn
alveolus (pl. alveoli)	alveol/o	ăl-vē-ōl-ō
anterior	anter/o	ăn-ter-ō
anus	an/o	ā-nō
	proct/o	prŏk-tō
aorta	aort/o	ā-or-tō
arm	brachi/o	brăk-ē-ō
around	circum-	sĕr-kŭm
	peri-	pĕr-ĭ
arteriole	arteriol/o	ar-tĕr-ĭ-ōl-ō
artery (little)	arteriol/o	ar-tĕr-ĭ-ōl-ō
atrium	atri/o	ā-trē-ō
attraction for	-phil	fĭl
	-philia	fĭl-ē-ăh

English	Combining form	Pronunciation
away from	ab-	ăb
back	dors/o	dor-sō
backbone	poster/o	pŏs-tĕr-ō
	spondyl/o	spŏn-dĭl-ō
	vertebr/o	vĕr-tĕ-brō
backward	post-	pōst
	postero-	pŏs-tĕr-ō
	retro-	rĕt-rō
backward	bacteri/o	băk-tē-rē-ō
bacteria	dys-	dĭs
bad	mal-	măl
basic	bas/o	bā-sō
before	ante-	ăn-tē
	anter/o	ăn-tĕr-ō
	pre-	prē
	pro-	prō
beginning	-arche	ăr-kē
beginning process	-genesis	jĕn-ĕ-sĭs
behind	post-	pōst
	postero-	pŏs-tĕr-ō
	retro-	rĕt-rō
belly	celi/o	sē-lē-ō
	ventr/o	vĕn-trō
belly-side	ventr/o	vĕn-trō
below	hypo-	hī-pō
	infra-	ĭn-frăh
	sub-	sŭb

Continued on the following page(s)

Medical Word Elements for English Terms *Continued*

ENGLISH TERM	MEDICAL WORD ELEMENT	PRONUNCIATION
beneath	hypo-	hī·pō
	infra-	ĭn·frah
	sub-	sŭb
beside	para-	păr·ăh
between	inter-	ĭn·tĕr
beyond	hyper-	hī·pĕr
	meta-	mĕt·ah
	para-	păr·ăh
	ultra-	ŭl·trah
bile	chol/e	kō·lē
bile duct	choledoch/o	kō·lē·dō·kō
bile vessel	cholangi/o	kō·lăn·jē·ō
biliary system	bil/i	bĭl·ē
binding	-desis	dē·sĭs
birth	nat/a	nā·tă
black	melan/o	mĕl·ah·nō
bladder	cyst/o	sĭs·tō
	vesic/o	vĕs·ĭ·kō
blood	hem/o	hēm·ō
	hemat/o	hēm·ăh·tō
blood condition (of)	-emia	ē·mē·ăh

Term	Combining form	Pronunciation
blood vessel	hemangi/o	hē-mǎn-jē-ō
blue	cyan/o	sī-ǎn-ō
body	somat/o	sō-mǎt-ō
bone	oste/o	ǒs-tē-ō
bone marrow	myel/o	mī-ě-lō
borne	-phoresis	fō-rē-sǐs
both	ambi-	ǎm-bǐ
both sides	ambi-	ǎm-bǐ
brain	encephal/o	ěn-sěf-ah-lō
brain covering	mening/o	mě-nǐng-gō
	meningi/o	mě-nǐn-jē-ō
break down	-lysis	lǐ-sǐs
breaking of	-clasis	klǎh-sǐs
breast	mamm/o	mǎ-mō
	mast/o	mǎs-tō
breastbone	stern/o	stěr-nō
breathe	pneumat/o	nū-mǎh-tō
	spir/o	spī-rō
breathing	-pnea	nē-ah
bronchus (pl. bronchi)	bronch/o	brǒng-kō
	bronchi/o	brǒng-kē-ō
burst forth (of)	-rrhage	rǐj
	-rrhagia	rā-jē-ǎh
calcaneum	calcane/o	kǎl-kā-nē-ō
calcium	calc/o	kǎl-kō
calculus	-lith	lǐth
cancer	carcin/o	kǎr-sǐn-ō

Continued on the following page(s)

Medical Word Elements for English Terms *Continued*

ENGLISH TERM	MEDICAL WORD ELEMENT	PRONUNCIATION
carbon dioxide, CO_2	-capnia	kăp-nē-ah
carpus	carp/o	kăr-pō
carried	-phoresis	fō-rē-sĭs
cartilage	chondr/o	kŏn-drō
cavity(ies)	-porosis	pō-rō-sĭs
	sinus/o	sī-nŭs-ō
cell	cyt/o	sī-tō
cerebellum	cerebell/o	sĕr-ē-bĕl-lō
cerebrum	cerebr/o	sĕr-ē-brō
cervix	cervic/o	sĕr-vĭ-kō
chamber	thalam/o	thăl-ăh-mō
change	meta-	mĕt-ah
cheek	bucc/o	bŭk-ō
chemical	chem/o	kē-mō
chest	pector/o	pĕk-tō-rō
	steth/o	stĕth-ō
	thorac/o	thŏr-ăh-kō
	-thorax	thō-răks
childbirth	-tocia	tō-sē-ăh
choroid	choroid/o	kō-roid-ō
clot	thromb/o	thrŏm-bō

ciliary body	cycl/o	sī-klō
coal	anthrac/o	ăn-thrah-kō
cold	cry/o	krī-ō
colon	col/o	kō-lō
color	-chrome	krōm
	chrom/o	krōm-ō
condition (of)	-ia	ē-ah
	-iasis	ī-ă-sĭs
	-ism	ĭzm
	-y	ē
condition of calculi	-lithiasis	lĭth-ī-ăh-sĭs
condyle	condyl/o	kŏn-dĭ-lō
constriction	-stenosis	stĕ-nō-sĭs
contraction, involuntary	-spasm	spăzm
control	-stasis	stā-sĭs
cornea	corne/o	kōr-nē-nō
	kerat/o	kĕr-ah-tō
correct measure	emmetr/o	ĕm-ĕ-trō
cranium	crani/o	krā-nē-ō
crush	-tripsy	trĭp-sē
cut into	-tomy	tō-mē
dawn-colored	eosin/o	ē-ō-sĭn-ō
decrease	-penia	pē-nē-ăh
deficiency	-penia	pē-nē-ăh
destroy	-lysis	lĭ-sĭs
development	-plasia	plā-zē-ăh
	-plasm	plăzm

Continued on the following page(s)

899

Medical Word Elements for English Terms *Continued*

ENGLISH TERM	MEDICAL WORD ELEMENT	PRONUNCIATION
diaphragm	-trophy	trō-fē
different	phren/o	frĕn-ō
difficult	heter/o	hĕt-ĕr-ō
digit (finger or toe)	dys-	dis
dilation	dactyl/o	dăk-tĭ-lō
dim	-ectasis	ĕk-tăh-sĭs
discharge	ambly/o	ăm-blē-ō
discharge of pus	-rrhea	rē-ah
disease	-pyorrhea	pī-ō-re-ah
distant	-pathy	păh-thē
double	dist/o	dĭs-tō
dropping	diplo-	dĭp-lō
drug	-ptosis	tō-sĭs
dry	chem/o	kē-mō
	ichthy/o	ĭk-thē-ō
	xer/o	zē-rō
dull	ambly/o	ăm-blē-ō
duodenum	duoden/o	dū-ŏd-ē-nō
dust	coni/o	kō-nē-ō
ear	ot/o	ō-tō
eardrum	myring/o	mē-rĭng-gō

	tympan/o	tĭm-păh-nō
easy	eu-	ū
eat	phag/o	făg-ō
eating	-phagia	fā-jē-ăh
egg	oo/o	ō-ō
elderly	presby/o	prĕz-bē-ō
embolus	embol/o	ĕm-bŏl-ō
embryonic	-blast	blăst
	blast/o	blăs-tō
enlargement	-megaly	mĕg-ăh-lē
epididymis	epididym/o	ĕp-ĭ-dĭd-i-mō
epiglottis	epiglott/o	ĕp-ĭ-glŏt-ō
equal	is/o	ī-sō
esophagus	esophag/o	ē-zŏf-ah-gō
eustachian tube	salping/o	săl-pĭn-gō/săl-pĭn-jō
examination, visual	-scopy	skō-pē
excess	ultra-	ŭl-trah
excessive	hyper-	hī-per
excision	-ectomy	ĕk-tō-mē
expansion	-ectasis	ĕk-tăh-sĭs
extremity	acr/o	ăk-rō
eye	ocul/o	ŏk-ū-lō
	ophthalm/o	ŏf-thăl-mō
	opt/o	ŏp-tō
eyelid	blephar/o	blĕf-ah-rō
falling	-ptosis	tō-sĭs
fallopian tubes	salping/o	săl-pĭng-gō

Continued on the following page(s)

Medical Word Elements for English Terms *Continued*

ENGLISH TERM	MEDICAL WORD ELEMENT	PRONUNCIATION
false	-salpinx	săl-pǐnks
fat	pseudo-	soo-dō
	adip/o	ăd-ǐ-pō
		lǐ-pō
fatty	steat/o	stē-ăh-tō
fatty degeneration	steat/o	stē-ăh-tō
fatty deposit	ather/o	ăth-ěr-ō
fear (of)	ather/o	ăth-ěr-ō
	-phobia	fō-bē-ăh
feeling	-esthesia	ěs-thē-zē-ah
female	gynec/o	gī-ně-kō
femur	femor/o	fěm-ō-rō
fibula	fibul/o	fǐb-ū-lō
finger	dactyl/o	dăk-tǐ-lō
first	primi-	prī-mǐ
fixation	-pexy	pěk-sē
flesh	sarc/o	săr-kō
flow	-rrhea	rē-ăh
foot	ped/i	pěd-ē
	pod/o	pō-dō
	-iasis	ī-ă-sǐs
formation	-plasia	plā-zē-ăh

	-plasm	plăzm
	-plasty	plăs-tē
	-poiesis	poi-ē-sĭs
formation of calculi	-lithiasis	lĭth-ĭ-ă-sĭs
forming a new opening	-stomy	stō-mē
four	quadri-	kwŏd
	quadri-	kwŏd-rĭ
from	ab-	ăb
front	anter/o	ăn-tēr-ō
fungus	myc/o	mī-kō
fungal infection	-mycosis	mī-kō-sĭs
fusion	-desis	dē-sĭs
gall	chol/e	kō-lē
gallbladder	cholecyst/o	kō-lē-sĭs-tō
ganglion (knot)	gangli/o	găng-glē-ō
	ganglion/o	găng-glē-ŏn-ō
germ cell	-blast	blăst
	blast/o	blăs-tō
gland	aden/o	ăd-ĕn-ō
glans penis	balan/o	băh-lăn-ō
globe	spher/o	sfē-rō
glomerulus	glomerul/o	glō-mĕr-ū-lō
glue	gli/o	glē-ō
good	eu-	ū
granule	granul/o	grăn-ū-lō
gray	glauc/o	glaw-kō
	polio-	pō-lē-ō

903

Continued on the following page(s)

Medical Word Elements for English Terms *Continued*

ENGLISH TERM	MEDICAL WORD ELEMENT	PRONUNCIATION
green	chlor/o	klōr-ō
growth	-physis	fī-sĭs
	-plasia	plā-zē-ăh
	-plasm	plăzm
gum	gingiv/o	jĭn-jĭ-vō
hair	pil/o	pī-lō
	trich/o	trĭk-ō
half	hemi-	hĕm-ē
	semi-	sĕm-ē
hard	kerat/o	kĕr-ăh-tō
	scirrh/o	skĭr-rō
	scler/o	sklē-rō
hardening	-sclerosis	sklē-rō-sĭs
head	cephal/o	sĕf-ăl-ō
hearing	audi/o	aw-dē-ō
	-cusis	kū-sĭs
heart	cardi/o	kăr-dē-ō
	coron/o	kōr-ō-nō
heat	therm/o	thĕr-mō
heavy	pachy/o	păk-ē-ō
heel bone	calcane/o	kăl-kă-nē-ō

hernia	-cele	sēl
hidden	crypt/o	krip-tō
horny, hornlike, horny substance	kerat/o	kĕr-ăh-tō
humerus	humer/o	hū-mĕr-ō
hydrochloric acid	-chlorhydria	klōr-hī-drē-ah
ileum	ile/o	ĭl-ē-ō
ilium	ili/o	ĭl-ē-ō
ill	mal-	măl
imperfect	atel/o	ăt-ē-lō
in	endo-	ĕn-dō
	intra-	ĭn-trah
in addition to	epi-	ĕp-ĭ
in front of	ante-	ăn-tē
	anter/o	ăn-tĕr-ō
	pre-	prē
	pro-	prō
incision	-tomy	tō-mē
incomplete	atel/o	ăt-ē-lō
increase	-osis	ō-sis
inflammation	-itis	ī-tis
ingesting	-phagia	fā-jē-ăh
inner ear	labyrinth/o	lăb-ĭ-rin-thō
instrument to cut	-tome	tōm
instrument for measuring	-meter	mē-tĕr
instrument to measure pressure	-manometer	măn-ŏm-ĕt-ĕr
instrument to view or examine	-scope	skōp
instrument used for recording	-graph	grăf

Continued on the following page(s)

905

Medical Word Elements for English Terms *Continued*

ENGLISH TERM	MEDICAL WORD ELEMENT	PRONUNCIATION
intestines	enter/o	ĕn-tĕr-ō
involuntary contraction	-spasm	spăzm
iris	ir/o	ĭr-ō
	irid/o	ĭr-ĭ-dō
iron	sider/o	sĭd-ĕr-ō
irregular	poikil/o	poi-kĭ-lō
ischium	ischi/o	ĭs-kē-ō
jejunum	jejun/o	jē-joo-nō
joint	arthr/o	ăr-thrō
kidney	nephr/o	nĕf-rō
	ren/o	rē-nō
kneecap	patell/o	pah-tĕl-ō
labor	-tocia	tō-sē-ah
labyrinth	labyrinth/o	lăb-ĭ-rĭn-thō
lack of	a-	ah
	an-	ăn
	ar-	ăr
	-penia	pē-nē-ăh

lamina	lamin/o	lăm-ĭ-nō
large	macro-	măk-rō
larynx	laryng/o	lah-rĭng-ō
left	sinistr/o	sĭn-ĭs-trō
lens	phak/o	fā-kō
lese	hypo-	hī-pō
likeness	home/o	hō-mē-ō
lip	cheil/o	kī-lō
little	labi/o	lā-bē-ō
	-icle	ĭk-ăl
	-ole	ōl
	-ula	ūlă
little	-ule	yool
little belly	ventricul/o	věn-trĭk-ū-lō
liver	hepat/o	hěp-ăh-tō
lobe	lob/o	lō-bō
loins	lumb/o	lŭm-bō
lung	pneum/o	nū-mō
	pneumon/o	nū-môn-ō
	pulmon/o	pŭl-môn-ō
lymph	lymph/o	lĭm-fō
lymph tissue	lymph/o	lĭm-fō
male	andr/o	ăn-drō
many	multi-	mŭl-tē
	poly-	pōl-ē
mass	onc/o	ông-kō
mastoid process	mastoid/o	măs-toi-dō

Continued on the following page(s)

907

Medical Word Elements for English Terms *Continued*

ENGLISH TERM	MEDICAL WORD ELEMENT	PRONUNCIATION
maze	labyrinth/o	lăb-ĭ-rĭn-thō
measure	-meter	mē-tĕr
measuring (act of)	-metry	mĕt-rē
medulla	medull/o	mĕd-ū-lō
meninges	mening/o	mē-nĭng-gō
	meningi/o	mē-nĭn-jē-ō
menses	men/o	mĕn-ō
menstruation	men/o	mĕn-ō
mesh (immature RBC)	reticul/o	rē-tĭk-ū-lō
metacarpus (bones of the hand)	metacarp/o	mĕt-ah-kăr-pō
middle	medi-	mē-dē
	mes/o-	mĕs-ō
	mid-	mid
milk	galact/o	gă-lăk-tō
	lact/o	lăk-tō
mind	phren/o	frĕn-ō
minute	-icle	ĭk-ăl
	-ole	ōl
	-ula	ū-lă
	-ule	yool
mouth	or/o	ŏr-ō

Meaning	Element	Pronunciation
	stomat/o	stō-mah-tō
	-stomy	stō-mē
movement	kinesi/o	kĭ-nē-sē-ō
	-kinesia	ki-nē-zē-ăh
much	multi-	mŭl-tē
	poly-	pŏl-ē
muscle	my/o	mī-ō
muscular coordination	-taxia	tăk-sē-ah
nail	onych/o	ŏn-ĭ-kō
	ungu/o	ŭng-gwō
narrowing	-stenosis	stē-nō-sĭs
near	ad-	ăd
	proxim/o	prŏk-sĭm-ō
neck	cervic/o	sĕr-vĭ-kō
nerve	neur/o	nū-rō
net (immature RBC)	reticul/o	rē-tĭk-ū-lō
neuron	neur/o	nū-rō
neutral dye	neutr/o	nū-trō
new	ne/o	nē-ō
night	noct/o	nŏk-tō
nipple-like protuberance or elevation	papill/o	păp-ĭ-lō
nipple	thel/o	thē-lō
nose	nas/o	nā-zō
	rhin/o	rī-nō
not	a-	ah
	an-	ăn
	ar-	ăr

Continued on the following page(s)

Medical Word Elements for English Terms *Continued*

ENGLISH TERM	MEDICAL WORD ELEMENT	PRONUNCIATION
	im-	ĭm
	in-	ĭn
nourishment	-trophy	trō-fē
nucleus	kary/o	kăr-ē-ō
	nucle/o	nū-klē-ō
old age	presby/o	prĕs-bē-ō
on both sides	amphi-	ăm-fī
one	mono-	mŏn-ō
	uni-	yoo-nē
one who	-er	ĕr
one who specializes	-ist	ĭst
organ	viscer/o	vĭs-ĕr-ō
origin	-genesis	gĕn-ĕ-sĭs
out	ec-	ĕk
	ex-	ĕks
out from	ec-	ĕk
	ex-	ĕks
	ecto-	ĕk-tō
outside	exo-	ĕks-ō
	extern/o	ĕks-tĕr-nō
	extra-	ĕks-trah

Term	Combining form	Pronunciation
ovary	oophor/o	ō-ŏf-ō-rō
over	ovari/o	ō-vār-ē-ō
	epi-	ĕp-ĭ
oviduct(s)	hyper-	hī-pĕr
	meta-	mĕt-ah
	salping/o	săl-pĭng-gō
	-salpinx	săl-pĭnks
ovum	oo/o	ō-ō
oxygen, O₂	ox/o	ŏks-ō
	oxy/o	ŏks-ĭ-ō
pain	-algesia	ăl-gē-sē-ah
	-algia	ăl-jē-ah
	-dynia	dĭn-ē-ah
pain	dys-	dĭs
painful		
pancreas	pancreat/o	păn-krē-ăt-ō
paralysis	-plegia	plē-jē-ah
paralysis, partial or incomplete	-paresis	pah-rē-sĭs
parathyroid glands	parathyroid/o	păr-ah-thī-roid-dō
partial	hemi-	hĕm-ē
	semi-	sĕm-ē
patella	patell/o	pah-tĕl-ō
pelvis	pelv/i	pĕl-vē
perineum	perine/o	pĕr-ĭ-nē-ō
peritoneum	peritone/o	pĕr-ĭ-tō-nē-ō
pertaining to	-ac	ăk
	-al	ăl
	-ar	ĕr
	-ary	ĕr-ē

Continued on the following page(s)

Medical Word Elements for English Terms *Continued*

ENGLISH TERM	MEDICAL WORD ELEMENT	PRONUNCIATION
	-ic	ĭk
	-ical	ĭk-ăl
	-ory	ŏr-ē
	-ous	ŭs
	-tic	tĭk
pertaining to a meal	-prandial	prăn-dē-ăl
phalanges (bones of fingers and toes)	phalang/o	făl-ăn-jō
pharynx	pharyng/o	făh-rǐng-gō
plastic repair	-plasty	plăs-tē
plate	-plakia	plăk-ē-ah
platelet	thrombocyt/o	thrŏm-bō-sĭ-tō
pleura	pleur/o	ploo-rō
plug	embol/o	ĕm-bōl-o
poison	-toxic	tŏks-ĭk
	tox/o	tŏks-ō
poor	mal-	măl
pores	-porosis	pō-rō-sĭs
posterior	poster/o	pŏs-tĕr-ō
pregnancy	-cyesis	sī-ē-sĭs
	-gravida	grăv-ĭ-dah

presence of calculi	-lithiasis	lĭth-ī-ă-sĭs
pressure	-tension	tĕn-shŭn
primitive	-blast	blăst
	blast/o	blăs-tō
process	-ia	ē-ăh
	-y	ē
production	-poiesis	poi-ē-sĭs
prolapse	-ptosis	tō-sĭs
prostate	prostat/o	prŏs-tăh-tō
protected	immun/o	ĭm-ū-nō
protection	-phylaxis	fĭ-lăk-sĭs
protein	-globin	glō-bĭn
pubis anterior	pub/o	pū-bō
pulse	sphygm/o	sfĭg-mō
pupil	cor/e	kō-rē
	core/o	kō-rē-ō
	pupill/o	pū-pĭ-lō
purple	purpur/o	pŭr-pū-rō
purulent discharge	-pyorrhea	pī-ō-rē-ah
pus	py/o	pī-ō
pylorus	pylor/o	pī-lō-rō
rapid	tachy-	tăk-ē
record	-gram	grăm
recording (instrument used for)	-graph	grăf
recording (process of)	-graphy	grȧ-fē
rectum	proct/o	prŏk-tō
	rect/o	rĕk-tō

Continued on the following page(s)

Medical Word Elements for English Terms *Continued*

ENGLISH TERM	MEDICAL WORD ELEMENT	PRONUNCIATION
red	eosin/o	ē-ŏ-sĭn-ō
	erythem/o	ĕr-ĭ-thē-mō
	erythr/o	ē-rĭth-rō
	rube/o	roo-bē-ō
red cell	erythrocyt/o	ē-rĭth-rō-sī-tō
refracture	-clasis	klăh-sis
relating to	-ac	ăk
	-al	ăl
	-ar	ĕr
	-ary	ĕr-ē
	-ic	ĭk
	-ical	ĭk-ăl
	-ory	ŏr-ē
	-ous	ŭs
	-tic	tĭk
removal	-ectomy	ĕk-tō-mē
renal pelvis	pyel/o	pī-ē-lō
resemblance	home/o	hō-mē-ō
resemble	-oid	oid
retina	retin/o	rĕt-ĭ-nō
ribs	cost/o	kŏs-tō

right	dextr/o	dĕks-trō
rod	rhabd/o	răb-dō
rosy	eosin/o	ē-ō-sĭn-ō
round	spher/o	sfē-rō
rupture	-rrhexis	rek-sĭs
sac of fluid	cyst/o	sĭs-tō
safe	immun/o	ĭm-ū-nō
saliva	sial/o	sī-ăh-lō
salivary gland	sial/o	sī-ăh-lō
same	homo-	hō-mō
scale	squam/o	skwā-mō
scaly	ichthy/o	ĭk-thē-ō
scanty	olig/o	ō-lĭg-ō
sclera	scler/o	sklē-rō
sebum	seb/o	sēb-ō
seizure	-lepsy	lĕp-sē
seminal vesicle	vesicul/o	vē-sĭk-ū-lō
sensation	-esthesia	ĕs-thē-zē-ah
separate	-lysis	lī-sĭs
sex glands	gonad/o	gō-năd-ō
shape	morph/o	mōr-fō
side	later/o	lăt-ĕr-ō
sigmoid colon	sigmoid/o	sĭg-moid-dō
sinus	sinus/o	sī-nŭs-ō
skeletal (striated) muscle	rhabdomy/o	răb-dō-mī-ō
skin	cutane/o	kū-tā-nē-ō
	derm/o	dĕr-mō

Continued on the following page(s)

915

Medical Word Elements for English Terms *Continued*

ENGLISH TERM	MEDICAL WORD ELEMENT	PRONUNCIATION
skull, skull bones	dermat/o	děr-mah-tō
	crani/o	krā-nē-ō
sleep	narc/o	năr-kō
slow	brady-	brăd-ē
small	-icle	ĭk-ăl
	-ole	ōl
	micro-	mī-krō
	-ula	ūlă
	-ule	yool
smell	-smia	ŏz-mē-ah
smooth (visceral) muscle	leiomy/o	lī-ō-mī-ō
softening	-malacia	mah-lā-shē-ăh
speech	-phasia	fā-zē-ăh
sperm	spermat/o	spěr-mah-tō
sphincter	sphincter/o	sfĭngk-těr-ō
spinal column	rach/o	răk-ō
	rachi/o	răk-ē-ō
spinal cord	myel/o	mī-ē-lō
spitting	-ptysis	tĭ-sĭs
spleen	splen/o	splē-nō
stabilization	-desis	dē-sĭs

standing still	-stasis	stā-sĭs
stapes	staped/o	stā-pē-dō
state of being	-ism	ĭzm
sternum	stern/o	stĕr-nō
stiff joint	ankyl/o	ăng-kĭ-lō
stimulate	-tropin	trō-pĭn
stomach	gastr/o	găs-trō
stone	-lith	lĭth
stop	-stasis	stā-sĭs
straight	orth/o	ŏr-thō
striated (skeletal) muscle	rhabdomy/o	răb-dō-mĭ-ō
stroke	-plegia	plē-jē-ăh
study of	-logy	lō-jē
sugar	gluc/o	gloo-kō
	glucos/o	gloo-kō-sō
	glyc/o	glī-kō
surgical puncture	-centesis	sĕn-tē-sĭs
surgical repair	-plasty	plăs-tē
suspension	-pexy	pĕk-sē
suture	-rrhaphy	răf-ē
swallow	phag/o	fāg-ō
swallowing	-phagia	fā-jē-ăh
sweat	hidr/o	hī-drō
sweetness	gluc/o	gloo-kō
	glyc/o	glī-kō
swelling	-cele	sēl

tawny cirrh/o sĭr-rō

Continued on the following page(s)

917

Medical Word Elements for English Terms *Continued*

ENGLISH TERM	MEDICAL WORD ELEMENT	PRONUNCIATION
tear	dacry/o	dăk-rē-ō
	lacrim/o	lăk-ri-mō
tear gland	dacryoaden/o	dăk-rē-ō-ăd-ĕn-ō
tendon	ten/o	tĕn-ō
	tend/o	tĕnd-ō
	tendin/o	tĕn-din-ō
testes	orch/o	ŏr-kō
	orchi/o	ŏr-kē-ō
	orchid/o	ŏr-ki-dō
	test/o	tĕs-tō
thalamus	thalam/o	thăl-ah-mō
thick	pachy/o	păk-ē-ō
thigh bone	femor/o	fĕm-ō-rō
thirst	-dipsia	dĭp-sē-ah
three	tri-	trī
throat	pharyng/o	făr-ing-ō
thrombocyte	thrombocyt/o	thŏm-bō-si-tō
through	-dia	dē-ah
	trans-	trănz
thymus	thym/o	thī-mō
thyroid	thyr/o	thī-rō

Term	Combining form / Affix	Pronunciation
tibia	thyroid/o	thī·roi·dō
tissue	tibi/o	tĭb·ē·ō
to	hist/o	hĭs·tō
to bear	ad-	ăd
to break	-para	păr·ah
to grow	-clast	klăst
to love	-physis	fĭ·sĭs
	-phil	fĭl
	-philia	fĭl·ē·ăh
to measure	-metry	-mĕt·rē
to produce	-gen	jĕn
to secrete	-crine	krĭn or krīn
to the left of	sinistr/o	sĭn·ĭs·trō
to the right of	dextr/o	dĕks·trō
	syn-	sĭn
toe	dactyl/o	dăk·tĭ·lō
together	sym-	sĭm
tone	ton/o	tōn·ō
tongue	gloss/o	glŏs·ō
	lingu/o	lĭng·gwō
tonsil	tonsill/o	tŏn·sĭ·lō
tooth	dent/o	dĕnt·ō
	odont/o	ō·dŏn·tō
toward	ad-	ăd
trachea	trache/o	trā·kē·ō
treatment	-therapy	thĕr·ăh·pē
tumor	-oma	ō·măh
	onc/o	ŏng·kō

Continued on the following page(s)

ENGLISH TERM	MEDICAL WORD ELEMENT	PRONUNCIATION
turning	-tropia	trō-pē-ah
twitching	-spasm	spăzm
two	bi-	bī
	di-	dī
tympanic membrane	myring/o	mē-rĭng-gō
	tympan/o	tĭm-pah-nō
under	hypo-	hī-pō
	infra-	ĭn-frăh
	sub-	sŭb
union	sym-	sĭm
	syn-	sĭn
upon	epi-	ĕp-ĭ
ureter	ureter/o	ū-rē-tĕr-ō
urethra	urethr/o	ū-rē-thrō
urine	ur/o	ū-rō
	-uria	ū-rē-ah
uterine tubes	salping/o	săl-pĭng-gō
	-salpinx	săl-pĭnks
uterus	hyster/o	hĭs-tĕr-ō
	metr/o	mĕ-trō

	uter/o	ū-tĕr-ō
vagina	colp/o	kŏl-pō
	vagin/o	vă-jĭn-ō
varied	poikil/o	poi-kĭl-lō
vas deferens	vas/o	vah-sō
vein	phleb/o	flĕb-ō
	ven/o	vē-nō
ventricles	ventricul/o	vĕn-trĭk-ū-lō
venule	venul/o	vĕn-ū-lō
vertebrae	rach/o	răk-ō
	rachi/o	răk-ē-ō
	spondyl/o	spŏn-dĭ-lō
	vertebr/o	vĕr-tĕ-brō
vessel	angi/o	ăn-jē-ō
	vas/o	vă-zō
vision	-opia	ō-pē-ah
	-opsia	ŏp-sē-ah
visual examination	-scopy	skō-pē
voice	-phonia	fō-nē-ah
vomit	-emesis	ĕ-mĕ-sĭs
vulva	episi/o	ĕ-pĭz-ē-ō
	vulv/o	vŭl-vō
water	aque/o	ă-kwē-ō
	hydr/o	hī-drō
white	leuc/o	loo-kō
	leuk/o	loo-kō

Continued on the following page(s)

921

| Medical Word Elements for English Terms *Continued* | | |

ENGLISH TERM	MEDICAL WORD ELEMENT	PRONUNCIATION
white cell	leukocyt/o	loo-kō-sī-tō
white protein	albumin/o	ăl-bŭ-mĭn-ō
within	endo-	ĕn-dō
without	intra-	ĭn-trah
	a-	ah
	an-	ăn
	ar-	ăr
without granules	agranul/o	ā-grăn-ū-lō
without strength	-asthenia	ăs-thē-nē-ăh
woman	gynec/o	gī-nĕ-kō
womb	hyster/o	hĭs-ter-ō
	metr/o	mĕ-trō
wrist	uter/o	ū-tĕr-ō
a writing	carp/o	kar-pō
	-gram	grăm
yellow	cirrh/o	sĭr-rō
	xanth/o	zăn-thō

Reference

1. Gylys, BA and Wedding, ME: Medical Terminology: A Systems Approach, ed 2. FA Davis, Philadelphia, 1988.

KÜBLER-ROSS'S STAGES OF DYING

In 1969 Dr. Elisabeth Kübler-Ross published *On Death and Dying*. Since that date the renewed interest in the field of thanatology has led to many theories and models from dozens of volumes. However, in Kübler-Ross's first work, she described five stages of dying. They are not universally accepted but are an excellent conceptual model that can be used when working with terminal patients.

First Stage: Denial and Isolation

In this early period, patients may attempt to deny the diagnosis, shop for other doctors, or simply believe that they will defy the prognosis. Kübler-Ross considers it a healthy stage with great value as a buffer against the sudden realization of impending death. The isolation may arise from our inability to deal with such a person or their lack of desire to face challenges to the denial.

Second Stage: Anger

To understand this stage, Kübler-Ross suggests imagining how we would feel if all our plans and all our dreams collapsed, we were denied a future that we had saved for, or we were denied the chance to finish raising our children. The anger is coupled with resentment and may be expressed toward anyone near the patient. Anger may be most severe in patients who have had a lot of control over their lives. For them, the loss of control may be equally as disastrous as the death to come.

Third Stage: Bargaining

This is the period when the patient may attempt to deal with the medical team or supernatural forces. Kübler-Ross compares it to the childhood habit of seeking favors or privileges by swearing to be good, doing the dishes, or never hitting someone again. In a very real sense the child, like the patient, tries to gain control by offering something. In this stage patients may bargain for time, the use of body parts, or for life itself. The stage may be especially significant if patients reveal an inner guilt about themselves. It may be during this period that patients show that they will give up a behavior for which they feel they are now being punished.

Fourth Stage: Depression

This stage sets in as the patient realizes loss. Life is not what it was before the illness and never will be again. If accompanied by guilt and shame, this can be especially painful. Kübler-Ross suggests that it may be possible to alleviate some of the guilt and shame, when unrealistic, but otherwise this is a step toward acceptance. Depression, she says, may be functional and should not be denied by attempts to "look at the sunny side." Expressions of sorrow may be vital so that a patient may enter the final stage.

Fifth Stage: Acceptance

Kübler-Ross says that those who have been given help through the previous stages will arrive at acceptance. They have expressed sorrow and anger and can now deal with the fate ahead. This, she says, is marked by a period of quiet expectation, during which the patient is tired and rests frequently. It is compared to the sleep of a newborn, but in reverse. As the patient finds peace and acceptance, there may be withdrawal from previous interests. Kübler-Ross says that some — a few — never reach this stage and fight to the end. She says that such patients reach a point where they can no longer fight; although they might never peacefully accept, they too reach a point of giving in.

Reference

1. Kübler-Ross, E: On Death and Dying. MacMillan, New York, 1970.

alternate forms reliability (parallel forms reliability): *bility*.

assessment: To measure, quantify, or place a value upon something; often confused with *evaluation* (see *evaluation*).

attribute: A variable; a quality that is measured.

classification (categorization): Assignment of an entity to a group. Assignment must be based on rules; groups must be defined so that they allow all entities to belong to a group (classes or categories are exhaustive) and only one possible group (classes or categories are mutually exclusive).

clinical decision making: Determinations made that relate to direct patient care, indirect patient care, acceptance of patients for treatment, and whether patients should be referred to other practitioners. (This definition is modified from that presented by Charles Magistro at a conference on Clinical Decision Making held under APTA auspices in October 1988 in Lakes of the Ozarks, Missouri.) Diagnoses are a form of clinical decision making. When direct supporting evidence for a clinical decision is lacking, such decisions are based on clinical opinions.

clinical opinion: The belief or idea that a professional holds regarding a patient. This opinion may be based on the use of tests and measurements but cannot be directly supported by evidence relating to those tests and measurements. Clinical opinions should be based on the therapist's evaluation of all available information; clinical decisions based on a therapist's synthesis of information are based on clinical opinions.

concurrent validity: See *validity*.

construct: A concept that has been developed for the purpose of measurement. Support for the construct is through logical argumentation based on theoretical and research evidence.

construct validity: See *validity*.

content validity: See *validity*.

criterion-based (related) validity: See *validity*.

data: Synonymous with measurements (see *measurement*).

derived measurement: A measurement that is obtained as the result of a mathematical operation.

evaluation: A judgment based on a measurement; often confused with assessment and examination (see *assessment* and *examination*).

examination: A test or a battery of tests used for the purpose of obtaining data (see *assessment* and *evaluation*).

false negatives: The number of persons who test negatively for some attribute but in fact have that attribute (see *true negative*).

false positives: The number of persons who test positively for some attribute but in fact do not have that attribute (see *true positive*).

instrument: A machine, questionnaire, or any device that is used as part of a test to obtain a measurement.

intertester reliability: See *reliability*.

intratester: See *reliability*.

measure: The act of obtaining a measurement (data).

measurement: The numeral assigned to an object or event or the classification (categorization) of objects, events, or persons according to rules.

normalization: A process that yields a new measurement that is mathematically derived to change the distribution of measurements.

objective measurement: A measurement that is not affected by some aspect of the person obtaining the measurement; the opposite of a subjective measurement (see *subjective measurement*).

operational definition: a set of procedures that guides the process of obtaining a measurement. It should include descriptions of the conditions under which a measurement can be taken, what attributes of an entity are measured, and what actions must be taken in order to obtain the measurement.

parallel (alternate) forms reliability: See *reliability*.

practicality of a test: The usefulness of a test based on issues relating to personnel, time, equipment, cost of administration, and impact on the person taking a test.

predictive validity: See *validity*.

predictive value of a measurement: The degree of certainty that can be associated with a positive or negative finding. The predictive value of a positive measurement is the ratio formed by dividing the number of true positives by all positive findings; the predictive value of a negative measurement is the ratio formed by dividing the number of true negatives by the number of all negative findings.

prescriptive validity: See *validity*.

primary purveyor: See *purveyor*.

purveyor: Any person or organization that offers or promotes the use of a test or any person or organization that develops a test.

> **primary purveyor:** Persons who promote or require the use of tests. This includes persons within clinical institutions who require the use of specific tests. Persons who conduct continuing education courses in which a major component involves the advo-

cacy of the use of specific testing procedures are primary purveyors. Persons who sell instruments that may be used for testing but who do not describe or advocate specific testing procedures are not purveyors (see *purveyor, secondary purveyor,* and *tertiary purveyor*). Any person or organization that offers or promotes the use of a test by selling testing equipment, manuals, books, or similar materials is a primary purveyor. In the case of books that serve as test manuals, the primary purveyor is the author.

secondary purveyor: Any researcher or other person who publishes a scholarly work that examines aspects of tests and who in that scholarly work suggests (advocates) that a test be used (see *tertiary purveyor*).

tertiary purveyor: Any person who teaches or prepares instructional material that describes specific tests or specific uses of measurements. This includes, but is not limited to, persons teaching in academic institutions, clinical educators, and continuing educators who are not acting in the role of primary or secondary purveyors.

reactivity: The degree to which the process of taking a test affects a measurement or other measurements in the future or otherwise affects the person taking the test.

reliability: The consistency of a measurement; the repeatability of measurements; the degree to which measurements are error-free.

intertester reliability: The consistency of measurements when more than one person takes measurements; indicates agreement or consistency of measurements taken by different examiners.

intratester reliability: The consistency of measurements when one person takes repeated measurements separated in time; indicates stability (reliability) over time.

parallel (alternate) forms reliability: The consistency or agreement of measurements obtained with different forms of a test; indicates whether measurements obtained with different tests can be used interchangeably.

score (grade): The numeric (quantitative) or verbal (qualitative) descriptor used to characterize the results of a test. A score is a measurement (see *measurement*).

secondary purveyor: See *purveyor*.

sensitivity of a test: An indication of how well a test identifies people who should have a positive finding. The numerical representation of this is a ratio formed by taking the number of persons with true-positive response on a test and dividing this number by the number of persons who should have had a positive response (i.e., the number of persons who are known to have properties that would indicate that they should test positive).

specificity of a test: An indication of how well a test identifies people who should have a negative finding. The numerical representation of this is a ratio formed by taking the number of persons with a true-negative response on a test and dividing this number by the number of persons who should have had a negative response (i.e., the number of persons who are known to have properties that would indicate that they should test negative).

standardization: A process by which a score is converted (transformed) into another score by using measures of central tendency and variability; a commonly used standardization (transformation) is the z-score.

subjective measurement: A measurement that is affected by some aspect of the person obtaining the measurement; the opposite of an objective measurement (see *objective measurement*).

tertiary purveyor: See *purveyor*.

test: A procedure or set of procedures that is used to obtain measurements (data). The procedures may require the use of instruments.

test manual: A booklet prepared by a primary test purveyor. It guides the process of obtaining a measurement and provides documentation and justification for the test.

test setting: Environment in which a test is given. It refers to the physical setting and the characteristics of that setting.

test user: One who chooses tests, interprets scores, or makes decisions based on test scores. (This definition is from Standards for Educational and Psychological Tests. American Psychological Association, Washington, DC, 1974, page 1.)

transformation of data: The use of standardization or normalization procedures for the purpose of changing the value or distribution of a measurement.

true negatives: The number of persons who test negatively for some attribute and who do not have that attribute (see *false negatives*).

true positives: The number of persons who test positively for some attribute and who have that attribute (see *false positives*).

validity: The degree to which a useful interpretation can be inferred from a measurement.

> **concurrent validity:** A form of criterion-based validity in which an inference is justified by comparing a measurement to supporting evidence that was obtained at approximately the same time.

> **construct validity:** The conceptual (theoretical) basis for using a measurement to make inferences. Evidence for construct validity is

through logical argumentation based on theoretical and research evidence.

content validity: A form of validity that deals with the extent to which a measurement reflects all the meaningful elements of a construct and no extraneous elements.

criterion-based (related) validity: Three forms of criterion-based validity exist: concurrent validity, predictive validity, and prescriptive validity. The common element is that with each of these forms of validity the correctness of an inference can be tested by comparing a measurement with either a different measurement or data obtained by other forms of testing.

predictive validity: A form of criterion-based validity in which an inference is justified by comparing a measurement to supporting evidence that is obtained at a later point in time; examines the justification of using a measurement to say something about future events or conditions.

prescriptive validity: A form of criterion-based validity in which the inference of a measurement is justified based on the successful determination of the type of treatment a person will receive. The inference is justified based on the outcome of the chosen treatment.

SYMPTOMS AND SIGNS OF DRUG ABUSE*†

DRUG	ACUTE INTOXICATION AND OVERDOSE	WITHDRAWAL SYNDROME
CNS Stimulants: Cocaine, amphetamine, dextroamphetamine, methylphenidate, phenmetrazine, phenylpropanolamine, STP‡, MDMA§, Bromo-DMA‖, diethylpropion, most amphetaminelike antiobesity drugs	*Vital signs:* temperature elevated; heart rate increased; respirations shallow; BP elevated. *Mental status:* sensorium hyperacute or confused; paranoid ideation; hallucinations; delirium; impulsivity; agitation; hyperactivity; sterotypy. *Physical Exam:* pupils dilated and reactive; tendon reflexes hyperactive; cardiac arrhythmias; dry mouth; sweating; tremors; convulsions; coma; stroke.	Muscular aches; abdominal pain; chills, tremors; voracious hunger; anxiety; prolonged sleep: lack of energy; profound depression, sometimes suicidal; exhaustion
Opioids: heroin, morphine, codeine, meperidine, methadone, hydromorphone, opium, pentazocine, propoxyphene, fentanyl, sufentanil	*Vital signs:* temperature decreased; respiration depressed; BP decreased, sometimes shock. *Mental status:* euphoria; stupor. *Physical exam:* pupils constricted (may be dilated with meperidine or extreme hypoxia); reflexes diminished to absent; pulmonary edema; constipation; convulsions with propoxyphene or meperidine; cardiac arrhythmias with propoxyphene; coma.	Pupils dilated; pulse rapid; gooseflesh; lacrimation; abdominal cramps; muscle jerks; "flu" syndrome; vomiting; diarrhea; tremulousness; yawning; anxiety

CNS depressants: barbiturates, benzodiazepines, glutethimide, meprobamate, methaqualone, ethchlorvynol, chloral hydrate, methyprylon, paraldehyde	*Vital signs:* respiration depressed; BP decreased, sometimes shock. *Mental status:* drowsiness or coma; confusion; delirium. *Physical exam:* pupils dilated with glutethimide or in severe poisoning; tendon reflexes depressed; slurred speech; nystagmus; convulsions or hyperirritability with methaqualone; signs of anticholinergic poisoning with glutethimide; cardiac arrhythmias with chloral hydrate.	Tremulousness; insomnia; sweating; fever; clonic blink reflex; anxiety; cardiovascular collapse; agitation; delirium; hallucinations; disorientation; convulsions; shock
Hallucinogens: LSD**, psilocybin, mescaline, PCP‡‡	*Vital signs:* temperature elevated; heart rate increased; BP elevated. *Mental status:* euphoria; anxiety or panic; paranoia; sensorium often clear; affect inappropriate; illusions; time and visual distortions; visual hallucinations; depersonalization; with PCP hypertensive encephalopathy. *Physical exam:* pupils dilated (normal or small with PCP); tendon reflexes hyperactive; with PCP cyclic coma or extreme hyperactivity, drooling, blank stare, mutism, amnesia, analgesia, nystagmus (sometimes vertical), gait	None

931

Continued on the following page(s)

SYMPTOMS AND SIGNS OF DRUG ABUSE*† *Continued*

DRUG	ACUTE INTOXICATION AND OVERDOSE	WITHDRAWAL SYNDROME
	ataxia, muscle rigidity, impulsive or violent behavior; violent, scatological, pressured speech.	
Cannabis group: marijuana, hashish, THC‡‡; hash oil, sinsemilla	*Vital signs:* heart rate increased; BP decreased on standing. *Mental status:* anorexia, then increased appetite; euphoria; anxiety; sensorium often clear; dreamy; fantasy state; time-space distortions; hallucinations may be rare. *Physical exam:* pupils unchanged; conjunctiva injected; tachycardia, ataxia, and pallor in children.	Nonspecific symptoms including anorexia, nausea, insomnia, restlessness, irritability, anxiety, depression
Anticholinergics: atropine, belladonna, henbane, scopolamine, trihexyphenidyl, benztropine mesylate, procyclidine, propantheline bromide; jimson weed seed	*Vital signs:* temperature elevated; heart rate increased; possibly decreased BP. *Mental status:* drowsiness or coma; sensorium clouded; amnesia; disorientation; visual hallucinations; body image alterations; confusion; with propantheline restlessness, excitement. *Physical exam:* pupils	Gastrointestinal and musculoskeletal symptoms

dilated and fixed; decreased bowel sounds; flushed, dry skin and mucous membranes; violent behavior, convulsions; with propantheline circulatory failure, respiratory failure, paralysis, coma.

*Mixed intoxications produce complex combinations of signs and symptoms.
†From The Medical Letter, Vol. 29, Sept. 11, 1987, with permission.
‡STP (2,5-dimethoxy-4-methylamphetamine)
§MDMA (3,4-methylenedioxymethamphetamine)
¶Bromo-DMA (4-Bromo-2,5-dimethoxyamphetamine)
**LSD (D-lysergic acid diethylamide)
††PCP (phencyclidine)
‡‡THC (delta-9-tetrahydrocannabinol)
From the Medical Letter, Vol. 29, Sept. 11, 1987, with permission.

RESOURCE PHONE NUMBERS: HELPLINES
(listed by disability or disease alphabetically)

The telephone numbers and addresses listed are subject to periodic change. All hours listed are Eastern Standard Time. Information and referral services are indicated by *I&R*.

Acne
800-235-ACNE (M–F 10–8)
  Acne Research Center: Information on acne and its treatment.

AIDS
(also see *AIDS* section in this book) 800-342-AIDS (24 hr)
  Public Health Service: Information on history and prevention.

Alcohol
800-ALCOHOL (24 hr)
  Doctor's Hospital of Worcester: Alcohol and drug counseling I&R

Alzheimer's Disease
800-621-0379; 800-572-6037 in IL (M–F 9–5)
  Alzheimer's Disease and Related Disorders Association: Local chapter and support group referral. Information about publications.

Anorexia
(201) 836-1800
  American Anorexia/Bulimia Association, Inc.
(614) 436-1112
  National Anorexic Aid Society, Inc.

Blind
800-424-8666 (M–F 9–5)
  American Council of the Blind: I&R on issues of visually impaired; publications; advice on legal questions Electronic Reading (Optacon): (415) 493-2626
  Free cassettes: 800-221-4792, (609) 452-0606 in AK, HI, NJ (M–F 9–5). Library Services: 800-424-9100, (202) 287-5100 in DC (M–F 8–4:30).

Bulimia
(201) 836-1800
  American Anorexia/Bulimia Association, Inc.

Cancer
800-4-CANCER (M–F 9–4:30)
  National Cancer Institute: Cancer-related I&R
  Counseling: 800-525-3777 (M–F 11:30–8).

Celiac Sprue
(515) 270-9689
  Celiac Sprue Association—U.S.

Child Abuse
800-422-4453 (24 hr)
> Child Help U.S.A: Information, crisis counseling, referral to local agencies for child abuse reports.
> Self-help groups: 800-421-0353; 800-352-0386 in CA (M–F 8:30–5)

Cocaine
800-COCAINE (24 hr)
> Fair Oaks Hospital, Summit, NJ: I&R about addiction and treatment.

Communicable Diseases
(404) 329-3311 (day); (404) 329-3644 (evening).
> Centers for Disease Control: Information concerning communicable diseases and epidemics.

Cornelia de Lange Syndrome
800-223-8355
> Cornelia de Lange Syndrome Foundation: Phone or mail response to messages. Printed materials.

Cystic Fibrosis
800-FIGHT-CF (M–F 8:30–5:30)
> Cystic Fibrosis Foundation: Medical, fund-raising information; referral to local chapters or hospitals with CF center.

Diabetes, Juvenile
800-223-1138; (212) 889-7575 in NY (M–F 9–5)
> Juvenile Diabetes Foundation: Referrals to physicians and clinics. Brochures; answers questions.

Disabled, Job Accommodation
800-526-7234 (M–F 8:30–4:30)
> Affiliated with President's Committee on Employment of the Handicapped: Information on all types of accommodations made and equipment available to assist handicapped persons to obtain employment.
> Software: 800-327-5892 (M–F 8–5)
> Special Education Software Center: Sends information matching software to hardware of handicapped pertinent to level of handicap.
> Special Projects: 800-248-ABLE (M–F 9–5:30)
> National Organization on Disability: Information on community, corporate, and national human service organization projects to aid the handicapped. Volunteer opportunities and networking of disabled with local contacts.

Disabled, Postsecondary Education
800-54-HEATH (M–F 9–5)
> Heath Resource Center: I&R on postsecondary education and training programs for handicapped.

Diving Accidents
(919) 684-8111
  Divers Alert Network (DAN).

Down's Syndrome
800-221-4602
  National Down Syndrome Society: Information on early intervention, referral to self-help groups.

Drug Abuse
800-554-KIDS; (301) 585-KIDS in MID (M–F 9–5)
  National Federation of Parents for Drug-Free Youth: Referrals to parent support groups and to alcohol and drug abuse centers.
  Information, referral: 800-241-7946 (M–F 8:30–5).
  Prevention: 800-638-2045; (301— 443-2450 in MD (M–F 8–4:30).

Drug Abuse, Confidential Referral Service
800-662-HELP (24 hr)
  National Institute of Drug abuse.

Dyslexia
800-ABCD-123 (M–F 9–5)
  Orton Dyslexia Society: Information and guidelines for seeking help/networks callers with members.

Gay/Lesbian Concerns
800-221-7044 (M–F 3–9)
  National Gay/Lesbian Task Force: Information about AIDS, assistance for victims of anti-gay violence, and gay/lesbian concerns of any kind.

Health
800-336-4797 (M–F 8:30–5)
  National Health Information Clearinghouse: Information on health-related organizations and programs; Recorded information: 800-621-8094.

Hearing/Communication Handicaps
800-424-8576, (703) 642-0580 in VA (M–F 9–5)
  Better Hearing Institute: Information on hearing problems, available hearing help, and prevention of deafness. Captioned films for the deaf: 800-237-6213 (M–F 9–5). Career advice: 800-638-8255; (301) 897-8682 in MD, TTY/TDD (M–F 8:30–4:30)
  Research: 800-835-DEAF (M–F 9–5).

Heart
800-241-6993 (M–F 9–4)
  Heart Line: Answers questions about cardiovascular disease; printed materials.

Hemophilia
(212) 219-8180
  National Hemophilia Foundations.

Herpes
800-638-0742; 800-492-0359 in MD
U.S. Department of Health and Human Services: Information on hospitals participating in Hill-Burton Hospital Free Care Program only.

Hospital Care, Children
800-237-5055; 800-282-9161 in FL (M–F 8–5)
Shriner Hospital for Crippled Children: Information on free hospital care available to children under 18 needing orthopedic care and burn treatment.

Hospital Emergency Telephone
800-451-0525; (617) 923-4141 in AK, HI, MA (M–F 9–5)
Lifeline Systems, Inc.: Information on emergency telephone system for elderly and handicapped people to maintain direct line to local hospitals.

Kidney
800-638-8299; 800-492-8361 in MD (M–F 8–5:30)
American Kidney Fund: Financial assistance for kidney patients; information on kidney-related diseases and organ donation.

Lupus
800-558-0121 (M–F 10–5:30)
Lupus Foundation of America: Referral to chapters; printed information; bibliography of books by doctors and patients on lupus.

Medical Information
800-621-8094
American Medical Association.

Medic Alert
800-344-3226; 800-469-1020 in CA, (209) 668-3333 in AK, HI (24 hr)
Medic Alert Foundation: Identity bracelets and/or necklaces. Maintains computerized file of individuals' medical records.

Medicare
800-462-9306 (M–F 9–4:30)
Information on benefits and payments.

Missing Children
800-843-5678 (M–F 7 A.M.–midnight; Sat 10–6)
National Center for Missing and Exploited Children: For reported sightings of missing children. Educational materials available.
Referral: 800-235-3535 (24 hr).
The Missing Children Network: Referral to network of participating missing child/person organizations.
Report sightings: 800-426-5678, (914) 255-1848 in NY (M–F 9–9) (call collect only to identify msising child).

National Self-Help Clearinghouse at the City University of New York
(212) 840-1259
Up-to-date listing of mutual-aid organizations throughout the nation.

Organ Donation
800-528-2971; (713) 528-2971 in TX (24 hr)
　Living Bank: Registry and referral service for people wanting to commit any or all organs, bones, tissue, or entire body for research or transplantation.
800-24-DONOR; 804-289-5380
　United Network for Organ Sharing (UNOS): Information on donors or organ sharing.

Parkinson's Disease
800-327-4545; 800-433-7022 in FL; (305) 547-6666 in Miami (M–F 8–5)
　National Parkinson Foundation: Answers nonmedical questions, written information on request.
　Information: 800-344-7872 (M–F 10–7)
　Information and counseling, limited referral.

Pesticides
800-858-7378 (24 hr)
　Environmental Protection Agency: Gathers and disseminates information.

Phobias
(301) 231-9350
　Phobia Society of America: Information about phobias and assistance in finding experts throughout the country. Sponsors meetings to inform professionals about research findings dealing with disorders.

Rare Disorders
(203) 746-6518
　National Organization for Rare Disorders: Clearinghouse for information about rare disorders and orphan drugs.

Rehabilitation
800-34-NARIC (Voice/TDD) (M–F 9–5)
　National Rehabilitation Information Center: I&R about research, assistive devices, and other resources for any type of disability.

Respiratory
800-222-LUNG (M–F 10:30–7)
　National Asthma Center, National Jewish Hospital: Information and literature, referral for lung disease.

Retinitis Pigmentosa
800-638-2300;(301) 225-9400 in MD (M–F 8:30–5)
　National Retinitis Pigmentosa Foundation: I&R to medical centers, RP chapters.

Reye's Syndrome
800-233-7393 (M–F 8:30–5)
　National Reye's Syndrome Foundation: Printed information on symptoms; referral for treatment, networking.

Runaways
800-621-4000 (24 hr)
   National Runaways Switchboard, MetroHelp, Inc.: Phone counseling, locate residential facilities, relay message to parents on request. Similar service: 800-231-6946 (24 hr).

Sexual Addiction
800-622-9494
   National Association on Sex Addiction Problems.

Snake Antivenim
800-522-4611
   Oklahoma Poison Information Center.

Special Education
800-345-TECH (M–F 1–6)
   Center for Special Education Technology Information Exchange, Special Education Program, U.S. Dept. of Education: Information on computer-based video and audio technology for special education needs.

Spina Bifida
800-621-3141 (M–F 9–5)
   Spina Bifida Association of America: Referral to chapters; printed information.

Spinal Cord Injury
800-526-3456; 800-638-1733 in MD (M–F 8–4)
   Maryland Institute for Emergency Medical Service Systems, Univ. of Maryland: I&R for people with spinal cord injuries and their families. Peer support network Equipment, programs: 800-624-1698 (M–F 11:30–8).

Stuttering
800-221-2483; (212) 532-1460 in NY (M–F 9–5)
   National Center for Stuttering: Information and advice.

Surgery, Second Opinion
800-638-6833 (7 days, 8 A.M.–midnight)
   U.S. Dept. of Health and Human Services: Information on locating a doctor for a second opinion for nonemergency surgery.

Venereal Disease
800-227-8922 (M–F 2 A.M.–2 P.M.)
   American Society Health Organization: Consultation, I&R on all aspects of sexually transmitted diseases.

From Taber's Cyclopedic Medical Dictionary, ed 16. FA Davis, Philadelphia, 1989, p 2301.

TRANSLATIONS

ENGLISH

Hello. I want to help you. I do not speak (English) but will use this book to ask you some questions. I will not be able to understand your spoken answers. Please respond by shaking your head or raising one finger to indicate "no"; nod your head or raise two fingers to indicate "yes."

SPANISH

Translation	*Phonetic*
Saludos. Quiero ayudarlo. Yo no hablo español, pero voy a usar este libro para hacerle algunas preguntas. No voy a poder entender sus respuestas; por eso haga el favor de contestar, negando con la cabeza o levantando un dedo para indicar "no" y afirmando con la cabeza o levantando dos dedos para indicar "sí."	Sah-loo′dohs. Ki-air′oh ah-joo-dar′loh. Joh noh ah′bloh es′pan-yohl, pair′oh voy ah oo-sawr′ es′tay lee′broh pahr′ah ah-sair′lay ahl-goo′nahs pray-goon′tahs. Noh voy ah poh-dair′ en-ten-dair′ soos res-poo-es′rahs; pore es-soh ah′gah el fah-vohr′ day kohn-tes-tahr′, nay-gahn′doh kohn lah kah-bay′thah oh lay-vahn-tahn′doh oon day′doh pahr′ah een-dee-kahr′ noh ee ah-feer-manh′doh kohn lah kah-bay′thah oh lay-vahn-tahn′doh dohs day′dohs pahr′a een-dee-kahr′ see.

ITALIAN

Translation	*Phonetic*
Buon giorno. La voglio aiutare. Io non parlo italiano, ma userò questro libro per farle qualche domanda. Non potrò comprendere le Sue domande. Per favore risponda con un cenno di testa. Alzi un dito per indicare 'no'; muova la Sua testa su e giu o alzi due dita per indicare 'si.'	Bwon jih-or′noh. Lah vol′yoh ah-yoo-tar′day. Ee′oh nohn par′loh ee-towl-ee-ah′noh mah oo-say′roh kwes′toh lee′broh pehr fahr′lay kwall′kay doh-mahn′dah. Non poh′throh kohm-prehn′deh-ray lay soo′ee doh-mahn′day. Pehr fah-vohr′ay ray-spohn′dah kohn oon chay′noh dee tes′tah. Ahlt′zih oon dee′toh pehr in-dee-kar′ay noh; moo-eh′vah lah soo′ah tes′tah soo eh joo oh alht′zih doo′ay dee′tay pehr in-dee-kar′ay see.

Translation

Bonjour. Je veux bien vous aider. Je ne parle pas français mais tout en me servant de ce livre je vais vous poser des questions. Je ne comprendrai pas ce que vous dites en français. Je vous en prie, pour répondre: pour indiquer "non", secouez la tête ou levez un seul doigt; pour indiquer "oui", faites un signe de tête ou levez deux doigts.

Phonetic

Bon-zhoor'. Zheh voo bih-ehn' voo ay-day'. Zheh neh parl pah frahn-say' may too ahn meh sehr-vahn' d' seh lee'vrah zheh vay voo poh-say' day kehs-tih-on'. Zheh neh kahm-prahn'dry pah seh keh voo deet ahn frahn-say'. Zheh voo ahn pree, por ray-pahn'drah; por ahn-dee-kay nohn, seh-kway' lah teht oo leh-vay' oon sool dwoit; por ahn-dee-kay wee', fayt oon seen deh teht oo leh-vay' duh dwoit

Translation

Hallo! Ich mochte Ihnen helfen. Ich spreche kein Deutsch, aber ich werde dieses Buch benützten um Sie einiges zu fragen. Ich werde Ihre Antworten nicht verstehen. Deshalb antworten Sie mir indem Sie Ihren Kopf schütteln oder heben Sie Ihren Finger um "nein" auszudrücken; nicken Sie mit dem Kopf oder heben Sie zwei Finger um "ja" auszudrücken.

Phonetic

Ha-loh! Ich möhh'tuh ee'nuhn hel'fuhn. Ich shpre'huh kīn doitsh, ah'buhr ich ver'duh dee'zuhs bookh bā-nüt'zuhn um zee ī'ni-guhs tsoo frah'guhn. Ich ver'duh ee'ruh ant'vor-tuhn nihht fer-shtay'uhn. Dās-halb' ant'vor-tuhn zee meer in-dām' zee ee'ruhn kopf shü'tln ō'der hāb'uhn zee ee'ruhn fing'uhr um nīn ows'tsoo-drük-uhn; nick'uhn zee mit dām kopf ō'der hāb'uhn zee tsvī fing'uhr um ya ows'tsoo-drük-uhn.

Common Physical Therapy Directions

ENGLISH	SPANISH	FRENCH	ITALIAN	GERMAN
General Expressions				
You are not going to fall	No vas a caer	Vous n'allez pas tomber	Non va cadere	Sie werden nicht fallen
Don't be afraid	No tengas miedo	N'ayez pas peur	Non abbia paura	Haben Sie keine Angst
That doesn't hurt you	No te duele	Cela ne fait pas mal	Questro non le fa male	Es wird Ihnen nicht weh tun
Don't cry	No llores	Ne pleurez pas	Non pianga	Nicht weinen
Don't worry	No tengas cuidado	Ne vous inquiétez pas	Non tema	Machen Sie sich keine Sorgen
Sit up	Siéntete	Asseyez-vous	Si metta a sedere	Aufsetzen
Stand up	Párete	Levez-vous	Si alzi	Aufstehen
Walk	Ande	Marchez	Cammini	Gehen
Roll over	Ruédete	Tournez-vous	Si giri	Umdrehen
Lie on your face on the table	Acuéstete con la boca para abajo en la mesa	Couchez-vous à plat ventre sur la table	Si corichi con la faccia voltata verso la tavola	Legen Sie sich auf den Bauch
Lie on your back on the table	Acuéstete con la boca para arriba en la mesa	Couchez-vous sur le dos sur la table	Si corichi sulla tavola	Lagen Sie sich auf den Rücken

English	Spanish	French	Italian	German
Lie on your side	Acuéstete de lado	Couchez-vous sur le côté	Si corichi sul fianco	Legen Sie sich auf die Seite
Lie on your other side	Acuéstete al otro lado	Couchez-vous de l'autre côté	Si corichi sul altro fianco	Legen Sie sich auf die andere Seite
This way	Así	Ainsi	Cosí	Hierhin
Again	Otra vez	Encore	Di nuovo	Noch einmal
Hold it	Detenlo	Restez ainsi	Lo tenga	Halten
With force (against resistance)	Con fuerza	Avec force	Con forza	Mit Kraft
Push down with your hands to lift your body	Empuje para abajo con las manos para levanter el cuerpo	Appuyez vous sur les mains et soulevez votre corps	Faccia forza sulle mani a fine di alzare ilcorpo	Stemmen Sie mit den Händen
Slowly	Despácio	Lentement	Adagio	Langsam
Not so fast	No tan récio	Pas si vite	Non cosí in fretta	Nicht so schnell
Rest	Descánsete	Reposez-vous	Si riposi	Ausruhen

Anatomical Names

English	Spanish	French	Italian	German
Neck	El cuello	Le cou	Il collo	Hals
Abdomen	El abdomen	L'abdomen	Il addome	Leib
Chest	El pecho	La poitrine	Il petto	Brust
Back	La espalda	Le dos	La schiena	Rücken
Spine	El espinazo	L'épine dorsale	La spina dorsale	Rückengrad
Face	La cara	Le visage	La faccia	Gesicht

Continued on the following page(s)

943

Common Physical Therapy Directions *Continued*

ENGLISH	SPANISH	FRENCH	ITALIAN	GERMAN
Thumb	El dedo grande	Le pouce	Il pollice	Daumen
Buttocks	Las nalgas	Les fesses	Le natiche	Popo
Knee	La rodilla	Le genou	Il ginocchio	Knei
Heel	El talón	Le talon	Il tallone	Absatz
Shoulder	El hombro	L'épaule	La spalla	Schulter
Arm	El brazo	Le bras	Il braccio	Arm
Elbow	El codo	Le coude	Il gomito	Elbogen
Wrist	La muñeca	Le poignet	Il polso	Gelenk
Hand	La mano	La main	La mano	Hand
Fingers	Los dedos	Les doigts	Le dita	Fingers
Hip	La cadera	La hanche	L'anca	Hüfte
Leg	La pierna	La jambe	La gamba	Bein
Face and Neck				
Lift your head	Levante la cabeza	Levez la tête	Alzi la testa	Kopf heben
Open your mouth	Abra la boca	Ouvrez la bouche	Apra la bocca	Mund öffnen—
Close your mouth	Cierre la boca	Fermez la bouche	Chiuda la bocca	Mund schliessen
Open your eyes	Abra los ojos	Ouvrez les yeux	Apra gli occhi	Augen öffnen

English	Spanish	French	Italian	German
Close your eyes	Cierre los ojos	Fermez les yeux	Chiuda gli occhi	Augen schleissen
Wrinkle your nose	Arruque la nariz	Plissez le nez	Corrughi il naso	Nase runzeln
Smile	Deme una sonrisa	Souriez	Sorrida	Lächeln

Upper Extremity

English	Spanish	French	Italian	German
Raise your arm	Levante el brazo	Levez le bras	Alzi il braccio	Armheben
Move your arm out to the side	Mueva el brazo para afuera	Ecartez le bras du corps	Muova il braccio di alto	Arm seitheben
Move your arm back to your side	Mueva el brazo para adentro	Ramenez le bras vers le corps	Muova il braccio verso il fianco	Arm anlegen
Bend your elbow	Doble el codo	Pliez le coude	Pieghi il gomito	Ellbogen bewegen
Straighten your elbow	Enderece el codo	Redressez le coude	Estenda il gomito	Ellbogen streden
Turn your hand over	Voltee la mano	Retournez la main	Giri la mano	Hand drehen
Bend your fingers	Doble los dedos	Pliez les doigts	Pieghi le dita	Finger bewegen
Straighten your fingers	Enderece los dedos	Redressez les doigts	Estenda le dita	Finger strecken
Bend your wrist (flexion)	Doble la muñeca	Pliez le poignet	Pieghi il polso	Handgelenk beugen
Lift your hand (extension)	Levante la mano	Relevez la main	Alzi la mano	Hand strecken
Pull your shoulders together	Junte los hombros	Redressez les épaules	Tiri le spalle	Schultern zusammenziehen
Lift your shoulder	Levante el hombro	Levez l'épaule	Alzi la spalla	Schultern heben

Continued on the following page(s)

Common Physical Therapy Directions *Continued*

ENGLISH	SPANISH	FRENCH	ITALIAN	GERMAN
Lower Extremity				
Bend your hip	Doble la cadera	Pliez la hanche	Pieghi l anca	Hüfte beugen
Lift your leg	Levante la pierna	Levez la jambe	Alzi la gamba	Bein anheben
Bend your knee	Doble la rodilla	Pliez le genou	Pieghi il ginocchio	Knie beugen
Straighten your knee	Enderece la rodilla	Redressez le genou	Estenda il ginocchio	Knie strecken
Roll your leg in	Ruede la pierna para adentro	Faites tourner la jambe en-dedans	Giri la gamba in dentro	Bein einwärts drehen
Roll your leg out	Rueda la pierna para afuera	Faites tourner la jambe en-dehors	Giri la gamba in fuori	Bein auswärts drehen
Lift your foot	Levante el pie	Levez le pied	Alzi il piede	Fuss hoch heben
Push your foot down	Empuje el pie para abajo	Poussez le pied contre en-bas	Spinga il piede in giu	Fuss herunterdrehen
Lift your toes	Levante los dedos	Levez les orteils	Alzi le dita del piede	Zehen strecken
Bend your toes	Doble los dedos	Pliez les orteils	Pieghi le dita del piede	Zehen beugen
Pull your foot in	Mueva el pie para adentro	Tournez le pied en-dedans	Muova il piede in dentro	Fuss nach innen ziehen
Pull your foot out	Mueva el pie para afuera	Tournez le pied en-dehors	Muova il piede in fuori	Fuss nach aussen ziehen

THE INTERPRETER IN FIVE LANGUAGES

General

Basic Questions and Replies

ENGLISH	SPANISH	ITALIAN	FRENCH	GERMAN
Good morning.	Buenos días.	Buon giorno.	Bonjour.	Guten Morgen.
What is your name?	¿Cómo se llama?	Come si chiama Lei?	Quel est votre nom?	Wie heissen Sie?
How old are you?	¿Cuántos años tiene?	Quanti anni ha?	Quel âge avez-vous?	Wie alt sind Sie?
Do you understand me?	¿Me entiende?	Mi capisce?	Me comprenez-vous?	Verstehen Sie mich?
Answer only	Conteste solamente . . .	Risponda solamente . . .	Répondez seulement . . .	Antworten Sie nur
Yes No	Sí No	Sì No	Oui Non	Ja Nein
What do you say?	¿Qué dice?	Cosa dice?	Que dites-vous?	Was sagen Sie?
Speak slower.	Hable más despacio.	Parli più adaggio.	Parlez plus lentement.	Sprechen Sie langsamer.
Say it once again.	Repítalo, por favor.	Lo dica ancora unà volta.	Répétez ça.	Wiederholen Sie das.
Don't be afraid.	No tenga miedo.	Non abbia paura.	N'ayez pas peur.	Haben Sie keine Angst.
Try to recollect.	Trate de recordar.	Cerchi di ricordarsi.	Cherchez à vous en rappeler.	Versuchen Sie sich zu erinnern.

Continued on the following page(s)

947

Basic Questions and Replies *Continued*

ENGLISH	SPANISH	ITALIAN	FRENCH	GERMAN
You cannot remember?	¿No recuerda?	Non si ricorda?	Ne vous en souvenez pas?	Können Sie sich nicht erinnern?
Come to my office.	Venga a mi oficina.	Venga al mio ufficio.	Venez à mon bureau.	Kommen Sie in mein sprechzimmer
Please remove all your clothes.	Por favor, desvístase completamente.	Per cortesia, si spogli.	Veuillex-vous déshabiller.	Ziehen Sie sich bitte ganz aus.
You will?	¿Usted quiere?	Desidera?	Vous voulez bien?	Sie wollen?
You will not?	¿No quiere usted?	Non desidera?	Vous ne voulez pas?	Sie wollen nicht?
You don't know?	¿No sabe?	Non sa?	Vous ne savez pas?	Wissen Sie nicht?
Is it impossible?	¿Es imposible?	È impossibile?	C'est impossible?	Ist es unmöglich?
It is necessary.	Es necesario.	È necessario.	C'est nécessaire.	Es ist unbedingt nötig.
That is right.	Está bien.	Va bene.	C'est bien.	Das ist richtig.
Show me . . .	Enséñeme . . .	Mi faccia vedere	Montrez-moi . . .	Zeigen Sie mir . . .
Here There	Aquí Allí	Qui Qua	Ici Là	Hier Da
Which side?	¿En qué lado?	Quale lato?	Quel côté?	Auf welcher Seite?
Since when?	¿Desde cuándo?	Da quando?	Depuis quand?	Seit wann?
Right	Derecha	A destra	A droit	Rechts

English	Spanish	Italian	French	German
Left	Izquierda	A sinistra	A gauche	Links
More or less	Más o menos	Più o meno	Plus ou moins	Mehr oder weniger
How long?	¿Cuánto tiempo?	Da quanto tempo?	Combien de temps?	Wie lange?
Not much	No mucho	Non molto	Pas beaucoup	Nicht viel
Try again.	Trate otra vez.	Provi di nuovo.	Essayez encore une fois.	Versuchen Sie es noch ein mal.
Never	Nunca	Mai	Jamais	Niemals
Never mind.	Olvídelo.	Non importa.	Ça ne fait rien.	Lassen Sie es gut sein.
That will do.	Suficiente.	Basta così.	Ça suffit.	Das ist genug.
About how much daily?	¿Más o menos qué cantidad diariamente?	Circa quanto al giorno?	A peu près combien par jour?	Ungefähr wie viel täglich?
So much?	¿Tanto?	Tanto?	Autant?	So viel?
You must be very careful.	Tiene que tener mucho cuidado.	Deve usare molte precauzioni.	Vous devez prendre garde.	Sie müssen sehr vorsichtig sien.

SEASONS

English	Spanish	Italian	French	German
In the spring.	En la primavera.	Nella primavera.	Au printemps.	Im Frühjahr.
In summer.	En el verano.	Nell' estate.	En été.	Im Sommer.
In autumn.	En el otoño.	Nell' autunno.	En automne.	Im Herbst.
In winter.	En el invierno.	Nell' inverno.	En hiver.	Im Winter.

Continued on the following page(s)

949

MONTHS

ENGLISH	SPANISH	ITALIAN	FRENCH	GERMAN
The months	Los meses	I mesi	Les mois	Die Monate
January	enero	gennaio	janvier	Januar
February	febrero	febbraio	février	Februar
March	marzo	marzo	mars	März
April	abril	aprile	avril	April
May	mayo	maggio	mai	Mai
June	junio	giugno	juin	Juni
July	julio	luglio	juillet	Juli
August	agosto	agosto	août	August
September	septiembre	settembre	septembre	September
October	octubre	ottobre	octobre	Oktober
November	noviembre	novembre	novembre	November
December	diciembre	dicembre	décembre	Dezember

DAYS OF THE WEEK

Sunday	domingo	domenica	dimanche	Sonntag
Monday	lunes	lunedì	lundi	Montag
Tuesday	martes	martedì	mardi	Dienstag
Wednesday	miércoles	mercoledì	mercredi	Mittwoch
Thursday	jueves	giovedì	jeudi	Donnerstag
Friday	viernes	venerdì	vendredi	Freitag
Saturday	sábado	sabato	samedi	Sonnabend

NUMBERS AND TIME OF DAY (Office Hours, Age, Diagnosis, Treatment)

One	Uno	Uno	Un	Eins
Two	Dos	Due	Deux	Zwei
Three	Tres	Tre	Trois	Drei
Four	Cuatro	Quattro	Quatre	Vier
Five	Cinco	Cinque	Cinq	Fünf
Six	Seis	Sei	Six	Sechs
Seven	Siete	Sette	Sept	Sieben
Eight	Ocho	Otto	Huit	Acht
Nine	Nueve	Nove	Neuf	Neun
Ten	Diez	Dieci	Dix	Zehn
Twenty	Veinte	Venti	Vingt	Zwanzig

Continued on the following page(s)

951

Basic Questions and Replies *Continued*

ENGLISH	SPANISH	ITALIAN	FRENCH	GERMAN
Thirty	Treinta	Trenta	Trente	Dreissig
Forty	Cuarenta	Quaranta	Quarante	Vierzig
Fifty	Cincuenta	Cinquanta	Cinquante	Fünfzig
Sixty	Sesenta	Sessanta	Soixante	Sechzig
Seventy	Setenta	Settanta	Soixante-dix	Siebzig
At 10:00	A las diez	Alle dieci	A dix heures	Um zehn Uhr
At 2:30	A las dos y media	Alle due e mezzo	A deux heures et demie	Um halb drei
Early in the morning	Temprano por la mañana	Di buon mattino	De bon matin	Frühmorgens
In the daytime	En el día	Durante il giorno	Pendant la journée	Bei Tag
At noon	A mediodía	A mezzo giorno	A midi	Mittags
At bedtime	Al acostarse	All' ora di coricarsi	A l'heure de se coucher	Vor dem Schlafengehen
At night	Por la noche	Alla sera	Le soir	Abends

English	Spanish	Italian	French	German
Before meals	Antes de las comidas	Prima del pasto	Avant les repas	Vor den Mahlzeiten
After meals	Después de las comidas	Dopo il pasto	Après les repas	Nach den Mahlzeiten
Today	Hoy	Oggi	Aujourd'hui	Heute
Tomorrow	Mañana	Domani	Demain	Morgen
Every day	Todos los días	Ogni giorno	Chaque jour	Jeden Tag
Every hour	Cada hora	Ogni ora	Chaque heure	Jede Stunde
How long have you felt this way?	¿Desde cuándo se siente así?	Da quanto tempo si siente cosi?	Depuis quand vous sentez-vous comme ça?	Seit wann fühlen Sie sich so?
It came all of a sudden?	¿Vino de repente?	Venne tutto ad un tratto?	Ça vous est arrivé tout à coup?	Ist es ganz plötzlich gekommen?
For how many days or weeks?	¿Cuántos días o semanas?	Da quanti giorni o settimane?	Depuis combien de jours ou semaines?	Seit wievielen Tagen oder Wochen?
Do they come every day?	¿Los tiene todos los días?	Le vengono tutti i giorni?	Ça vous gêne tous le jours?	Kommt es jeden Tag?
At the same hour?	¿A la misma hora?	Alla stessa ora?	A la même heure?	Zur selben Stunde?
At intervals?	¿De vez en cuando?	Ad intervalli?	De temps à autre?	Dann und wann?
It will be too late.	Será demasiado tarde.	Sarà troppo tardi.	Çe sera trop tard.	Es wird zu spät sein.
		COLORS		
Black	Negro	Nero	Noir	Schwartz
Blue	Azul	Blu	Bleu	Blau

953

Continued on the following page(s)

Basic Questions and Replies *Continued*

ENGLISH	SPANISH	ITALIAN	FRENCH	GERMAN
Green	Verde	Verde	Vert	Grün
Pink	Rosado	Rosa	Rose	Rosa
Red	Rojo	Rosso	Rouge	Rot
White	Blanco	Bianco	Blanc	Weiss
Yellow	Amarillo	Giallo	Jaune	Gelb

WORK HISTORY

ENGLISH	SPANISH	ITALIAN	FRENCH	GERMAN
What work do you do?	¿Cuál es su ocupación?	Che lavoro fa?	Quelle est votre profession?	Was ist Ihr Beruf?
Is it heavy physical work?	¿Es un trabajo corporal pesado?	È un pesante lavoro manuale?	Est-ce que c'est un travail physiquement fatigant?	Ist es eine schwere körperliche Arbeit?
What work have you done?	¿Qué trabajo ha hecho?	Che lavoro ha fatto?	A quoi avez-vous travaillé?	Welche Arbeit haben Sie getan?

History

FAMILY

Are you married?	¿Es usted casado?	È sposato?	Etes-vous marié?	Sind Sie verheiratet?
A widower?	¿Viudo?	È vedovo?	Veuf?	Ein Witwer?
A widow?	¿Viuda?	È vedova?	Veuve?	Eine Witwe?
Do you have children?	¿Tiene usted hijos/	Ha bambini?	Avez-vous des enfants?	Haben Sie Kinder?
Are they still living?	¿Viven todavía?	Vivono ancora?	Sont-ils encore vivants?	Leben sie noch?
Do you have any sisters?	¿Tiene hermanas?	Ha sorelle?	Avez-vous des soeurs?	Haben Sie Schwestern?
Do you have any brothers?	¿Tiene hermanos?	Ha fratelli?	Avez-vous des frères?	Haben Sie Brüder?
Of what did your mother die?	¿De qué murió su madre?	Di checosa è morta Sua mamma?	De quoi est morte votre mère?	Woran ist Ihre Mutter gestorben?
And your father?	¿Y su padre?	E Suo padre?	Et votre père?	Und Ihr Vate?
Your grandfather?	¿Su abuelo?	Suo nonno?	Votre grand-père?	Ihr Grossvater?
Your grandmother?	¿Su abuela?	Sua nonna?	Votre grand-mère?	Ihre Grossmutter?

GENERAL

Do you have . . . ?	¿Tiene . . . ?	Ha Lei	Avez-vous . . . ?	Haben Sie . . . ?
Have you ever had . . . ?	¿Há tenido . . . ?	Ha mai avuto . . . ?	Avez-vous jamais eu . . . ?	Haben Sie je . . . gehabt?

Continued on the following page(s)

Basic Questions and Replies *Continued*

ENGLISH	SPANISH	ITALIAN	FRENCH	GERMAN
Chills	Escalofrios	I brividi	Les frissons	Ein Fieberfrösteln
An attack of fever	Un ataque de calentura	Un attacco di febbre	Une attaque de fièvre	Ein Fieberanfall
Toothache	Dolor de muelas	Mal di denti	Le mal aux dents	Zahnschmerzen
Hemorrhage	Hemorragia	Emorragia	De hémorragie	Die Blutergüsse
Nosebleeds	Hemorragia por la nariz	Emorragia nasale	Saignements de nez	Das Nasenbluten
Unusual vaginal bleeding	Hemorragia vaginal fuera de los periodos	Perdite di sangue irregulari dalla vagina	Du saignement vaginal anormal	Jemals unregelmässiges bluten aus der Scheide
When did you last have a period?	¿Cuándo tuvo usted su última menstruación?	Quando ha avuto l'ultima volta le menstruazione?	Quand avez-vous eu vos régles pour la dernière fois?	Wann war die letze Menstruation?
Do you take birth control pills?	¿Toma. usted píldoras anticonceptvas	Prende pillole contro la gravibanza	Est-ce que vous prenez des	Nehmen Sie Geburtskontroll-

English			médicaments anticonceptionnels?	pillen?
Hoarseness	Ronquera	Raucedine	Enrouement	Heiserkeit

DISEASES

English	Spanish	Italian	French	German
What diseases have you had?	¿Qué enfermedades ha tenido?	Che malattie ha avuto?	Quelles maladies avez-vous eues?	Welche Krankheiten haben Sie gehabt?
Allergy	Alergia	Allergie	Une maladie allergique	Überempfind-lichkeiten
Anemia	Anemia	Anemia	L'anémie	Blutarmut
Bleeding tendency	Tendencia a sangrar	Tendenza alle emorragie	Une tendance à saigner	Neigung zum Bluten
Cancer	Cáncer	Cancro	Le cancer	Krebs
Chickenpox	Varicela	Varicella	La varicelle	Windpocken
Diabetes	Diabetes	Diabete	Le diabète	Zuckerkranckheit
Diphtheria	Difteria	Difterite	La diphthérie	Diphtherie
German measles	Rubéola	Rosolia	Rubéole	Röteln
Gonorrhea	Gonorrea	Gonorrea	La gonorrhée	Gonorrhöe, Tripper
Heart disease	Enfermedad del corazón	Malattia di cuore	Une maladie de coeur	Herzkrankheit
High blood pressure	Presión sanguínea elevada	Pressione alta del sangue	La tension arterielle trop élevée	Hohen Blutdruck
Influenza	Gripe (influenza)	Influenza	La grippe	Grippe

Continued on the following page(s)

Basic Questions and Replies *Continued*			
ENGLISH	SPANISH	ITALIAN	FRENCH	GERMAN
Lead poisoning	Envenenamiento con polmo	Avvelenamento da piombo	Empoisonnement causé par le plomb	Bleivergiftung
Liver disease	Enfermedad del hígado	Una malattia del fegato	Une maladie de foie	Eine Leberkrankheit
Malaria	Malaria (paludismo)	Malaria	La malaria	Malaria
Measles	Sarampión	Morbillo	La rougeole	Die Masern
Mental disease	Enfermedades mentales	Malattie mentali	Une maladie mentale	Geisteskrankheit
Mumps	Paperas	Orecchioni	Les oreillons	Mumps
Nervous disease	Enfermedades nerviosas	Malattie nervose	Une maladie nerveuse	Nervenkrankheit
Pleurisy	Pleuresía	Pleurite	Une pleurésie	Rippenfellentzündung
Pneumonia	Pulmonía	Polmonite	Pneumonie	Die Lungenentzündung
Rheumatic fever	Reumatismo (fiebre reumática)	Febbre reumatica	La fièvre rhumatismale	Rheumatisches Fieber

Rheumatism	Reumatismo	Reumatismo	Le rhumatisme	Der Rheumatismus
Scarlet fever	Escarlatina	Febre scarlattina	La fièvre scarlatine	Das Scharlachfieber
Smallpox	Viruela	Vaiolo	La variole	Pocken
Syphilis	Sífilis	Sifilide (lue)	La syphilis	Syphilis
Tuberculosis	Tuberculosis	Tuberculosi	Tuberculose	Die Tuberkulose
Typhoid fever	Tifoidea	Febre il tifo	La fièvre typhoide	Der Typhus

Examination

GENERAL

English	Spanish	Italian	French	German
How do you feel?	¿Cómo se siente?	Come stà?	Comment vous sentez-vous?	Wie fühlen Sie sich?
Good	Bien	Bene	Bien	Gut
Bad	Mal	Male	Mal	Schlecht
Let me see . . .	Déjeme ver . . .	Mi lasci vedere . . .	Permettez-moi de voir . . .	Lassen Sie mich sehen . . .
Let me feel your pulse.	Déjeme tomarle el pulso.	Mi lasci sentire il polso.	Permettez-moi de vous tâter le pouls.	Lassen Sie mich Ihren Puls fühlen.
Whisper: one, two, three.	Repita en voz baja: uno, dos, tres.	Dica piano: uno, due, tre.	Dites tout bas: un, deux, trois.	Flüstern Sie: eins, zwei, drei.
Say it out loud.	Dígalo en voz alta.	Lo dica ad alta voce.	Dites-le à voix haute.	Sagen Sie es laut.
Sit down.	Siéntese.	Si sieda.	Asseyez-vous.	Setzen Sie sich.
Stand up.	Levántese.	Si alzi.	Levez-vous.	Stehen Sie auf.

Continued on the following page(s)

Basic Questions and Replies *Continued*

ENGLISH	SPANISH	ITALIAN	FRENCH	GERMAN
Can you not rise quicker?	¿No puede levantarse más rápidamente?	Non si può alzare un po' più presto?	Vous ne pouvez pas vous lever plus vite?	Können Sie sich nicht schneller erheben?
Walk a little way.	Ande algunos pasos.	Cammini un po'.	Faites quelques pas.	Gehen Sie einige Schritte.
Return; go backwards.	Vuelva; ande para atrás.	Ritorni; cammini all' indietro.	Revenez; allez à retours.	Kommen Sie zurück; gehen Sie rückwärts.
Do you feel like falling?	¿Le parece que se va a caer?	Si sente come se dovesse cadere?	Vous sentez vous comme si vous allez tomber?	Ist es Ihnen als ob Sie fallen werden?
Do you feel dizzy?	¿Tiene usted vértigo?	Ha delle vertigini?	Avez-vous le vertige?	Ist Ihnen schwindlig?
Are you tired?	¿Está usted cansado?	Si sente molto stanco?	Êtes vous fatigué?	Sind Sie müde?
Have you slept well?	¿Ha dormido bien?	Ha dormito bene?	Avez-vous bien dormi?	Haben Sie gut geschlafen?
Have you any difficulty in breathing?	¿Tiene dificultad al respirar?	Ha difficoltà di respirare?	C'est difficile à respirer?	Fällt Ihnen das Atemholen schwer?

English	Spanish	Italian	French	German
Have you lost weight?	¿Ha perdido usted peso?	É dimagrito?	Avez-vous maigri?	Haben Sie abgenommen?
Since when have you had this eruption?	¿Desde cuándo tiene esta erupción?	Da quanto ha questa eruzione?	Depuis quand avez-vous cette éruption?	Seit wann haben Sie diesen Ausschlag?
Do you sweat much at night?	¿Suda mucho por la noche?	Suda molto alla notte?	Transpirez-vous beaucoup pendant la nuit?	Schwitzen Sie viel in der Nacht?
Are you warm?	¿Tiene calor?	Ha caldo?	Avez-vous chaud?	Ist Ihnen heiss?
Are you cold?	¿Tiene frío?	Ha freddo?	Avez-vous froid?	Isst Ihnen kalt?
Have you been exposed much to the wet weather?	¿Ha estado expuesto a la intemperie?	Si è mai esposto all' umidità?	Avez-vous été longtemp sous la pluie?	Sind Sie dem feuchten Wetter ausgesetzt gewesen?
Can you eat?	¿Puede comer?	Può mangiare?	Pouvez-vous manger?	Können Sie essen?
Have you a good appetite?	¿Tiene usted buen apetito?	Ha buon appetito?	Avez-vous un bon appétit?	Haben Sie guten Appetit?
Are you thirsty?	¿Tiene sed?	Ha sete?	Avez-vous soif?	Haben Sie Durst?
Do you still feel very weak?	¿Se siente muy débil todavía?	Si sente ancora molto débol?	Vous sentez-vous encore très faible?	Fühlen Sie sich noch sehr schwach?
Had you been drinking?	¿Había tomado alguna bebida alcohólica?	Ha bevüto?	Est-ce que vous-aviez bu quelque chose d'alcoolique?	Waren Sie angetrunken/

Continued on the following page(s)

Basic Questions and Replies *Continued*

ENGLISH	SPANISH	ITALIAN	FRENCH	GERMAN
Are you a drinking man?	¿Toma usted bebidas alcohólicas habitualmente?	Ha l'abitudine di bere?	Buvez-vous des choses alcooliques d'habitude?	Sind Sie ein Trinker?
Are you nervous?	¿Está usted nervioso?	É nervoso?	Etes-vous nerveux?	Sind Sie nervös?
When were you first taken sick?	¿Cuándo le empezó esta enfermedad?	Quando si è ammalato la prima volta?	Quand êtes-vous tombé malade d'abord?	Wann hat diese Krankheit begonnen?
How did this illness begin?	¿Cómo empezó esta enfermedad?	Come ha incominciato questa malattia?	Comment cette maladie a-t-elle commencé?	Wie hat diese Krankheit begonnen?
Did you take anything for it?	¿Tomó algo para mejorarla?	Ha preso qual cosa per curarsi?	Avez-vous pris quelque chose pour cela?	Haben Sie etwas dafür genommen/
Have you taken the medicine?	¿Ha tomado usted la medicina?	Ha preso la medicina?	Avez-vous pris la medicament?	Haben Sie die Medizin genommen?
A wound	Una herida	Una piaga	Une plaïe	Eine Wunde

PAIN

English	Spanish	Italian	French	German
Did you prick yourself with a pin?	¿Se ha pinchado con un alfiler?	Si è punto con una spilla?	Vous êtes-vous piqué avec une épingle?	Haben Sie sich mit einer Stecknadel gestochen/
Did you burn yourself?	¿Se quemó?	Si è bruciato?	Vous êtes-vous brulé?	Haben Sie sich verbrannt?
Did you sprain your foot?	¿Se torció el pie?	Si ha dislocato un piede?	Vous êtes-vous fait une entorse au pied?	Haben Sie Ihren Fuss verstaucht?
Have you any pain?	¿Tiene dolor?	Ha dolori?	Avez-vous mal quelque?	Haben Sie Schmerzen?
Where does it hurt?	¿Dónde le duele?	Dove la duele?	Où avez-vous mal?	Wo haben Sie Schmerzen?
Do you have pain here?	¿Le duele aquí?	Ha dolori qui?	Avez-vous mal par ici?	Haben Sie Schmerzen hier?
Do you have a pain in your side?	¿Le duele el costado?	Avete dolori al fianco?	Avez-vous mal au côté?	Haben Sie Seitenstechen?
Show me where.	Enséñeme dónde.	Mi mostri dove.	Montrez-moi où.	Zeigen Sie mir wo.
What did you feel in the beginning?	¿Qué sentía cuando empezó?	Che sentiva al principio?	Qu'avez-vous senti au commencement?	Was haben Sie anfangs gespürt?
Shooting pains?	¿Dolores agudos?	Dei dolori acuti?	Des élancements?	Stechende Schmerzen?
As if one were pricking you with pins?	¿Como si estuvieran pinchándole con alfileres?	Come se fosero delle spille?	Comme si l'on vous piquâit avec des épingles?	Als ob man Sie mit Stecknadeln stäche?

Continued on the following page(s)

Basic Questions and Replies *Continued*

ENGLISH	SPANISH	ITALIAN	FRENCH	GERMAN
Did you feel much pain at the time?	¿Sintió mucho dolor entonces?	Avete sentito molto dolore allora?	Est-ce que ça vous a fait beaucoup de mal alors?	Haben Sie gleich damals arge Schmerzen gespürt?
Is it worse now?	¿Está peor ahora?	È peggio ora?	Est-ce que c'est encore pire maintenant?	Ist es jetzt schlimmer?
Does it still pain you?	¿Le duele todavía?	Fa male ancora?	Est-ce que ça vous fait mal toujours?	Schmerzt er noch?
Do you still have that heavy pain?	¿Le duele mucho todavía?	Ha ancora quel dolore pesante?	Avez-vous toujours la douleur pesante?	Haben Sie noch den drückenden Schmerz?
Does it pain you to breathe?	¿Le duele al respirar?	La fa male respirare?	Votre respiration est-elle douloureuse?	Spüren Sie Schmerzen beim Atmen?
HEAD				
How does your head feel?	¿Cómo siente la cabeza?	Come si sente la testa?	Comment va votre tête?	Wie geht es Ihrem Kopf?

Your memory	Su memoria	La sua memoria	Votre mémoire	Ihr Gedächtnis
Is it good?	¿Es buena?	È buona?	Est-elle bonne?	Ist es gut?
Have you any pain in the head?	¿Le duele la cabeza?	Ha dolor di testa?	Avez-vous mal à la tête?	Haben Sie Kopfschmerzen?
Did you fall and how did you fall?	¿Se cayó, y cómo se cayó?	È caduto, e come è caduto?	Etes-vous tombé et comment êtes-vous tombé?	Sind Sie gefallen und wie sind Sie gefallen?
Did you faint?	¿Se desmayó?	È svenuto?	Vous êtes-vous évanoui?	Sind Sie ohnmächtig geworden?
Have you ever had fainting spells?	¿Ha tenido desmayos alguna vez?	È mai svenuto regolarmente?	Avez-vous jamais eu des évanouissements?	Haben Sie jemals Ohnmachtsanfälle gehabt?

EARS

Do you have ringing in the ears?	¿Le pitan los oídos?	Le tentennano le orecchie?	Avez-vous des bourdonnements d'oreilles?	Haben Sie Ohrenbrausen?
Do you have discharge from the ears?	¿Le supuran los oídos?	Le esce materia dalle orecchie?	Est-ce que vous avez un écoulement des oreilles?	Eitern Ihre Ohren?
The hearing	El oído	L'udito	L'ouïe	Das Gehör
Is it affected?	¿Está afectado?	È compromesso?	Est-elle changée?	Ist es angegriffen?

Continued on the following page(s)

Basic Questions and Replies *Continued*

ENGLISH	SPANISH	ITALIAN	FRENCH	GERMAN
		EYES		
Look up.	Mire para arriba.	Guardi sù.	Regardez en haut.	Schauen Sie hinauf.
Look down.	Mire para abajo.	Guardi giu.	Regardez en bas.	Schauen Sie hinunter.
Look toward your nose.	Mire la nariz.	Si guardi il naso.	Regardez le nez.	Schauen Sie auf Ihre Nase.
Look at me.	Mireme.	Mi guardi.	Regardez-moi.	Sehen Sie mich an.
Can you see what is on the wall?	¿Puede ver lo que está en la pared?	Può vedere cosa c'e sui muro?	Pouvez-vous voir ce qu'il y a contre le mur?	Können Sie sehen was hier an der Wand ist?
You cannot?	¿No puede?	Non può?	Vous ne pouvez pas?	Können Sie es nicht erkennen?
Can you see it now?	¿Puede verlo ahora?	Può vederlo adesso?	Le voyez-vous maintenant?	Können Sie es jetzt sehen?
And now?	¿Y ahora?	Ed ora?	Et maintenant?	Und nun?
What is it?	¿Qué es ésto?	Che cosa è?	Qu'est-ce que c'est?	Was ist es?

English	Spanish	Italian	French	German
Tell me what number it is?	Dígame qué número es éste.	Mi dica che numero è.	Dites-moi quel est le numéro.	Sagen Sie mir welche Nummer es ist.
Tell me what letter it is.	Dígame qué letra es ésta.	Mi dica che lettera è.	Dites-moi quelle est la lettre.	Nennen Sir mir diesen Buchstaben.
Do you see things through a mist?	¿Ve las cosas a travès de una niebla?	Vede le cose come se fossero fra la nebbia?	Voyez-vous les choses à travers d'un brouillard?	Sehen Sie alles durch einen Nebel?
Can you see clearly?	¿Puede ver claramente?	Può vedere chiaro?	Pouvez-vous voir clairement?	Sehen Sie deutlich?
Better at a distance?	¿Mejor a cierta distancia?	Meglio a distanza?	Mieux à distance?	Besser aus der Entfernung?
Do your eyes water a good deal?	¿Le lagrimean mucho los ojos?	Le lacrimano molto gli occhi?	Est-ce que les yeux vous coulent beaucoup?	Tränen Ihre Augen stark?
Can't you open your eye?	¿No puede abrir el ojo?	Non puo aprire l'occhio?	Ne pouvez-vous pas ouvrir l'oeil?	Können Sie Ihr Auge nicht öffnen?
Did anything get into your eye?	¿Le entró algo en el ojo?	Le è entrata qualche cosa nell'occhio?	Est-ce que quelque chose est entré dans l'oeil?	Ist Ihnen etwas ins Auge geflogen?
Do you sometimes see things double?	¿Ve las cosas doble algunas veces.	Vede qualche volta le cose doppie?	Est-ce que la vue est double parfois?	Sehen Sie manchmal doppelt?
Does the eyeball feel as if it were swollen?	¿Le parece que ele ojo está hinchado?	Le sembra che l'occhio sia gonfio?	L'oeil vous semble-t-il gonflé?	Fühlt sich das Auge wie geschwollan?

Continued on the following page(s)

Basic Questions and Replies *Continued*

ENGLISH	SPANISH	ITALIAN	FRENCH	GERMAN
You must be careful not to go out yet.	Tenga cuidado de no salir todavía.	Deve aver cura a non andar fuori.	Gardez vous de sortir maintenant.	Sie dürfen durchaus noch nicht ausgehen.
Since when has your eyesight failed you?	¿Desde cuando ha disminuido su vista?	Da quanto tempo la sua vista È diminuita?	Depuis quand votre vue s'est-elle diminuée?	Seit wann hat Ihre Sehkraft nachgelassen?
THROAT AND MOUTH				
Cough.	Tosa.	Tossisca.	Toussez.	Husten Sie.
Cough again.	Tosa otra vez.	Tossisca ancora.	Toussez encore une fois.	Husten Sie noch einmal.
Open your mouth.	Abra la boca.	Apra la bocca.	Ouvrez la bouche.	Öffnen Sie den Mund.
Does it hurt you to open your mouth?	¿Le duele al abrir la boca?	Le fa male aprir la bocca?	Ouvrir la bouche vous fait-il mal?	Spüren Sie Schmerzen wenn Sie den Mund öffnen?

English	Spanish	Italian	French	German
Since when do you cough?	¿Desde cuándo tose usted?	Da quando ha la tosse?	Depuis quand avez-vous la toux?	Seit wann husten Sie?
You cough a little?	¿Tose poco?	Tossisce poco?	Toussez-vous un peu?	Husten Sie manchmal?
Take a deep breath.	Respire profundamente.	Prenda un gran respiro.	Respirez profondement.	Atmen Sie tief.
Do you expectorate much?	¿Escupe mucho?	Sputa molto?	Crachez-vous beaucoup?	Spucken Sie viel aus?
What's the color of your expectorations?	¿De qué color es el esputo?	Di che color lo sputo?	De quelle sont vos crachats?	Welche Farbe hat der Speichel?
Does your tongue feel swollen?	¿Siente usted la lengua hinchada?	Ha la lingua gonfia?	Est-ce que la langue vous paraît gonflée?	Fühlt sich Ihre Zunge wie geschwollenan?
Do you have a sore throat?	¿Le duele la garganta?	Ha mal di gola?	Avez-vous mal à la gorge?	Haben Sie Halsschmerzen?
Does it hurt to swallow?	¿Le duele al tragar?	Quando ingoia le fa male?	Ça vous fait mal à avaler?	Spüren Sie Schmerzen beim Schlucken?

ARMS AND HANDS

English	Spanish	Italian	French	German
Let me see your hand.	Enséñeme la mano.	Mi faccia vedere la sua mano.	Montrez-moi la main.	Zeigen Sie mir Ihre Hand.
Have you no power in it?	¿No tiene fuerza enla mano?	Non ha forzan ella mano?	Est-elle complètement inerte?	Ist sie ganz kraftlos?
Grasp my hand.	Apriet mi mano.	Mi stringa la mano.	Serrez-moi la main.	Drücken Sie mir die Hand.

Continued on the following page(s)

Basic Questions and Replies *Continued*

ENGLISH	SPANISH	ITALIAN	FRENCH	GERMAN
Can you not do it better than that?	¿No puede hacerlo más fuerte?	Non può far meglio?	Vous ne pouvez-pas serrer plus fort que cela?	Können Sie nicht fester greifen?
Your arm feels paralyzed?	¿Parece que el brazo está paralizado?	Si sente il braccio paralizzato?	Est-ce que vle bras vous paraît paralysé?	Ihr Arm erscheint Ihnen gelähmt?
Raise it more.	Más alto.	Ancora di più.	Plus haut.	Höher.
Now the other.	Ahora el otro.	Adesso l'altro.	Maintenant l'autre.	Jetzt den andern.
Since when is your arm so powerless?	Desde cuándo no tiene fuerza en el brazo?	Da quando il suo braccio è senza forza?	Depuis quand votre bras a-t-il perdu la force?	Seit wann ist Ihr Arm so kraftlos?
Had you been sleeping on your arm?	¿Ha dormido encima del brazo?	Ha dormito col braccio sotto la testa?	Vous êtes-vous endormi sur le bras?	Sind Sie auf Ihrem Arm eingeschlafen?

970

GASTROINTESTINAL

Do you have stomach cramps?	¿Tiene calambres en el estómago?	Ha dei dolori acuti allo stomaco?	Avez-vous des crampes de l'estomac?	Haben Sie Magenkrämpfe?
Since when is your tongue that color?	¿Desde cuándo tiene la lengua de ese color?	Da quando la sua lingua è di questo colore?	Depuis quand votre langue a-t-elle cette couleur?	Seit wann hat Ihre Zunge diese Farbe?
Have you a pain in the pit of your stomach?	¿Tiene dolor en la boca del estómago?	Ha dei dolori alla bocca dello stomaco?	Est-ce que ça vous fait mal dans le creux de l'estomac?	Haben Sie Schmerzen in der Magengrube?
Nausea	Náusea	La nausa	La nausée	Die Übelkeit
Does eating make you vomit?	¿El comer le hace vomitar?	Vomita dopo aver manginto?	Rendez-vous ce que vous mangez?	Erbrechen Sie nachdem Sie gegessen haben?
How are your stools?	¿Cómo son sus defecaciones?	Come va di corpo?	Comment allez-vous à la selle?	Wie ist der Stuhlgang?
Are they regular?	¿Son regulares?	Va regolarmente?	Allez-vous à la selle régulièrement?	Ist er regelmassig?
Have you noticed their color?	¿Se ha fijado en el color?	Si è accorto di che colore?	Avez-vous remarqué la couleur de vos selles?	Haben Sie auf die Farbe geachtet?
Are you constipated?	¿Está estreñido?	È stitico?	Etes-vous constipé?	Leiden Sie an Verstopfung?
Do you have diarrhea?	¿Tiene diarrea?	Ha diarrea?	Avez-vous la diarrhée?	Haben Sie Durchfall?

Continued on the following page(s)

971

Basic Questions and Replies *Continued*

ENGLISH	SPANISH	ITALIAN	FRENCH	GERMAN
Do you pass any blood?	¿Con sangre?	Passa sangue?	Y-a-t-il du sang?	Ist Blut im Stuhl?
Have you vomited?	¿Ha vomitado?	Ha vomitato?	Avez-vous vomi?	Haben Sie erbrochen?
Do you still vomit?	¿Vomita todavía?	Vomita ancora?	Vomissez-vous encore?	Erbrechen Sie noch immer?
Do you vomit blood?	¿Vomita sangre?	Vomita sangue?	Vomissez-vous du sang?	Erbrechen Sie Blut?
Is it of a dark or bright red color?	¿Es de color rojo oscuro o claro?	È di colore rosso chiaro o rosso scuro?	La couleur du sang est elle foncée ou claire?	Ist es dunkel oder hellrot?
		KIDNEYS		
Have you any difficulty passing water?	¿Tiene dificultad en orinar?	Ha della difficoltà nell' urinare?	Avez-vous de la difficult ga uriner?	Haben Sie chwierigkeiten beim Wasserlassen?

972

English	Spanish	Italian	French	German
Do you pass water involuntarily?	¿Orina sin querer?	Urina involontariamente?	Urinez-vous involontairement?	Lassen Sie den Harn ohne es zu wollen?
Are any of your limbs swollen?	¿Estan hinchados alguno de sus miembros?	Si sente gonfio in qualche parte?	Avez-vous des membres gonflés?	Ist irgendeines Ihrer Glieder geschwollen?
How long have they been swollen like this?	¿Desde cuándo estan hinchados así?	Da quanto tempo che li ha cosi gonfi?	Depuis quand sont-ils gonflés comme ça?	Seit wann sind sie so angeschwollen?
Were they ever swollen before?	¿Han estado hinchados alguna vez antes?	Sono stati mai gonfi prima?	Ont-ils jamais été gonflés autrefois?	Sind sie je früher so angeschwollen gewesen?

Treatment

GENERAL

English	Spanish	Italian	French	German
It is nothing serious.	No es nada grave.	Non è nulla.	Ce n'est rien de grave.	Es ist nichts ernstliches.
You will get better.	Usted se mejorará.	Si sentirà meglio.	Vous vous remettrez.	Es wird besser werden.
Do exactly as I tell you.	Haga exactamente lo que le digo.	Faccia estattamente ciò che Le dico.	Faites exactement ce que je vous dis.	Tun Sie genau was ich Ihnen sage.
Take a bath.	Tome un baño.	Si faccia un bagno.	Prenez un bain.	Nehmen Sie ein bad

Continued on the following page(s)

973

Basic Questions and Replies *Continued*

ENGLISH	SPANISH	ITALIAN	FRENCH	GERMAN
A sponge bath	Un baño de esponja	Un bagno con la spugna	Un bain à l'éponge	Ein Schwamm bad
Bathe with hot water.	Báñese con agua caliente.	Faccia il bagno con acqua calda.	Bagnez-vous dans de l'eau chaude.	Baden Sie mit heissem Wasser.
Bathe with cold water.	Báñese con agua fría.	Si faccia il bagno con acqua fredda.	Baignez-vous dans de l'eau froide.	Baden Sie mit kaltem Wasser.
Bathe with alcohol.	Báñese con alcohol.	Si bagni con alcool.	Baignez-vous avec de l'alcool.	Reiben Sie sich alkoholab.
Paint the swelling with this.	Pinte la hinchazón con esto.	Deve pitturare il gonfiore con questo.	Badigeonnez l'enflure avecceci.	Pinseln Sie die Geschwulst damit.
I will use electricity.	Usaré electricidad.	Userò dell'elettricità.	Je ferai un traitment a la electricité.	Ich werde elektrischen Strom anwenden.

English	Spanish	Italian	French	German
Apply bandage to . . .	Ponga un vendaje a . . .	Si metta una fasciatura . . .	Mettez un bandage à . . .	Verbinden Sie . . .
Apply ointment.	Aplíquese ungüento.	Applichi un unguento.	Appliquez un onguent.	Verwenden Sie Salbe.
Keep very quiet.	Estése muy quieto.	Sia tranquillo.	Restez tranquille.	Verhalten Sie sich sehr ruhig.
You must not speak.	No debe hablar.	Non deve parlare.	Vous ne devez pas parler.	Sie dürfen nicht sprechen.

GLOSSARY OF TERMS USED TO DESCRIBE INSTRUMENTS
In Alphabetical Order

AAMI: Association for Advancement of Medical Instrumentation.

address buss: The conductors within a computer that pass power or data back and forth.

address code: A numerical code used to describe a location within a computer memory where a unit of information is stored.

ASCII: American Standard Code for Information Interchange, a code standardizing control commands and alphanumeric data units in computers.

assembly language: A system of computer programming codes characteristic to a given class of computers (determined by the type of microprocessor used in the computer).

astable multivibrator: A form of square wave or rectangular wave generator that yields a continuous output when power is applied. They are used to provide timing pulses in all types of devices, particularly TENS units and other stimulators.

Bandwidth: The range of frequencies within which performance (in respect to a specific characteristic) falls within specified limits.

barrier layer cell: An optical sensor that is sometimes used in colorimeters (also called *photovoltaic cell*).

BASIC: A computer programming language (Beginners All purpoSe Instructional Code).

baud rate: The units describing the rate at which data are transmitted by a computer (usually by a modem or a serial communications device).

binary code: A term used to describe a computer's machine-level programming language. The language consists of ones and zeroes.

bit: The smallest unit of information or data handled by a computer.

bode plot: A graph used to describe the frequency-gain characteristic of an electronic amplifier.

boolean algebra: The basis for the laws governing the design of computer logic circuits.

bridge amplifier: A specialized type of amplifier that is often used to amplify the difference between two signals, where one signal usually serves as the reference (a form of differential amplifier).

bridge circuit: A term used most often to describe a Wheatstone bridge measuring circuit or a bridge amplifier; often used as part of the circuitry of a strain gauge.

bridge rectifier: An electronic rectifier using four diodes in a bridge design to convert AC current into DC current.

buss: A general term in electronics used to describe a common conductor that connects parts of a device.

byte: The term used to describe the number of bits of data that defines a given computer's word size. A byte can be 4, 8, 16, 32, or 64 bits in length. (Note that an 8-bit byte can encode up to 256 different characters.)

CMRR (common mode rejection ratio): The ability of an amplifier to amplify a signal in the presence of electrical noise; the higher the number, the less the noise amplification.

computer interface: Describes a circuit or part that is used to connect a computer to an external device such as a printer or modem.

decibel: A unit of audio power that is also used to describe the gain or attenuation of an electronic circuit by the following formulae:

$$\text{Power in db} = 20 \log (V \text{ out}/V \text{ in})$$

$$\text{Power in db} = 10 \log (P \text{ out}/P \text{ in})$$

A gain of 100 in an amplifier is equivalent to a gain of 40 db.

detector (optical): A sensor that yields an output voltage or current that is proportional to the intensity of the light striking it. It may be a light-sensitive resistor (LSR), a photodiode, or a photomultiplier tube.

differential amplifier: A specialized type of amplifier that is used to amplify the difference between two signals. One signal usually serves as the reference. A bridge amplifier is a form of differential amplifier.

digital computer: A computer that processes information in the form of discrete digits or units.

digital-to-analog convertor: Converts digital data into analog data (the opposite of an analog-to-digital converter, or ADC).

distortion: A term used to describe variations in the amplitude or frequency of a signal brought about by overdriving an amplifier.

electrode (surface): Usually a metal element that detects bioelectrical (chemoelectrical) activity; surface electrodes, which are placed on the skin, are usually silver or silver chloride (Ag/AgCl).

file: A term used to describe data stored as a single unit by a computer.

filter: A circuit that allows only a single frequency or band (range) of frequencies to pass.

flip-flop: A computer circuit that yields as an output one of two possible conditions: either high (1) or low (0). These are used in memory circuits and counters (also called *bistable multivibrator*).

full-wave rectifier: An electronic circuit found in most instrument power supplies; converts AC voltage into DC voltage.

gain: The term used in electronics to describe the amplification factor of a given circuit (the ratio of voltage in to voltage out); also used to describe the sensitivity of the amplifier setting.

gate: A term used to describe the smallest possible decision-making (logic) circuit in a computer.

hexidecimal: A numbering system in computers that uses base eight, rather than base two (binary) or base ten (decimal).

inductor: An electronic component used in filter circuits and transformers that employs electromagnetic induction.

integrator: An electronic circuit that yields as an output the mathematical integral (total) of the input signal.

interface: A device or part of a computer that allows two normally incompatible circuits or parts to function together so as to pass data back and forth.

modem (modulator-demodulator): A device that allows computers to transmit and receive data in a serial fashion over phone lines.

modulation: An electronics term that describes the manner in which a signal is used to vary either the amplitude, frequency, or phase of a normally constant carrier signal. It is a method of coding information onto a carrier.

multiplexor: A circuit used in computers and instruments that allows a single processor to sample multiple channels by sequencing them.

multivibrator: A class of electronic circuits that provides a square wave output. They may be free running or may require a trigger.

noise: An unwanted signal or distortion of a signal due to electromagnetic or thermal effects.

null: A condition in which a measuring circuit is balanced and yields zero output.

offset voltage: The term used to describe the unwanted DC voltage at the input end of a signal-processing circuit. This voltage must be "offset" before the output yields zero reference (i.e., a true zero). An offset voltage is most often encountered when using a transducer that cannot be zeroed.

one shot: A circuit that yields a single preset pulse when triggered (also called a *monostable multivibrator*).

open circuit: A circuit in which the normal path for current has been broken. No current may flow in an open circuit.

oscillator: A circuit used to generate a continuous output signal in the form of a sine wave, or, in the case of relaxation oscillators, a rectangular or square wave.

parallel circuit: A circuit in which there is more than one path in which current may flow.

peak detector: A circuit that detects the maximum value of a signal, even though that signal may vary continuously.

peak-to-peak amplitude: The amplitude of a signal voltage from the most positive point to the most negative.

potentiometer (POT): A variable resistor most often used as an operator-adjustable control on instruments.

potentiometry: The measurement of a half-cell potential at zero current; the basis upon which many chemical sensors (electrodes) operate.

power: In electronics it is the product of the current times voltage. It is a measure of the amount of energy dissipated by a circuit (measured in units of watts).

RAM (random access memory): The portion of a computer's memory that holds temporary information (a program or data). This information is lost when the computer loses power.

range: A measure of the frequency range of an amplifier; the range of voltages that can be read by a voltmeter.

resonance: A condition in which an electrical circuit exhibits zero reactance and is therefore capable of filtering a given frequency, or in the case of an amplifier is capable of being driven into oscillation if positive feedback is present.

ROM (read only memory): The portion of a computer's memory that contains permanent information that cannot be changed by the user through programming. This information is stored in a way that it remains even if the computer loses power.

SCR (silicon-controlled rectifier): A triggered rectifier used to control large amounts of current; used in motors.

semiconductor: The term used to describe electronic components that are manufactured from a silicon chip, such as transistors, diodes, and integrated circuits.

sensitivity: The ability of a device to detect a small amount of voltage; usually given in ohms per volt when describing a voltmeter. The greater the ratio of ohms per volt, the better the sensitivity.

sensor: That part of a measurement instrument that senses activity to be measured; usually they are in the form of transducers.

series circuit: A circuit in which the current can follow only one path.

short circuit: A circuit in which the normal path for current flow has been passed (replaced) by a path of lower resistance. This results in excess circuit current, and often the device containing the circuit is damaged.

signal-to-noise ratio: The ratio of signal voltage to noise voltage. It is used to describe the sensitivity of an amplifier or measuring device; the greater the signal-to-noise ratio, the better.

span (chart recorder): The voltage required by a recorder to cause the pen to deflect fully across the chart paper.

strain gauge: A transducer that employs a resistive element to change an applied force into a resistance change and into a voltage (used in force measuring devices).

thermistor: A thermally sensitive resistor often used as the active element in some temperature-monitoring applications.

transducer: A device that transforms energy of one form into energy of another form. A light bulb, a photodiode, a car, and a stereo speaker are all transducers.

zener diode: A two-element device in the form of diode that functions, when reversed biased, as a simple voltage regulator. It is most often used to provide small reference voltages.

References

1. IEEE Standard Dictionary of Electrical and Electronic Terms.
2. Buschraums Complete Handbook of Practical Electronic Reference Data.

Index

An italic page number indicates a figure; a "T" following a page number indicates a table.

palmar, 77-78
Interosseous ligaments
  of tarsometatarsal joints, dorsal and
      plantar, 57
  of wrist, 54
Interosseous nerve. *See* Anterior
      interosseous nerve
      syndrome; Posterior
      interosseous nerve
      entrapment
Interpeak interval, 355
Interphalangeal ligaments, volar and
      collateral, 54
Interpotential interval, 355
Interscapular reflex, test for, 328
Interspinous ligament, 58
Intertarsal joints, ligaments of, 56-57
Intertester reliability, 927
Intertransversarii muscle, 78
Intracranial hemorrhage
  compression head injury and,
      649
  intraventricular, 649
Intratester reliability, 927
Intraventricular hemorrhage, 649
Intrinsic-plus test, 127
Inverse square law, electromagnetic
      modalities and, 629
Inversion of muscle action, 741
Iodines
  iodophors, disinfection by, 781
  tincture of, disinfection by,
      781
Ionizing radiation, disinfection by,
      780
IPSP. *See* Inhibitory postsynaptic
      potential, 354
Irregular potential, 368
IRV. *See* Inspiratory reserve volume,
      354
Ischiocavernosus muscle, 78
Ischiofemoral ligament, 55
Ischium, ligaments of, 55
Isokinetic contraction, 742
Isokinetic movement, 741
Isolation precautions, 774-779
Isologous graft, 766
Isometric contraction, 737, 738, 742
Isotonic contraction, 742-743
Italian language, English translations
      and, 940
  basic questions and replies and,
      947-975
  common physical therapy
      directions and, 942-946
Iterative discharge, 366

Jacksonian epilepsy, 376, 377
Jakob test, 134
Jaw reflex, test for, 326
Jerk sign, 134
Jitter, 356
Jogging, energy requirements for,
      569
Joint(s)
  anterior view of, *50*
  capsular patterns of, 141-142
  classification of, 47-51
  close-packed positions of, 52
  loose-packed positions of, 53
  posterior view of, *51*
Joint forces, gait and, 730
Joint motion
  Maitland's grade of movement and,
      145
  terminology for
    Kaltenborn terms and, 143
    Macconnaill terms and, 143-144
    Maitland terms and, 145
Jolly test, 356
Jugular foramen
  anterior compartment of, 11, 15
  middle compartment of, 12, 15
  posterior compartment of, 12, 15
Junctional rhythm, 530, *530*
Juvenile rheumatoid arthritis,
      diagnostic criteria for,
      166-167

Kaltenborn Terms, 143
Kendall and McCreary
  MMT positions, 115, 116
  MMT grades, 115, 116
Kernig's sign, 128
Kidney, helpline for, 937
Kinematics, 741
Kinesiological electromyography,
      747-748
  temporal processing of signal and,
      746
  terminology and, 749
Kinesiology
  terminology and, 739-745
  types of muscle contractions and,
      737-738
Kinetic energy, 741
Kinetics, 741
Kitchens, specifications for
      accommodation of
      handicapped persons and,
      826
Kleiger test, 137
Kleist hooking sign, test for, 333

Timing, for emphasis, 427
Tinel's sign, 127, 277
Tissue approximation end-feel, 138
Tissue tension tests, of Cyriax,
    138–139
  significance of diagnostic
    movements in, 140
TLC. See Total lung capacity, 598
TLR. See Symmetrical tonic
    labyrinthine reflex, 652
Toe(s), muscles moving, 104–105
Toe out or in, degree of, gait and,
    730
Toilets, specifications for
    accommodation of
    handicapped persons and,
    826
Token tests, of language
    comprehension, 406
Tonic-clonic seizures, 376, 378
  electroencephalographic pattern
    and, *375*
Torkildsen shunt, 385
Torque, 744
  gait and, 731
Total lung capacity (TLC), 598
Tracheal breath sounds, 594
Trachoma, method of transmission of,
    772–773
Traction, 427
Traction reflex, test for, 651
Trail Making Test, 457
Train of positive sharp waves,
    363–364
Train of stimuli, 371
Training heart rate (THR), 575
Trans-A-Chair, 820–821
Transcortical aphasia, 403
Transcutaneous electrical nerve
    stimulation (TENS)
  characteristics of, 641
  motor points and, 643, *643–645*
  reaction to degeneration and, 642
  rheobase and chronaxie and, 642
Transducer, 980
Transformation, of data, 928
Translations, 940–975
Transposition of the great vessels, 559
Transverse humeral ligament test, 125
Transverse ligament
  of hip, 55
  of pubis, 55
Transversus abdominus muscle, 89
Transversus menti muscle, 89
Transversus perinei profundus
    muscle, 89

Transversus perinei superficialis
    muscle, 89
Transversus thoracis muscle, 89
Trapezium bone, articulations of, 29
Trapezius muscle, 89–90
Trapezoid bone, articulations of, 29
Treadmill ergometer, oxygen
    requirements for, 580–581
Treadmill protocols, in cardiac
    rehabilitation, 578–579
Tremor
  intentional, tests for, 420
  postural, tests for, 420
  resting, tests for, 420
Trendelenburg gait, 728
Trendelenburg's test, 132
Trepidation sign, test for, 336
Triangularis bone, articulations of, 29
Triceps brachii muscle, 90
Triceps reflex, test for, 327
Trigeminal nerve
  distribution of, 224–225
  functional components of, 219
  testing of, 228
Trigeminy, ventricular, 537, *538*
Trigger points, 170
  of hand, *175*
  of head and neck, *171–174*
  of trunk and lower extremities,
    176–181
Triglycerides, burns and, 762
Triphasic action potential, 371
Triple discharge, 371–372
Triplegia, spastic, cerebral palsy and,
    395
Triplet, 371–372
Triquetrum bone, articulations of,
    29
Trochlear nerve
  distribution of, 224
  functional components of, 219
  testing of, 228
Trochoid joints, 47
Trömner's reflex, test for, 332
True negatives, 928
True positives, 928
Trunk
  arteries of, 475–479
  trigger points of, *176–181*
Tuberculosis
  bovine, method of transmission of,
    772–773
  human, method of transmission of,
    772–773
Tubs, specifications for
    accommodation of

Credits

Illustrations appearing on pages 184 to 189, 191 to 209, and 229 are from Manter and Gatz's Essentials of Clinical Neuroanatomy and Neurophysiology by Sid Gilman, M.D. and Sarah Winans Newman, Ph.D. Artwork by Margaret Croup Brudon.

AAEE Glossary of Terms in Clinical Electromyography, AAEM's Glossary of Terms in Clinical Electromyography (Muscle & Nerve 1987, 10: G1–G60). Approval for inclusion of the glossary in this book in no way implies review or endorsement by the AAEM of material contained in this book. (pp. 341–372)

Rancho Los Amigos Cognitive Functioning Scale, Adult Brain Injury Services of the Rancho Los Amigos Medical Center, Downey, California. (p. 412)

Cardiac and Noncardiac Drug Interventions and Their Possible Effect on Exercise Regimens. From American College of Sport Medicine: Guidelines for Graded Exercise Testing and Exercise Prescription, ed. 2. Lea & Febiger, Philadelphia, 1980. (pp. 564-66)

Approximate Energy Requirements in METs for Horizontal and Grade Walking. From American College of Sport Medicine: Guidelines for Graded Exercise Testing and Exercise Prescription, ed. 2. Lea & Febiger, Philadelphia, 1980. (p. 568)

Approximate Energy Requirements in METs for Horizontal and Uphill Jogging/Running. From American College of Sport Medicine: Guidelines for Graded Exercise Testing and Exercise Prescription, ed. 2. Lea & Febiger, Philadelphia, 1980. (p. 569)

Approximate Energy Expenditure in METs During Bicycle Ergometry. From American College of Sport Medicine: Guidelines for Graded Exercise Testing and Exercise Prescription, ed. 2. Lea & Febiger, Philadelphia, 1980. (p. 570)

Indications for Stopping an Exercise Test. From American College of Sport Medicine: Guidelines for Graded Exercise Testing and Exercise Prescription, ed. 2. Lea & Febiger, Philadelphia, 1980. (p. 582)

Criteria for an Abnormal Exercise Test. From American College of Sport Medicine: Guidelines for Graded Exercise Testing and Exercise Prescription, ed. 2. Lea & Febiger, Philadelphia, 1980. (p. 582)

Contraindications for Entry into Inpatient and Outpatient Exercise Programs. From American College of Sport Medicine: Guidelines for Graded Exercise Testing and Exercise Prescription, ed. 2. Lea & Febiger, Philadelphia, 1980. (p. 583)

Criteria for Termination of an Inpatient Exercise Session. From American College of Sport Medicine: Guidelines for Graded Exercise Testing and Exercise Prescription, ed. 2. Lea & Febiger, Philadelphia, 1980. (p. 583)

Oxygen Requirements for Step, Treadmill, and Bicycle Ergometer—The Exercise Standards Book, 1979. American Heart Association. Reproduced with permission. (pp. 580–81)

Spirograms and Lung Volumes. The Merck Manual of Diagnosis and Therapy. ed. 15. pp. 568-87, edited by Robert Berkow. Copyright 1987 by Merck & Co., Inc. Used with permission. (p. 599)

Normal and Abnormal Electroencephalogram Wave Patterns, *The Merck Manual of Diagnosis and Therapy,* ed. 13. pp. 1408-1409 edited by Robert Berkow. Copyright 1977 by Merck & Co., Inc. Used with permission. (p. 375)

Braintree Hospital Cognitive Continuum, Braintree Hospital, Braintree, Mass. (p. 414)

Drugs Used in the Treatment of Parkinson's Syndrome. From Chusid, JG: Correlative Neuroanatomy and Functional Neurology, ed. 19. Lange Medical Publications, Los Altos, CA 1985. (pp. 408-09)

Summary of Isolation Precautions: Protective Asepsis. Adapted from JS Garner and BP Simmons: CDC guidelines for isolation precautions in hospitals. *Infective Control,* July/August 1983, 4(4): 258-60. Used by permission. (pp. 774-779)

Nonsteroidal Anti-Inflammatory Drugs Used for Arthritis. Modified from Simon, LS, and Mills, JA: Drug Therapy: Nonsteroidal Anti-inflammatory Drugs (two parts). N Engl J Med 302:1179, 1237, 1980. From Goldenberg, DL and Cohen, AS: Drugs in the Rheumatic Diseases. Grune and Stratton, Orlando, 1986. (pp. 168-69)

Normal Development: Postural Control. From Keogh, J and Sugden, D: Movement Skill Development, Macmillan, New York, 1985 with permission. (p. 655)

Variations in Blood Pressure with Age. From Kozier and Erb: Techniques of Clinical Nursing. Addison-Wesley, Redwood City, CA, 1989, p. 487, with permission. (p. 516)

Values for Electrodiagnostic Testing. From Motor and Sensory Conduction in the Musculocutaneous Nerve, J Neurol Neurology Psychiat 37:890-899, 1976. (p. 270)

Common Physical Therapy Directions Reprinted from Physical Therapy with permission of the American Physical Therapy Association. (pp. 942-46)

Contribution of the Epiphyses to Bone Growth. From Rang, M: The Growth Plate and Its Disorders. Williams & Wilkins, Baltimore, 1969. (p. 158)

Classification of Epiphysical Plate Injuries. Salters, R B: Textbook of Disorders and Injuries of the Musculoskeletal System. ed. 2. Williams & Wilkins, Baltimore, 1983. (Type I, P. 153, Type II, p. 154, Type III, p. 155, Type IV, p. 156, Type V, p. 156, Type VI, p. 157)

Symptoms and Signs of Drug Abuse. From the Medical Letter, Vol. 29, Sept. 11, 1987, with permission. (pp. 930-933)

Elevation of Enzymes Following Acute Myocardial Infarction. From Warren and Lewis: Diagnostic Procedures in Cardiology. Year Book Medical Publishers, Chicago, 1985, p. 214 with permission. (p. 554)

Sample In-Patient Rehabilitation: Seven-Step Myocardial Infarction Program, Wenger, N: Rehabilitation of the Coronary Patient, ed. 2. John Wiley & Sons, New York, 1984. (p. 562)

ENGLISH-TO-METRIC CONVERSIONS

Note: To convert a metric measurement into an English measurement, divide by the factor shown in the tables that follow.

Area

To obtain square meters, multiply:

Sq inches	$\times\ 6.4516^{-4}$
Sq feet	$\times\ 0.092903$
Sq yards	$\times\ 0.8361274$
Sq miles	$\times\ 2.589,988$
Acres	$\times\ 4.046,856$
Sq millimeters	$\times\ 1.0^{-6}$
Sq centimeters	$\times\ 1.0^{-4}$
Sq meters	$\times\ 1.0$
Sq kilometers	$\times\ 1,000,000$
Hectares	$\times\ 10,000$

Length

To obtain meters, multiply:

Inches	$\times\ 0.0254$
Feet	$\times\ 0.3048$
Statute miles	$\times\ 1609.344$
Nautical miles	$\times\ 1852$
Millimeters	$\times\ 0.001$
Centimeters	$\times\ 0.01$
Meters	$\times\ 1.0$
Kilometers	$\times\ 1000$
Newtons	$\times\ 101.9716$

Volume and Capacity

To obtain cubic meters, multiply:

Cubic inches	$\times\ 1.6387^{-5}$
Cubic feet	$\times\ 0.0283168$
Cubic yards	$\times\ 0.7645549$
Ounces	$\times\ 2.9574^{-5}$
Quarts	$\times\ 9.4635^{-4}$
U.S. gallons	$\times\ 0.0037854$
Imperial gallons	$\times\ 0.0045461$
Cubic cm	$\times\ 1.0^{-6}$
Cubic meters	$\times\ 1.0$
Liters	$\times\ 0.001$